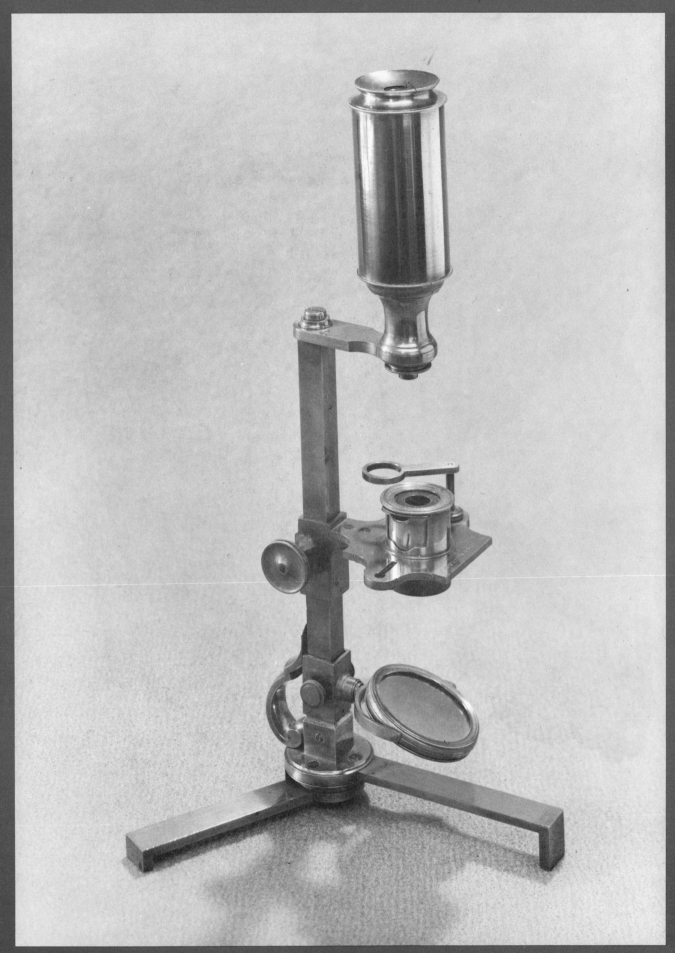

Wm. Harris Holborn, c. 1798, *London*

Histologic Diagnosis of Inflammatory Skin Diseases

A METHOD BY PATTERN ANALYSIS

Illustrative Compositions
LEON TERMIN, M.D.

with the technical assistance of
JUDITH TERMIN DE ROSE

Photomicrography
WILLIAM H. ATKINSON, R.B.P.

LEA & FEBIGER · PHILADELPHIA

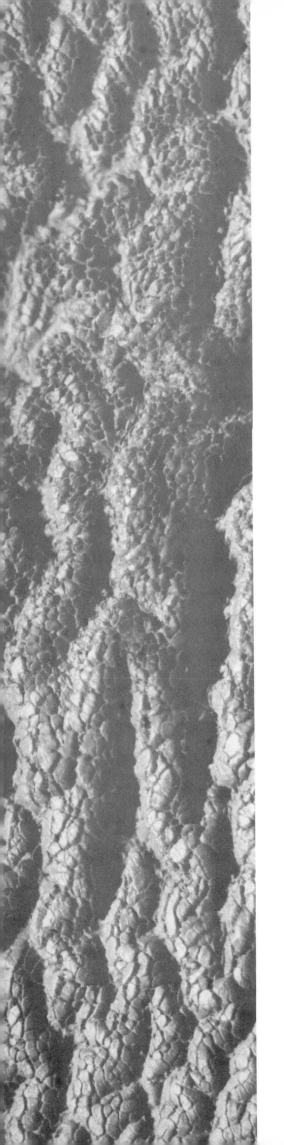

A. Bernard Ackerman, M.D.

Professor of Dermatology and Pathology, Director of Dermatopathology,
New York University School of Medicine, Adjunct Professor of Pathology,
New York University College of Dentistry, Consultant Dermatopathologist,
Department of Pathology Memorial Sloan-Kettering Cancer Center, New York

Histologic
Diagnosis
of
Inflammatory
Skin
Diseases

A Method by Pattern Analysis

CREDITS

Chapter 1 is adapted by permission from Chapter 1, Structure and Function of the Skin, in *Dermatology*, 2nd edition, edited by S. L. Moschella, D. M. Pillsbury, and H. J. Hurley, Jr., copyright 1975, W. B. Saunders Company.

Parts of Chapter 4 are adapted by permission from Biopsy: Why, Where, When, How in The Journal of Dermatologic Surgery, *1:1*, copyright 1975.

Figure 7–10 is reproduced by permission from *Scabies* by Milton Orkin, copyright 1977, J. B. Lippincott Company.

Figure 2, Plate 4, and Figures 10-51A and 12-65 are reproduced by permission from Archives of Dermatology, *107*:375-376, copyright 1973, American Medical Association.

Library of Congress Cataloging in Publication Data

Ackerman, A. Bernard, 1936–
    Histologic diagnosis of inflammatory skin diseases.
    Bibliography.
    Includes index.
    1. Skin—Inflammation—Diagnosis.   2. Histology, Pathological.   I. Title. [DNLM:
1. Histological technics.   2. Dermatitis—Diagnosis. WR140 A182h]
RL231.A23   616.5'07'583   76-49437
ISBN 0-8121-0581-8

Published in Great Britain by Henry Kimpton Publishers, London
PRINTED IN THE UNITED STATES OF AMERICA

Print Number 2

To my nuclear family, my father Leon, mother Elizabeth,
brother Jim, and sister Sue,
and to my extended family, my students, teachers, and colleagues,
with affection and gratitude

Preface

DERMATOPATHOLOGY is a continuously evolving, but still youthful discipline. Its late nineteenth century pioneers were Europeans, namely, Albert Jesionek, Josef Kyrle, Paul Unna, Achille Civatte, and Felix Pinkus. Oskar Gans' classic text in German appeared in 1925. The first original American textbook by Walter Lever appeared in 1949, followed by those of Arthur Allen in 1962, Hamilton Montgomery in 1967, Hermann Pinkus and Amir Mehregan in 1969, and James Graham, Waine Johnson, and Elson Helwig in 1972.

Long recognized clinical conditions are continually being defined and redefined histologically, and seemingly new skin diseases are constantly developing and being discovered. For example, prior to 1943, any bullous disease that ended fatally was called "pemphigus." In that year Civatte perceptively separated pemphigus vulgaris from other bullous eruptions on histologic grounds. And it was not until 1956 that toxic epidermal necrolysis was described by Lyell and subcorneal pustular dermatosis by Sneddon and Wilkinson. In 1957, Pierard called attention to characteristic histologic features of dermatitis herpetiformis, a disease previously considered to be microscopically nondiagnostic. As late as 1970, Grover described "transient acantholytic dermatosis," a papulovesicular disease with histologic features that must be differentiated from those of keratosis follicularis (Darier's disease), familial benign chronic pemphigus (Hailey-Hailey disease), and pemphigus. Only recently has it been generally appreciated that neoplasms that appear to be malignant by histologic criteria may be biologically benign. In 1948 Spitz distinguished benign juvenile melanoma from malignant melanoma, and in 1968 Macaulay described lymphomatoid papulosis, a benign simulator of malignant lymphoma.

The first principle in the classic method of elucidating pathology is application of detailed knowledge of both gross and microscopic features as they develop over time. This approach should be especially applicable to the body's exteriorized organ, the skin. Nevertheless, the study of skin diseases is not to this day pursued in this traditional unified fashion. Gross pathologic changes in skin are still almost exclusively in the discipline of practicing dermatologists, whereas microscopic matters have been left to general pathologists or a small group of dermatopathologists.

It would be unthinkable for a general pathologist to cut sections of a diseased liver for histologic study without first describing its gross aspects. The dermatologist routinely examines gross specimens of the skin (clinical lesions) and advances to biopsy only in exceptional cases, because so many skin diseases are clinically diagnostic and do not require biopsy for confirmation. For this reason the dermatologist perforce has become the gross pathologist of the skin par excellence. Why is the general pathologist not a student of gross pathology of the skin? The reasons are several: (1) residency training in general pathology does not include rotation through dermatologic clinics where gross aspects of skin diseases are studied in the living patient and where nuances of color, form, and substance can be learned; (2) the amount of skin tissue submitted to pathology laboratories is almost always relatively minute (curettings, slices or shaves, punched out specimens, and small excisions), and these do not permit visual reconstruction of the original clinical lesions; and (3) the forbidding dermatologic nomenclature, including names of diseases like "pityriasis lichenoides et varioliformis acuta," "telangiectasia macularis eruptiva perstans," and "hyperkeratosis follicularis et parafollicularis in cutem penetrans," must intimidate even the most curious and courageous general pathologist.

Unfortunately, lack of familiarity with the gross appearance of skin diseases limits the capability of the general pathologist to acquire expertise with respect to microscopy of the skin. Thus, inflammatory diseases of the skin that are histologically distinguishable and diagnosable are too often diagnosed as "chronic nonspecific dermatitis." Cutaneous neoplasms, especially of the adnexa, can be baffling and frustrating to the point of intellectual surrender. Consequently, the general pathologist not uncommonly leafs through the pages of a modern standard textbook of dermatopathology hoping to happen upon a histologic picture that resembles the perplexing one under his own microscope. Usually, the cursory search proves vain.

Thus, there is a need for a textbook that weds the gross and microscopic features of skin diseases and simultaneously provides a logical, systematic, and reproducible method of histologic diagnosis. This book endeavors to fill that need in part and to serve all students of skin disease, be they dermatologists, pathologists, surgeons, residents, or medical students. The concern is with inflammatory skin diseases, because as a group these conditions pose the greatest diagnostic difficulty and have hitherto not been presented in a comprehensive or discriminating fashion. The attention devoted to each disease is roughly proportional to the frequency with which each is encountered in the Western world or to the relative medical importance of each of them. Common conditions like contact dermatitis and psoriasis and those with internal organ concomitants like lupus erythematosus, for example, are considered at length. Less emphasis is accorded the rare and esoteric.

It is difficult to decide whether some diseases are truly inflammatory or neoplastic (e.g., angiolymphoid hyperplasia with eosinophils, nonlipid reticuloendotheliosis or Letterer-Siwe disease, and reticulohistiocytoma). The reader may disagree with some of my conclusions about them.

The approach to histologic diagnosis of inflammatory skin diseases herein presented presumes a rudimentary knowledge of general pathology and hardly any of dermatology. The method is based upon diagnosis by pattern, rather than by presumption of cause or mechanism (see Chapter 5, Diagnosis by Histopathologic Patterns). The crucial characteristics for histologic diagnosis of many inflammatory skin diseases have been recorded in outline form. Diagnostic features are further emphasized by photomicrographic and schematic illustrations. Clinical features are explained in terms of histologic findings. In this way the pathologic process can be viewed as a dynamic continuum. The limitations of this method for a comprehensive understanding of a total disease process are obvious. A biopsy *in parte*, like a snapshot, records a partial truth, that is, one perception of an event at a moment in its history. Histologic sections, 5 microns thin, cut from an originally minuscule specimen that previously has run a chemical gauntlet, further narrow the pathologist's overview. What is needed to understand truly the sequence of events that constitutes the lesion is a histologic motion picture from inception of the disease to date of examination. The time-lapse footage, composed of sequential biopsies, would be short for a wheal, but long for a lesion of discoid lupus erythematosus or necrobiosis lipoidica. Furthermore, an attempt should be made in the mind's eye to reconstruct tridimensionally what one sees histologically as a vertical plane.

An attempt has been made to compensate for the inherent inadequacy of judgments based on relatively few, randomly obtained biopsies by including a summation. The summation, which places the diagnostic features of each disease into a larger framework of its reconstructed history, indicates unusual or exceptional features and elaborates upon noteworthy aspects, such as a cause and pathogenesis when they are known.

The student is encouraged to read each of the first five chapters consecutively in order to become familiar with terminology and concepts and thus to be better prepared for the succeeding chapters. Space has been left for the reader's own observations, some of which may differ from the author's. The reader is encouraged to participate in this adventure in learning about skin disease and to make this book as much his as the author's.

The language of this text is that of general pathology as well as of dermatology. For example, "epidermal hyperplasia" is used in lieu of "acanthosis," and "dermatitis" is used to mean "inflammation of the skin." Usages that are parochial, in my opinion, and muddle, rather than clarify, thinking are eschewed. The term *eczema* is never used, because so frequently the word conveys entirely different meanings to equally competent dermatologists. Fanciful expressions like "alteration cavitaire," "festooning," "corps ronds," and "grains" are avoided, as are words in the vocabulary of classic pathology that tend to be misconstrued, e.g., "leukoplakia," "dysplasia," and "necrobiosis" (except in the disease "necrobiosis lipoidica"). Inflammatory cells are individually named, rather than misleadingly designated "acute" or "chronic" in conglomeration (e.g., lymphocytes are dominant in an acute condition like urticaria, and neutrophils in a chronic condition like erythema elevatum diutinum). In lieu of eponyms, such as microabscess of Munro, microabscess of Pautrier, spongiform pustule of Kogoj, and Civatte bodies, the actual cytologic and morphologic changes are described.

This book is intended to be of practical assistance in the histologic diagnosis of inflammatory skin diseases and is not a reference textbook for those interested in an exhaustive review of the literature about each subject. Such compendia already exist. This book, except for the first two chapters, represents a distillation of my own experience, a personal judgment about pathologic processes in skin as witnessed by me. For this reason no references are given. Additional readings are suggested at the end of Chapters 1 and 2. Some inflammatory conditions (e.g., disseminated lipogranulomatosis, yaws, and anthrax) will not be discussed at all, only because such cases have yet to come to my personal attention. To discourse on them would be copying from secondary sources, a practice I have avoided. I would be grateful to colleagues who would permit me to study their slides of diseases that have not been included here, but which they think should be.

No exposition of any subject is really and entirely one's own. Each of us perceives from a position to which we have been led by those who have explored before us. My own thinking has been vastly enriched by teachers, students, and colleagues.

In particular, I am thankful for having had the opportunity to take residency training in dermatology at Columbia University, Harvard University, and the University of Pennsylvania. I am greatly indebted to Carl Nelson, who exemplifies the best of the careful, concerned, conservative approach to the study of skin disease, and to Albert Kligman, who by instruction and example makes the skin into a playground where any lively intellect can unlock secrets if only he would cavort daringly, imaginatively, and skeptically.

The influence of my teacher, Wallace Clark, on my thinking about pathologic processes in skin cannot be overemphasized or adequately acknowledged. It was he who taught me to classify skin disease on the basis of distinctive histologic patterns. His other students will recognize the impact of some of his precepts upon these pages: insistence upon precise clinicopathologic correlation; emphasis on biologic behavior; abhorrence of clichés like "junctional activity," "liquefaction degeneration," and "toxic hyalin;" contention that "diseases don't read the textbooks;" and protestation that "special stains only make what you don't know a different color."

More recently, as a counterweight to these iconoclastic teachings, Arkadi Rywlin, schooled in Europe and in the Virchowian tradition, has kindled in me esteem for the principles of classic pathology. For years now he has been an ever-ready consultant as well as a staunch friend.

Harvey Blank created a department of dermatology at the University of Miami School of Medicine in which those prepared in mind could flourish. I was there for four years. Much of the material presented in these pages is a condensation of my thinking during that seminal period in Miami.

This work was completed at the Skin and Cancer Unit of New York University School of Medicine. There, Rudolf Baer provided an idyllic setting for me and for dermatopathology, physically and spiritually. I am grateful to him for this, and particularly for being the kind of person he is.

No acknowledgment can adequately express the debt that I owe to my students, residents in dermatology and pathology, and fellows in dermatopathology (especially Marc Chalet, Dong

Chang, Richard Connors, Robert Greenberg, Paul Kechijian, John Maize, John Niven, Cleire Paniago-Pereira, Harold Rabinovitz, Ken Raiten, Michael Schwartz, Thomas Wade, Anna Ragaz, and Elaine Waldo) who as a group reviewed the manuscript with me chapter by chapter. Their contributions were more than simply a curious and critical approach to dermatopathology. This book in large measure represents the dividends of their emotional investment in me. Additional thanks are due John Niven for his invaluable assistance in the study of the panniculitides.

Lewis Shapiro, one of my teachers and now a close colleague, kindly permitted me to utilize his extensive collection of histologic slides of the panniculitides, and my Munich colleagues, Gerd Plewig, Helmut Wolff, and Otto Braun-Falco, graciously lent me several tissue blocks. Individual slides have also been kindly given to me by Dan Hellerman, William Hamilton, and Lynn From. David Bickers, a young colleague, read the entire manuscript and made helpful suggestions. Sections of this book have been read by many friends and colleagues at different times. Let it be known to them that they have my appreciation and grateful thanks.

Gary Wagner, while a resident in dermatology at the University of Minnesota, developed a method for making impressions of the skin surface by using a polysulfide rubber base dental impression material. He kindly permitted me to use some of his magnificent and artistic photographs on the title page and in Chapter 1.

For nearly eight years now, I have been fortunate in having the help of two exceptional persons in the production of this book, namely, William Atkinson for the photography and Dr. Leo Termin for the illustrations. Bill did not merely "shoot" thousands of photomicrographs; he "posed" each specimen and reproduced every one of them as "still life." He did not merely click the shutter of his camera; he studied his "subjects" and brought out their quality starkly and realistically. And, if Bill is in the tradition of the great camera artists, Dr. Termin is equally in the tradition of the great graphic artists. Leo is not just a superb medical illustrator because he is skillful with the tools of the craft but because he brings to his artistry the broad knowledge he has as the fine general pathologist he is.

The unsung heroes and heroines of this endeavor are the histology technicians of our laboratory who, in preparation for photography, cut tissue blocks over and over again until flawless sections were obtained.

With me in "the agony and the ecstasy" have been my secretaries, Anne Trivoluzzi, Linda Pivovarnik, and Judy Baker, who typed and retyped the manuscript, my administrative assistant,

Joyce Curwen, who helped to collate the written and pictorial parts, Louise Fred who honed the syntax, and Isabelle Clouser, Thomas Colaiezzi, and Kenneth Bussy of Lea & Febiger who put it all together as a book. Special thanks are also due to Howard N. King whose imagination and esthetic sense were invaluable in the design of this book. The pharmaceutical companies, Reed and Carnrick and Westwood, and the Samuel Penneys Foundation helped to defray the cost of color photography. I am very grateful to all of them.

This series of acknowledgments would not be complete without a special note of thanks to my linguistic luminary, Morris Leider. He gave me generously of his time and literary talent, carefully, thoughtfully, and critically reviewing the entire manuscript with me word by word from title to index. He also argued and made suggestions about the technical matter.

These colleagues, and others, helped to lay the foundation for this approach to the diagnosis and understanding of inflammatory skin diseases. I have attempted to erect girders; it is for the reader to fashion the rest.

Disce, doce, dilige.

A. BERNARD ACKERMAN, M.D.

New York, New York

Contents

Histologic Diagnosis of Inflammatory Skin Diseases

A METHOD BY PATTERN ANALYSIS

Skin: Structure and Function

Skin:

Structure *and* Function

UNDERSTANDING pathologic processes in skin, as in any organ, requires thorough grounding in normal structure and function. For inflammatory skin diseases, this is especially true of the vasculature, in particular, the blood vessels.

Embryonic Development

All constituents of human skin are derived from either ectoderm or mesoderm. The epithelial structures (epidermis, pilosebaceous-apocrine unit, eccrine unit, and nails) are ectodermal derivatives. Nerves and melanocytes arise from neuroectoderm. Mesenchymal structures (collagen and elastic fibers; blood vessels, muscles, and fat) originate from mesoderm. The dermis will be considered first, because inflammation predominantly takes place there. Initially, embryonal dermis consists of stellate mesenchymal cells suspended in a matrix of acid mucopolysaccharides. At approximately 6 weeks of embryonic development, the first delicate collagen fibers appear; by 12 weeks, collagen bundles can be recognized; and by 24 weeks, elastic fibers are also present within this myxomatous matrix. The collagen fibers in the upper part of the dermis are arranged in thinner bundles than they are in the deeper part. Eventually, as the fibrillar component steadily increases and the cellular content declines proportionately, the dermis acquires features typical of connective tissue.

Blood vessels are formed within the dermis from mesenchymal cells rich in alkaline phosphatase. A vascular network begins to organize about the twelfth week. Characteristic venous and arterial plexuses are not apparent until the final weeks of fetal development. Beneath the dermis, mesenchymal cells surrounding newly formed blood vessels differentiate into lipid-filled cells to form the subcutaneous fat.

Cutaneous nerves originate from the neural crest and are detectable in the embryonic dermis at about 5 weeks. In succeeding weeks, an elaborate neural network develops. Deeper nerve trunks send out ascending branches that terminate as slender fibrils in the papillary dermis, and Meissner's corpuscles appear at the tips of the papillae in acral areas, such as fingers. Pacini's corpuscles later appear, deep in the dermis and in the subcutaneous fat.

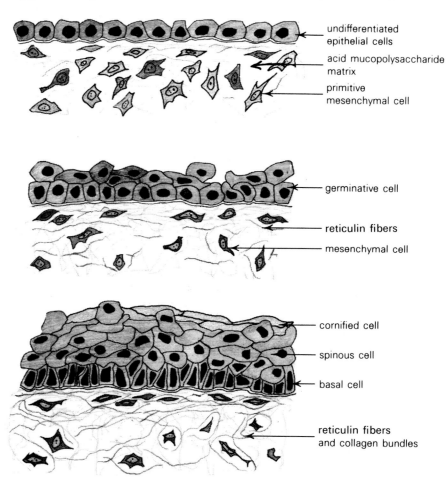

FIG 1-1. Histogenesis of epidermis from single layer of undifferentiated epithelial cells into multilayered cornifying epithelium.

The epidermis, which develops from the surface ectoderm, consists of a single layer of undifferentiated cells in a 3-week-old embryo (Fig. 1-1). By 4 weeks, it has an inner germinative layer of cuboidal cells with dark, compact nuclei and an outer layer of slightly flatter cells. About this time, dendritic cells (melanocytes) derived from the neural crest appear at the base of the epidermis. Between the fourteenth and sixteenth weeks, several layers of glycogen-rich, pale cells come into being in the intermediate zone. Under the light microscope, these cells appear to be joined together by delicate bridges that resemble spines. Granules (keratohyaline) become increasingly prominent in the upper part of the spinous zone. After the seventeenth week, when the germinative cells become columnar and the surface cells lose their nuclei and begin to cornify, the fetal epidermis begins to resemble the neonatal epidermis. From below upward, there are basal, spinous, granular, and cornified layers. The epidermis is a characteristic epithelium with contiguous cells and little extracellular material.

In the early stages of development, the interface between the epidermis and dermis is flat. At about 10 weeks, this boundary becomes wavy. The dermal papillae arise as nipple-shaped insertions of connective tissue into hollows of the epidermal undersurface. The papillae contain both terminal capillary loops and sensory nerve endings. A basement membrane, contributed partly by the adjacent epidermal cells, develops at the junction between the dermis and epidermis.

The first indication of impending hair follicle differentiation is seen at 10 weeks when nubbins of mesenchymal cells aggregate beneath discrete foci of closely crowded, elongated germinative epidermal cells (Fig. 1-2). These rapidly dividing epidermal cells grow downward as solid, slanting epithelial columns that penetrate through the developing dermis and reach into the subcutaneous fat. The germinative cells also proliferate upward and by piercing the epidermis establish the funnel-shaped opening of the hair canal which later will house the hair shaft. The descending columns of epithelial cells advance as if in pursuit of the nubbins of mesenchymal cells mentioned above. The base of the epithelial column becomes bulbous as it finally catches and partially encloses the nubbin that by now has become a spade-shaped ball of vascular connective tissue that will serve as the hair papilla. Continuous with the papilla is the fibrous sheath that envelops the entire follicle. Around the papilla in crescent-shaped array are the germinative, or matrix, cells of the hair follicle. This hair unit of papilla and matrix cells is analogous to the epidermal unit formed by the papillary dermis and the basal cells. Damage to the hair papilla or matrix will be reflected in an altered hair shaft.

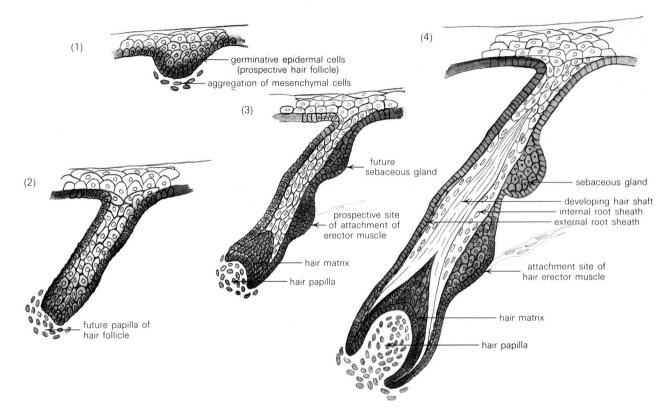

FIG 1-2. Beginning of pilosebaceous unit with massing of primitive mesenchymal cells, which become papilla of hair follicle, and above which epidermal cells become eventual hair follicle. Sebaceous gland and attachment site of hair erector muscle then develop from epithelium of hair follicle.

The cells of the hair matrix proliferate and mature into the several concentrically arranged cellular tubes that in conglomeration constitute the hair and its follicle. From inside outward, they are the hair cortex, hair cuticle, inner root-sheath cuticle, Huxley's layer, Henle's layer, and outer root sheath (trichilemmal sheath). The hair cortex (shaft), in the center of the follicle, is pushed upward by the stream of cornifying cells supplied by the matrix. By the thirteenth week, wisps of hair emerge from ostia on the eyebrow, upper lip, and chin. These hairs (lanugo) eventually cover the whole skin surface, except for the palms, soles, terminal phalanges of the digits, and the glans penis.

As it slants downward into the dermis, the prospective hair follicle is cylindrical. Near the sixteenth week, epithelial cells crowd together at three discrete loci on the side of the follicle that forms the widest angle with the epidermis. These three buds of epithelial cells expand outward into the mesenchyme. The lowest of these linearly arranged outgrowths forms a bulge that becomes the inferior attachment site of the erector muscle of the hair. This smooth muscle bundle develops from elongated mesenchymal cells and extends from the bulge to the superior attachment site beneath the epidermis. As its cells become laden with lipid, the middle bud develops into the lobulated sebaceous gland. The sebaceous gland connects to the central hair canal by a narrow duct. The uppermost outgrowth of the follicular epithelial cells forms the apocrine gland, which grows down into the subcutaneous fat as a solid cord of cells that, by 24 weeks, becomes coiled. A lumen, formed by a cleft between the cells, usually opens into the hair canal above. Less commonly, the lumen of the apocrine duct empties directly onto the skin surface. The anlagen of apocrine glands probably develop in all hair follicles, but most of them regress before birth. Those that persist are situated mainly in the axillary and genital regions.

Initially, the epidermis that will become the future nail unit is indistinguishable from the surrounding surface epithelium (Fig. 1-3). At 10 weeks, a smooth, shiny quadrangular area, demarcated laterally and proximally by a continuous shallow groove, can be recognized on the distal dorsal surface of each digit. The epidermis in this circumscribed area consists of three layers: surface, intermediate, and germinative. At 11 weeks, the column of germinative and intermediate cells, the anlage of the nail matrix, grows proximally and slants downward for a short distance into the dermis. The acute angle formed between the matrix and the surface epidermis becomes the proximal nail fold. Later, the distal boundary of the matrix will be represented by the lunula, a whitish half-moon-shaped area that extends beyond the proximal nail fold. The lunula is best seen in the thumbnail.

At 13 weeks, four layers can be recognized in the epidermis of the prospective nail area: basal, spinous, granular, and cornified. This area, now called the nail bed, loses its granular layer by the twentieth week. At 14 weeks, the proximal part of the nail bed acquires an additional cover of cornified cells, the nail plate or actual nail. The nail plate is produced by the matrix, without an intermediary granular layer. The cornified layer that extends from the undersurface of the proximal nail fold onto the surface of the newly formed nail plate is called the cuticle. By 16 weeks, the nail plate has advanced from the matrix distally to cover one half of the nail bed and has completely covered it by 19 weeks, at which age the fetal nail resembles that of the adult.

The germinative cells of the epidermis, hair, and nail come to the same end. They become cornified cells composed mainly of keratin, a fibrous protein. All epithelial cells in skin that become keratin are called keratinocytes.

Eccrine sweat glands develop first on the palms and soles of 10-week-old embryos as focal massings of germinative cells at the bases of the epidermal ridges (Fig. 1-4). These apparently occur without the development of mesenchymal papillae. Slender col-

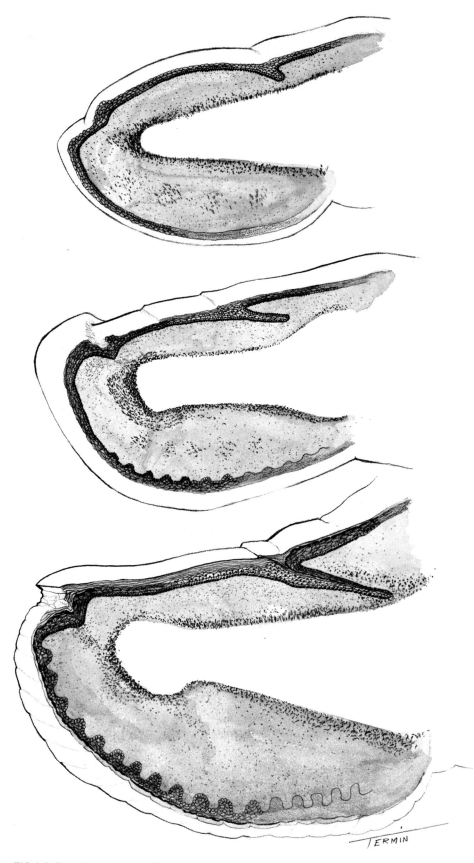

FIG 1-3. Evolution of nail unit in a fashion similar to that of hair follicle. Nail plate, hair shaft, and epidermal cornified layer are end products of germinative cells of nail and hair matrices and basal layer of epidermis.

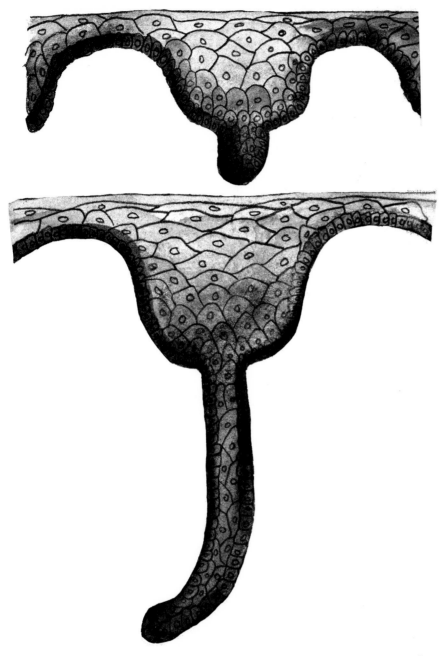

FIG. 1-4. Development of eccrine sweat unit from undifferentiated epidermal cells at base of rete ridge.

umns of glycogen-filled epithelial cells project perpendicularly downward into the dermis and upward through the epidermis. The outer layers of these columns are continuous with the germinative layer of the epidermis, whereas the inner cores connect with the intermediate layer. When the epithelial downgrowths reach the subcutaneous fat, their deepest portions become coiled. Lumens form about the thirtieth week. From the base upward, a mature eccrine sweat unit consists of a coiled secretory gland, a coiled intradermal duct, a straight intradermal duct, and a spiraled intraepidermal duct.

Topography and Regional Variation

The surface of the skin is intricate and varied. Regional differences in skin structure represent either adaptations to particular functions or the vestiges of prehuman life. The reader should inspect his own skin as a demonstration model while perusing the following paragraphs.

The skin of infants is traversed by a subtle maze of markings that develops during the third and fourth months of fetal life and becomes increasingly prominent during childhood. The designs remain unchanged throughout life and are nearly indestructible. Swirled patterns typify palms and soles. Small, roughly diamond-shaped outlines crisscross the rest of the body surface and are particularly well seen in the skin over the volar aspect of the wrist and elbows, in the antecubital fossae, and between the knuckles (Fig. 1-5). The developmental conditions that determine the orientation of the surface ridges are unknown, but they are thought to result from (1) epidermal rete ridges-dermal papillae

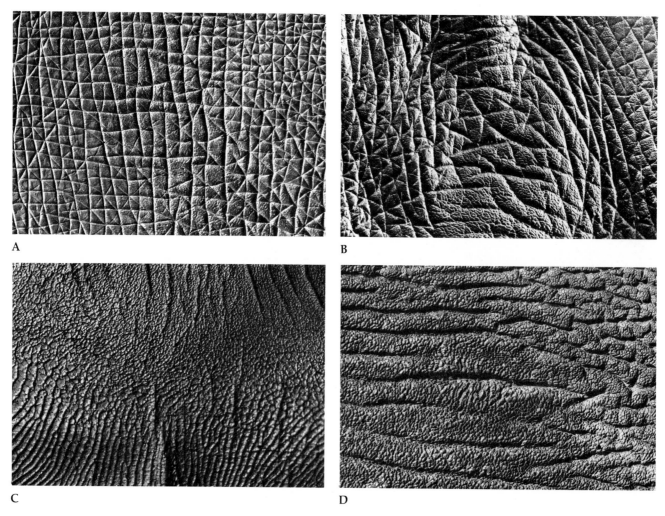

A

B

C

D

FIG. 1-5. Normal skin. A, Lateral ankle. B, Knuckle. C, Left index finger. D, Knee. (Courtesy Gary Wagner.)

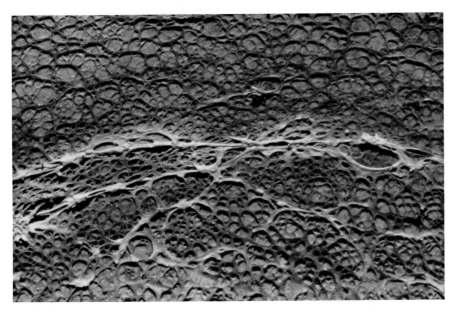

FIG. 1-6. Moldings of various sizes and shapes on undersurface of epidermis at junction of nipple and areola of a woman. (Courtesy William Montagna, Ph.D.)

configuration, (2) arrangement of underlying collagen bundles, and (3) pull of muscle and fascia on the dermis. Just as the epidermal surface is marked by diverse figurations, so too is the epidermal undersurface of different body regions distinguished by varied contours (Fig. 1-6).

The etchings that cover the entire surfaces of the palms and soles, excluding flexion and other secondary creases, are collectively termed "dermatoglyphic patterns" (Fig. 1-7). Parallel ridges and furrows form whorls, loops, and arches on the fingertips in a

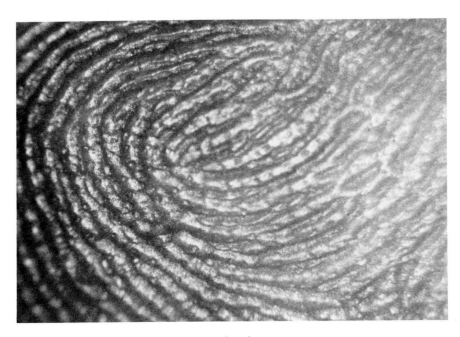

FIG. 1-7. Dermatoglyphic pattern on a thumb.

pattern so highly individualistic that fingerprinting has been used as a reliable method for personal identification, even permitting the distinction between identical twins. There are noticeable differences in dermatoglyphic patterns on the palms and fingers of the same person. Statistically, the patterns of women contain fewer whorls and more arches than those of men. The study of dermatoglyphics has enabled early detection of genetic abnormalities, such as Down's syndrome, and of defects caused in utero by infectious agents, such as the virus of rubella. Histologically, palmar and plantar skin is characterized by a thick cornified layer, prominent rete and papillae, numerous nerve endings and eccrine sweat units, and the absence of hair follicles. The corrugated palmar skin, like the tread of a tire, is well suited for grasping and gripping. The exquisite tactile sensibility of the fingertips was utilized by Braille in his reading system for the blind.

The dense, luxurious pelage that covers the scalp is reflected microscopically in numerous deeply rooted hair follicles. In man, hair is largely ornamental, whereas in other mammals hair serves primarily as a furry blanket to conserve heat. Although on casual observation man is an apparently naked animal, except for the scalp, pubes, axillae, beard, mustache, and chest, in actuality the entire body surface, excluding acral volar skin and mucocutaneous junctions, is dotted by hairs, many of them fine and tiny. The follicular ostia from which these extremely fine vellus hairs emerge are easily detectable on the forearm. Vellus hairs on the face of women, such as those above the lip, are usually inconspicuous until menopause, when hormonal changes can cause them to enlarge.

The taut skin of the back, composed of a thick dermis with broad collagen bundles, is well constructed to withstand the stress of man's upright posture. In contrast, the distensible skin of the eyelids, with its thin dermis, is aptly designed for the rapid movements necessary to protect the eyes. In general, skin is elastic.

At the body openings, skin is continuous with mucous membrane. Mucocutaneous junctions occur at the eyelids, nares, mouth, vulva, prepuce, clitoris, and anus. Histologically, skin differs from mucous membrane by possessing a cornified layer of cells without nuclei (Fig. 1-8).

Other regions of the skin also have distinguishing features: the greasy middle third of the face, especially in adolescents, results from secretions of the numerous large sebaceous glands associated with small hair follicles having prominent follicular orifices (sebaceous follicles) (Fig. 1-9); the helix of the ear is covered by many tiny vellus hairs, seen microscopically as closely set minute hair

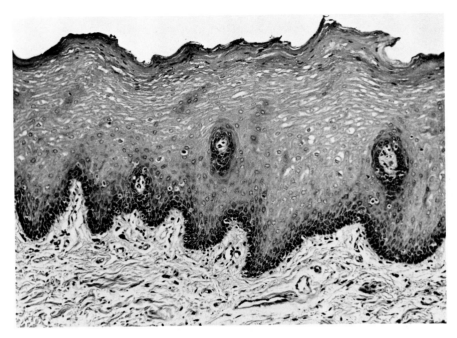

FIG. 1-8. Mucous membranes. Unlike skin, nuclei are within cells of slightly cornified surface. ($\times$ 187.)

follicles in a dermis having few sweat glands (Fig. 1-10); pigmented zones like the areola contain increased amounts of epidermal melanin; the hairy, sweaty axilla is an adnexal potpourri of hair follicles and sebaceous glands and myriads of apocrine and eccrine glands; and erectile tissues, such as nipples, clitoris, and penis, are endowed with highly vascularized smooth muscles. A consequence of man's upright posture is elevated hydrostatic pressure, and in the blood vessels of the legs, especially below the knee, this results in thick-walled superficial dermal blood vessels having plump endothelial cells (Fig. 1-11). The vasculature of the skin also eloquently reflects intense emotions, betraying shame and anger (reddening) and fear (pallor). Telltale signs of anxiety are cold hands and sweaty palms (clammy palms).

The Dermis

The skin is composed of three anatomically distinct layers. From the surface downward, these are the epidermis, the dermis, and the subcutaneous fat.

The dermis is mostly composed of dense, relatively noncellular fibroelastic tissue within which are embedded the pilosebaceous, apocrine, and eccrine units, blood vessels, lymphatics, muscles, and nerves. The dermis is 15 to 40 times thicker than the epidermis, depending upon its location, but its energy needs are low. The dermis rests on a thick pad of fat.

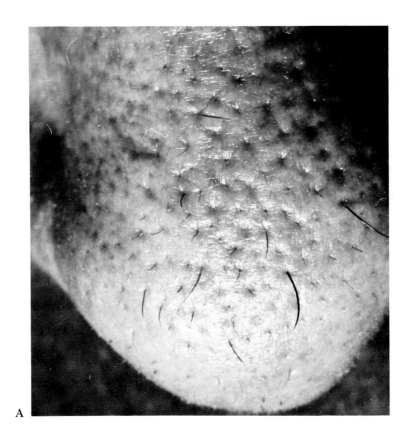

A

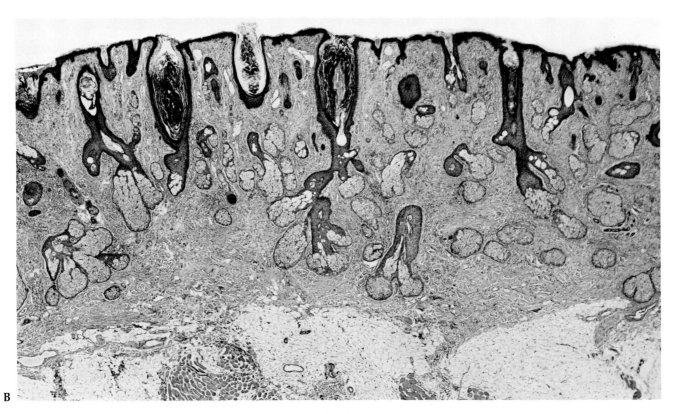

B

FIG. 1-9. Sebaceous follicles in skin of nose, a region characterized by prominent, patulous follicular ostia. A, clinical view. B, Histologic view. Note numerous large sebaceous glands attached to vellus follicles whose hair bulbs are situated high in dermis (× 22).

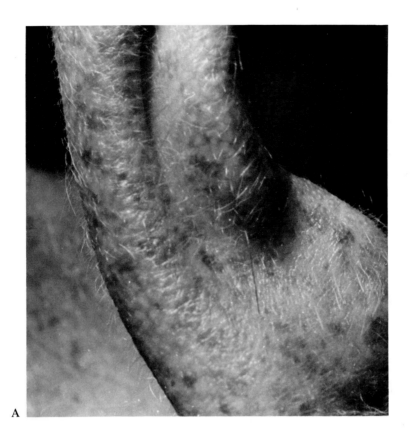

A

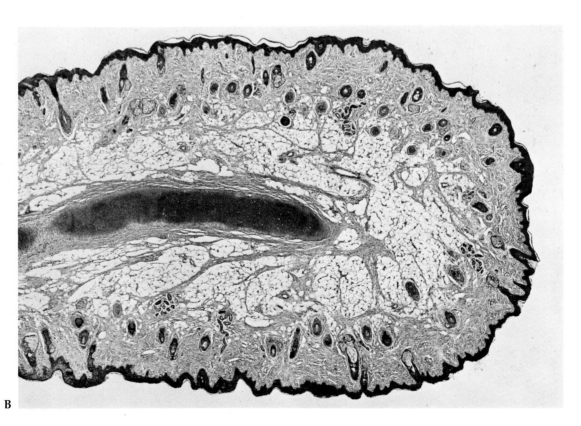

B

FIG. 1-10. Vellus hairs on pinna of ear. A, Clinical view. B, Histologic view. (×27.)

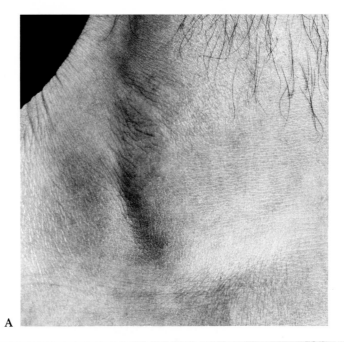

A

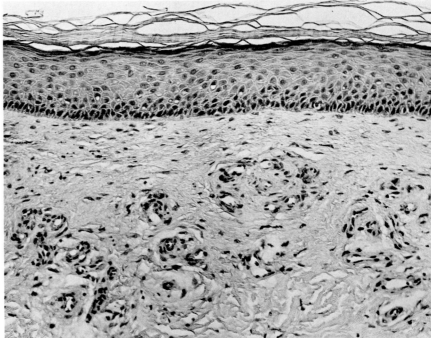

B

FIG. 1-11. Superficial dermal blood vessels near ankle. They have thick walls with plump endothelial cells. A, Clinical view. B, Histologic view. (× 250.)

Embryologically, primitive mesenchymal cells of the meso-derm give rise to the following dermal components:

1. Cells
    a) fibroblasts (fibrocytes)
    b) endothelial and perithelial cells
    c) myocytes (myoblasts)
    d) mast cells

2. Fibers
    a) collagen, including reticulin
    b) elastic

3. Ground substance
    a) hyaluronic acid
    b) chondroitin sulfate
    c) dermatan sulfate

The Cells, Fibers, and Ground Substance

The fully formed dermis can be conveniently divided into two distinct compartments: (1) the thin zone immediately beneath the epidermis (papillary dermis) and around adnexa (periadnexal dermis) and (2) the thick reticular dermis.

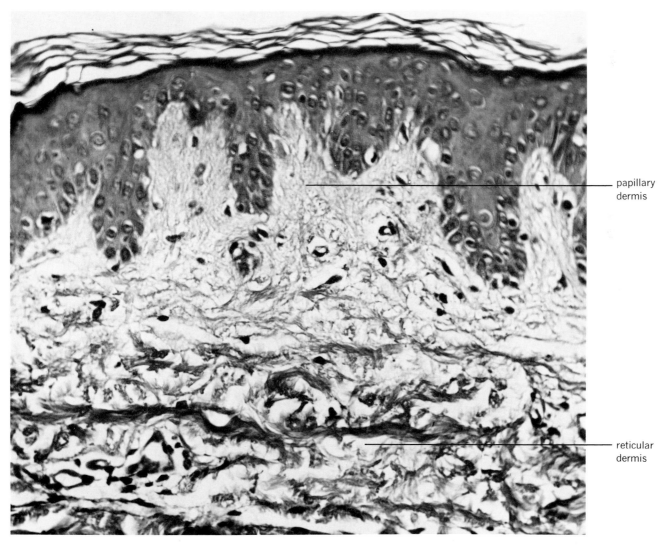

papillary dermis

reticular dermis

FIG. 1-12. Superficial (papillary) dermis. It is composed of thin, haphazardly arranged collagen fibers, in contrast to deeper (reticular) dermis, which is composed of thick collagen bundles. ($\times$ 374.)

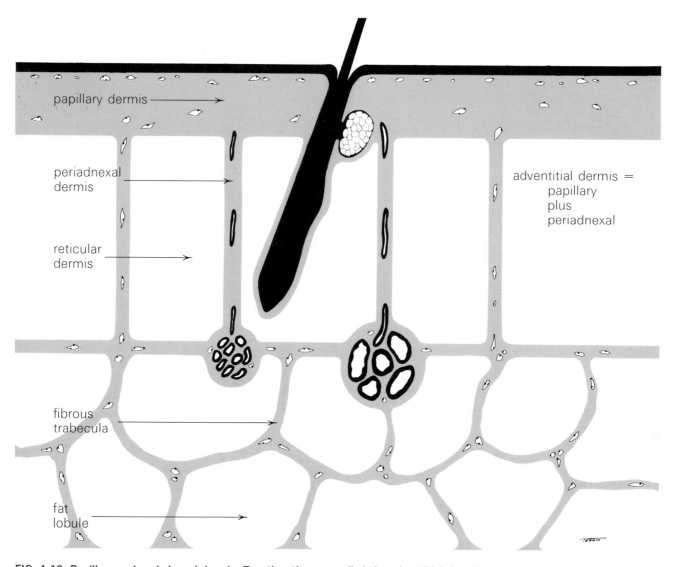

papillary dermis

periadnexal dermis

adventitial dermis = papillary plus periadnexal

reticular dermis

fibrous trabecula

fat lobule

FIG. 1-13. Papillary and periadnexal dermis. Together they are called the adventitial dermis and have similar appearances and functions.

The combined anatomic unit of papillary and periadnexal dermis is called the "adventitial dermis." It is characterized by thin, haphazardly arranged collagen fibers, delicate branching elastic fibers, numerous elongated, plump, and stellate-shaped fibroblasts, abundant ground substance, and plentiful capillaries linked to superficial arterial and venous plexuses (Fig. 1-12). The papillary dermis and epidermis together form a morphologic and functional unit, whose intimacy is reflected in their joint alteration by common inflammatory diseases. A similar relationship exists between periadnexal connective tissue and its adjacent epithelium.

The larger component of the dermis (reticular dermis) extends from the base of the papillary dermis to the subcutaneous fat (Fig. 1-13). It is composed of thick collagen bundles mostly arranged parallel to the skin surface in an orthogonal wickerwork. A network of coarse wiry elastic fibers enmeshes the collagen bundles.

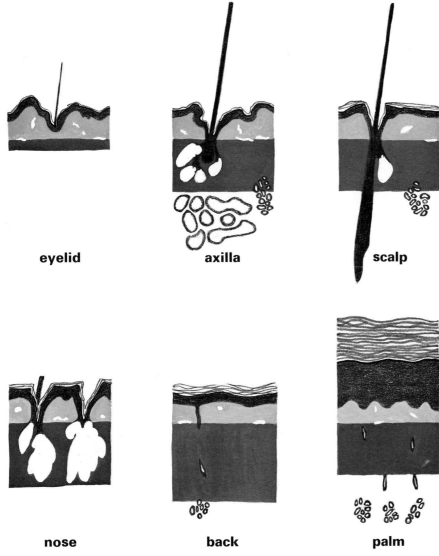

eyelid　　　　**axilla**　　　　**scalp**

nose　　　　**back**　　　　**palm**

FIG. 1-14. Variation in thicknesses of epidermis and dermis in different regions.

Proportionally, there are fewer fibroblasts and blood vessels and less ground substance in the broad reticular dermis than in the narrow adventitial dermis. Occasionally, cells of the subcutaneous fat (lipocytes) can be found within the dermis, and striated muscle is commonly seen in the dermis of facial skin.

The dermis varies in thickness in different regions, being thinnest in the eyelids and thickest in the back (Fig. 1-14). The total thickness of the papillary dermis increases when the skin is subjected to long-standing rubbing (lichen simplex chronicus), and the entire reticular dermis thickens in the disease scleredema. Individual collagen bundles become thinner in an atrophic scar and wider in a keloid. Like other tissues, the dermis decreases in thickness with advancing age.

The fibroblast is the builder cell of the dermis. It produces all the fibrillar components, as well as the ground substance. As seen

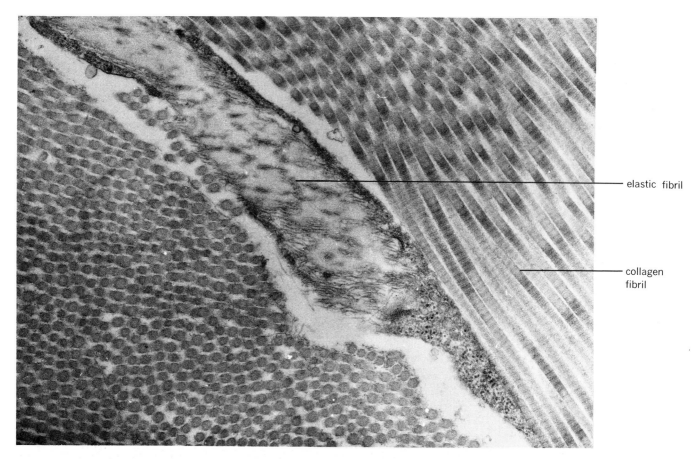

elastic fibril

collagen fibril

FIG. 1-15. Longitudinally cut collagen microfibrils. An elastic fibril consists of noncollagenous microfibrils embedded in homogeneous elastin. (× 55,000.) (Courtesy of Richard Wood, Ph.D.)

with the light microscope, the fibroblast has a spindle or stellate-shaped nucleus and indistinct cytoplasm. The electron microscope discloses that the cytoplasm of the fibroblast contains well-developed rough endoplasmic reticulum, mitochondria, and a distinct Golgi apparatus. These are features of a metabolically active cell, and it is likely that the fibroblast not only synthesizes the substance of connective tissue, but catabolizes it as well.

The fibrous proteins of connective tissue are formed from relatively small, soluble monomeric units synthesized on ribosomes within the cell and conveyed to the outside where they are polymerized. Collagen and elastic fibers are fashioned, in their final form, outside the fibroblast.

Contemporary nomenclature distinguishes among fibers that can be seen with the naked eye, fibrils that can be seen with the light microscope, and microfibrils that can be seen only with the electron microscope.

The collagen of the dermis consists of two genetically different types. Type I collagen forms thick fibers which are arranged in a dense orthogonal network in the reticular dermis. Type I fibers have a width of up to 20 μm and a high mechanical stability.

Electron-microscopically, the type I fibrils show distinct cross-bands 68 nm apart (Fig. 1-15). In contrast, type III collagen, formerly called "reticulin," is found principally in the adventitial dermis and consists of thin fibers, loosely arranged. Type III fibers have a diameter of about 1.5 μm, are not visible with hematoxylin-and-eosin stains, but are blackened by silver stains (argyrophilic). Type III collagen fibers are prominent within and beneath the epidermal basement membrane, where they intermingle with type I collagen fibers. In this zone, type III collagen fibers and finer filaments coursing in and through the basal lamina apparently help anchor the epidermis to the dermis. This narrow subepidermal zone of densely packed type III collagen fibers separates the elastic fibers of the papillary dermis from the epidermis. In the papillary dermis, elastic fibers are thin and mostly oriented perpendicularly to the epidermis. In the reticular dermis, elastic fibers are thicker and seemingly arranged mostly parallel to the skin surface (Fig. 1-16).

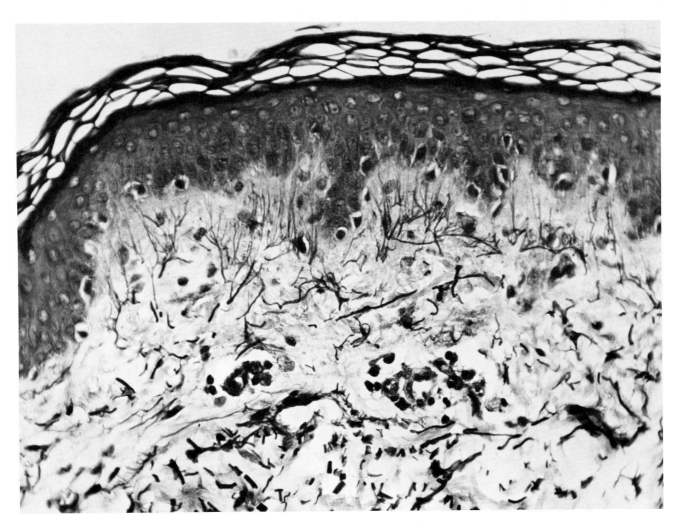

FIG. 1-16. Elastic fibers. In the papillary dermis they are thin and, in the main, are oriented perpendicularly to epidermis, whereas in reticular dermis, elastic fibers are thicker and tend to be arranged parallel to skin surface. (Elastic tissue stain.)

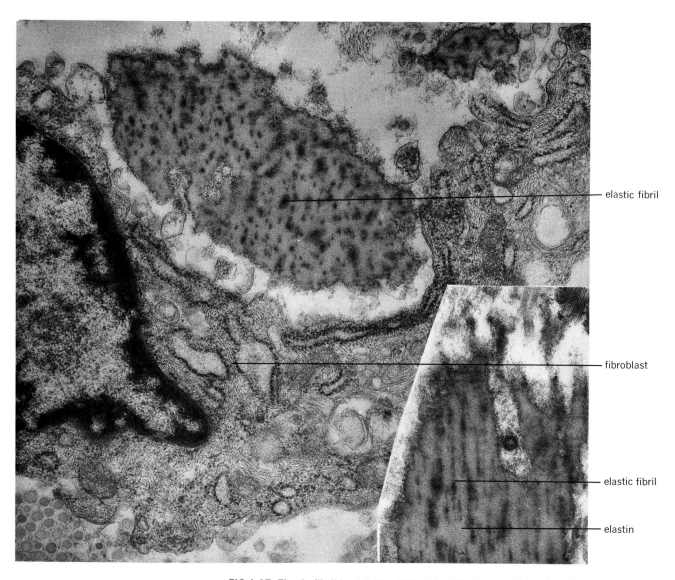

elastic fibril

fibroblast

elastic fibril

elastin

FIG 1-17. Elastic fibril in vicinity of fibroblast that has well-developed, rough-surfaced endoplasmic reticulum. In inset, an elastic fibril is seen to consist of microfibrils and homogeneous elastin. ($\times$ 22,500, insert $\times$ 41,750.) (Courtesy Ken Hashimoto, M.D.)

Immature elastic fibers are aggregates of protein microfibrils grouped cylindrically along the surface of the fibroblast (Fig. 1-17). Later, a second protein, elastin, is synthesized and secreted by the cell into the preformed tube of microfibrils. Elastic fibers then consist of microfibrils about 11 nm in diameter and elastin, with a molecular weight of 40,000. The two major fibrous components of the skin are closely associated with each other, elastic fibers being found only where there are collagen fibers. Collagen presumably provides the skin with tensile strength, whereas elastin returns the skin to its original dimensions after stretching. Diminution or absence of elastic fibers allows the skin to bulge in atrophic conditions such as striae and the anetodermas. The abundance of elastic fibers is peculiar to human skin.

Fibroblasts also give rise to ground substance, the extracellular mucinous matrix of the dermis. In routine histologic sections, the ground substance is invisible, appearing as empty spaces between collagen bundles. Special stains, such as alcian blue and colloidal iron, reveal ground substance in normal skin, especially in the adventitial dermis. The ground substance accounts for a substantial portion of the volume. Acid mucopolysaccharides—particularly hyaluronic acid, chondroitin sulfate, and dermatan sulfate—are the major elements of the ground substance. Other components of the ground substance are neutral mucopolysaccharides, proteins, and electrolytes. The ground substance is concentrated in the papillae of anagen hair follicles and around eccrine sweat glands. Ground substance has great capacity to bind water. It also contributes to the malleability of the skin.

In certain pathologic states, the amount of acid mucopolysaccharides in the dermis increases. This deposit is widespread in myxedema and is localized in focal mucinosis.

In addition to fibroblasts, there are other important wandering cells in the dermis. Scattered among the fibers are histiocytes, distinguished from fibroblasts, not always by histologic appearance, but by function. These are the scavengers of the dermis that engulf hemosiderin, melanin, lipid, and miscellaneous debris.

Mast cells, located primarily around blood vessels, can be recognized in hematoxylin-and-eosin-stained tissue sections by their darkly basophilic ovoid nuclei and granular amphophilic cytoplasm. They are discussed in Chapter 2.

The Vasculature

Vascular structures of skin are derived from primitive mesenchymal cells. A lining of endothelial cells is common to all parts of the vascular system. In the smallest cutaneous capillaries a single endothelial cell may encircle the entire circumference of the vessel. In larger capillaries a single layer of four to five flat endothelial cells, whose serrated edges interdigitate with each other, curves around the lumen (Fig. 1-18). Capillary endothelial cells are ensheathed by thin collagen or reticulin fibers. Arterioles have an intima of endothelial cells, a media containing smooth muscle cells, and an adventitia composed of collagen and elastic fibers. An internal elastic membrane is present beneath the endothelium of larger arterioles. Arteries that supply the skin are located in the subcutaneous fat, and they have both an internal and an external elastic membrane. Venules consist only of endothelium sur-

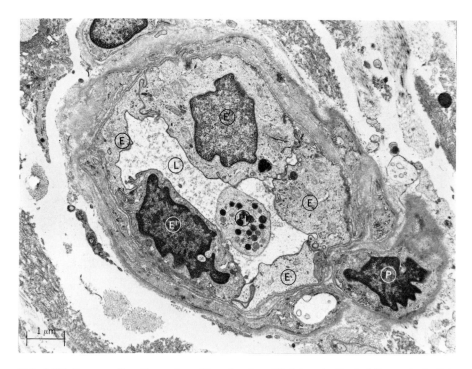

FIG. 1-18. Cross section through capillary in adventitial dermis. Part of five endothelial cells are pictured (E, E'), in two of which nuclei are seen (E'). Basement membrane is seen surrounding endothelial cells and pericyte (P). Within lumen (L) is a platelet (Pl). (× 9000.) (Courtesy Helmut Wolff, M.D.).

rounded by a thin zone of collagen fibers. In progressively larger venules, smooth muscles, elastic fibers, and an external elastic membrane appear. Pericytes lie just outside the endothelial cells of the microvasculature.

It is through the capillaries and venules that oxygen, water, nutrients, and hormones are distributed from the blood to the tissues, and carbon dioxide and other products of skin metabolism are collected for transmission to the excretory organs. The endothelium of capillaries and venules functions as a porous membrane, permeable to water and crystalloids, but relatively impermeable to larger molecules. Venules also are of primary importance in changes associated with inflammation.

The architecture of the dermal vasculature is a three-dimensional network of two plexuses that parallel the skin surface (Fig. 1-19). One plexus of arterioles and venules arranged in parallel is in the lower reticular dermis (deep plexus); the other courses beneath the papillary dermis in the upper reticular dermis (superficial plexus). The division into superficial and deep vascular plexuses provides a working concept for the study of inflammatory diseases in skin and is not meant to be an absolutely strict anatomic representation.

Perpendicularly oriented communicating blood vessels connect the deep and superficial plexuses. The deeper blood vessels have

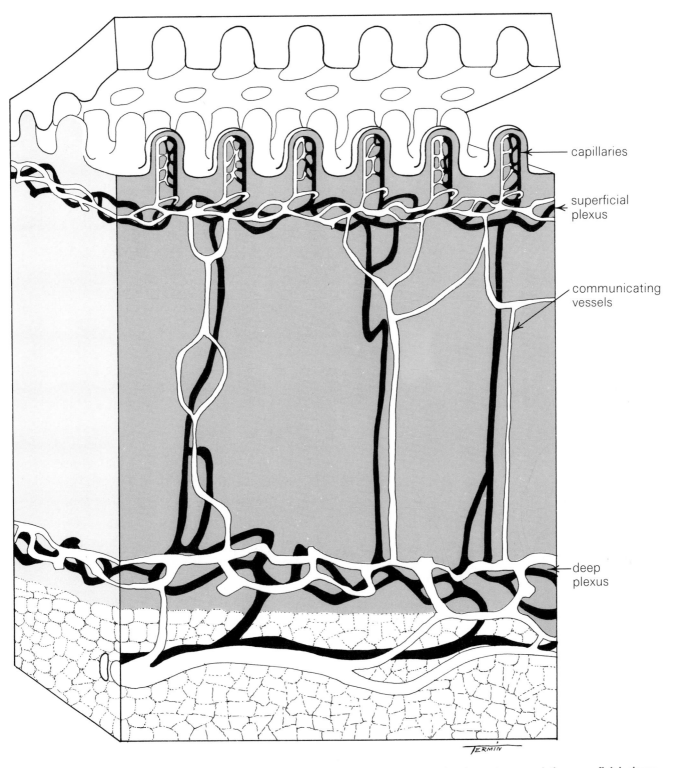

capillaries

superficial
plexus

communicating
vessels

deep
plexus

FIG. 1-19. Dermal vasculature. A network of two plexuses parallels skin surface: the deep plexus and the superficial plexus, connected by perpendicularly oriented communicating blood vessels. Rich capillary bed emanating from relatively straight, large conduits of two parallel plexuses and their communicating vessels provides microcirculation within dermis, especially adventitial dermis.

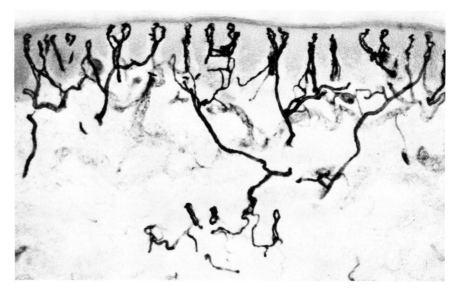

FIG. 1-20. Arcades of capillaries looping upward into papillae from subpapillary plexus. Alkaline phosphatase preparation. (Courtesy William Montagna, Ph.D.)

larger diameters. From the subpapillary plexus, arcades of capillaries loop upward into the papillae (Fig. 1-20). There are about 40 to 70 of these loops per square millimeter of skin surface. Each loop of these capillary "candelabra" consists of an ascending arterial limb and a descending venous one. The venous portion empties into the postcapillary venules of the superficial plexus and successively into the communicating venules, the venules of the deep plexus, and the small veins of the subcutis. Similar vessels to those in the dermal papillae infuse the periadnexal dermis. The rich blood supply of the adventitial dermis constitutes a microcirculation, in contrast to the relatively straight, large conduits of the two parallel plexuses and their communicating vessels. Abundant alkaline phosphatase activity can be demonstrated in the endothelial cells of the capillaries in the adventitial dermis (Figs. 1-21, 1-22).

Arteriovenous anastomoses are present in skin, especially in the digits. These specialized segments, known as Sucquet-Hoyer canals, are interposed between arterioles and venules (Fig. 1-23). They are surrounded by three to six rows of uniform, ovoid smooth-muscle cells that serve as sphincters. Each of these shunts, known as a "glomus," enables blood to bypass the capillaries and thus accelerates blood flow through the acral skin. Both the glomera and the arterioles are under the control of the sympathetic nervous system. A small nerve is associated with every glomus. Arterioles also respond to a variety of pharmacologic agents, e.g., epinephrine, vasopressin, and angiotensin cause vasoconstriction, whereas histamine, ethanol, acetylcholine, and prostaglandins of the E series cause vasodilation.

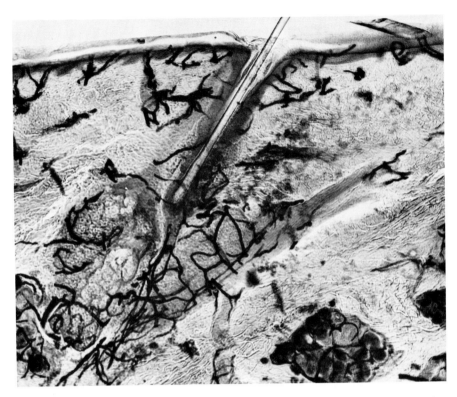

FIG. 1-21. Abundant capillaries in adventitial dermis, here shown enveloping sebaceous and eccrine glands. Alkaline phosphatase preparation. (Courtesy William Montagna, Ph.D.)

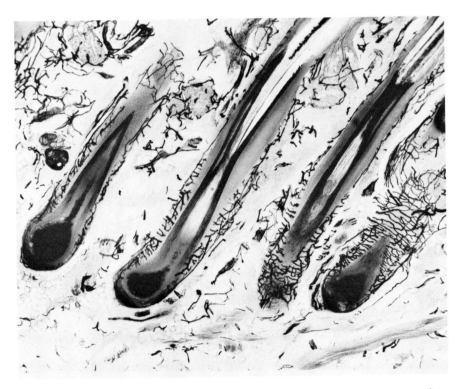

FIG. 1-22. Rich capillary supply to hair follicles. Alkaline phosphatase preparation.
(Courtesy William Montagna, Ph.D.)

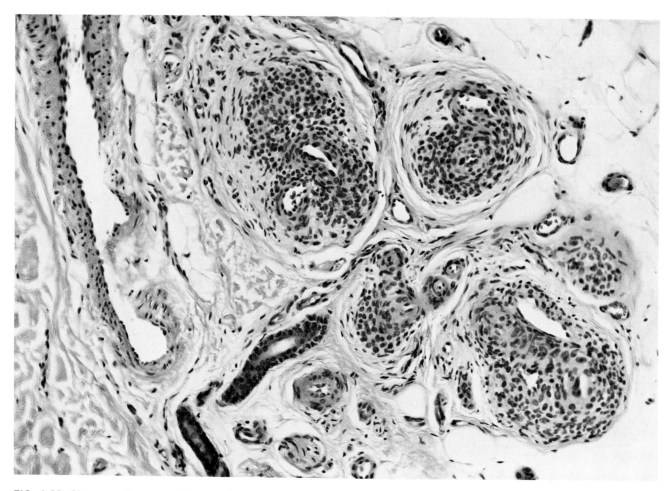

FIG. 1-23. Glomus cells surrounding arterioles and venules of specialized shunts known as glomus bodies or Sucquet-Hoyer canals. (× 187.)

Thermoregulation is a cardinal function of the cutaneous vasculature. Blood vessels in the skin maintain the body at a constant temperature by buffering the effect of wide variations in environmental and internal temperatures. Blood flow through the dermis varies in response to changes in the core temperature of the body and the temperature of the external environment. The control of dermal blood flow is partly directed by the hypothalamus and is mediated by the sympathetic nervous system.

Another function of the dermal blood vessels is to bring nutriments to the skin. The plentiful capillaries of the adventitial dermis supply epithelial structures whose oxidative requirements are greater than those of connective tissue. The total volume of blood that circulates through the dermis is requisite for thermoregulation but is considerably greater than necessary simply to nurture the skin.

Dermal blood vessels play the central role in inflammatory skin diseases. The microcirculatory unit of the papillary dermis participates in skin diseases characterized by erythema. These include all the common inflammatory eruptions whose red color is imparted by blood. The entire dermal vasculature presumably reacts, albeit to a lesser degree, in these inflammatory disorders.

Skin also harbors an elaborate network of lymphatics that parallels the major vascular plexuses but is independent of them. Like capillaries, the walls of lymphatics are constructed of a single-layered endothelium, but unlike capillaries the lymphatics have no pericytes, an absent or fragmentary basal lamina, and intercellular lateral gaps. Larger lymphatics can sometimes be distinguished from capillaries by the presence of valves. One terminus of a lymphatic tube ends blindly; the other empties into a lymphatic plexus. Lymphatics filter and transport a large portion of the capillary transudate, called "lymph," and return it to the venous system.

The Subcutaneous Fat

Subcutaneous fat, like the dermis, is derived from the mesenchyme, and fibroblast-like mesenchymal cells give rise to lipocytes, as well as to fibrocytes. Lipocytes manufacture so much fat in their cytoplasm that it displaces, presses, and flattens the nucleus against the periphery of the cell. Electron microscopy of lipocytes demonstrates that their cytoplasm contains relatively few mitochondria, but many free ribosomes. Human fat consists largely of triglycerides.

Strands of collagen divide the population of lipocytes into lobules. These fibrous elements, known as trabeculae or septa, house the major vascular networks, lymphatics, and nerves (Fig. 1-24). Lipomas, benign tumors of normal-appearing fat cells, are recognized histologically by the absence of a normal trabeculated framework. The coiled secretory tubules of eccrine and apocrine glands, as well as the bulbs of scalp hair follicles, may be found in the subcutis.

The subcutaneous fat varies in thickness from one part of the body to another, tending to be especially broad in the waists of the middle-aged and nearly nonexistent in the eyelid, penis, and scrotum. There are also regional differences between the sexes in deposition of fat, most notable in the rounded contours of the female torso. In both sexes the subcutaneous fat functions as a heat insulator, shock absorber, and nutritional depot which is mobilized during starvation. It also facilitates mobility of skin over underlying structures, a function notably lost in scleroderma where the fat is largely replaced by collagen. (The vasculature of the subcutaneous fat is discussed in Chapter 14.)

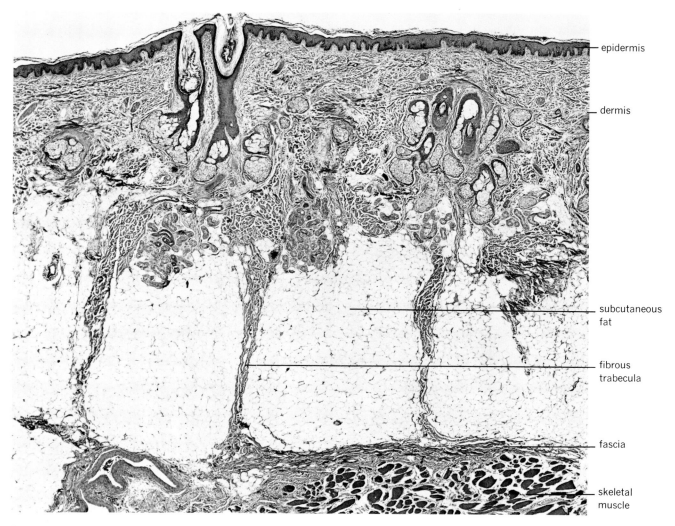

epidermis

dermis

subcutaneous fat

fibrous trabecula

fascia

skeletal muscle

FIG. 1-24. Strands of collagen termed trabeculae dividing conglomerations of subcutaneous fat cells into lobules. These fibrous septa also house major vascular networks, lymphatics, and nerves. (× 25.)

In humans, as in many species of vertebrates, there is a second type of adipose tissue, namely, brown fat, which differs in form and function from the previously discussed white fat. Whereas white (unilocular) lipocytes are characterized by large size (up to 120 μ in diameter), oval to round shape, and a single large lipid inclusion which displaces the nucleus to the periphery of the cell, brown (multilocular) fat cells are typically smaller (25 to 40 μ in diameter), polygonal in shape, and possess many small lipid inclusions within granular cytoplasms. Whereas white fat constitutes the bulk of all adipose tissue and is in general distributed throughout the body as well as the skin, brown fat occurs only at certain sites in embryos such as the interscapular region. However, brown fat is not an embryonic form of white fat, but exists as a distinct entity. It is especially prominent in rodents and hibernating animals where it is thought to function as a heat-producing tissue. Hibernoma is a benign neoplasm composed of cells that resemble those of brown fat.

The skin is a major sensory organ, serving to receive a barrage of stimuli and to perceive man's environment. In a sense, the skin is a specialized neural structure, the terminus of the peripheral nervous system. The sensations of touch, pressure, temperature, pain, and itch are received by millions of microscopic dermal nerve endings (Fig. 1-25). They are most numerous on hairless parts (palms, soles, fingers) and mucocutaneous areas, especially oral and minor genital lips, glans penis, nipples, and clitoris, the erogenous zones. These tiny end organs terminate principally in the papillary dermis and around hair follicles. Sensory receptors may be free or encapsulated, myelinated or unmyelinated, and are visualized with difficulty by hematoxylin and eosin staining. Fine nerve endings require special staining with silver, methylene blue, or cholinesterase methods.

The sensations of temperature, pain, and itch are gathered by tiny unmyelinated nerves that end in the papillary dermis and surround the hair follicles. Stimuli received by these nerve endings are transmitted to the central nervous system by relatively slow conducting unmyelinated fibers (C-fibers).

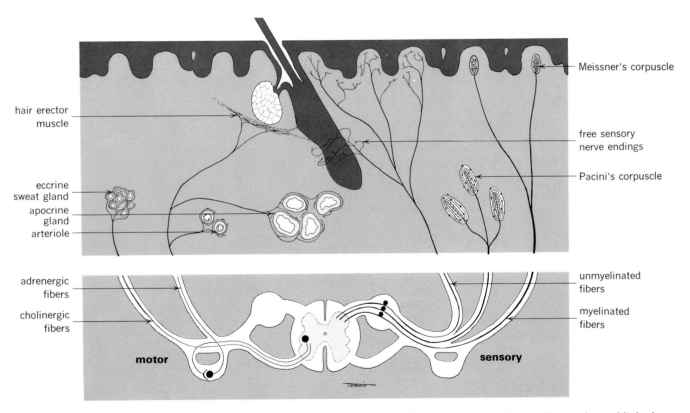

FIG. 1-25. Unmyelinated cutaneous nerve endings that transmit sensations of touch, pressure, temperature, pain, and itch via dorsal root ganglia to central nervous system. All motor fibers in skin are supplied by autonomic nervous system. Adrenergic fibers activate arterioles, glomus body, hair erector muscle, and apocrine glands; cholinergic fibers stimulate eccrine sweat glands.

Of all the sensations mediated by nerve fibers in the skin, itch is among the most distressing. Itching is most simply defined as the sensation that provokes the desire to scratch and is probably a type of mild pain. The sensation of itching is believed to be carried on C-fibers, whereas the sensation of pain travels on both C-fibers and small unmyelinated A-fibers. The nerve impulse frequency in itching is appreciably lower than in pain. By scratching, especially furiously, the pruritic patient substitutes pain for itch, replacing the slower maddening impulses with faster more tolerable ones.

The sensations of touch and pressure are recorded by the specialized corpuscles of Meissner and Pacini. Anatomically, one can recognize Meissner's corpuscles in the papillary dermis on palms and soles as encapsulated nerve endings consisting of a cylindrical connective-tissue unit within which myelinated and unmyelinated nerve fibers are ramified. Pacini's corpuscles are found principally on weight-bearing surfaces in the deep portion of the dermis and in the subcutis. They are large encapsulated end organs composed of thin lamellae of fibrous tissue arranged in concentric fashion around the myelinated and unmyelinated nerve fibers. The impulses originating at these mechanoreceptors pass into myelinated fibers and are swiftly transmitted to the central nervous system.

The sympathetic division of the autonomic nervous system supplies neuroeffector fibers to the skin. Sympathetic postganglionic fibers travel in mixed peripheral nerves and arborize into terminal autonomic plexuses that innervate cutaneous blood vessels, arrector pili muscles, apocrine glands, and eccrine glands. Stimulation of adrenergic fibers produces vasoconstriction by activating alpha-receptors on vascular smooth muscle. A similar mechanism causes contraction of hair erector muscles, pulling hair follicles into an upright position and producing "goose flesh."

Apocrine and eccrine glands have both adrenergic and cholinergic innervation. However, apocrine secretion is thought to result primarily from adrenergic activity. Cholinergic stimulation is mainly responsible for widespread eccrine sweating important in regulation of temperature, whereas adrenergic mechanisms cause localized perspiration on the palms and soles during periods of emotional stress.

Sebaceous gland secretion is not under direct neural control but depends upon circulating hormones. Epithelial and neural elements in skin arise from the same embryonal ectoderm and function together in a communication and control system designed to protect the organism and maintain internal homeostasis in a constantly changing environment. The afferent limb of this system is the area of cutaneous sensibility, and the efferent limb controls sweating, contraction of hair erector muscles, and vascular activity.

The Epidermis

The epidermis has an average thickness about equal to that of the paper of this page and is the thinnest layer, varying from 0.04 mm on the eyelids to 1.6 mm on the palms. It is a stratified squamous epithelium with a high metabolic rate. The epidermis is populated by four types of cells: keratinocytes, melanocytes, Langerhans' cells, and Merkel cells.

The Keratinocyte

The epidermis is composed mostly of keratinocytes. Its cells differentiate as they rise to the surface, and as they die they produce a cornified external membrane. In older estimates the process of differentiation whereby germinative keratinocytes move upward to become fully cornified cells was given to be 14 days. Newer studies suggest that the process takes about 31 days. Then an additional 14 days are spent in transit through the cornified layer until the keratinocytes are shed. Thus, the time required for a keratinocyte to traverse the entire epidermis is between 28 and 45 days. The rate of epidermopoiesis varies slightly from one body site to another. Dead epidermal cells are constantly being shed from the body surface, and new cells are continually being generated by mitosis in the germinative zone. In health, cell birth (replication) is in equilibrium with cell death (desquamation).

The replication of epidermal cells (mitosis) normally occurs at the basal layer of the epidermis and, in very thick epidermis, in the next cell layer as well. In the basal layer, 3 to 5% of the cells are synthesizing DNA at any given time, but only about one per 1000 basal cells is then in mitosis. The daughter cells from each division may either remain in the basal layer or migrate upward and differentiate; about 50% remain and 50% move up. In pathologic processes such as psoriasis or in the process of stripping the cornified layer with adhesive tape, an increased rate of mitoses in the basal zone results in replacement of the entire epidermal population in 24 to 72 hours. A similar phenomenon may account for the peeling following sunburn.

During their upward migration toward maturation, keratinocytes undergo characteristic changes. One can recognize basal, spinous, granular, and cornified layers. These strata reflect stages in the conversion of a germinative keratinocyte to the end product of epidermal differentiation, the cornified keratinocyte. The four layers are not independent of one another but are interrelated as continuous phases in the life histories of epidermal cells. During

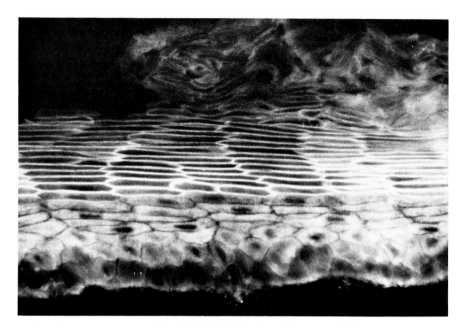

FIG. 1-26. Arrangement of cells in cornified layer in vertical columns like stacked pie plates. The photograph is of a cryostat section of guinea-pig skin treated with 0.1 N sodium hydroxide. (Courtesy Enno Christophers, M.D.)

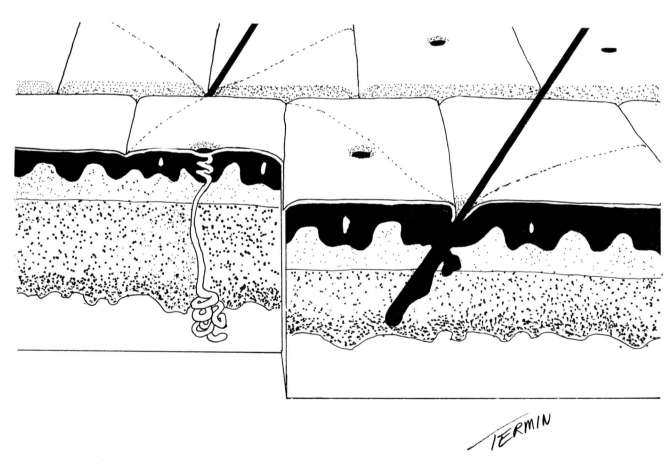

TERMIN

FIG. 1-27. Keratinocytes of the epidermis. Adnexal keratinocytes rise through epidermis en route to skin surface. Keratinocytes of hair follicle and sweat duct within epidermis exist in intimate association with rest of epidermal keratinocytes.

the process of keratinization, living germinative basal cells are transformed by a series of biochemical events into dead cornified cells (Fig. 1-26).

Three biologically separate species of keratinocytes live together in association within the epidermis. Epidermal keratinocytes predominate, but adnexal keratinocytes (intraepidermal hair-follicle or acrotrichial keratinocytes and intraepidermal sweat-duct or acrosyringial keratinocytes) course through the epidermis en route to the skin surface (Fig. 1-27).

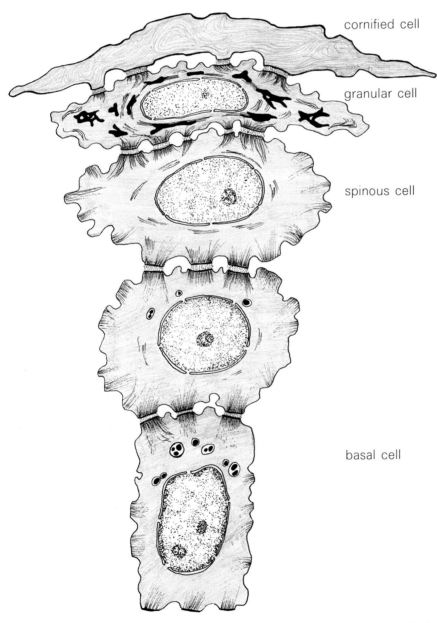

cornified cell

granular cell

spinous cell

basal cell

FIG. 1-28. Basal, spinous, and granular cells: stages in conversion of germinative keratinocytes to end stage of epidermal differentiation, namely, cornified keratinocytes. Columnar basal cells thus end up as horizontally aligned, thin, flat cornified cells.

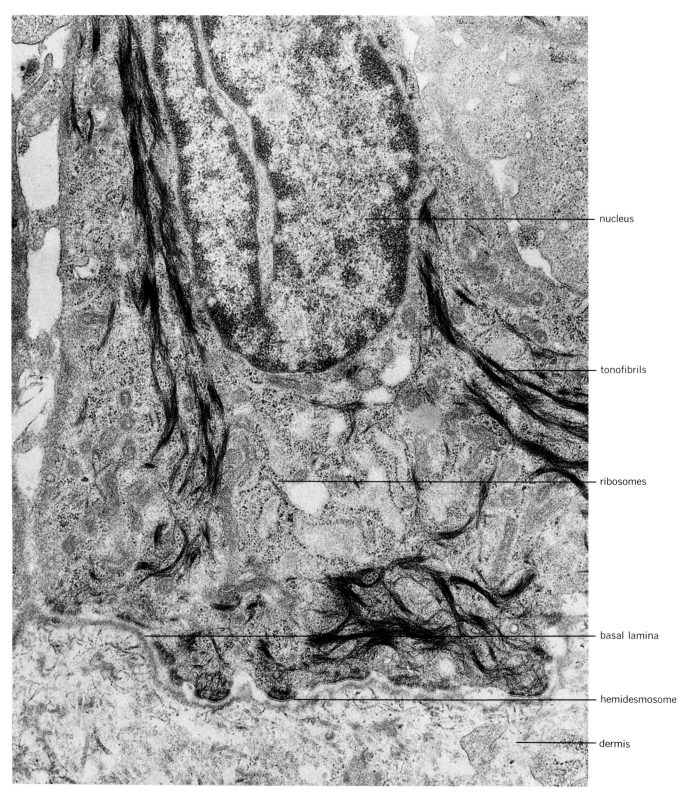

nucleus

tonofibrils

ribosomes

basal lamina

hemidesmosome

dermis

FIG. 1-29. Cytoplasm of a basal cell. Note numerous mitochondria and ribosomes, but relatively few tonofibrils, which are fundamental markers of keratinocytes. In photomicrograph a basal cell is seen situated upon basal lamina and is connected to it by a number of hemidesmosomes. (× 25,000.) (Courtesy Ken Hashimoto, M.D.)

Basal keratinocytes, cuboid or columnar in shape, arranged in a single row, contain relatively large oval nuclei and slightly more basophilic cytoplasm than the keratinocytes above them (Fig. 1-28). The polygonal-shaped cells of the suprabasal spinous layer assume a gradually more flattened configuration as they approach the skin surface. The spinous keratinocytes are named for the delicate spines that, with light microscopy, are seen to cross the narrow intercellular spaces between them. Toward the surface are flattened diamond-shaped cells filled with coarse, irregularly shaped, darkly basophilic granules (keratohyaline granules). The outermost layer of the epidermis is formed by flat, anucleated, eosinophilic-staining, cornified cells. As they ascend, the vertically oriented, columnar basal cells are transformed into horizontally aligned, thin, cornified cells. Each pancake-shaped cornified cell covers the area occupied by about 25 basal cells.

With the electron microscope, one can obtain a more detailed view of the structural alterations of keratinocytes during ascent. The cytoplasm of basal cells is packed with ribosomes, which impart basophilia to hematoxylin-and-eosin-stained sections, an indication that the cells synthesize protein. Tonofibrils, composed of bundles of fibrous protein threads, 4 to 5 nm in width, are also present in the cytoplasm of basal cells. Tonofibrils are fundamental structures of all keratinocytes. The nuclei of basal cells are large, with prominent chromatin networks and one or more nucleoli. Each cell is enclosed by a well-defined, highly convoluted cell membrane (Fig. 1-29). As the offspring of basal keratinocytes journey upward, the number of tonofibrils progressively increases, tonofilaments thicken to 7 nm, and the number of ribosomes decreases (Fig. 1-30). The tonofibrils are responsible for the eosinophilia of cornified cells being stained with hematoxylin and eosin. At the top of the spinous layer, granules with a highly ordered lamellar internal structure appear near Golgi complexes and then scatter throughout the cytoplasm. Next, dense osmiophilic bodies that lack internal structure (keratohyalin granules) appear in what becomes the granular layer (Fig. 1-31). As the osmiophilic bodies and tonofibrils accumulate, the nucleus and most of the intracellular organelles disappear. The lamellar granules move to the region of the plasma membrane and are discharged into the intercellular space, presumably acting as a cementing substance for adherence of cornified cells. Concurrently, the thickness of the cell membranes in the cornified layer doubles, presumably due to deposits upon them (Fig. 1-32).

In summary, cornified cells of the epidermis bear little resemblance to their progenitor basal cells. Nuclei and organelles are absent. The cell is filled with closely packed tonofibrils encased in

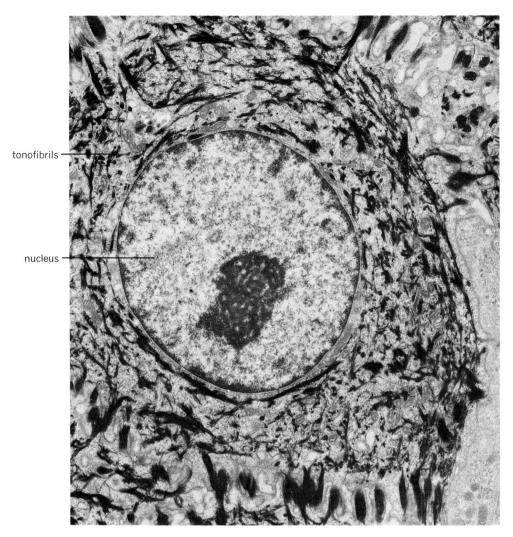

tonofibrils —

nucleus —

FIG. 1-30. Cytoplasm of spinous cell almost entirely filled with tonofibrils, except for a small number of mitochondria and free, scattered ribosomes. Tonofibrils surround nucleus and radiate toward periphery, particularly converging upon desmosomes. (× 9500.) (Courtesy Ken Hashimoto, M.D.)

a protein matrix. During differentiation, among other changes, keratinocytes (1) change shape (flatten), (2) lose organelles, (3) form fibrous proteins, (4) become dehydrated, and (5) acquire thickened cell membranes.

The same type of tough fibrous protein that constitutes the cornified cells of skin also forms the major component of claws and armor of reptiles, feathers and beaks of birds, and hooves, horns, hair, and nails of mammals. This protein, keratin, possesses enormously versatile properties. The principal differences among these various cornified end products of keratinocytic differentiation appear to be (1) the mode of packing of the tonofibrils and (2) the amount and constitution of the sulfur-rich matrix in which they are embedded. By electron microscopic examination, the tonofibrils themselves seem to possess a remarkably uniform structure.

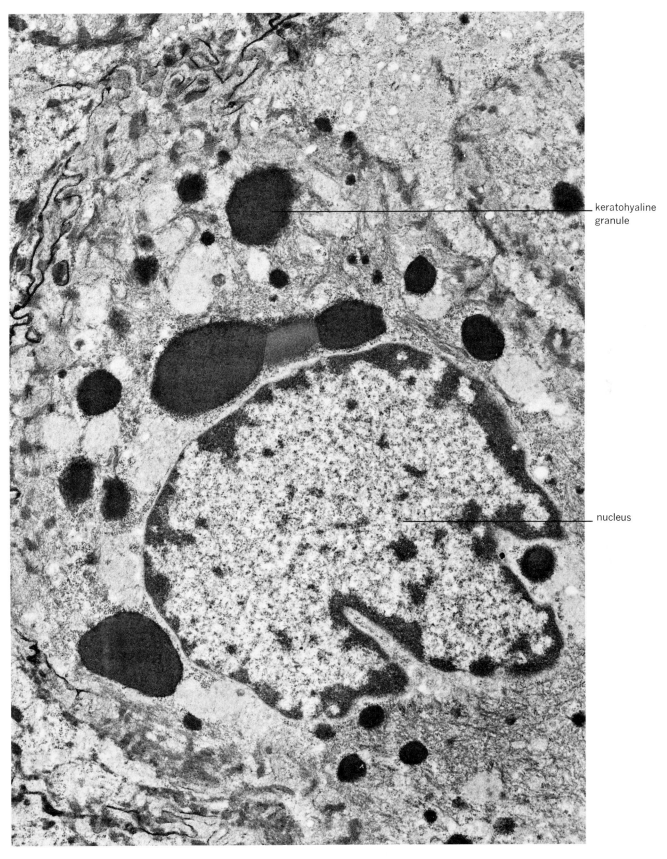

keratohyaline
granule

nucleus

FIG. 1-31. Granular layer. Cytoplasm of cell contains keratohyaline granules, as well as tonofibrils and a few ribosomes. Smaller keratohyaline granules represent immature forms, whereas larger ones often result from fusion of granules. ($\times$ 11,500.) (Courtesy Ken Hashimoto, M.D.)

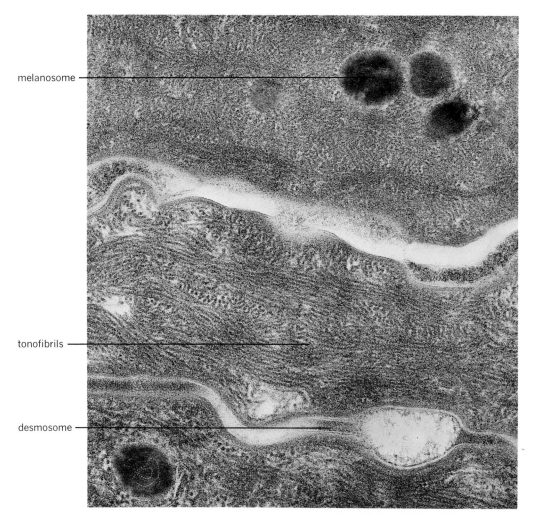

melanosome

tonofibrils

desmosome

FIG. 1-32. Cornified cells attached by vestigial desmosomes. Cornified cell is a package of tonofibrils encased in protein matrix. Nucleus and cytoplasmic organelles have degenerated and been lost during maturation. Melanosomes, which are organelles that produce melanin, are found within keratinocytes at all levels of epidermis, including cornified layer. ($\times$ 75,000.) (Courtesy Ken Hashimoto, M.D.)

Epidermal cells are joined to one another by specialized intercellular attachment devices called desmosomes (Fig. 1-33), characteristic of all epithelia, and by intercellular substance. The desmosomes are formed by multilayered, electron-dense materials that occur on both sides of adjacent cell membranes. Tonofibrils sweep across the interior of the cell where some loop and attach to the plasma membrane at the desmosome. Desmosomes provide firm mechanical attachment between adjacent cells, but they break and re-form during the process of keratinocytic migration and maturation. Cleavage between desmosomes in the cornified layer results in the invisible shedding of dead keratinocytes.

Immediately beneath the basal layer a thin zone containing neutral mucopolysaccharide, the basement membrane, can be demonstrated with the light microscope, especially by the periodic acid-Schiff (PAS) stain (Fig. 1-34). The basement membrane is

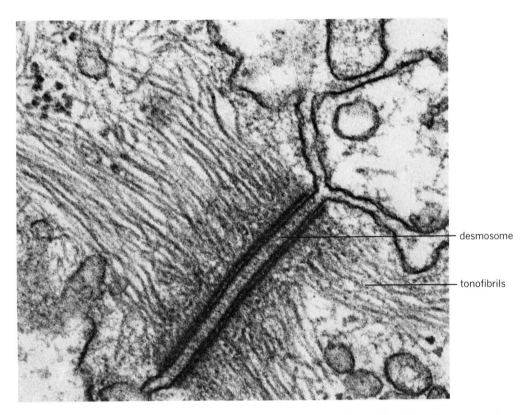

desmosome

tonofibrils

FIG. 1-33. Looping of tonofibrils at desmosome between adjacent keratinocytes (× 132,000.) (Courtesy Douglas E. Kelly, Ph.D.)

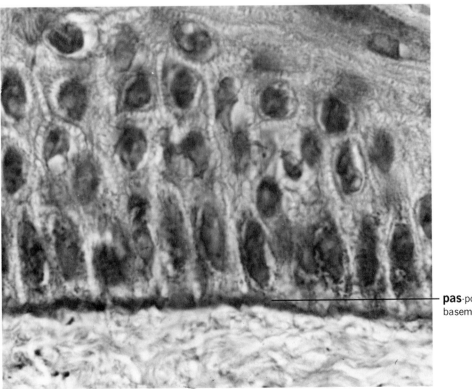

pas-positive
basement membrane

FIG. 1-34. Basement membrane. With light microscope, it is seen to be a band of PAS-positive, neutral mucopolysaccharide lying immediately beneath basal-cell layer of epidermis.

usually not evident with hematoxylin and eosin stain. With the electron microscope, individual components of the basement membrane can be visualized: a basal lamina parallels the lower border of the basal-cell plasma membrane, from which it is separated by a thin electron-lucent intermembranous space (lamina lucida). Beneath the basal lamina are fibers of the papillary dermis. Hemidesomosomes attach the basal-cell plasma membrane to the basal lamina (Fig. 1-35).

There are no blood vessels within the epidermis, nourishment being provided wholly by transudation of nutrients from capillaries in the papillary dermis. For this reason, incising the epidermis alone will not cause bleeding.

The cornified layer, situated at the interface between man and his environment, serves as a shield without which life is not possible. This thin, flexible, transparent covering of cornified cells functions as (1) *a major barrier*, possessing the critical properties of resistance against damaging corrosives, physical toughness that mutes the injurious effects of friction, high electrical impedance that restricts passage of electrical current, and a relatively dry surface that retards proliferation of microorganisms; and (2) *a rate-limiting membrane* for passage of water and other molecules between the "wet" internal environment of the body and the "dry" external environment.

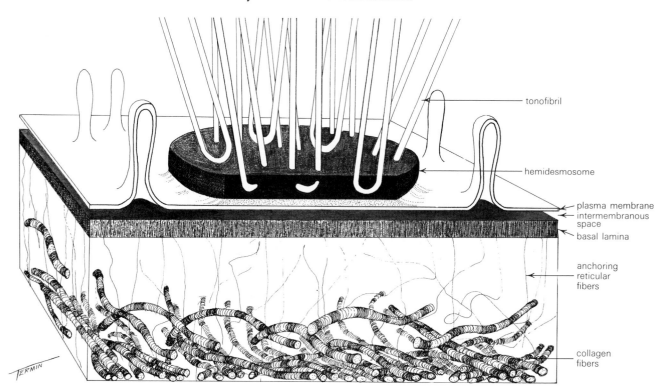

FIG. 1-35. Components of basement membrane. A basal lamina parallels lower border of basal-cell plasma membrane, from which it is separated by a thin, electron-lucent, intermembranous space (lamina lucida). Beneath basal lamina are fibers of papillary dermis. Hemidesmosomes attach basal-cell plasma membrane to basal lamina. (Drawing after that of Douglas E. Kelly, Ph.D.)

All of the cellular strata of the cornified layer, approximately 15 to 40 cells in number, depending upon the site, contribute to its barrier function. Although this layer is an effective barrier against excessive penetration of most substances, it is not a perfect barrier. The ability of molecules to diffuse through the cornified layer enables development of allergic contact dermatitis.

Unique permeability properties of the cornified layer underlie its essential function in the maintenance of the body's water content and electrolyte concentration. When the cornified layer is altered, water loss and percutaneous absorption are increased; if the injury to the cornified layer is severe and widespread, death may result from dehydration or toxicity.

The Melanocyte

Melanocytes are dendritic cells that synthesize and secrete melanin pigment. They are derived from the neural crest and migrate to the epidermis, mucous-membrane epithelium, dermis, hair follicles, leptomeninges, uveal tract, retina, and other tissues irregularly (Fig. 1-36). In the skin, melanocytes are situated at the

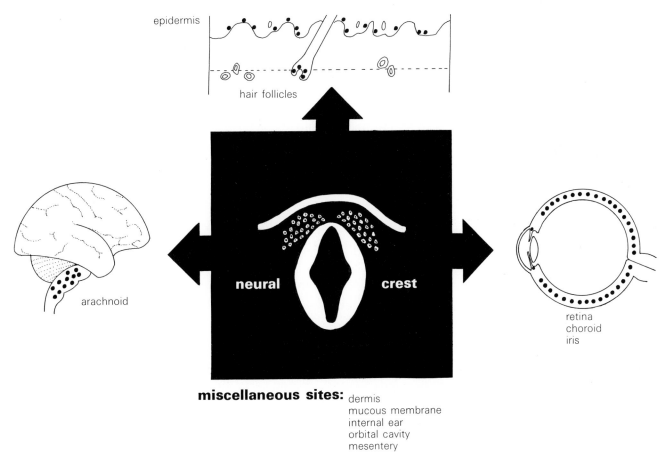

FIG. 1-36. Melanocytes (black dots). Melanocytes are derived from primordial neural crest and migrate to skin, mucous membranes, ocular structures, leptomeninges, and other tissues.

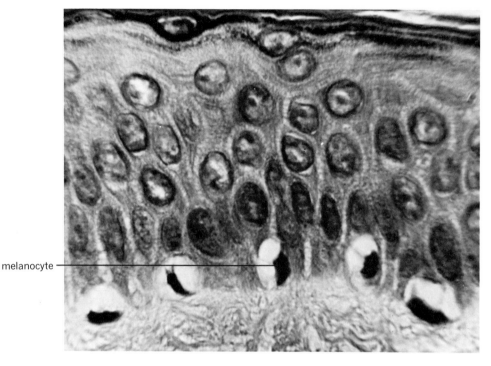

melanocyte

FIG. 1-37. Epidermal melanocytes. With the light microscope, they appear as clear cells in and immediately beneath basal-cell layer. Vacuity is an artifact of fixation caused by collapse of cytoplasm of cells around nucleus. Note that nuclei of melanocytes are smaller and more deeply basophilic than are those of contiguous keratinocytes. (× 1350.)

dermoepidermal junction, except for those that remain behind in the dermis. Dermal melanocytes are seen in blue sacral patches (Mongolian spots) and other blue nevi.

Melanocytes are present in the epidermis of all regions of the body, but their concentration varies. The ratio of melanocytes to keratinocytes in the basal layer varies from 1:4 to 1:10, depending upon the region; for example, they are more abundant on the cheek than on the trunk. With advancing age, the ratio of melanocytes to keratinocytes shifts in favor of the latter. The relative number of melanocytes is the same for both sexes and for all races. Differences in coloration among the races result not from differences in the number of melanocytes but from the way melanin is packaged. The intensity of skin coloration is further determined by the total number, size, and intracellular distribution of melanin granules within epidermal keratinocytes.

With the light microscope, epidermal melanocytes appear as clear cells in and immediately beneath the basal-cell layer (Fig. 1-37). The clear space is an artifact of fixation due to the collapse of the melanocytic cytoplasm around the nucleus. The nucleus of the melanocyte is smaller and more deeply basophilic than that of the keratinocyte. Although all levels of the epidermis, including the cornified layer, contain melanin pigment, the basal layer is the

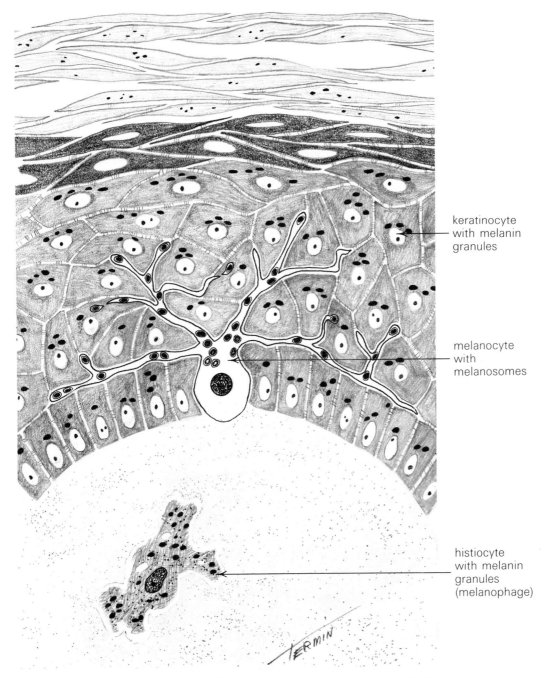

labels:
keratinocyte
with melanin
granules

melanocyte
with
melanosomes

histiocyte
with melanin
granules
(melanophage)

FIG. 1-38. Dendrites of a melanocyte. Note extension in all directions, especially along basal-cell layer and upward between keratinocytes in spinous-cell layer. Once melanin is formed, it is transferred from melanocytes into keratinocytes by apocopation.

most heavily pigmented. Melanocytes can be better seen by staining with silver salts, which combine with the melanin pigment to form a black deposit. Melanin granules are concentrated in umbrellalike array above each keratinocyte nucleus on the side toward the skin surface. The dendrites of melanocytes extend in all directions, laterally along the basal layer, downward toward the dermis, and upward between the keratinocytes in the spinous layer (Figs. 1-38, 1-39).

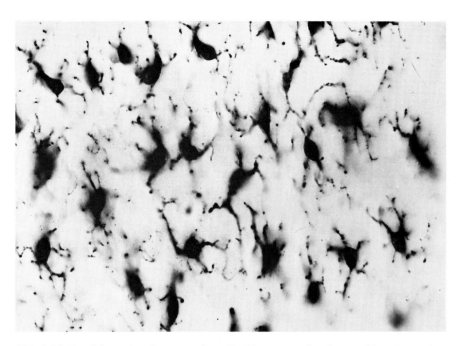

FIG. 1-39. Dendrites of melanocytes in split-skin preparation from a Rhesus monkey that had been irradiated 28 days. (DOPA stain.) (Courtesy William Montagna, Ph.D.)

Seen under the electron microscope, the melanocyte appears to be a protein-synthesizing cell with large mitochondria, rough endoplasmic reticulum containing many ribosomes, prominent Golgi apparatus, and no tonofibrils or desmosomes. Inside the cytoplasm of melanocytes are special organelles, called "melanosomes" (Fig. 1-40). These are spherical or ellipsoid membrane-bounded particles with a highly organized internal structure composed of longitudinally oriented concentric lamellae with a characteristic periodicity (Figs. 1-41, 1-42).

Melanosomes are the site of melanin formation. Once melanin is formed, it is transferred from melanocytes into keratinocytes by apocopation. The keratinocytes actively engulf the melanin-filled tips of melanocytic dendrites, resulting in the discharge of melanin granules into both epidermal and hair keratinocytes. Thus, melanin-making cells (melanocytes) and melanin-taking cells (keratinocytes) constitute a biologic unit. The interdependence and interaction of melanocytes and keratinocytes is witnessed in a variety of pathologic processes. These processes range from blockage of melanosome transfer in certain keratinocytic hyperplasias and neoplasias to excessive transfer of melanosomes in postinflammatory hyperpigmentation. Once transferred to the keratinocyte, the fully melanized melanosomes are partially degraded by lysosomal enzymes and shed as cornified cells are desquamated. Exposure to ultraviolet light expedites the formation and delivery of melanosomes to keratinocytes. This results in tanning.

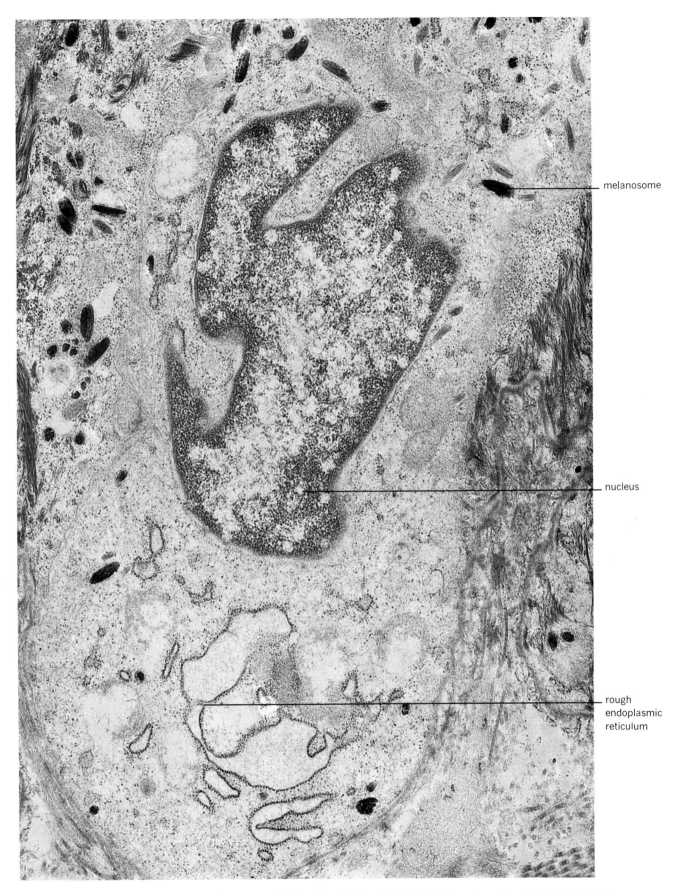

melanosome

nucleus

rough
endoplasmic
reticulum

FIG. 1-40. Melanocyte. It contains melanosomes, but no tonofibrils. (× 17,000.) (Courtesy Ken Hashimoto, M.D.)

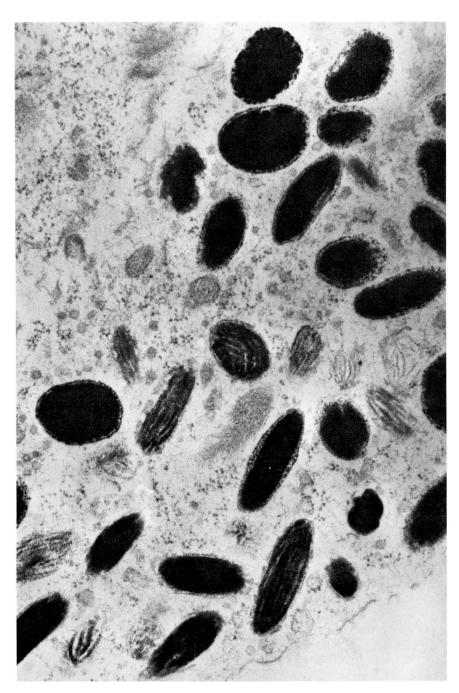

FIG. 1-41. Spherical and elliptical membrane-bounded melanosomes at various stages of development. (Courtesy Alvin Zelickson, M.D.)

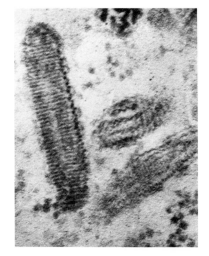

FIG. 1-42. Melanosomes. Internal structures composed of longitudinally oriented, concentric lamellae with characteristic periodicities are highly organized. ($\times$ 929,000.) (Courtesy Alvin Zelickson, M.D.)

The principal function of melanin in the skin is to screen the skin from the sun's harmful ultraviolet rays by absorbing their radiant energy. Melanosomes both scatter and absorb the ultraviolet light. The damaging effects of sunlight on unpigmented skin are evident in the fair-skinned and especially in albinos. In albinism, melanocytes are present, but the melanosomes lack the enzyme tyrosinase requisite for melanin production. Solar keratoses and all forms of skin cancer readily develop in albinos who are exposed to the sun's rays.

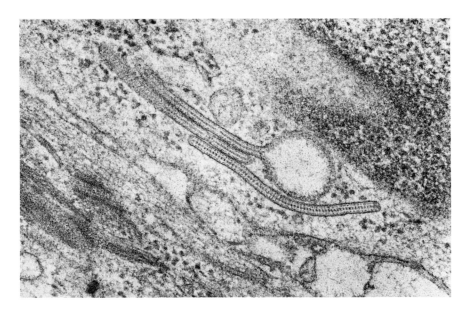

FIG. 1-43. Langerhans' granules with tennis-racquet configuration resulting from vesicular dilatation at one end of organelle. ($\times$ 82,600.) (Courtesy Alvin Zelickson, M.D.)

The Langerhans' Cell

In addition to melanocytes, other dendritic clear cells are found within the normal epidermis as early as the fourteenth week of fetal life. These cells, called Langerhans' cells, are often referred to as "high-level dendritic cells" because they usually reside in the upper part of the epidermis. Unlike melanocytes, they do not possess tyrosinase (as evidenced by their negative staining reaction with DOPA), do not increase in number after stimulation by ultraviolet light, are relatively constant in number from one region of the body to another, and are stained by gold chloride. Langerhans' cells are increased in number in vitiligo, a condition characterized by the virtual absence of melanocytes.

Electron microscopy is reliable for distinguishing Langerhans' cells from melanocytes. Langerhans' cells have a convoluted, notched nucleus and contain characteristic granules with a "tennis-racket" configuration resulting from vesicular dilatation at one end of the organelle (Fig. 1-43). Langerhans' cells, like other nonmelanin-making cells, such as keratinocytes and histiocytes, may also possess melanin granules. These granules are contributed solely by melanocytes, the only cells known to be capable of melanin synthesis. The function of Langerhans' cells is thought to be that of monocytic macrophage.

Merkel's Cell

Merkel's cell, found in the basal cell layer of the epidermis in glabrous skin and in the hair disk in hairy skin, is a clear cell best distinguished from melanocytes by distinctive electron-dense cytoplasmic granules as seen with the electron microscope. It functions as a touch receptor and is associated with fine unmyelinated nerves.

The Hair Follicle

Man is, at the same time, a naked and a hairy animal. Only the palms, soles, and a few other areas do not contain hair. Over most of the body surface the hairs are vestigial. Even the apparently hairless baby is covered with inconspicuous hairs. The protective value of hair, so important in furry animals against heat loss in the cold and against sunburn in the tropics, is insignificant in man. However, an adaptive value of hair is as an ornament, a means of sexual attraction.

The fetus is covered by wisps of lightly pigmented hairs, called "lanugo." Similar fine hairs that cover most of the body in youngsters and adults are termed "vellus." Even when an individual seems bald, vellus hairs are actually present. In the adult, the coarse pigmented hairs, named "terminal hairs," are most fully developed on the scalp, the beard, and the pubic and axillary regions. A single scalp follicle may initially produce a lanugo hair, later a terminal hair, and finally, with baldness, a vellus hair.

Hair is different, morphologically and biologically, on different parts of the body. Hairs vary in structure, length, rate of growth, and responses to various stimuli. For instance, sex hormones do not directly govern the development of eyelashes and eyebrows, yet body, axillary, pubic, and facial hairs are directly dependent upon hormonal stimulation for their adult characteristics. These latter hairs are part of the ensemble composing the secondary sexual characteristics. They wax and wane in time with the physiologic flow of sex hormones, becoming prominent at puberty and regressing with senescence.

Morphologic and quantitative differences in hair exist among the races. Caucasoids are hairiest; Mongoloids, least hairy; Negroids fall in between. Morphologically, hairs can be divided into four major categories: straight, wavy, helical, and spiral. Mongoloid hairs are straight, because the hair follicle is oriented at right angles to the skin surface. Negroid hairs are spiral because of curved hair follicles that have concavities facing the skin surface, and the hair shafts are ovoid rather than round. Caucasoid hairs may be any of these types. In terms of biophysics and biochemistry, there are no significant differences in hair properties among the races.

The hair follicle and its hair are fundamentally one structure derived from undifferentiated cells of the fetal epidermis. In longitudinal sections, the hair follicle can be divided anatomically into three segments: (1) infundibulum, the upper, funnel-shaped invagination that extends from the follicular orifice above to the entrance of the sebaceous duct below, (2) isthmus, the short midsection of the follicle bounded superiorly by the sebaceous duct and inferiorly by the insertion of the hair-erector muscle, and (3) inferior segment, extending from the muscle insertion to the base of the follicle (Fig. 1-44).

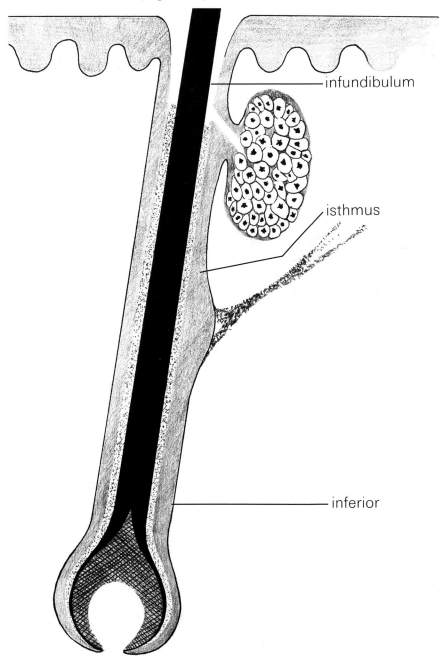

infundibulum

isthmus

inferior

FIG. 1-44. Three I's of follicular structure: infundibulum, isthmus, and inferior segment.

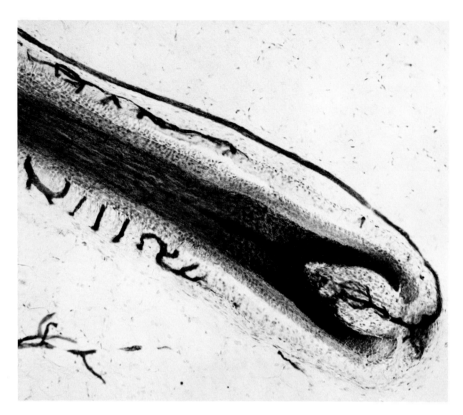

FIG. 1-45. Ovoid connective tissue papilla at base of hair follicle is richly vascular. Alkaline phosphatase preparation. (Courtesy William Montagna, Ph.D.)

At the expanded lower part of the follicle is the hair bulb, which encloses an ovoid, vascular connective-tissue papilla (Fig. 1-45). The round, uniform-appearing matrix cells of the bulb have a similar relationship to the hair papilla as have the basal cells of the epidermis to the papillary dermis. Through a narrow outlet at the distal end of the bulb, the papilla emerges to become contiguous with the connective tissue sheath that envelops the entire follicle (periadnexal dermis). Concentric circular and longitudinal layers of collagen fibers, with their associated fibroblasts, comprise the outermost fibrous sheath. A glassy, PAS-positive basement membrane, composed of type III collagen fibers and neutral mucopolysaccharides, separates the fibrous sheath from the follicular epithelium of the outer root sheath. A thin rim of epithelial cells in the outer root sheath encloses the hair bulb (Fig. 1-46). Most of the mitotic activity occurs within the matrix cells in the bottom half of the bulb and, to a lesser extent, in the outer root sheath. Dendritic melanocytes are interspersed among matrix cells in the upper half of the hair bulb (Fig. 1-47).

Unlike epidermal germinative cells, which produce only one population (spinous cells), the cells of the hair matrix differentiate along six separate lines. These changes are first detected near the base of the bulb. Here the plump matrix cells give rise to elon-

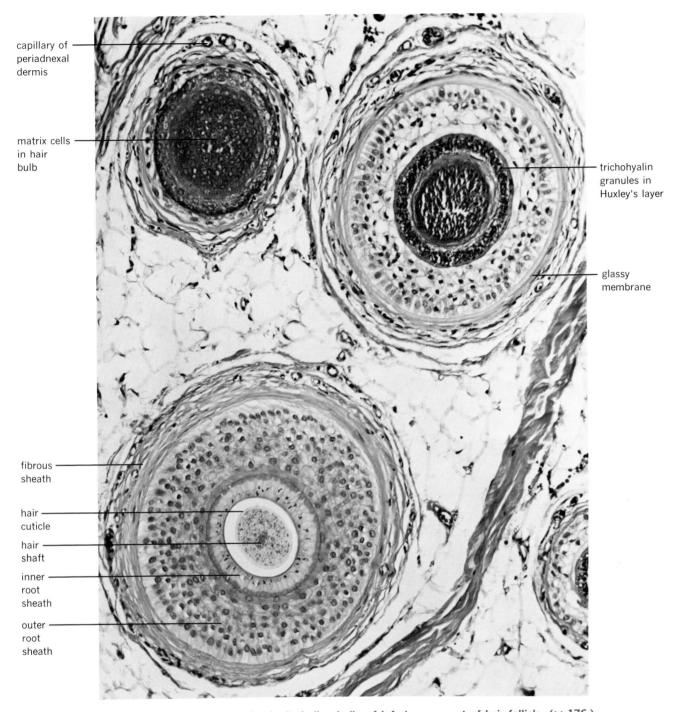

capillary of
periadnexal
dermis

matrix cells
in hair
bulb

trichohyalin
granules in
Huxley's layer

glassy
membrane

fibrous
sheath

hair
cuticle

hair
shaft

inner
root
sheath

outer
root
sheath

FIG. 1-46. Cross sections through different levels, including bulb, of inferior segment of hair follicle. (× 176.)

gated cells that form the 3 concentric layers of the inner root sheath and the 3 concentric layers of the hair itself (Figs. 1-48, 1-49). From the outside inward, these are (1) Henle's layer, the first to cornify and but one cell thick, (2) Huxley's layer, characterized by brightly eosinophilic-staining trichohyaline granules and two cells thick, (3) cuticle of the inner root sheath, (4) cuticle of the hair, (5) hair cortex, and (6) hair medulla (except for lanugo and vellus hairs). Enveloping this central core is the pale-staining,

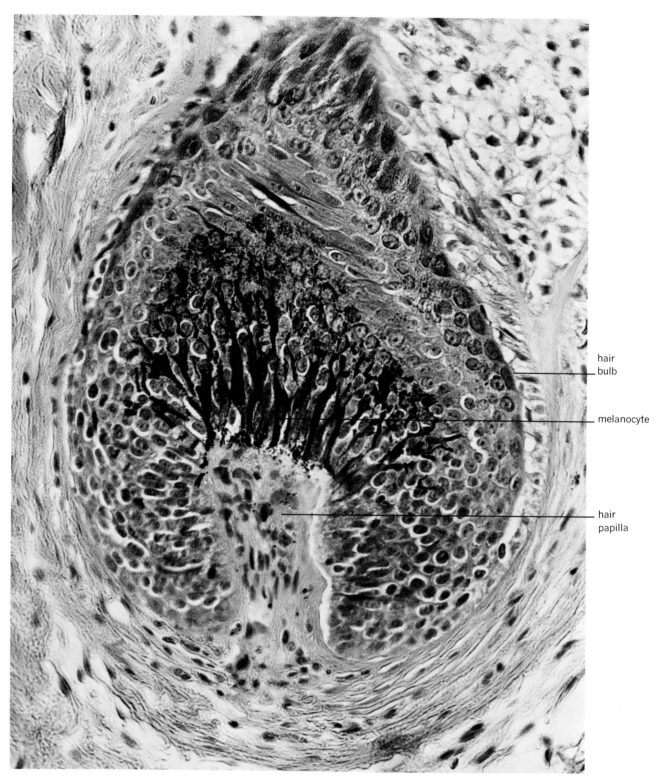

hair
bulb

melanocyte

hair
papilla

FIG. 1-47. Dendritic melanocytes situated in upper half of hair bulb. (× 352.)

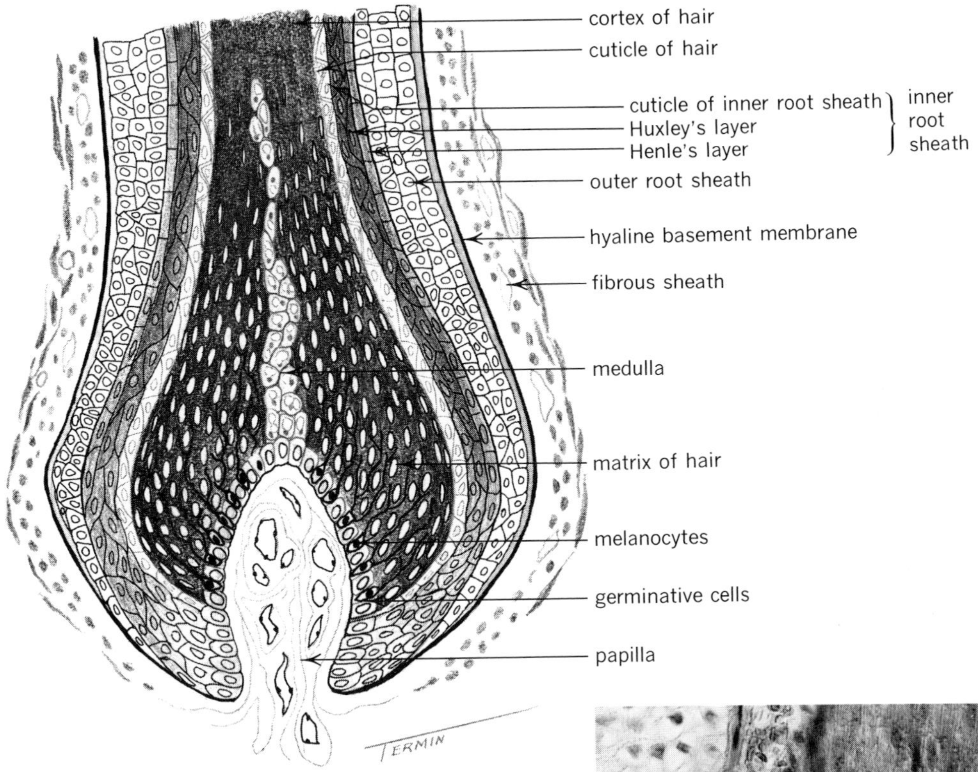
cortex of hair
cuticle of hair
cuticle of inner root sheath
Huxley's layer
Henle's layer
inner root sheath
outer root sheath
hyaline basement membrane
fibrous sheath
medulla
matrix of hair
melanocytes
germinative cells
papilla
TERMIN

A

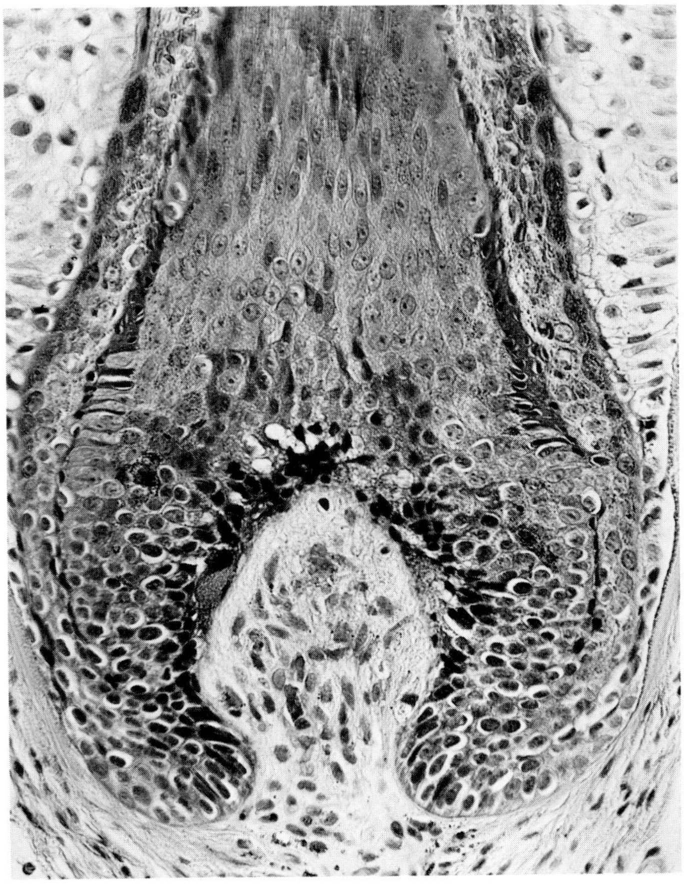

B

FIG. 1-48. Differentiation of cells of hair matrix along six separate lines of development. A, schematic view: from outside inward, Henle's layer, only one cell thick and the first to cornify; Huxley's layer, characterized by brightly eosinophilic-staining tricho-hyaline granules and but two cells thick; cuticle of inner root sheath; cuticle of hair; hair cortex; and hair medulla. Surrounding central core of these products of matrix is pale-staining, relatively broad, outer root sheath. Through narrow outlet at distal end of bulb, papilla emerges to become continuous with connective tissue sheath that envelops entire follicle. B, photomicrograph of hair matrix. (× 374.)

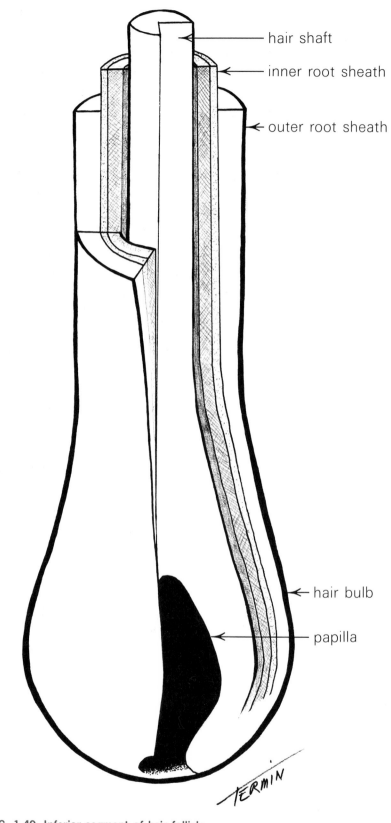

hair shaft

inner root sheath

outer root sheath

hair bulb

papilla

FIG. 1-49. Inferior segment of hair follicle.

relatively broad outer root sheath composed of glycogen-filled cells. The mechanism whereby a similar appearing population of hair matrix cells produces six morphologically different end products in concentric arrangement is unknown. It has been proposed that cells at equal radial distance from the base of the egg-shaped papilla undergo the same type of differentiation.

The matrix cells form a pool of undifferentiated cells with intense metabolic activity. The mitotic rate of the active hair matrix is greater, with the possible exception of bone marrow, than that of any other normal tissue. A complete cycle of reduplication occurs every 12 to 24 hours. The matrix products, inner root sheath and hair, move upward, gliding over the passive, relatively stationary outer root sheath. In contrast, the cuticle of the inner root sheath interdigitates with the cuticle of the hair so that hair and inner root sheath ascend together at the same pace.

An anatomic change occurs at the isthmus, which is delimited below by the insertion of the hair-erector muscle to which it is bound by elastic tissue (Fig. 1-50). The entire follicle beneath the isthmus, the inferior segment, can be considered temporary because it disappears during the involutional stage of the hair cycle and reforms again during the growth phase. The upper segments, isthmus and infundibulum, are permanent. At the isthmus, the cells of the inner root sheath disintegrate, and the outer root sheath, no longer in contact with an inner root sheath, begins to cornify (Fig. 1-51).

Another anatomic boundary of the hair follicle is marked by the entry of the sebaceous duct into the follicular wall. This point forms the upper limit of the isthmus and the lower pole of the infundibulum. The infundibulum passes through the epidermis (acrotrichium) and opens onto the skin surface. Infundibular epithelium is morphologically identical to that of the epidermis with which it is continuous, even to the presence of keratohyaline granules and a basket-weave pattern to the cornified layer. However, infundibular keratinocytes are biologically different from epidermal keratinocytes, a phenomenon well illustrated in a solar keratosis, where proliferation of atypical epidermal keratinocytes bypasses the normal appearing keratinocytes of intraepidermal adnexa. Follicular infundibula, especially on the face, scalp, and upper trunk, harbor a potpourri of microorganisms including bacteria (Staphylococcus epidermidis and Propionibacterium acnes), yeasts (Pityrosporum ovale and Pityrosporon orbiculare), and a mite, Demodex folliculorum (Fig. 1-52). Some bacteria and yeasts are also found in the interfollicular cornified layer of the epidermis, and all of these organisms can be found in the sebaceous duct.

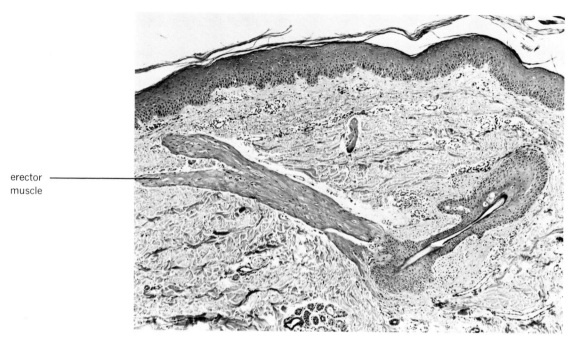

erector
muscle

FIG. 1-50. Hair erector muscle dwarfing telogen hair follicle, to which it is attached at "the bulge." In telogen, entire follicle beneath insertion of hair erector muscle (inferior segment) disappears. (× 81.)

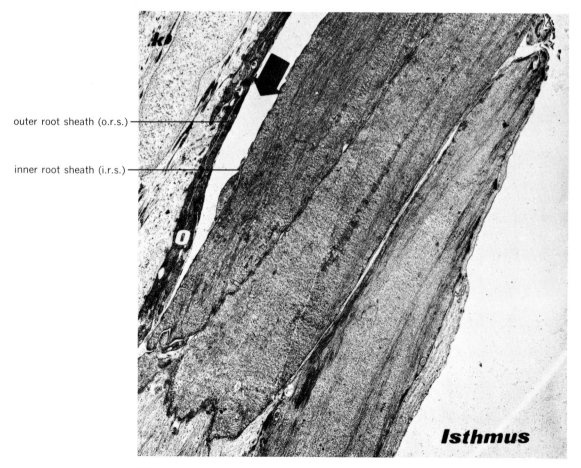

outer root sheath (o.r.s.)

inner root sheath (i.r.s.)

Isthmus

FIG. 1-51. Hair of human embryo. At isthmus, inner root sheath detaches from outer root sheath, which then begins to cornify. (× 10,000.) (Courtesy Ken Hashimoto, M.D.)

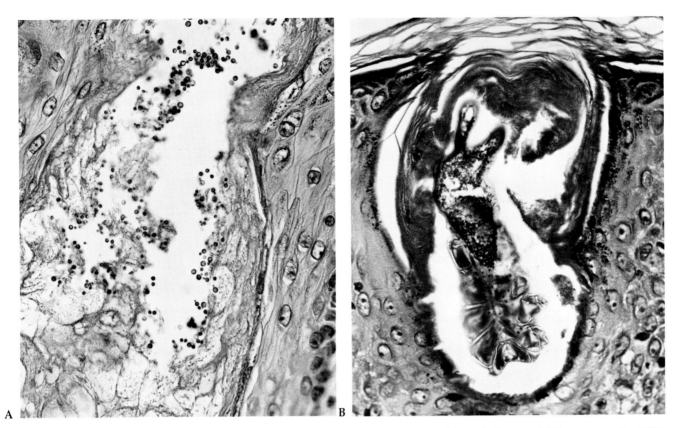

A

B

FIG. 1-52. Common inhabitants of follicular infundibulum of pilosebaceous units of face. A, Spores of Pityrosporon. (× 623.) B, The mite Demodex folliculorum (× 670.)

The hair shaft is a cornified structure that protrudes from the follicle above the surface of the skin. It has three components; an outer cuticle, next a cortex, and then an inner medulla. The medulla in human hair is discontinuous and sometimes absent. Fetal and vellus hairs have no medulla. Medullary cells are loosely aggregated, in contrast to the tightly packed, fusiform keratinocytes of the cortex. Cortical cells are aligned with their long axes parallel to the shaft of the hair. The outermost cuticular squames overlap each other to form an imbricated cylinder around the cortex (Fig. 1-53).

The color of hair depends primarily upon the amount and distribution of melanin within the hair shaft. In blond hair the bulbar melanocytes produce fewer melanosomes or incompletely melanized melanosomes, resulting in a lightly pigmented hair shaft. Gray hair is a consequence of the relative absence of melanosomes in the hair shaft secondary to a diminished number of melanocytes in the hair bulb. The melanin in red hair is chemically distinct from that of black hair, and the melanosomes therein are spherical rather than ellipsoidal. Melanocytes are absent in the snow-white hair of the aged. Melanocytes are present, but devoid of tyrosinase, in hair bulbs of albinos.

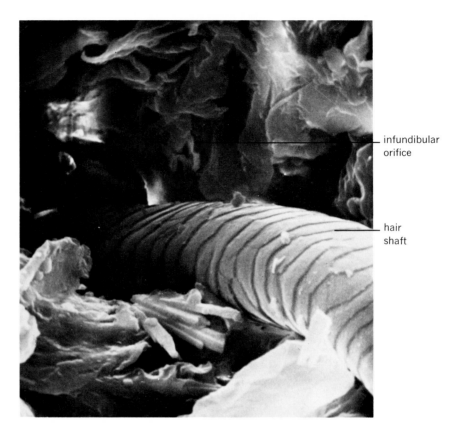

infundibular
orifice

hair
shaft

FIG. 1-53. Exterior cuticular squames of hair shaft. With scanning electron microscope, they can be seen to overlap and form an imbricated capsule around cortex.
(Courtesy Christopher Papa, M.D.)

The growth of hair is cyclical. The three phases in the life cycle
of a hair are (1) the growing (anagen), (2) the involuting (catagen),
and (3) the resting (telogen) (Fig. 1-54).

At the end of the active growth phase, a remarkable series of
involutional changes occur in the hair bulb. Catagen is heralded by
loss of metachromasia of the hair papilla, and the glycogen-filled
outer root sheath retracts into a cornifying epithelial sac around
the bulbous lower end of the hair shaft, forming a club hair.
Melanocytes of the hair bulb stop synthesizing melanin, causing
the expanded end of the club hair to turn white. A thin column of
epithelial cells, probably contributed by the matrix below and the
outer root sheath above, replaces the entire inferior segment of the
follicle. This epithelial column connects the papilla to the cornifying epithelial sac that encloses the club hair. The epithelial stalk
is surrounded by an enormously thickened and corrugated glassy
basement membrane (Fig. 1-55). Eventually, the club hair ascends
to lie at the level of insertion of the pilary muscle.

During telogen, the club hair remains within its cornified sac,
and the subjacent attached column of epithelial cells shrinks
upward. As this strand shortens, it is followed upward by the
liberated papilla that migrates closely behind. Left in the wake of

this shortened epithelial column is a streamer of fibrous connective tissue (Fig. 1-56). The epithelial column comes to rest as a ball of undifferentiated cells on the undersurface of the epithelial sac of the club hair. The melanocytes in the hair apparatus remain inactive and then return to function with the renewal of anagen.

The anagen phase of the cycle begins with a resumption of contiguity between the papilla and the undifferentiated cells that partially enclose it. A new hair matrix is formed, and papilla and matrix then descend together along the preformed fibrous-sheath pathway. An epithelial column then develops, and at the lower end a new bulb forms. The differentiated matrix cells of the bulb generate a new inner root sheath and hair. These events recapitulate the formation of the original hair from undifferentiated cells in the fetal epidermis. The new hair formed by the matrix pushes

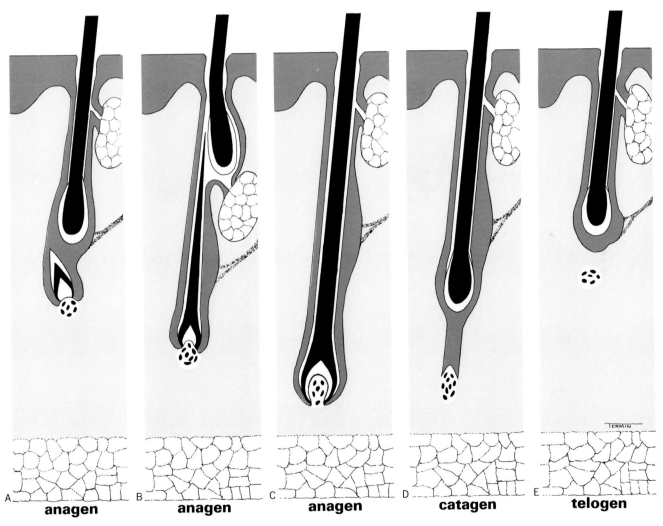

A	B	C	D	E
anagen	**anagen**	**anagen**	**catagen**	**telogen**

FIG. 1-54. Phases in life cycle of a hair. A, Anagen begins with renewal of intimate relationship between papilla and undifferentiated cells that partially enclose it. B, As anagen proceeds, matrix cells generate a new hair that pushes upward toward surface and in the process dislodges old club hair. C, Mature anagen hair follicle consists of infundibular, isthmic, and inferior segments. D, During catagen, entire inferior segment of follicle shrivels into thin cord of epithelial cells and is followed upward by papilla. E, During telogen, club hair rests in its cornified sac at level of hair erector muscle.

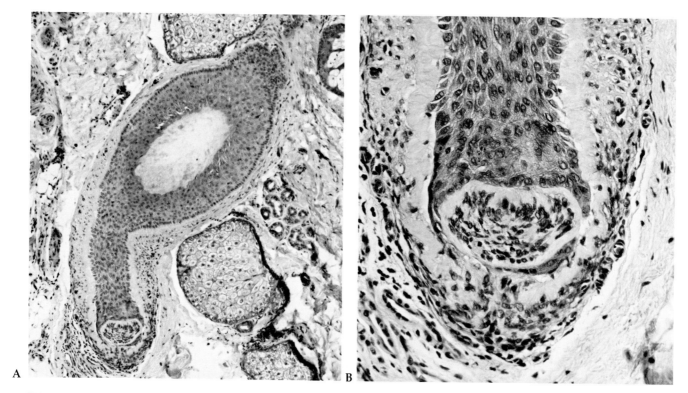

FIG. 1-55. Catagen hair follicle. Note the enormously thickened and corrugated glassy basement membrane. (A, × 120; B, × 410.)

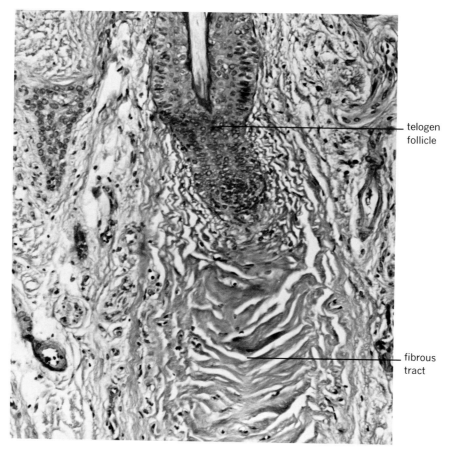

telogen follicle

fibrous tract

FIG. 1-56. Telogen. A fibrous connective tissue streamer is left in wake of inferior segment of hair follicle as it rises upward in position. (× 241.)

upward toward the surface, dislodging the old resting hair in the process. For a time there may be two hairs in a single follicle, the new hair and the old club hair. The root of the anagen hair is deeply pigmented and surrounded by a translucent sheath, whereas the bulbous tip of the telogen hair is unpigmented (Fig. 1-57). A graphic demonstration of these differences can be obtained by simply plucking hairs from your own scalp and eyebrows and comparing the roots.

Human hair follicles operate independently of one another, adjacent follicles being in different phases of the hair cycle. Hairs in humans are normally lost randomly and inconspicuously, whereas hairs in some animals are shed from body regions at one time (synchronous shedding) before a new crop is sprouted.

The time interval between the growing, declining, and resting phases is an important characteristic of the hair cycle. The hairs in different regions of the body have different intervals in anagen, which result in characteristic regional variation in the length of hairs. A scalp hair grows for 3 to 10 years, stops growing in a period of about 3 weeks, and rests for approximately 3 months. In healthy young adults, less than 10% of all scalp hairs are resting at any given time. The growing period of scalp hairs is much longer than those of hairs elsewhere on the body. As a rule, the growing phase of hairs on the extremities, trunk, and eyebrows does not exceed 6 months, and the duration of the resting phase is roughly the same. The final length attained by a hair varies directly with the duration of its growing period. The longest hairs on the scalp grow the longest time. Hair production is a continuous process in each of the approximately 100,000 anagen follicles on the average scalp. The protein-synthesizing capacity of the hair matrix is enormous when one considers that scalp hair is practically pure protein and grows at a rate of about 0.35 mm daily, resulting in the daily manufacture of approximately 100 feet of hair in total. Many factors, such as nutrition, general health, hormones, temperature, and light, control the growth of hair.

An array of curious abnormalities of the hair shaft results from still undefined disturbances of the hair matrix. Beaded, ringed, twisted, bamboo, and bayonet hairs are evidences of interferences, some of them genetic, others acquired, within the hair matrices.

Hair screens the nasal passages from irritants, the scalp from the sun's rays, and the eyes from the sunlight and droplets of sweat. It reduces friction in intertriginous regions. All hair follicles are associated with some sensory nerves (Fig. 1-58), a fact which suggests that hairs also participate in the cutaneous sensory system.

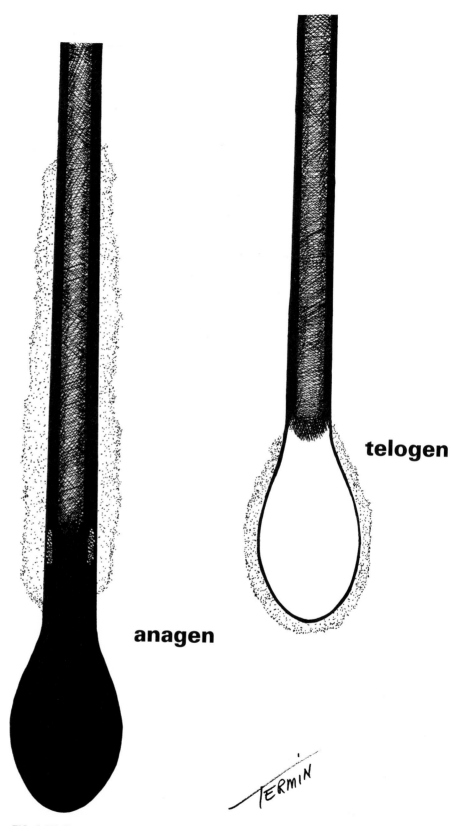

telogen

anagen

FIG. 1-57. Root of anagen hair. It is pigmented and surrounded by translucent sheath, whereas bulbous tip of telogen hair is unpigmented.

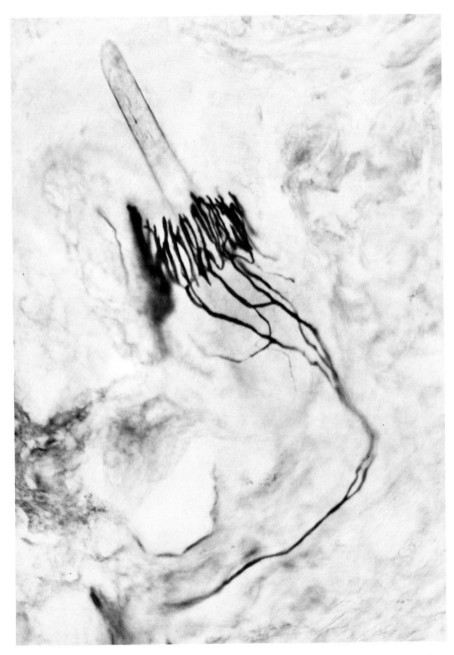

FIG. 1-58. End organ of vellus hair follicle demonstrated by silver impregnation after treatment with cholinesterase. (Courtesy William Montagna, Ph.D.)

The Sebaceous Gland

The sebaceous gland, specialized for lipid synthesis, arises embryologically as an epithelial bud from the outer root sheath at a point marking the junction of the future infundibulum and isthmus. Sebaceous glands are distributed over the entire body surface, except for the palms and soles. They are most populous and most productive on the face and scalp and largest on the back and forehead. Because of the mode of development, almost every

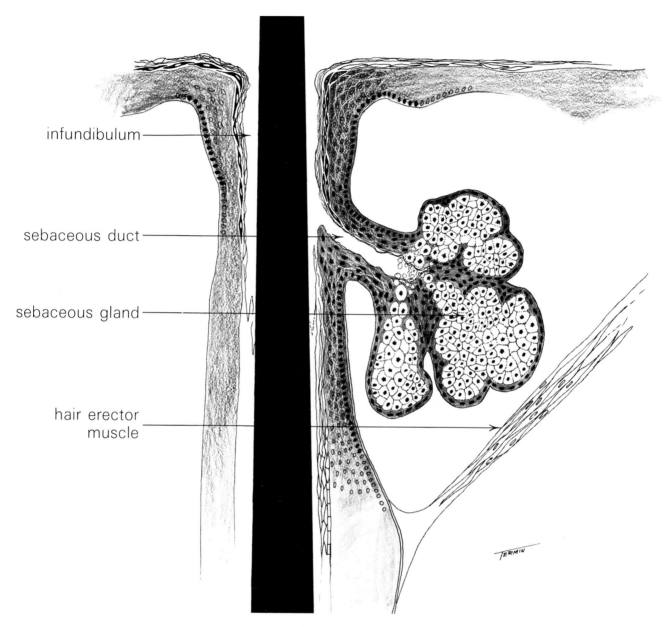

infundibulum

sebaceous duct

sebaceous gland

hair erector
muscle

FIG. 1-59. Schematic drawing to illustrate that almost every sebaceous gland is joined to a hair follicle.

sebaceous gland is joined to a hair follicle. As a rule, the size of sebaceous glands varies inversely as the diameter of the follicle with which it is associated, exceptions being the large glands adjoining sturdy follicles of the beard and scalp and the tiny glands attached to the vellus follicles. Some follicles contain puny hairs and amount to insignificant appendages of the sebaceous glands. Such sebaceous follicles are found on the face (excluding the beard) and on the upper part of the chest, shoulders, and back. In some places—namely, on the buccal mucosa and vermilion of the lip (Fordyce's spots), areolae of women (Montgomery's tubercles), prepuce (Tyson's glands), and the eyelids (Meibomian glands)—sebaceous glands are not associated at all with hairs.

The several lobules that comprise a sebaceous gland are enveloped by a thin, highly vascular, fibrous tissue capsule (periadnexal dermis) (Fig. 1-59). No motor nerves appear to be associated with the gland. The peripheral germinative cells are somewhat flattened or cuboidal and have large nuclei and homogeneous basophilic cytoplasm. Germinative cells of the sebaceous gland correspond to the basal cells of the epidermis. During differentiation, lipid droplets accumulate, eventually filling the cytoplasm of the cell. The more centrally located cells have a characteristic vacuolated cytoplasm and a scalloped nucleus, owing to compression by lipid globules (Fig. 1-60). The continuous

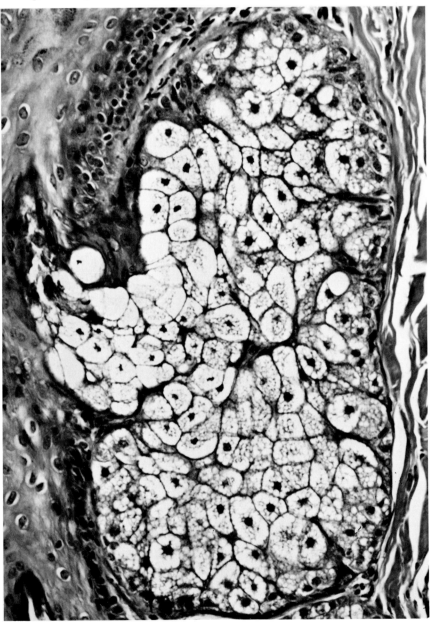

FIG. 1-60. Nuclei of cells of sebaceous gland nearest to peripheral germinative layer are round, but are scalloped as they differentiate, owing to compression by lipid droplets. ($\times$ 306.)

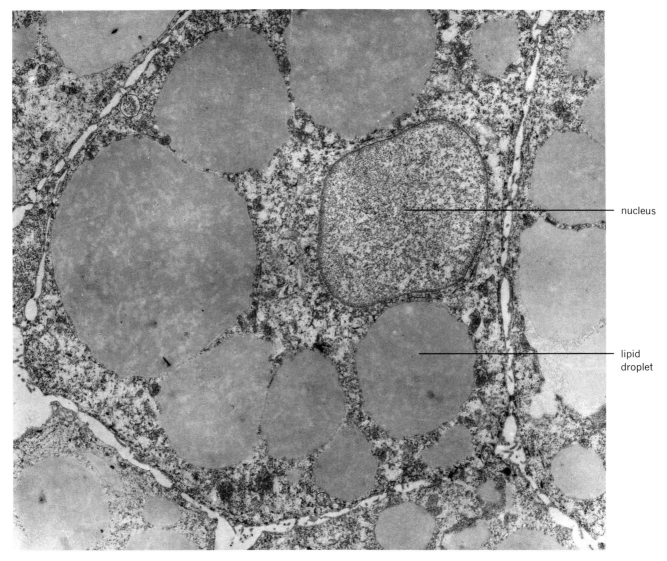

nucleus

lipid droplet

FIG. 1-61. Sebaceous gland cell filled with lipid. (× 14,500.) (Courtesy Ken Hashimoto, M.D.)

proliferation of undifferentiated peripheral cells gradually displaces the more differentiated vacuolated cells toward the center of the acinus. Finally, the boundaries of these bloated cells become indistinct, the cells disintegrate, and the mass of lipid and cellular debris (sebum) is discharged into the sebaceous duct, a short narrow common excretory duct connecting several sebaceous lobules with the wider follicular infundibulum. The sebaceous duct is lined by cornifying squamous epithelium.

The sebaceous gland is a holocrine gland because in the process of differentiation the entire cell is cast off in a manner analogous to the production of desquamating cornified cells by the epidermis. Furthermore, the term *sebum* given to the products of the sebaceous gland can be likened to *keratin;* both represent the composite end product of their specific tissue differentiations.

Histochemical and ultrastructural findings during sebaceous gland differentiation confirm and extend observations made with the light microscope (Fig. 1-61). The undifferentiated peripheral cells are glycogen laden and contain tonofilaments, rough and smooth endoplasmic reticulum, and many mitochondria. As differentiation proceeds, glycogen disappears, tonofibrils are displaced, and the cell cytoplasm fills with lipid vacuoles whose formation may be related to the numerous mitochondria, smooth endoplasmic reticulum, and large Golgi apparatus. Eventually, cell membranes become disorganized, the cell becomes fragmented, and the cellular components, including nuclear remnants, become dispersed.

Sebaceous glands are largely dependent upon androgens for development and activation. In the newborn, sebaceous glands are moderately well developed, attributable to the influence of maternal androgens transmitted placentally. The vernix caseosa is a mixture of fetal sebaceous material, lanugo hairs, and epidermal cornified cells. Early in infancy, sebaceous glands partially regress, only to enlarge again at puberty with the onset of increased androgenic activity. Androgens from the testes, ovaries, and, to a lesser extent, the adrenal glands are the major stimulants to the sebaceous gland. Androgens increase the size, the mitotic rate, and the amount of sebum of the sebaceous gland. Consequently, sebaceous glands are larger and more active in men than in women. Sebaceous glands have been shown not to depend upon neural control, despite the presence of minuscule nerves in the vicinity of the larger glands.

Whether the sebaceous gland serves a useful function in man is problematic. The gland has achieved a measure of notoriety for its probable role in the development of acne, the scourge of adolescence.

The Apocrine Gland

On the human body, the coiled, tubular apocrine glands are found in the axillae, areolae, mons pubis, labia minora, prepuce, scrotum, periumbilical and circumanal areas, external ear canal (ceruminous glands), and on the eyelids (Moll's glands). Apocrine glands may also be found on the face and scalp and in epithelial hamartomas such as nevus sebaceus and syringocystadenoma papilliferum. Apocrine glands produce a secretion whose function is not known. This product, acted upon by bacteria, is thought by some to have the effect of a pheromone.

In other mammals, such as dogs, monkeys, and apes, apocrine glands are distributed over the entire skin surface where they are believed to serve as identifying or sexual scent organs. Concomitant with the diminution in hair cover in man, there has been a decrease in the number of apocrine glands. During the fifth month of gestation, the human fetus has anlagen of apocrine glands in the entire skin. They largely regress, so that by term, apocrine glands remain only in the aforementioned sites. These glands remain small until early puberty, when they enlarge and begin to secrete their characteristic product.

There is wide ethnic variation in the number of apocrine glands. They are numerous in those of African descent, less numerous in Caucasians, and least in Japanese.

Histologically, the apocrine gland consists of two portions: (1) a coiled secretory gland situated in the lower reaches of the dermis or in the subcutaneous tissue and (2) a straight excretory duct that empties into the infundibular part of the hair follicle just above the entrance of the sebaceous duct (Fig. 1-62). Occasionally, apocrine ducts open directly onto the epidermis. In cross section, the apocrine secretory coil has a diameter several times wider than that of the eccrine coil (Fig. 1-63). These differences are best appreciated in the axilla, where apocrine glands are intermingled with eccrine glands in a ratio of about 1:1.

The lumen of the secretory coil is lined by one layer of cells ranging in shape from cuboidal to columnar, with round nuclei situated near the bases of the cells, and abundant, pale-staining, eosinophilic cytoplasm (Fig. 1-64). The convex apical borders of the secretory cells may project into the lumen to variable heights, depending on the stage in the secretory cycle of the cells. These secretory cells are surrounded by one layer of myoepithelial cells (Fig. 1-65), a PAS-positive basement membrane, and a network of elastic and type III collagen fibers.

The excretory duct is composed of two layers of cuboidal cells with an inner periluminal cuticle and no myoepithelial component. At its distal end, the apocrine duct merges with the epithelium of the outer root sheath.

With the electron microscope, the apocrine secretory cells are seen to contain organelles typical of secretory epithelia: many ribosomes, rough endoplasmic reticulum, mitochondria, lysosomes, and a prominent Golgi apparatus. Microvesicles present at the luminal border of the cells are indications of active secretion (Fig. 1-66). Histochemical stains show that secretory cells of apocrine glands also contain lipid, iron, lipofuscin, and PAS-positive, diastase-resistant granules. The type of secretion seen in apocrine glands was dubbed "apocrine" (*apo* meaning "off") because of the

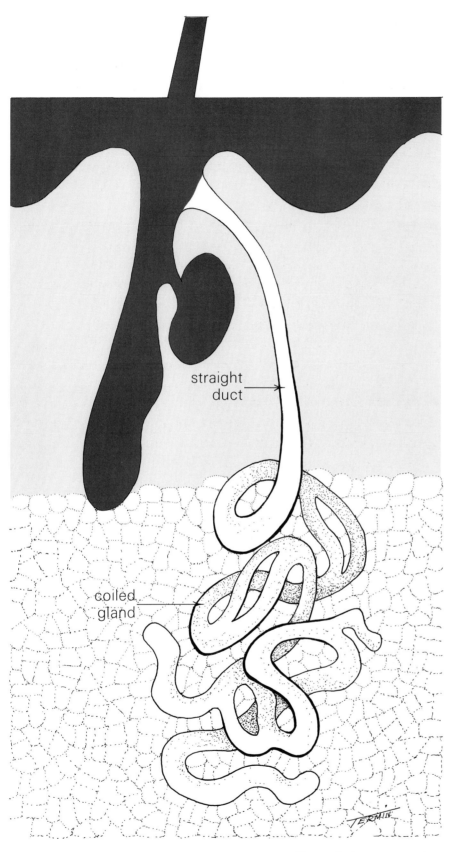

straight
duct

coiled
gland

TERMIN

FIG. 1-62. Apocrine gland consists of two portions: (1) a coiled secretory acinar structure housed in lower part of dermis or in subcutaneous fat and (2) a straight excretory duct that empties into infundibular part of hair follicle.

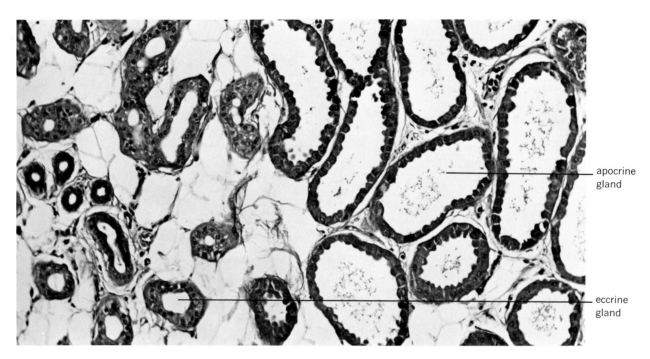

FIG. 1-63. Cross section of apocrine gland. The diameter is several times wider than that of eccrine gland. (× 176.)

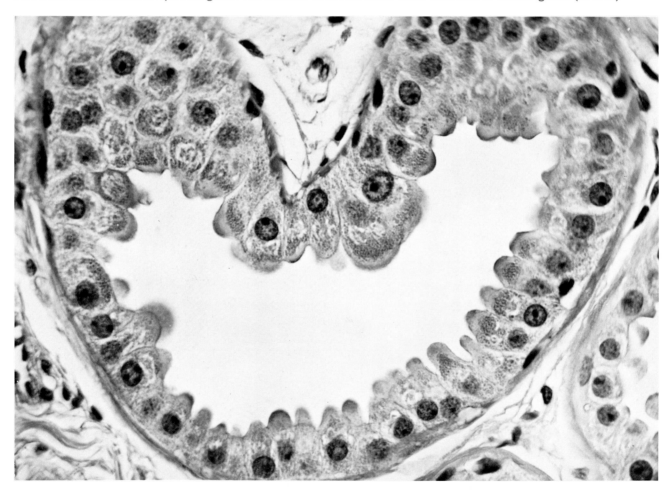

FIG. 1-64. Lumen of apocrine secretory coil lined by one layer of cells that are cuboidal or columnar in shape and have round nuclei near their bases and abundant, pale-staining, eosinophilic cytoplasm. Convex apical borders of cells project into lumen to various heights. (× 763)

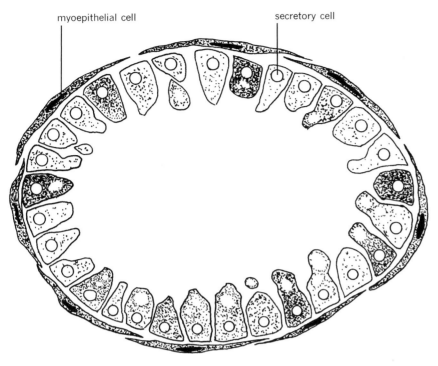

myoepithelial cell   secretory cell

FIG. 1-65. Secretory cells of apocrine gland surrounded by single layer of myoepithelial cells.

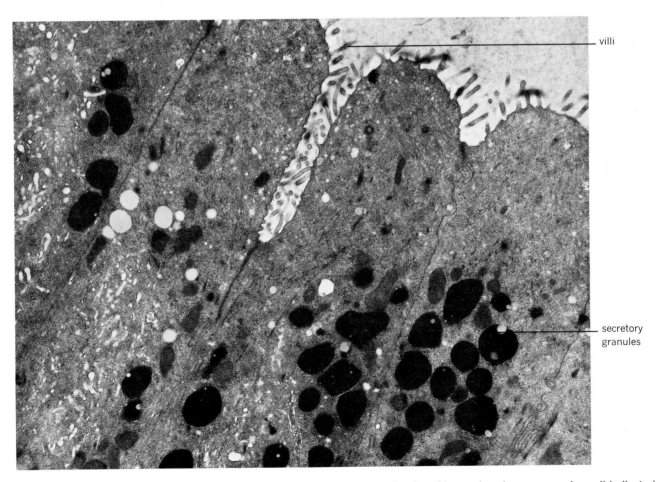

villi

secretory
granules

FIG. 1-66. Active secretory cell. Dense secretory granules and villi at free border of lumen in columnar apocrine cell indicate it is active. (× 7,500.) (Courtesy Ken Hashimoto, M.D.)

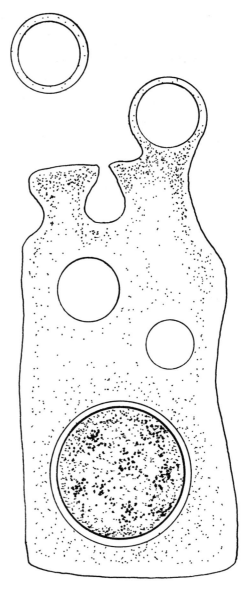

FIG. 1-67. Manner of secretion from apocrine glands by "pinching off" ("decapitation secretion") of apical cytoplasm into lumen.

appearance, under the light microscope, of pinching off (decapitation secretion) of apical cytoplasm into the lumen (Fig. 1-67). However, the exact mode of apocrine secretion is still unresolved.

There are two separate aspects to the production of apocrine sweat: (1) secretion and (2) excretion. Secretion by the apocrine gland is a continuous process, but excretion is episodic. Excretion occurs when the reservoir of apocrine secretion is propelled upward by peristaltic waves, presumably provided by the myoepithelial cell sheath. The myoepithelium is innervated by adrenergic and cholinergic sympathetic nerve fibers. Myoepithelial contraction and resultant apocrine excretion are induced by pharmacologic agents (pitocin and epinephrine) and by emotional stresses (fear and anger) that cause adrenergic sympathetic discharge.

The quantity of apocrine secretion is small, even in the axilla where sweat is mainly of eccrine-gland origin. After an apocrine gland empties, a refractory period ensues during which the duct refills with glandular secretion. Apocrine secretion has a milky color that fluoresces and contains proteins, carbohydrates, and fatty acids. Within the duct, apocrine secretion is sterile and odorless. The action of bacteria on apocrine secretion that has reached the skin surface causes the skin to become odorous (body odor). Many underarm deodorants, as advertised, contain antibacterial ingredients that eliminate the offending microorganisms.

The Eccrine Sweat Gland

Eccrine sweat units derive from the surface epidermis, independent of hair follicles, and descend through the dermis, coming to rest near the junction of the dermis and subcutaneous fat. Eccrine sweat units are present everywhere on human skin except at the mucocutaneous junctions. They are most highly concentrated in the palms, soles, forehead, and axillae and are least numerous on the arms and legs. It has been estimated that 3,000,000 eccrine sweat units are present at birth. Since no additional sweat glands are formed during life, the density is greatest in infant skin. Wide distribution of highly developed eccrine sweat units is unique to man. The eccrine sweat gland issues a hypotonic solution (sweat) that flows to the skin surface for cooling by evaporation in times of heat stress. It is the eccrine, rather than the apocrine, that is the true sweat gland in man. Eccrine sweat glands have been found only in higher primates and horses.

The sweat pores, or openings of the sweat ducts on the skin surface, are not visible to the naked eye. With a hand lens, tiny pits can be seen on the summit of the ridges on the palms and soles. These regularly arranged pits represent the orifices of the eccrine sweat ducts. Minute droplets of sweat can be detected in some of these depressions. Elsewhere on the body, sweat can be observed to emerge from the pores only after special preparation of the skin surface, such as with starch and iodine.

Each eccrine sweat unit is a simple hollow tube bounded distally by an opening onto the skin surface and proximally by a cul-de-sac (Fig. 1-68). Both ends of the tube are wound and connected by a straight duct. The proximal portion coils in irregular fashion, like a ball of yarn, whereas the distal portion spirals through the epidermis. The eccrine unit can be divided into a (1) coiled secretory gland, (2) coiled dermal duct, (3) straight dermal duct, and (4) spiraled intraepidermal duct (acrosyringium).

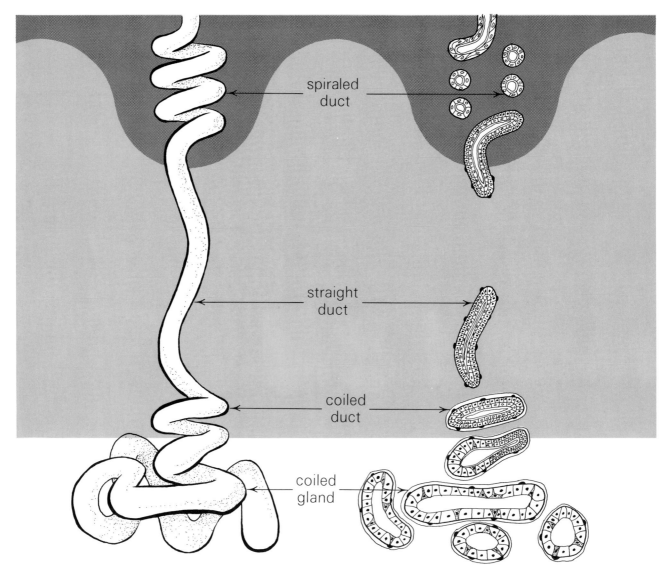

FIG. 1-68. Eccrine sweat unit. A simple hollow tube opens upon skin surface from intraepidermal spiral and ends in an irregularly coiled cul-de-sac deep in dermis or in subcutaneous fat. Both ends of the tube are connected by a straight duct.

The intradermal portions of the eccrine gland and duct are enclosed in a richly vascular connective tissue sheath (periadnexal dermis) that is separated from the tubal epithelium by a PAS-positive basement membrane.

The coiled secretory gland is composed of two layers of cells (Fig. 1-69): (1) a thin outer row of spindle cells (myoepithelium) and (2) an inner row of pyramidal epithelial cells (secretory epithelium). The single row of secretory cells that lines the lumen of the gland consists of two types of cells, distinguished by their staining characteristics. Small mucopolysaccharide-containing dark cells are crowded toward the lumen, and large glycogen-containing pale cells, are seen peripherally.

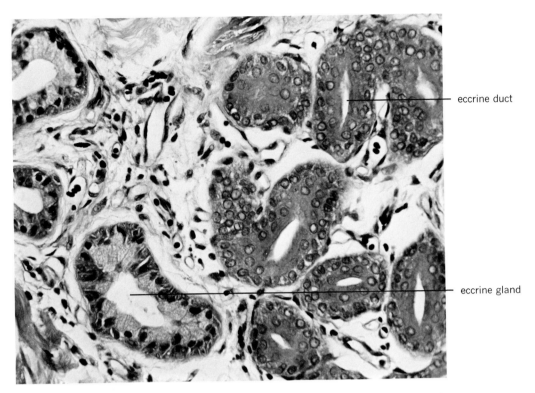

eccrine duct

eccrine gland

FIG. 1-69. Eccrine glands and ducts. Secretory portion of eccrine sweat gland is surrounded by basement membrane and consists of two layers of cells: (1) a thin outer row of myoepithelial cells and (2) an inner row of cuboidal epithelial secretory cells. Ductal portion is lined by two layers of smaller cuboidal epithelial cells with a luminal edge rimmed by homogeneous eosinophilic material. ($\times$ 440.)

The secretory gland is abundantly innervated by unmyelinated nerve fibers. The response of these fibers is mediated primarily by acetylcholine and inhibited by atropine. Actually, the eccrine sweat glands respond to both parasympathomimetic and sympathomimetic drugs, being more sensitive to parasympathomimetic ones.

The ductal epithelium is easily differentiated from the secretory epithelium. The eccrine dermal duct is lined by two layers of small, darkly basophilic staining, cuboidal epithelial cells. The luminal edge of these ductal cells is rimmed by a homogeneous eosinophilic cuticle. The duct narrows as it ascends from the coiled portion through the straight segment until the epidermis is reached. Here the duct again becomes coiled and widens as it spirals upward through the epidermis to open onto the skin surface. The intraepidermal keratinocytes of the eccrine duct differ morphologically and biologically from their neighboring epidermal keratinocytes, to which they are linked by desmosomes. Keratohyaline granules are present within the eccrine duct cells, and melanin granules are absent at almost all levels of the duct's twist throughout the epidermis. The keratinocytes of the intraepidermal sweat duct cornify independently. This difference is best

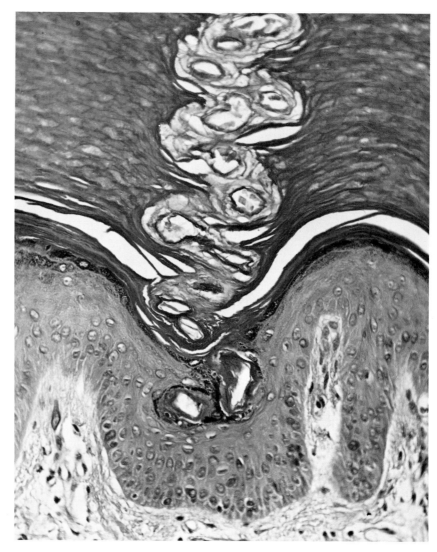

FIG. 1-70. Keratinocytes that form intraepidermal eccrine duct. They are morphologically and biologically different from their neighboring keratinocytes, as reflected in corkscrew pattern that is preserved even within cornified layer of this cross section from palm. ($\times$ 352.)

reflected in the corkscrew pattern preserved within the cornified layer, most evident on the palms and soles (Fig. 1-70). A cuticle lines the luminal border of the intraepidermal duct, just as it does that of the dermal duct.

The process of making sweat begins in the pale cells of the secretory gland in which there are abundant mitochondria and glycogen particles (Fig. 1-71). In these pale cells, active sweating is accompanied by dramatic changes indicative of intense metabolic activity. Within minutes after the onset of sweating, glycogen is consumed, and the number of other organelles is diminished. It is surmised that during this time anaerobic glycolysis depletes the cytoplasm of the pale cell, resulting in formation of lactate and hydrogen ions. These ions move into conduits, the intercellular canaliculi, which are lined by microvilli. In the canaliculi, hydrogen ions are removed by reaction with bicarbonate, and the lactate-containing solution flows from the canaliculi into the secretory lumen.

The precise role of the dark cells is unknown. Their cytoplasm contains abundant nucleic acids and vacuoles, but few mitochondria and no glycogen. During the process of active sweating, the numerous cytoplasmic vacuoles decrease in number and size. It has been suggested that the dark cells permit reabsorption of sodium, potassium, and chloride from the secretory lumen, but act as an impermeable membrane to lactate. Compared with plasma, the secretion formed in the lumen of the secretory coil by the combined efforts of pale and dark cells is isotonic, or slightly hypertonic.

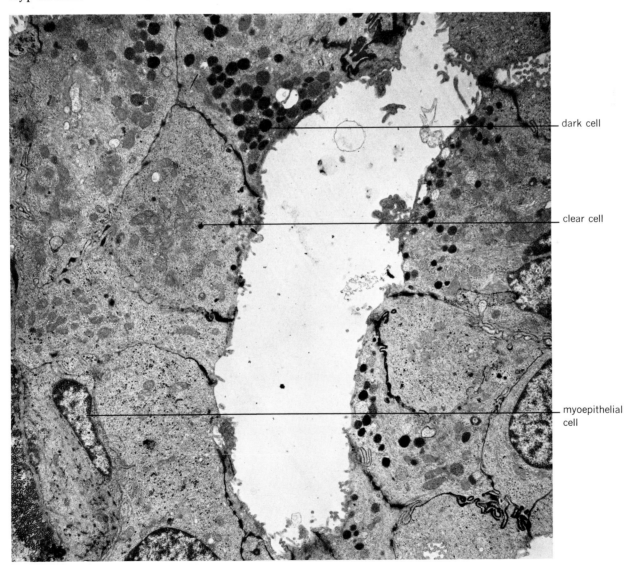

FIG. 1-71. Single row of secretory cells lining lumen of eccrine sweat gland. It consists of (1) clear cells that contain abundant glycogen and mitochondria and (2) dark cells that have dense granules. Luminal border bears numerous villi, and myoepithelial cells surround secretory cells. (× 7000.) (Courtesy Ken Hashimoto, M.D.)

Eccrine sweat is a colorless, odorless hypotonic solution composed of water, 99% by weight, and the remainder solutes, which in decreasing order are sodium, potassium, chloride, urea, protein, lipids, amino acids, calcium, phosphorus, and iron. All of the electrolytes present in plasma are found, to a lesser extent, in eccrine sweat. The specific gravity of sweat is approximately 1.005. Its pH is generally between 4.5 and 5.5, but as sweating progresses, the pH may increase to near neutrality.

Man is a warm-blooded animal, his internal body temperature remaining constant despite enormous changes in the temperature of his external environment. This feature of having a thermoregulatory system that sets a constant internal environment has enabled man to escape the rigid climatic limitations placed upon cold-blooded organisms. Unlike more furry mammals, man cannot rely upon hair for protection against cold. An arctic fox, clothed in its winter fur, rests comfortably at a temperature of $-50°C$ without increasing its resting rate of metabolism. Man, if unclothed, begins to shiver and raise his metabolic rate when air temperature falls to $28°C$. How does the body achieve thermal homeostasis? In large part the skin, its vasculature, and eccrine sweat glands are responsible. As the natural interface between the body and the external environment, the skin plays a passive role in all heat exchange, but, in addition, the skin has a specialized part to play as an active organ regulating heat exchange. The eccrine sweat units and the cutaneous blood vessels evolved as cardinal structures to serve this function. The eccrine sweat glands flood the skin surface with water for cooling, and the blood vessels dilate or constrict for dissipation or conservation of body heat. The capacity of the eccrine gland to make sweat for dissipation of excessive body heat is greatest in the human.

The Nail Unit

The nail unit consists of the nail (nail plate) and the tissues that surround it (Fig. 1-72). The nail is a hard, roughly rectangular, slightly convex, translucent plate, 0.5 to 0.75 mm thick, that covers the dorsal distal phalanges of the fingers and toes. It can be divided, longitudinally, into (1) a distal free edge which, if uncut and guarded, grows indefinitely, (2) a fixed portion lying upon the skin of its bed, and (3) a proximal edge that lies beneath the skin surface.

The nail plate, except for its free edge, inserts into grooves in the skin that are shallow laterally and deep proximally. The two

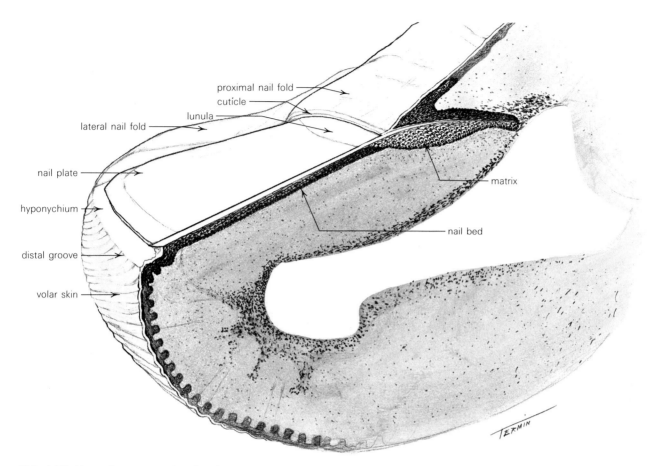

FIG. 1-72. Normal anatomy of nail unit.

lateral grooves are bounded by overhanging skin, the lateral nail folds, which continue proximally as the proximal nail fold.

The proximal edge of the nail plate fits snugly into a concavity that extends under the proximal nail fold for a distance of about 0.5 cm. The cornified layer of the proximal nail fold, the cuticle, emanates from the undersurface of the proximal nail fold and projects distally for a few millimeters beyond it onto the surface of the nail plate. Also found distal to the proximal nail fold is the lunula, a whitish crescent-shaped zone, almost always present on the thumbnail, usually absent on the fifth fingernail, and seen variably on the intervening fingernails.

The structure upon which the nail rests is the nail bed. It normally appears pink because of a blood-filled vascular network that is visible through the translucent plate. Compression of the nail plate forces blood out of the vessels and causes the nail bed to blanch. Distal to the nail bed is a narrow zone of skin, the hypo-nychium, which is contiguous with the volar skin of the fingertip. The hyponychium is divided from volar skin by the distal groove, a slightly elevated skin margin against which the free edge of the nail plate tends to abut.

Histologically, there are five epithelial components of the nail unit. Beginning with the superficial proximal skin and progressing around behind and under the nail to the distal edge, these are the (1) epidermis of the proximal nail fold, (2) epithelium of the nail matrix, (3) epithelium of the nail bed, (4) epidermis of the hyponychium, and (5) epidermis of the palms and soles.

The dorsal surface of the proximal nail fold possesses all four layers found in normal epidermis and an undulating epidermal rete-dermal papillae pattern. The ventral surface epithelium also cornifies by forming all the layers of normal epidermis, but its cornified layer extends outward over the surface of the fixed portion of the nail plate to constitute the cuticle.

Epithelium of the nail matrix consists of basal cells that differentiate into spinous cells and thence to the orthokeratotic cells that compose the nail plate. No granular zone is present in the nail matrix epithelium. The proximal boundary of the matrix is the ventral portion of the proximal nail fold, and the distal margin is the nail bed. The matrix, in sagittal sections, is the wedge-shaped blind end of the nail unit, and the crescent-shaped lunula represents the distal portion of the matrix.

Epithelium of the nail bed extends from the lunular border of the matrix to the epidermis of the hyponychium. The nail bed produces parakeratotic cells without the interposition of a granular layer. The few parakeratotic cells of nail bed origin are contiguous with the undersurface of the nail plate.

Epidermis of the hyponychium is situated between the nail bed and the distal groove. The hyponychium cornifies like volar epidermis with production of a granular layer and a thick, compact cornified layer.

Epidermis of the palms and soles begins with the distal groove and includes the tips of the digits. It is characterized by a well-developed rete-papillae pattern and a prominent granular and cornified layer.

The dermis beneath the epithelium of the nail unit is copiously supplied with capillaries and venules, especially within the papillae. In addition, there are special vascular shunts (glomus bodies) that aid in temperature regulation of the digits.

The epithelial kinetics of the nail unit revolve around the nail matrix. The proximal portion of the matrix is the predominant supplier of cornified cells that constitute the superior aspect of the nail plate, whereas the distal matrix (lunula) contributes the inferior portion of the plate. The nail plate is directed outward as a continuation of the angle assumed by the matrix, along guidelines provided by the proximal nail fold and the lateral nail grooves and folds.

Cornified cells of the nail bed are distinct from those of the nail plate, but both cornified products move outward together at the same pace. The forward growth of the nail plate is propelled by mitoses in the matrix, whereas cornified cells of the nail bed are carried outward by the movement of the plate, as well as by cell division occurring within the nail bed epithelium. Although no physiologic exchange exists between the undersurface of the nail plate and the nail bed on which it rests, the apposing surfaces are firmly attached. The cohesion is so great that when the nail is avulsed, the separation does not occur at the junction between the nail plate and the nail bed, but rather between the nail bed and the subjacent dermis. This cohesion results from the insertion of longitudinal parallel ridges and furrows between the nail bed epithelium and underlying connective tissue.

The nail plate is composed almost wholly of protein with a high sulfur content. Biochemically, protein of the nail plate appears to be similar to that in the cornified layer of the epidermis and in the hair shaft.

Like hair, the nail unit forms by invagination of the epidermis into the dermis. Each has a matrix that manufactures its own cornified end product: the hair shaft and the nail plate. The outer root sheath is comparable to the nail bed, and the inner root sheath is analogous to the cornified material supplied by the nail bed. The nail plate and the nail bed can be compared to the hair shaft and the internal root sheath. The cornified cells of both nail bed and hair root sheath disappear virtually unnoticed as they move outward.

Fingernails grow at about one-third the rate of hair, approximately 0.1 mm per day, whereas toenails grow more slowly. Thus, after avulsion, fingernails return to their former length in about 6 months, whereas toenails require about 12 months. Nails grow faster in summer than in winter (just as hair does) and more rapidly in children than in adults.

The nail plate grows continuously unless injured, either by physical force or by local or systemic disease. A transverse groove (Beau's line) reflects temporary malfunction of the matrix, such as in acute febrile illness. A longitudinal ridge or furrow implies focal damage to the matrix, and a longitudinal pigmented streak signals focal melanocytic hyperactivity, such as in a junctional type of melanocytic nevus. Pits, a mark of psoriasis, are evidences of pinpoint damage to the proximal matrix and represent loci where tiny clusters of parakeratotic cells have been shed from the surface of the nail plate. White spots (leukonychia) result from damage to the distal matrix and represent parakeratotic cells in the deeper portion of the nail plate. In lichen planus, focal scarring of the matrix produces a pterygium, whereas total scarring of the matrix results in anonychia. Subungual keratosis results from abnormal production of cornified cells by the nail bed. Dermatitis that chronically involves the proximal nail fold, as in candidiasis, may extend to the matrix, eventuating in cessation of nail growth and, ultimately, absence of the nails.

After this examination of the skin by reducing it to its components, it must be evident that the skin is a remarkably integrated organ in which epithelial and mesenchymal structures are delicately interrelated. It will hereafter be shown that inflammatory diseases of the human skin always entail some form of injury to blood vessels, especially those that course within the dermis. Vascular damage having occurred, reflections of it in the form of inflammatory-cell infiltrates may be seen in the epidermis, the dermis, or the subcutaneous fat, or all together. Most inflammatory processes in the dermis also affect the epidermis, and those in the fat, the dermis.

Suggested Readings

Embryology

Garber, B. B.: Control of epithelial development. Curr. Probl. Dermatol. *6*:154–190, 1976.

Flaxman, B. A., and Maderson, P. F. A.: Growth and differentiation of skin. J. Invest. Dermatol. *67*:8–14, 1976.

Topography and Regional Variation

Hashimoto, K.: Surface ultrastructure of human skin. Acta Derm. Venereol. (Stockh.) *55*(6):413–430, 1975.

Pinkus, H.: Die makroskopische Anatomie der Haut. *In* Jadassohn, J., Handbuch der Haut—und Geschlectskrankeiten, Normale und Pathologische Anatomie, Der Haut II. Berlin, Springer-Verlag, 1964.

Collagen

Bently, J. P.: Excelsior: A retrospective view of collagen. J. Invest. Dermatol. *67*:119–123, 1976.

Bornstein, P.: The biosynthesis of collagen. Annu. Rev. Biochem. *43*:567–603, 1974.

Pinnell, S.: Disorders of collagen. *In* Metabolic Basis of Inherited Disease edited by J. B. Stansbury, J. B. Wyngaarden, and D. S. Fredrickson. New York, McGraw-Hill, in press.

Shuster, S., Black, M. M., McVitie, E.: The influence of age and sex on skin thickness. Skin collagen and density. Br. J. Dermatol. *93*:639–643, 1975.

Stevanovic, D. V.: Elastotic degeneration: A light and electron microscopic study. Br. J. Dermatol. *94*:23–29, 1976.

Elastic Fibers

Breathnach, A. S.: An atlas of the ultrastructure of human skin. London, Churchill, 1971, p. 174.

Deutsh, T. A.: Elastic fibers in fetal dermis. J. Invest. Dermatol. *65*:320–323, 1975.

Gotte, L., Giro, M. G., Volpin, D., and Horne, R. W.: The ultrastructural organization of elastin. (J. Ultrasctruct. Res. *46*:23–33, 1974.

Ross, R., and Bornstein, P.: Elastic fibers in the body. Sci. Am. *224*:44–52, 1971.

The Vasculature

Montagna, W., and Parakkal, P. F.: Chapter 5, Blood supply. *In* The Structure and Function of the Skin. New York, Academic Press, 1974.

Ryan, T. J.: The blood vessels of the skin. J. Invest. Dermatol. *67*:110–118, 1976.

Yen, A.: Ultrastructure of the human dermal microcirculation: the horizontal plexus of the papillary dermis. J. Invest. Dermatol. *66*(3):131–142, 1976.

The Epidermal Keratinocyte

Bergstresser, P. R., and Taylor, J. R.: Epidermal 'turnover time'—a new examination. Br. J. Dermatol. 96:1–4, 1977.

Briggaman, R. A., and Wheeler, C. E.: The epidermal-dermal junction. J. Invest. Dermatol. 66:71, 1975.

Gelfant, S.: The cell cycle in psoriasis: a reappraisal. Br. J. Dermatol. 95:577–590, 1976.

Kefalides, N. A.: Basement membranes: structural and biosynthetic considerations. J. Invest. Dermatol., 65:85, 1975.

Matoltsy, A. G.: Keratinization. J. Invest. Dermatol. 67:20–25, 1976.

Wolff-Schreiner, E. C.: Ultrastructural cytochemistry of the epidermis. Int. J. Dermatol. 16:77–102, 1977.

The Melanocyte

Jimbow, K., Quevedo, W., Fitzpatrick, J. B., and Szabo, G.: Some aspects of melanin biology 1950–1975. J. Invest. Dermatol. 67:2–89, 1976.

Quevedo, W. C., et al.: Light and skin color. In Sunlight and Man edited by M. A. Pathak et al; T. B. Fitzpatrick, consulting editor. Tokyo, University of Tokyo Press, 1974, pp. 165–194.

The Langerhans Cell

Silberberg-Sinakin, J., et al.: Antigen-bearing Langerhans cells in skin, dermal lymphatics, and in lymph nodes. Cell. Immunol. 25:137–151, 1976.

Wolff, K.: The Langerhans Cell. Curr. Probl. Dermatol. 4:79–145, 1972.

The Merkel Cell

Mahrle, G., and Orfanos, C. E.: Merkel Cells as human cutaneous neuroreceptor cells. Arch. Dermatol. Forsch. 251:19–26, 1974.

Winkelmann, R. K., and Breathnach, A. S.: The Merkel Cell. J. Invest. Dermatol. 60:2–15, 1973.

The Nerves

Montagna, W.: Twenty-Sixth Symposium on the Biology of Skin: Morphology of cutaneous sensory receptors. J. Invest. Dermatol. 69(1):4, 1977.

The Subcutaneous Fat

Bloom, W., and Fawcett, D. W.: A Textbook of Histology, Chapter 7, Adipose tissue. Philadelphia, W. B. Saunders Company, 1975.

Hull, D., and Segall, M. M.: Distinction of brown from white adipose tissue. Nature, 212:469, 1966.

Napolitano, L.: The differentiation of white adipose cells. J. Cell Biol., *18:*663, 1963.

Napolitano, L.: Observations on the fine structure of adipose cells. N.Y. Acad. Sci., *131:*34, 1965.

Schamel, J., and Charvált, Z.: Fatty tissue in plastic surgery. Acta Chir. Plast. *6:*223–228, 1964.

The Hair Follicle

Biology and Disease of the Hair edited by K. Toda, Y. Ishibashi, Y. Hori, and F. Morikawa. Baltimore, University Park Press, 1976.

Ebling, F. J.: Hair. J. Invest. Dermatol. *67:*98–105, 1976.

Kollar, E. J.: The induction of hair follicles by embryonic dermal papillae. J. Invest. Dermatol. *55:*374–378, 1970.

Montagna, W., and Parrakkal, P. T.: The structure and function of skin, Third Edition. New York, Academic Press, 1974.

The Sebaceous Gland

Downing, D. T., and Strauss, J. S.: Syntheses and composition of surface lipids of human skin. *In* Advances in Biology of Skin, Vol XIV, Special Issue on Sebaceous Glands and Acne Vulgaris. J. Invest. Dermatol. *62:*228–244, 1974.

Nicolaides, N.: Skin lipids, their biochemical uniqueness. Science *186:*19–26, 1974.

Sansone-Bazzano, G., and Reisner, R. M.: Steroid pathways in sebaceous glands. *In* Advances in Biology of Skin, Vol. XIV, Special Issue on Sebaceous Glands and Acne Vulgaris. J. Invest. Dermatol. *62:*211–216, 1974.

Strauss, J. S., Pochi, P. E., and Downing, D. T.: The sebaceous glands: twenty-five years of progress. J. Invest. Dermatol. *67:*90–98, 1976.

The Apocrine Gland

Bell, M.: The ultrastructure of human axillary apocrine glands after epinephrine injection. J. Invest. Dermatol. *63:*147–159, 1974.

Robertshaw, D.: Neural and humoral control of apocrine glands. J. Invest. Dermatol. *63:*160–167, 1974.

The Eccrine Sweat Gland

Sato, K.: Sweat induction from an isolated eccrine sweat gland. Am. J. Physiol. *225:*1147–1152, 1973.

Wells, T. R., and Landing, B. H.: The helical course of the human eccrine sweat duct. J. Invest. Dermatol. *51:*177–185, 1968.

The Nail

Zaias, N.: Diseases of nails. *In* Clinical Dermatology edited by D. J. Demis, R. L. Dobson, and J. McGuire. New York, Harper and Row, 1976.

Inflammatory Cells: Structure and Function

Inflammatory Cells:

Structure *and* Function

2

THE HISTOLOGIC findings in cutaneous inflammation reflect structural, biochemical, and physiologic events that follow injury to the skin by various means—for example, by pathogens, immunogens, or foreign objects. Inflammation in skin is the result of a sequence of vascular responses to injury (transient vasoconstriction, arteriolar dilatation, increased rate of blood flow, capillary and venular dilatation, increased permeability, and serous exudation) that are accompanied by migration of leukocytes from blood vessels into the tissues. Leukocytes are inflammatory cells brought into tissues by chemotactic substances generated in the pathogenetic process. The histologic diagnosis of inflammatory skin diseases requires recognition of both the pattern in which the inflammatory cells are arranged and the individual cell types. In Chapter 5, the patterns formed by inflammatory cells in the skin will be described. The present chapter deals with the inflammatory cells themselves (the neutrophil, eosinophil, histiocyte, lymphocyte, mast cell, and basophil), where they come from, what they look like, and what they do. New discoveries about mechanisms of inflammation,

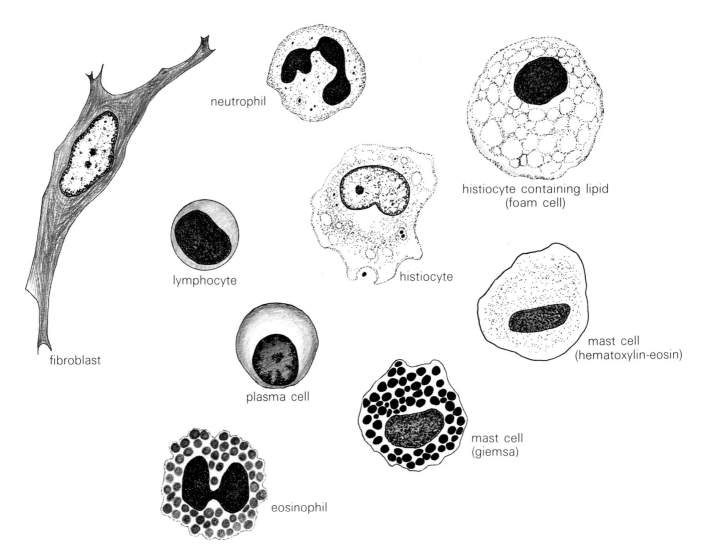

FIG. 2-1. Comparative cytology of inflammatory cells.

especially the immunologic, are being made so rapidly that some of the information in this chapter may be modified or perhaps superseded in the near future.

The Neutrophil

Neutrophils are the most numerous of the blood leukocytes, comprising 50% to 70% of the circulating white cells. The neutrophil is 10 to 12 microns in diameter and has a multilobed nucleus and a cytoplasm that contains delicate amphophilic granules that can be seen when they have been stained with hematoxylin and eosin. With the electron microscope, the granules have been identified as membrane-bound lysosomes (Fig. 2-2). Neutrophils are produced in the bone marrow, approximately 126 billion being generated each day in a 70-kg man. The neutrophil develops from a myeloblast through stages of promyelocyte, myelocyte, metamyelocyte, and band-shaped polymorphonuclear leukocyte, matures in 10 to 14 days, and then is released into the circulation where it spends approximately 7 hours before entering the extravascular tissues for its final few hours.

Leukocytes in small numbers migrate from the capillaries to the surrounding tissues under normal conditions, but injury intensifies this movement. Within minutes after injury, the blood flow usually slows, and the neutrophils stick to the endothelial lining of the capillaries. The neutrophils then insert pseudopods between endothelial cells, wriggle through the blood vessel wall, penetrate the basement membrane and perivascular connective tissue sheath, and enter the surrounding tissues.

Neutrophils function primarily as phagocytes. The sequence of events in phagocytosis is chemotaxis, adherence, engulfment, and digestion of foreign matter. Chemotaxis is a process by which certain biologically active substances direct migrating leukocytes

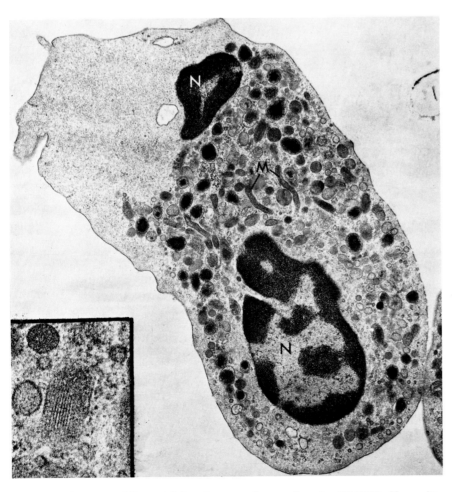

FIG. 2-2. A neutrophil containing lysosomal granules. ($\times$ 12,000.) M = mitochondria; N = nucleus. The inset shows the crystalline structure of a granule. ($\times$ 61,000). (Courtesy Dorothy Zucker-Franklin, M.D.)

toward injurious agents. Numerous agents or substances are chemotactic for neutrophils. Important among them are cleavage products resulting from the complement cascade.

The classic complement system, composed of many components, is conventionally designated C, and the individual complement components are represented by a suffix number (e.g., C1, C2). A bar above an individual complement component signifies that it is activated (e.g., $\overline{C1}$). Antigen-antibody interactions lead to formation of antigen-antibody complexes which, in turn, activate complement components C1, C4, and C2, in that order. The $\overline{C142}$ complex attacks C3 and C5, yielding C3a and C5a. These low-molecular-weight peptides are chemotactic for neutrophils, eosinophils, and monocytes. Activation of $\overline{C567}$ complex may also lead to the generation of chemotactic activity, but only for neutrophils. Some antigens, such as microbial polysaccharides, can generate C3a and C5a from C3 and C5 via the alternative, or properdin, pathway of complement activation, independent of the presence of antibodies. Furthermore, nonspecific proteases from bacteria or from damaged tissue can attack C3 and C5 directly and yield C3a and C5a.

In addition, the complement system is intimately interrelated with the kinin and clotting systems. Aggregating platelets can initiate chemotaxis by two mechanisms. One is the release of a platelet protein that cleaves a chemotactic factor from the fifth component of complement. The other results from activation of the Hageman factor, which generates kallikrein and plasminogen activator and initiates the clotting system. Both kallikrein and plasminogen activator have chemotactic activity. Additionally, ingestion of particulate matter by neutrophils causes them to release factors that directly call forth more neutrophils. The products of some bacteria also summon neutrophils. Neither kallikrein nor plasminogen is complement dependent. This series of chemotactins is in turn neutralized by other factors, still poorly defined, that would prevent a chain reaction of extensive tissue destruction.

Chemotactic factors seem to act on the plasma membrane of the neutrophil. A gradient of chemotactic-factor concentration is established that induces neutrophils to concentrate in sites of tissue damage. Chemotactic factors direct, rather than accelerate, the motion of these cells. Neutrophils enter the inflammatory site rapidly, whereas monocytes, which respond to the same chemotactic stimuli, do so more slowly. The presence of neutrophils, however, is *not* a requisite for the arrival of monocytes at a focus of injury. In fact, monocytes continue to appear in an inflammatory site long after neutrophils have ceased to arrive, perhaps because of the higher threshold of response of neutrophils to chemotactic factors and the accumulation of inhibitors of neutrophils motility.

The major task of the neutrophil is the ingestion and elimination of noxious material such as bacteria, fungi, immune complexes, foreign bodies, and tissues that have been injured or destroyed. The particles to be ingested and removed may have a special coating that enables neutrophils to recognize them. The process of coating is called opsonization. Uncoated bacteria, especially encapsulated ones, are resistant to phagocytosis. Once a bacterium has been coated by specific immunoglobulin and complement, it is readily ingested by neutrophils.

Phagocytosis is preceded by adhesion of the plasma membrane of the neutrophils to the membranes of bacteria by means of special receptors on the cell membrane for the Fc portion of IgG and the C3b fragment of C3. The neutrophil extends pseudopods which surround the bacterium and engulf it into a vacuole, called the phagocytic vacuole, almost simultaneously with particle uptake. The extent of degranulation seems to be roughly proportional to the amount of foreign material ingested. The neutrophil granules contain lysozyme, lactoferrin, phagocytin, hydrolytic enzymes, peroxidases, and cationic proteins. When phagocytosis occurs, hydrogen peroxide is formed within phagocytic vacuoles.

The neutrophil contains two types of granules, azurophilic and specific. The azurophilic granules are relatively large (800 nm) and dense. They constitute 25% of the granules in the neutrophil and contain at least 20 hydrolytic enzymes in addition to peroxidases. These hydrolases function at an acid pH to destroy bacteria and other foreign substances.

In contrast to the azurophilic granules, the specific granules are smaller (500 nm), less dense, and constitute 75% of the granules in neutrophils. Their major constituent is alkaline phosphatase. The specific granules do not contain lysosomal enzymes, and they function at a neutral or alkaline pH.

During phagocytosis, alkaline phosphatase is first released from the specific granules and is followed by peroxidases from the azurophilic granules. The combination of peroxidase-hydrogen peroxide and iodide is bactericidal and viricidal at pH 5 by causing iodination of the microorganism protein.

The Eosinophil

Eosinophils, like other granulocytes, originate in the bone marrow. After 3 or 4 days they are released into the blood stream, where they spend only 3 or 4 hours en route to completing the remaining 8 or so days of their life cycle in the tissues. There the eosinophil can be identified with the light microscope by the presence of a bilobed nucleus in a round cell whose cytoplasm contains numerous coarse granules that take up eosin and other acid dyes. The eosinophil granules have a characteristic ultrastructure (Figs. 2-3, 2-4). These membrane-bound granules are oval and have an electron-dense crystalline core oriented parallel to the long axis of the granule and a surrounding, less electron-dense, finely granular matrix. Chemically, the core of the eosinophil granule contains abundant phospholipid and a protein rich in arginine. The matrix of the granule contains cathepsin, ribonuclease, arylsulfatase, sulfatase, phospholipase D, and betaglucuronidase, in addition to other lysosomal enzymes and peroxidase.

In general, eosinophils function much like neutrophils. They have ameboid motion, respond to chemotactic stimuli, phagocytose matter, and undergo degranulation. There are several eosinophil chemotactic factors, each having a different chemical character and each arising under different circumstances. Eosinophils are strongly drawn to antigen-antibody complexes, especially those combined with activated complement. Eosinophils, like neutrophils, respond to a chemotactic factor generated during the interaction of antigen and antibodies of the IgG class and complement. Complement fragments cleaved during the ensuing complement cascade attract eosinophils and neutrophils, which account for the mixed inflammatory-cell population of the lesions in some immune-complex diseases. In skin, the prototype of such reactions is leukocytoclastic vasculitis.

Nonimmunologic molecular aggregates (e.g., proteins, polysaccharides, macromolecular simulators of antigen-antibody complexes, endotoxins manufactured by gram-negative bacteria, and tissue proteins denatured by injury) can also activate complement and thus generate an eosinophil chemotactic factor.

An important chemotactic factor, named eosinophil chemotactic factor of anaphylaxis (ECF-A), is released from mast cells during reactions between antigen and antibodies of the IgE class which are fixed on the surface of mast cells.

Eosinophils are highly phagocytic, capable of ingesting gram-positive and gram-negative bacteria, fungi, mycoplasma, immune complexes, mast cell granules, and inert particles. Most particles require opsonization to render them susceptible to phagocytosis by eosinophils. During phagocytosis, the degranulation of eosinophils is similar to that of neutrophils, but less complete. When viewed with the light microscope, an eosinophil that has full functional potential cannot always be readily distinguished from an eosinophil that is completely spent.

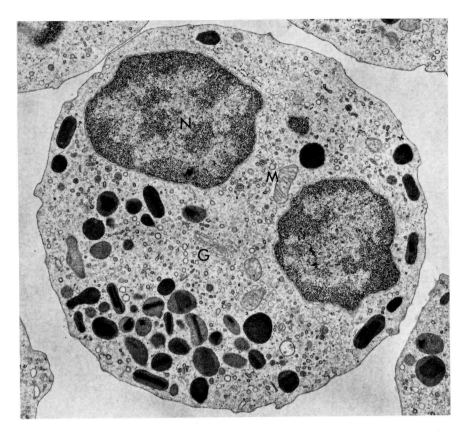

FIG. 2-3. An eosinophil containing granules that have an electron-dense core and a less electron-dense matrix. (× 9,500.) G = Golgi apparatus; M = mitochondria; N = nucleus. (Courtesy Dorothy Zucker-Franklin, M.D.)

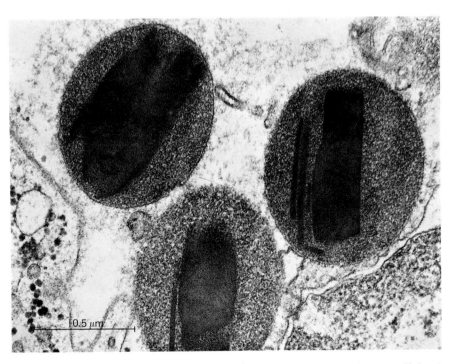

FIG. 2-4. Eosinophil granules at higher magnification (× 63,000). (Courtesy Helmut Wolff, M.D.)

Like neutrophils, eosinophils contain hydrolytic and proteolytic enzymes packaged in membrane-bound granules. The eosinophil, however, is less effective at bacterial phagocytosis than is the neutrophil; it lacks the neutrophil's degrading enzymes cathepsin and phagocytin; it has a chemically different peroxidase which is not bactericidal, and it does not produce the tissue necrosis that so often results from the neutrophil's proteolytic activity. Eosinophils are comparable to neutrophils in their capacity to phagocytose mycoplasma, immune complexes, and sensitized erythrocytes.

Although eosinophils share many functions with neutrophils, they have additional special roles. One example of the biochemical singularity of eosinophils is the presence of the enzyme arylsulfatase, which is not found in neutrophils, basophils, or platelets. Arylsulfatase inactivates slow-reacting substance of anaphylaxis (SRS-A) produced by mast cells. Another eosinophil enzyme, phospholipase D, inactivates platelet aggregating factor that is also generated by mast cells. In addition, an inhibitor derived from eosinophils prevents histamine release from human mast cells and basophils. Therefore, a significant role for the eosinophil in immediate hypersensitivity reaction is to regulate the mast cell by inactivating some of the mast cell's most potent products.

The Histiocyte

The histiocyte, also referred to as the macrophage, begins its existence as a promonocyte in the bone marrow, from which it is released within a few hours into the blood stream as a monocyte. The monocyte spends about 32 hours in the peripheral blood before moving to its final destination, the tissues. Cells whose progenitors are promonocytes are known by different names in different organs: Kupffer cells in the liver, alveolar macrophages in the lung, reticulum cells in the lymph nodes and spleen, microglial cells in the central nervous system, and histiocytes in the skin. This widely dispersed, but functionally integrated, system of cells is known as the "macrophage system" or the "reticuloendothelial system." Although these cells vary in appearance, they function similarly in defense against bacteria and other injurious agents.

Reticulum cells (fixed macrophages) are cytologically identical with histiocytes (free macrophages). The fixed macrophages may become free macrophages under certain conditions, such as tissue injury. The reticuloendothelial system is defined as an anatomic and physiologic unit composed of both the fixed and free macrophages. Both types of macrophages are present in the dermis, and therefore the skin contains part of the reticuloendothelial system.

Histiocytes are mononuclear cells that range in size from 15 to 25 microns. Their nuclei are generally larger and paler than those of lymphocytes and are gray-blue in sections stained with hematoxylin and eosin. Histiocyte nuclei may be round, reniform, deeply indented, or multilobed. The cytoplasm of the histiocyte is more abundant than that of the lymphocyte. Viewed with the electron microscope, the histiocyte cytoplasm contains a well-developed Golgi complex, mitochondria, small vacuoles, and lysosomal granules that increase in number when activated (Fig. 2-5).

In tissues the histiocyte often exists for months without undergoing a single cell division. The number of histiocytes in normal skin is small. In acute inflammatory reactions there is a prompt influx of monocytes from the blood. If the reaction persists for more than a few days, the histiocytes at the site begin to divide.

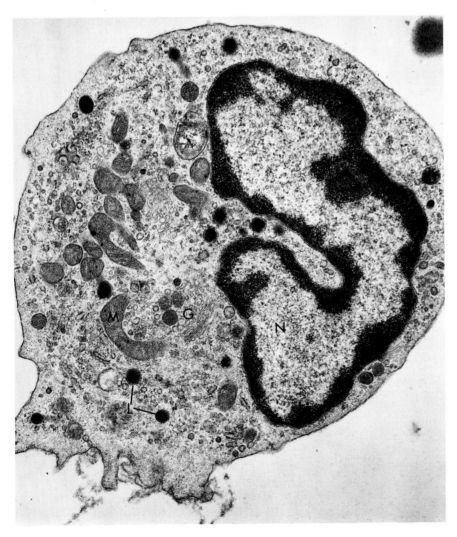

FIG. 2-5. A histiocyte containing lysosomes (L) and mitochondria (M). The Golgi apparatus (G) and nucleus (N) are also prominent. ($\times$ 22,000.) (Courtesy Dorothy Zucker-Franklin, M.D.)

In granulomatous reactions (i.e., those in which histiocytes predominate) the influx of newly-arrived blood monocytes accounts for only about 1% of all the histiocytes at the tissue site. The remaining histiocytes are the result of replication of histiocytes already on the scene. If the granulomatous response persists, the histiocytes become activated, enlarge, and appear to touch one another like epithelial cells, and hence are called epithelioid cells. Histiocytes may fuse to form multinucleated histiocytic cells (giant cells).

In acute inflammatory reactions, such as some infectious processes, the cytoplasm of activated histiocytes contains new granules, many of them lysosomal. These granules enhance the phagocytic and metabolic capabilities of the histiocytes, both specifically against the invading organism and nonspecifically against all other potential pathogens.

A major function of histiocytes is that of scavenger (Fig. 2-6). When histiocytes engulf opaque particles, the process is called phagocytosis (an eating process) in contrast to the ingestion of fluid droplets which is called pinocytosis (a drinking process). The initial step in phagocytosis is the attachment of the foreign material to the plasma membrane of the histiocyte. In order for phagocytosis to proceed effectively, the foreign object is usually coated with opsonins, such as IgM, IgG, and complement. Without this coating by antibody and complement, the foreign material simply remains on the surface of the histiocyte, rather than binding to specific receptors on the histiocyte membrane.

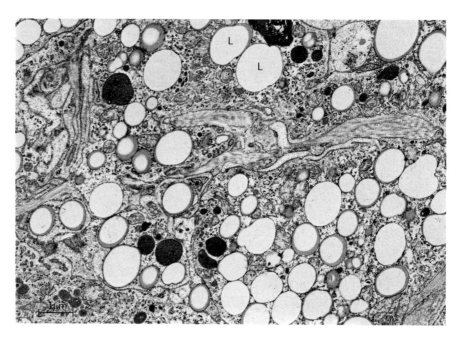

FIG. 2-6. Numerous lipid vacuoles (L) within the cytoplasm of a histiocyte (× 10,000.) (Courtesy Helmut Wolff, M.D.)

Pinocytosis, like phagocytosis, cannot proceed without specific binding of molecules to the histiocyte surface. The pinocytic activity of the cell can be increased by the presence of negatively charged molecules. Both phagocytosis and pinocytosis are energy-requiring processes. Once inside the histiocyte, the foreign material is enclosed within a vacuole that eventually fuses with lysosomes, forming a digestive vacuole. In the histiocyte, the enzymes for digestion of foreign materials include a variety of acid hydrolases, such as acid phosphatase, cathepsin, and beta glucuronidase. With histiocytic phagocytosis there is a striking increase both in cell volume and in the size of the Golgi apparatus, which is the site for active formation of many small lysosomes. During the intracellular digestion, lysosomes pour their hydrolytic enzymes into the phagocytic vacuoles. Thus, the number of lysosomes decreases during active phagocytosis. Their numbers increase again after the bulk of cellular debris and other foreign material has been eliminated.

Histiocytes also play a role in the immune response. They appear to have at least two functions in regard to antigen. One is the catabolism and elimination of potentially immunogenic molecules. This applies to approximately 90% of antigen molecules that are phagocytosed by the histiocyte. This clearance function of the histiocyte is critical because it prevents antigen overload, thus minimizing the chances of immune paralysis.

The other function of histiocytes in the immune response is the concentration and retention of a small amount of immunogen for subsequent presentation to the lymphocyte. About 7% of antigen molecules are not destroyed, but are concentrated and retained within the histiocytes. This retained antigen may possess immunogenicity for the lifetime of the histiocyte and may also be the antigen reservoir necessary for the maintenance of immune tolerance. The other 3 molecules per 100 molecules of antigen remain bound and unaltered on the histiocyte plasma membrane. These figures are averages because significant differences in the extent of degradation occur with different types of antigens. Hence, most immunogens are destroyed by histiocytes except for the small amount of them retained within the cell and an even smaller quantity that remains on the outside of the plasma membrane.

In cellular immune responses, the histiocytes become activated at the tissue site where antigen is localized. A cooperative effort ensues between activated histiocytes and specialized lymphocytes (committed T-lymphocytes). Once these committed T-lymphocytes have interacted with antigen processed by the histiocytes, they produce various lymphokines, which include chemotactic factors, migration-inhibiting and macrophage-activating factors, blastogenic factors, and cytotoxic factors. These factors, in large part, are directed toward the additional accumulation, retention, and activation of histiocytes. Thus, histiocytes act as effector cells under the direction of lymphocytes.

The Lymphocyte

Lymphocytes originate in the bone marrow as lymphoblasts and mature there into prolymphocytes. Once in the circulation as lymphocytes, some of these cells migrate into the thymus, where they reside for varying periods before being dispersed throughout the body. These thymus-influenced lymphocytes are known as T-lymphocytes and constitute about 80% of all circulating blood lymphocytes. Of the other 20% of circulating lymphocytes, the majority remain under the control of the bone marrow or other as yet undefined site(s) and are known as B- (or bursa-dependent) lymphocytes. A third, less well-understood population of lymphocytes that is now being recognized lacks the surface markers that have enabled identification of T- and B-lymphocytes.

T- and B-lymphocytes are indistinguishable by light microscopy. Both can be various sizes (small, 5 to 8 microns; medium, 8 to 12 microns; and large, 12 to 30 microns) with darkly staining or slightly indented round nuclei surrounded by a narrow rim of light-blue cytoplasm. These small, medium, and large lymphocytes are actually stages in a progression of sizes. Just as it is difficult to distinguish some circulating blood monocytes from circulating lymphocytes, so, too, it may be impossible to differentiate some histiocytes from lymphocytes in inflammatory skin diseases. Indeed, some mononuclear cells that would be classified as lymphocytes by cytologic criteria prove to be histiocytes by such functional criteria as the capacity to spread on glass and to ingest vital dyes.

The scanning electron microscope shows that, in vitro, T-lymphocytes usually have relatively smooth surfaces, whereas B-lymphocytes have rather villous surfaces. The transmission electron microscope shows that lymphocyte cytoplasm contains numerous free ribosomes, but sparse endoplasmic reticulum, few mitochondria, and a small Golgi complex (Fig. 2-7). When lymphocytes are stimulated by specific antigens, they develop prominent endoplasmic reticulum.

The lymphocyte is motile, but moves less quickly than the neutrophil. The life span of the lymphocyte varies greatly. In fact, some circulating small lymphocytes survive for many years.

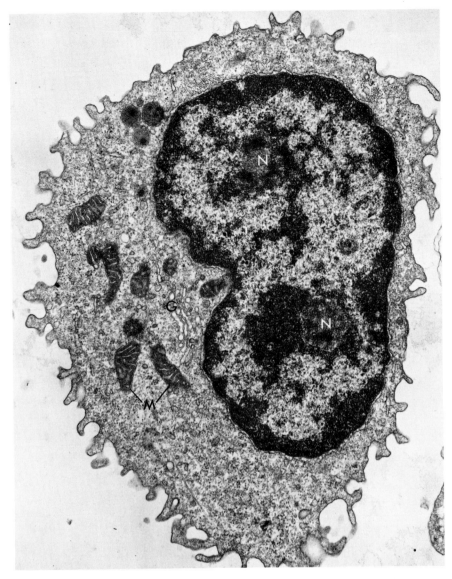

FIG. 2-7. A lymphocyte with numerous surface processes. G = Golgi apparatus; M = mitochondria; N = nucleus. (× 20,000.) (Courtesy of Dorothy Zucker-Franklin, M.D.)

Thymus-dependent lymphocytes are essential to cell-mediated immunity which consists of three interrelated but distinct phases. In the first phase, antigen is transported to immunologic centers where T-lymphocytes and macrophages reside. In the second phase, antigen is processed by macrophages and presented to uncommitted T-lymphocytes which then develop the capacity to recognize the antigen. The T-lymphocytes proliferate and release lymphokines, soluble protein mediators of the cell-mediated immune response. In the third phase, lymphokines recruit and activate other inflammatory cells, such as uncommitted lymphocytes and histiocytes, which digest and destroy the antigen. A few T-lymphocytes with the ability to specifically recognize antigen are able to muster a large number of other inflammatory cells to effectively eliminate foreign material.

Among the many functions of T-cells in cell-mediated immune reactions, as previously stated, is the recruitment of macrophages through the secretion of lymphokines. These soluble proteins are secreted by T-cells within hours after contact in vivo with specific antigens and in vitro with nonspecific, as well as specific, antigens. Among these lymphokines are macrophage-activating factor and migration-inhibiting factor. They enable a single lymphocyte to attract and activate as many as 1000 macrophages. Some lymphokines are lymphotoxins and chemotactins for the other inflammatory cells. Certain T-cells, the so-called killer T-cells, can also function as primary effector cells in the direct lytic destruction of cells bearing non-self antigen.

Transfer factor, another product of T-lymphocytes, is a substance that transfers T-cell-mediated immune capabilities to recipient T-lymphocytes. This capacity can be retained for approximately one year. The mode of action of transfer factor has not yet been elucidated, but therapeutic benefit with it has been achieved in patients suffering from lepromatous leprosy, mucocutaneous candidiasis, and the Wiskott-Aldrich syndrome. Prior to treatment with transfer factor, the lymphocytes of patients with Wiskott-Aldrich syndrome form few active T-rosettes. After successful treatment, the number of T-rosettes increases significantly.

T-lymphocytes play a crucial role in graft-versus-host reactions, allergic contact dermatitis, prevention of malignant neoplasia, and defense against bacteria, viruses, protozoa, and fungi. By contrast, B-lymphocytes are precursors of the antibody-producing plasma cells. B-lymphocytes are coated with immunoglobulins that can be readily demonstrated by immunofluorescent methods. In addition, the surface of the B-cell possesses receptor sites for fragments of the third component of complement (C3b and C3d), for antigen-antibody complexes (Fc fragment of IgG), and the Epstein-Barr virus. Such easily identified immunoglobulins are not present on the surfaces of T-cells. T-cells, however, have receptors for the direct formation of rosettes with normal sheep erythrocytes at low temperatures.

B-lymphocytes are found in bone marrow and in lymphoid organs. Although the majority of the lymphocytes in the thoracic duct are T-lymphocytes, B-lymphocytes also migrate from blood to tissues and vice versa through the thoracic duct. T-lymphocytes migrate from the blood to tissues, then via lymph into the lymph nodes and from there into the thoracic duct, and finally back into the blood. T-cells continuously recirculate between blood and lymph and intermittently into tissues and organs, including the skin. Skin lymphocytes arrive there from the blood, and after a sojourn in the tissues depart via the lymph stream.

Among the major functions of B- and T-lymphocytes are the recognition and elimination of antigens. Both B- and T-cells bind antigen to their surfaces. On B-cells, antigens are apparently bound to certain surface immunoglobulins.

B-cells function primarily to produce and secrete antibodies. Blastogenesis and mitosis occur when B-cells encounter antigen. T-helper-cells aid B-cells in the production of antibodies to certain antigens. The end result of B-lymphocyte maturation is the plasma cell. Plasma cells are rarely found in normal skin, but they are relatively plentiful in the lamina propria of normal mucous membranes. The distinctive features of plasma cells are seen when they are stained with hematoxylin and eosin. They are ovoid cells with eccentric round or oval nuclei and deeply purple cytoplasm. The nuclear chromatin is scattered in coarse clumps at the periphery of the nucleus, giving it a "clock-face" appearance. A pale-staining perinuclear area, or perinuclear halo can usually be detected. Older plasma cells often contain homogeneous eosinophilic globules of varying size within their cytoplasm. These accumulations of glycoprotein are known as Russell bodies.

Viewed with the electron microscope, the perinuclear halo of the plasma cell contains a pair of centrioles and a prominent Golgi apparatus. The remainder of the cytoplasm shows a highly developed rough endoplasmic reticulum (Fig. 2-8). This complex of

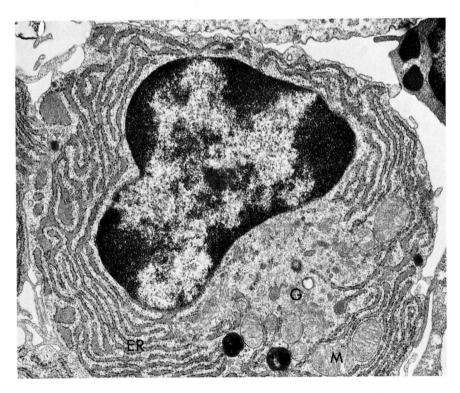

FIG. 2-8. A plasma cell replete with rough endoplasmic reticulum (ER). G = Golgi apparatus; M = mitochondria; N = nucleus. (× 11,500.) (Courtesy of Dorothy Zucker-Franklin, M.D.)

ribosomes and endoplasmic reticulum is the site of antibody synthesis in the plasma cell. Russell bodies can be recognized with the electron microscope as granular masses within the cisternae of the endoplasmic reticulum.

Immunoglobulins are secreted from plasma cells located both in lymphoid organs and in other tissues at sites of inflammation. Plasma cells seldom divide, are barely mobile, and do not ingest matter by phagocytosis.

The lymphocytes, therefore, are critical contributors to the inflammatory response. They function against pathogens and immunogens both directly, by producing specific substances that counter them, and indirectly, by producing substances that attract neutrophils, eosinophils, macrophages, and other lymphocytes to combat the injurious agents. Once at the reaction site, lymphocytes initiate a chain of biochemical events designed to eliminate or minimize the hazard to the host.

The Mast Cell

Mast cells—unlike neutrophils, eosinophils, histiocytes, and lymphocytes, all of which originate in the bone marrow—arise from undifferentiated mesenchymal cells. They are widely distributed in human connective tissue, including the dermis, especially around small blood vessels. In a sense, mast cells are the first line of cellular immunologic defense because they are the only effector cells that reside in the tissues. All the others arrive in the tissues via the blood.

Mast cells have a characteristic appearance when stained with hematoxylin and eosin and viewed through the light microscope. They vary in size from 8 to 15 microns and have a central dark-staining nucleus, varying from round to ovoid. Mast-cell cytoplasm is replete with tiny (0.6 to 0.7 microns) amphophilic granules. Viewed with the electron microscope, these granules are seen to be limited by a membrane (Fig. 2-9). The interior of the granules is composed of subunits consisting of lamellar whorls (Fig. 2-10). The endoplasmic reticulum is sparse, and the mitochondria are few, but the Golgi complex is well developed, and numerous villi project from the mast-cell surface (Fig. 2-11).

Mast-cell granules demonstrate metachromasia, by which is meant a reaction in which a dye selectively stains certain tissue substances in a color that differs from the color of the dye itself. The production of metachromasia results from the presence of free electronegative charges of a certain minimal density. Acid mucopolysaccharides, nucleic acids, and other acidic groups, if

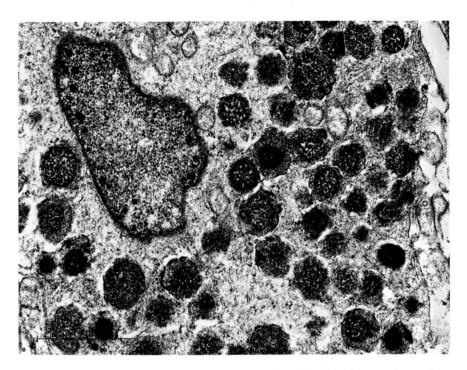

FIG. 2-9. A mast cell containing numerous granules (G) within the cytoplasm. N = nucleus. (× 31,000.) (Courtesy Helmut Wolff, M.D.)

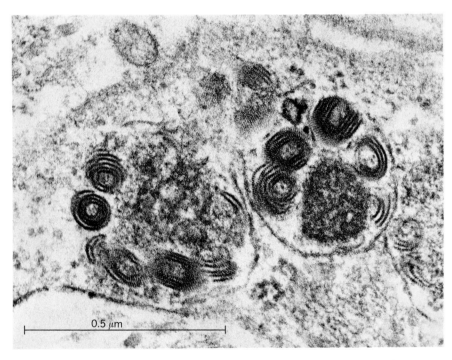

0.5 μm

FIG. 2-10. Mast-cell granules at higher magnification showing membrane-bound "scrolls" of fine crystalline structures and homogeneous material. (× 116,000.) (Courtesy Helmut Wolff, M.D.)

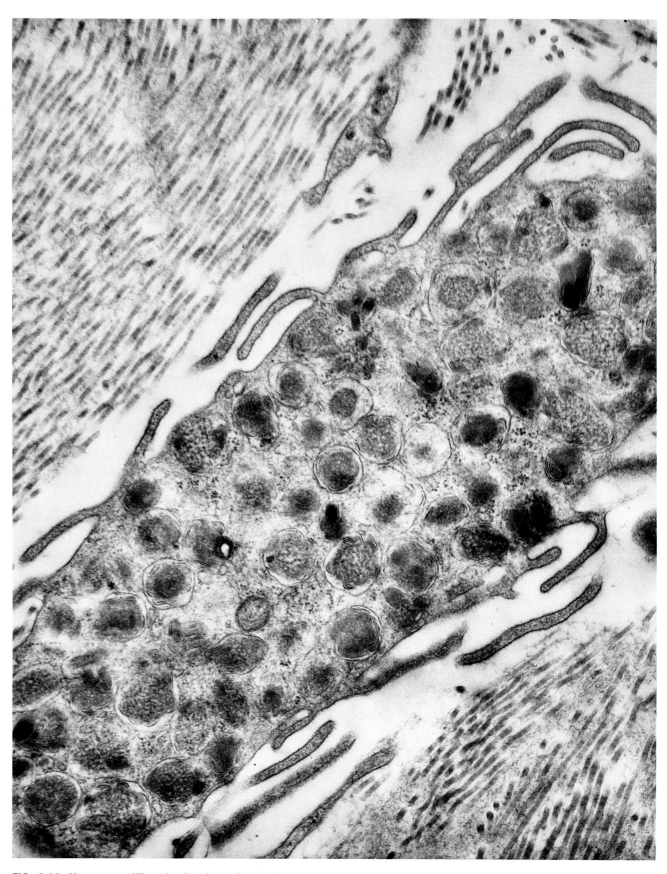

FIG. 2-11. Numerous villi projecting from the surface of a mast cell. (× 40,000.) (Courtesy Alvin Cox, M.D.)

present in sufficient quantity, will promote metachromasia. Mast-cell granules are metachromatically stained purple with basic dyes, such as toluidine blue and methylene blue. The metachromasia of mast-cell granules results from their content of the strongly acidic, sulfated mucopolysaccharide, heparin. Heparin is synthesized in the mast cell and is bound to protein. It constitutes 30% of the mast-cell granule by weight and is a major active biochemical substance in the granule. Tissue extracts containing heparin from mast cells can be shown to exert an anticoagulant effect. Nevertheless, for reasons unknown, local coagulation of blood is not prevented in pathologic conditions in which mast cells accumulate in skin.

Other mast cell mediators of acute inflammation are dependent for their release on immunoglobulin of the IgE type. IgE interaction with antigen on the surface of the mast cell leads to mast cell degranulation and release of chemical mediators of two general categories:

1. Preformed chemicals stored in mast cells (and basophils)

   a) Histamine
   b) Eosinophil chemotactic factor of anaphylaxis (ECF-A)
   c) Neutrophil chemotactic factor of anaphylaxis (NCF-A)

2. Newly formed chemicals generated immediately within mast cells (and basophils)

   a) Slow-reacting substance of anaphylaxis (SRS-A)
   b) Platelet-aggregating factor (PAF)

Histamine, present in mast cells and basophils, is a potent chemical mediator of inflammatory reactions. It acts to increase the permeability of postcapillary venules, thus allowing egress of serum and inflammatory cells. Antihistamines compete with histamine for specific receptors.

Eosinophil chemotactic factor of anaphylaxis (ECF-A) is even more active in attracting eosinophils than are the chemotactic factors derived from complement, kallikrein, and plasminogen activator, all of which are potent chemotactens for neutrophils. ECF-A is a mixture of two acidic peptides that function to bring eosinophils and to a lesser extent neutrophils, to the site of acute allergic reactions. Neutrophil chemotactic factor of anaphylaxis is the major mast cell chemotacten for neutrophils.

Slow-reacting substance of anaphylaxis (SRS-A), like histamine, causes increased vascular permeability. It is a chemically unique acidic sulfate ester. Interestingly, the eosinophil carries an enzyme, arylsulfatase, that specifically destroys the acidic sulfate ester of SRS-A. Unlike histamine, SRS-A is resistant to antihistamines.

During IgE-dependent reactions, histamine, being preformed and stored within the mast cells, begins to be released into the tissues in about 15 seconds, and the mast cell is completely depleted of histamine in about 2 hours. By contrast, SRS-A, which is made by the mast cell in response to the interaction of IgE and antigen on its surface, is not released from the mast cell for at least 5 minutes.

The factors released from mast cells have two general effects. The first is increased vascular permeability and consequent tissue edema. The second is activation of platelets, eosinophils, and neutrophils. Thus, mast cells are instrumental in bringing other inflammatory cells to the sites of IgE-mediated tissue injuries. Eosinophils modulate mast cell function by producing arylsulfatase, which inactivates both SRS-A and histamine, and phospholipase-D, which inactivates PAF. By inactivating the mast cell products—SRS-A, histamine, and PAF—the eosinophil helps to regulate the inflammatory reaction.

In addition to antigen-antibody reactions, degranulation of mast cells can be effected by several agents such as trauma (e.g., in urticaria pigmentosa), polymers (e.g., polysorbate 80), enzymes (e.g., chymotrypsin), and small molecular weight compounds (e.g., aspirin, morphine, polymyxin and 48/80).

Hyaluronic acid, a nonsulfated acid mucopolysaccharide, is also present in mast cells. Its role has not yet been defined, but it may convert edema fluid into a mucinous gel that then acts as a matrix for collagen deposition. In this way, hyaluronic acid would aid in the reparative phase of the inflammatory process.

The Basophil

In man, connective-tissue mast cells and blood basophils appear to be independent cell types, despite the similar staining properties of their granules. Morphologically, these two cells differ in the shape of their nuclei, the basophil nucleus being multilobed (Fig. 2-12) and the mast cell being single-lobed, and in the size of their granules, the basophil granules being slightly larger than those of the mast cell (Fig. 2-13). Despite some chemical differences, mast-cell and basophil granules have chemical similarities, and it is possible that their functions complement one another in allergic reactions. The basophil plays a role in certain types of delayed hypersensitivity reactions, such as allergic contact dermatitis, and

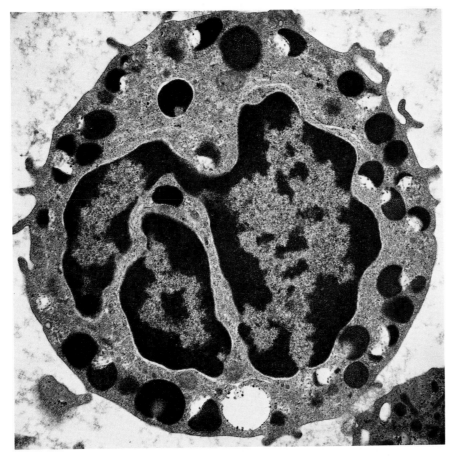

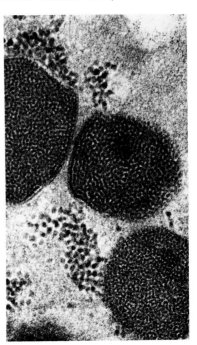

FIG. 2-13. Basophil granules at higher magnification showing concentric arrangement of intragranular particles in peripheral rows. (× 53.000.) (Courtesy Dorothy Zucker-Franklin, M.D.)

FIG. 2-12. A basophil with granules of various sizes. (× 20,000.) (Courtesy Dorothy Zucker-Franklin, M.D.)

will probably be shown to have a role in other inflammatory diseases of skin. Because basophils cannot be identified in sections stained with hematoxylin and eosin, but with special stains only, they are not crucial to my approach to the histologic diagnosis of inflammatory skin diseases.

Suggested Readings

General

Cochrane, C. G.: The participation of cells in the inflammatory injury of tissue. J. Invest. Dermatol. *64*:301–306, 1975.

Cohen, S.: Cell mediated immunity and the inflammatory system. Human Pathol. *7*:249–264, 1976.

Dvorak, H. F., et al.: Morphology of delayed type hypersensitivity reactions in man. Lab. Invest. *31*:111–130, 1974.

Fearon, D. T., and Austen, K. F.: Immunochemistry of the classical and alternate pathways of complement. *In* Immunochemistry, edited by L. E. Glynn and M. Steward. Chichester, England, John Wiley and Sons, Ltd., in press.

Götze, O., and Müller-Eberhard, H. J.: The role of properiden in the alternate pathway of complement activation. J. Exp. Med. *139*:44–57, 1974.

Jordan, R. E., and Provost, T. T.: The complement system and the skin. Yearbook of Dermatology, Chicago, Yearbook Medical Publishers, Inc., 1976, pp. 7–37.

Pike, J. E.: The prostaglandins. J. Invest. Dermatol. *67*:650–653, 1976.

Stossel, T. P.: Phagocytosis. Three parts. N. Engl. J. Med. *290*:717–723, 774–780, 833–839, 1974.

The Neutrophil

Cline, M. J.: The normal granulocyte in the white cell. Cambridge, Mass., Harvard University Press, 1975, pp. 5–103.

Goldstein, I. M.: Polymorphonuclear leukocyte lysosomes and immune tissue injury. Prog. Allergy *20*:301–340, 1976.

Senn, H. J., and Jungi, W. F.: Neutrophil migration in health and disease. Semien. Hematol. *12*:7–46, 1975.

Stossel, T. P.: Phagocytosis: Recognition and ingestion. Semien. Hematol. *12*:83–116, 1975.

The Eosinophil

Baehner, R. L., and Johnston, R. B. Jr.: Metabolic and bacteriocidal activities of human eosinophils. Br. J. Haematol. *20*:277–285, 1971.

Colley, O. G.: Eosinophils and immune mechanisms. J. Immunol. *110*:1419–1423, 1973.

Goetze, E. J., and Austen, K. F.: Eosinophil chemotactic factor of anaphylaxis (ECF-A): Cellular origin, structure, and function. *In* Monographs in Allergy edited by K. Rother. Basel, S. Karger, in press.

Hubscher, T.: Role of the eosinophil in the allergic reactions. J. Immunol. *114*:1379–1388, 1975.

Zucker-Franklin, D.: The properties of eosinophils. *In* Modern Concepts and Developments in Immediate Hypersensitivity edited by M. K. Bach. New York, Marcel Dekker, in press.

The Histiocyte

Adams, D. O.: The granulomatous inflammatory response. Am. J. Pathol. *84:*163–192, 1976.

Albrecht, R. M., et al.: Basic and clinical consideration of the monocyte-macrophage system in man. J. Pediatr. *88:*751–765, 1976.

Bellant, J. A., and Dayton, D. H.: The phagocytic cells in host resistance. New York, Raven Press Books, Ltd., 1975.

Unanue, E. R.: Secretory function of mononuclear phagocytes. Am. J. Pathol. *83:*395–418, 1976.

The Lymphocyte

Buckley, R. H.: The functions and measurement of human B- and T-lymphocytes. J. Invest. Dermatol. *67:*381–390, 1976.

Claudy, A. L., et al.: Morphological, immunological and immunocytochemical identification of lymphocytes extracted from cutaneous infiltrates. Clin. Exp. Immunol. *23:*61–68, 1976.

David, J. R.: Macrophage activation induced by lymphocyte mediators. Acta Endocrinol. *78:*1994–2245, 1975.

Lawrence, H. S.: Transfer factor in cellular immunity. Harvey Lect. *68:*239–350, 1974.

Mills, J. A., et al.: Lymphocyte physiology. Annu. Rev. Med. *22:*185–220, 1971.

Winkelstein, A., et al.: Lymphocyte biology. Bull. Rheum. Dis. *25:*185–220, 1971.

The Mast Cell

Soter, N. A., and Austen, K. F.: The diversity of mast cell-derived mediators: Implications for acute, subacute, and chronic cutaneous inflammatory disorders. J. Invest. Dermatol. *67:*313–319, 1976.

Definition of Terms

Histologic Terms

Epidermal changes

Dermal changes

Clinical Terms

Primary clinical lesions

Secondary clinical lesions

Confusing Terms

Definition
of Terms

3

LEARNING a new language or subject requires mastery of its basic vocabulary. Dermatopathology, as a gross and microscopic study of cutaneous diseases, has a specialized vocabulary. This chapter explains and illustrates those words and phrases that are essential to the language of dermatopathology.

Histologic Terms

Histologic terms used in dermatopathology may be subdivided into those describing phenomena occurring in the epidermis and those describing changes in the dermis.

Epidermal Changes

Hyperkeratosis: increased thickness of the cornified layer.

Hyperkeratosis may be "absolute," an actual increase in the thickness of the cornified layer, or "relative," an apparent increase in contrast to a thin spinous layer.

ORTHOKERATOSIS (Greek, "normal cornification"): hyperkeratosis composed of cells that have cornified completely (without retained nuclei). Strictly speaking, the word should be ortho-hyperkeratosis.

Three patterns of orthokeratosis may be seen:

1. Basket-weave, an exaggeration of the normal cornified layer (e.g., in tinea versicolor, Fig. 3-1A)

2. Compact (e.g., in lichen simplex chronicus, Fig. 3-1B)

3. Laminated (e.g., in ichthyosis vulgaris, Fig. 3-1C)

PARAKERATOSIS (Greek, "departure from the normal cornification"): hyperkeratosis in which pyknotic nuclei are retained in the cells, or squames, of the cornified layer (Fig. 3-1D).

Parakeratosis usually is seen in diseases having accelerated cell turnover. It occurs in processes that are inflammatory (e.g., psoriasis) and neoplastic (e.g., squamous-cell carcinoma). A diminished granular layer is frequently found beneath parakeratotic cells, presumably because the rapid turnover of epidermal cells precludes normal maturation.

① basket-weave orthokeratosis

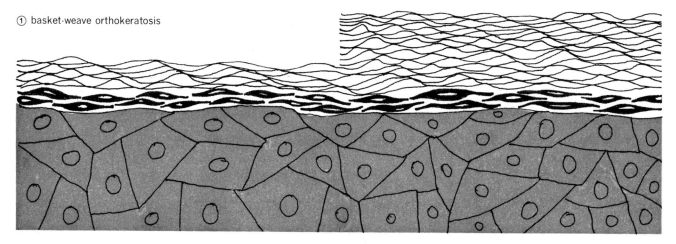

FIG. 3-1. A, Basket-weave orthokeratosis.

② compact orthokeratosis

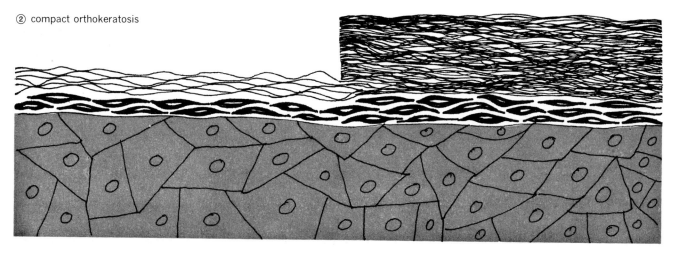

FIG. 3-1. B, Compact orthokeratosis.

Orthokeratosis may alternate with parakeratosis in both vertical and horizontal directions. Vertical alternation implies episodic changes in epidermopoiesis (e.g., in pustular psoriasis), and horizontal alternation results from focal changes in epidermopoiesis such as a sequel to spongiosis (e.g., in pityriasis rosea). Parakeratosis may be focal (e.g., in guttate psoriasis) as well as confluent (e.g., in psoriatic plaques). Parakeratosis may also be both vertically and horizontally focal in the same specimen (e.g., pityriasis rubra pilaris). Theoretically, cornified cells may be parakeratotic in the absence of hyperkeratosis, (e.g., exfoliative dermatitis where the cornified cells (squames) are constantly shed), but in actuality such instances are exceptional.

A scale-crust is a mixture of parakeratotic cells with plasma (homogeneous eosinophilic material) and occasionally white or red blood cells (Fig. 3-1E). Scale-crust may indicate previous spongiotic changes (e.g., seborrheic dermatitis) or result from external trauma (e.g., excoriation).

③ laminated orthokeratosis

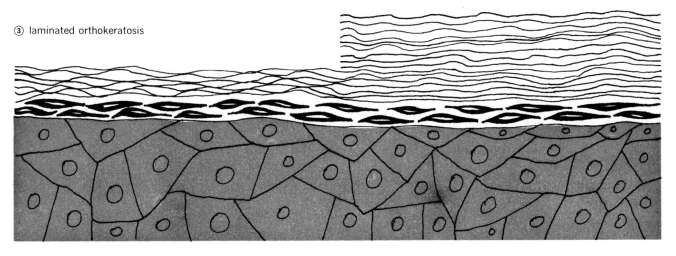

FIG. 3-1. C, Laminated orthokeratosis.

④ parakeratosis

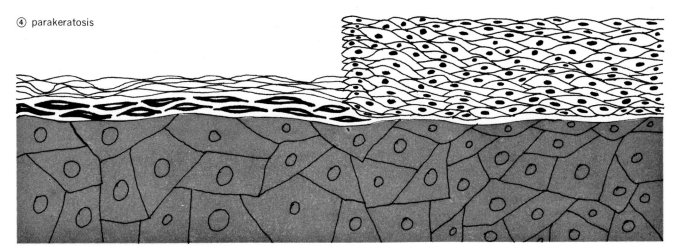

FIG. 3-1. D, Parakeratosis.

scale-crust

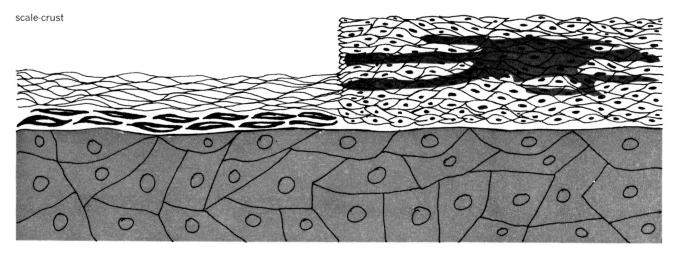

FIG. 3-1. E, Scale-crust.

hypergranulosis

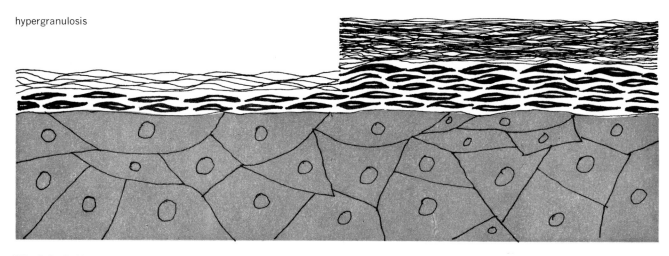

FIG. 3-2. A, Hypergranulosis.

hypogranulosis

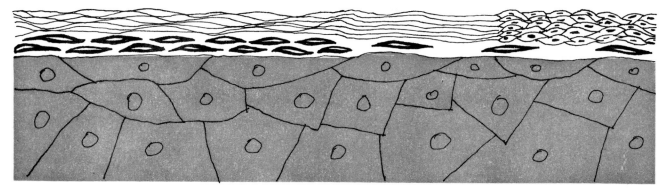

FIG. 3-2. B, Hypogranulosis.

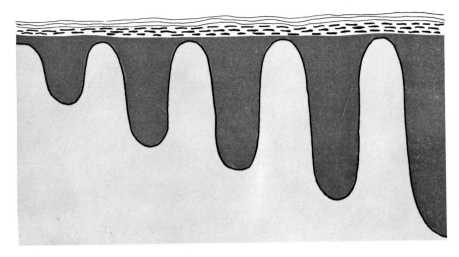

FIG. 3-3. Hyperplasia, downward growth.

Hypergranulosis: increased number of cells in the granular layer, usually associated with orthokeratosis (e.g., lichen planus) (Fig. 3-2A). An exception is ichthyosis vulgaris where orthokeratosis is associated with a diminished granular zone.

Hypogranulosis: decreased number of cells in the granular layer (e.g., ichthyosis vulgaris) (Fig. 3-2B).

Hyperplasia: increased number of cells that results in a thickened epidermis (Fig. 3-3).

The degree of thickening in hyperplasia may be slight, moderate, or extensive such as in the epidermis of halogenodermas and deep fungal infections. There are four major patterns of epidermal hyperplasia:

1. PSORIASIFORM: More or less evenly elongated rete ridges with preservation of the rete-papillae configuration (e.g., in psoriasis) (Fig. 3-4A).

2. IRREGULAR: uneven, elongated, pointed rete ridges and obliteration of the normal rete-papillae configuration (e.g., in lichen planus) (Fig. 3-4B).

3. PAPILLATED: digitate projections of epidermis above the skin surface (e.g., in verruca vulgaris) (Fig. 3-4C).

4. PSEUDOCARCINOMATOUS: epidermal hyperplasia that superficially resembles squamous-cell carcinoma.

Pseudocarcinomatous hyperplasia can be associated with inflammatory diseases (e.g., in deep fungal infections) and neoplastic ones (e.g., in granular cell tumors). (Fig. 3-4D).

Acanthosis (Greek, "a condition of spininess") refers specifically to a thickened spinous layer.

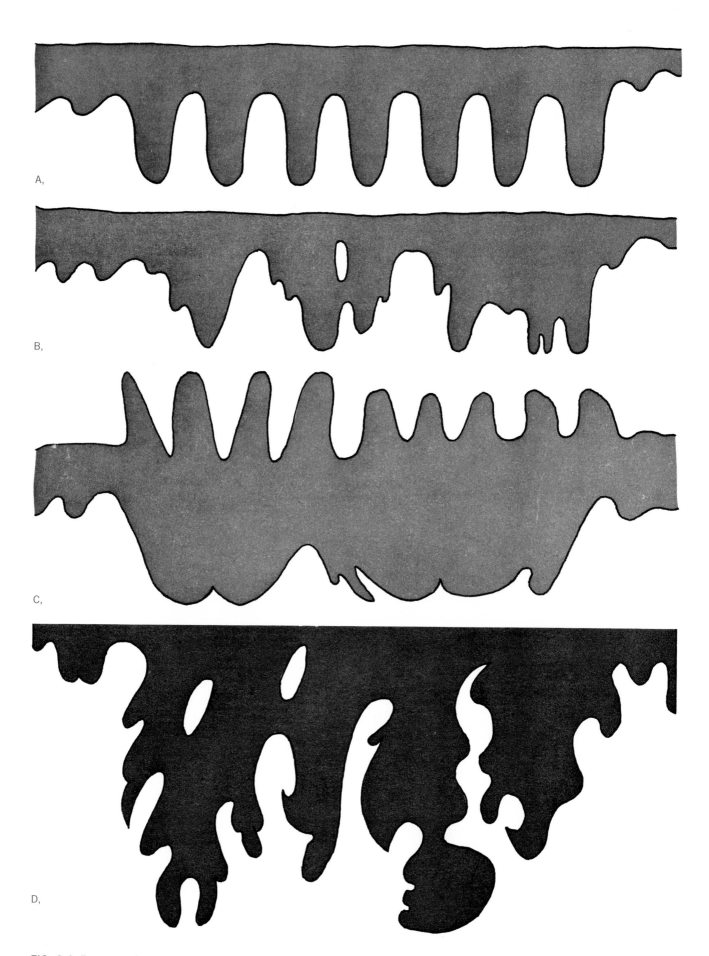

FIG. 3-4. Patterns of hyperplasia. A, Psoriasiform. B, Irregular. C, Papillated. D, Pseudocarcinomatous.

Hypoplasia: decreased number of cells that results in a thin epidermis (e.g., in chronic discoid lupus erythematosus).

Hypertrophy: increased size of spinous cells that results in a thickened epidermis.

Thickening of the epidermis may be due wholly to an increased number of cells (hyperplasia), as in psoriasis, or to an increase in size of cells (hypertrophy), as in lichen planus or lichen simplex chronicus.

Atrophy: decreased size of spinous cells that results in a thinner epidermis, usually with diminution or loss of the rete-papillae pattern (Fig. 3-5).

Spongiosis (intercellular edema): edema between the spinous cells results in widening of the intercellular spaces and a spongy appearance. Inflammatory cells, usually lymphocytes, are constant accompaniments of focal intercellular edema (Fig. 3-6A). Severe spongiosis may eventually lead to formation of an intraepidermal vesicle (e.g., in allergic contact dermatitis).

Ballooning (intracellular edema): increase in size of spinous cells, associated with pallor of their cytoplasm (Fig. 3-6B). Severe intracellular edema results in rupture of cell membranes and formation of multiloculated intraepidermal blisters (reticular alteration) (e.g., in herpesvirus vesicles). In addition to edema, large pale spinous cells may also be due to accumulation of glycogen, such as occurs following epidermal injury.

Acantholysis (Greek, "a loosening of spines"): loss of cohesion between epidermal cells that leads to formation of intraepidermal clefts, vesicles, or bullae (Fig. 3-7).

Acantholytic cells separate completely from their neighbors and in the process develop a round, uniformly staining nucleus rimmed by cytoplasm with condensation of eosinophilic material at the periphery (Fig. 3-8B). Acantholysis occurs in intraepidermal processes such as pemphigus, benign familial chronic pemphigus

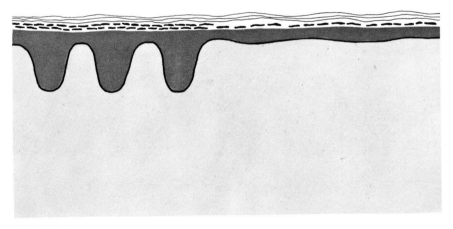

FIG. 3-5. Atrophy.

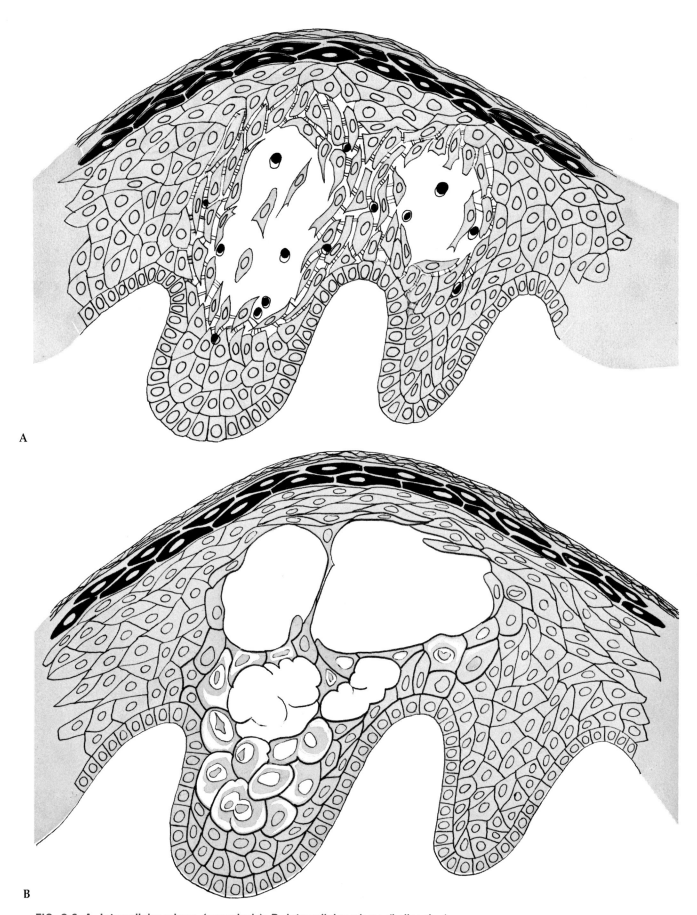

FIG. 3-6. A, Intercellular edema (spongiosis); B, intracellular edema (ballooning).

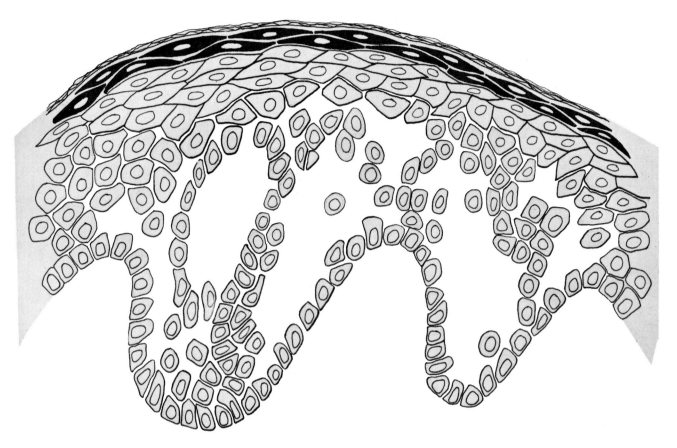

FIG. 3-7. Acantholysis.

(Hailey-Hailey disease), keratosis follicularis (Darier's disease) and its histologic analogues (focal acantholytic dyskeratosis), herpetic vesicles, staphylococcal scalded-skin syndrome, and all other subcorneal pustular diseases. In rare instances acantholytic cells can even be seen in the epidermis above the papillary abscesses in dermatitis herpetiformis, a subepidermal vesicular disease. Acantholytic cells may also occur in solar keratoses, pseudoglandular squamous-cell carcinomas, and, uncommonly, in keratoacanthomas. Acantholytic cells are not usually found in spongiotic conditions.

Spongiform pustule: accumulation of neutrophils within and between epidermal cells whose boundaries form a spongelike framework for the neutrophils (Fig. 3-9).

Spongiform pustules are sterile when they occur in pustular psoriasis and its variants (impetigo herpetiformis, acrodermatitis continua, keratoderma blenorrhagicum), but contain numerous spirochetes in rupial syphilis. Rarely do they accompany other inflammatory processes in which neutrophils predominate. Spongiform pustules are different from spongiotic vesicles.

Dyskeratotic cells: prematurely and therefore faultily cornified cells having eosinophilic cytoplasm and small, darkly-staining nuclei (Fig. 3-8C).

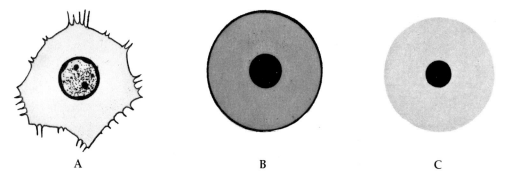

FIG. 3-8. A, Normal spinous cell; B, Acantholytic cell; C, Dyskeratotic or necrotic cell.

Cytologically, dyskeratotic cells are distinguished with difficulty from necrotic keratinocytes in sections stained by hematoxylin and eosin. This judgment usually depends upon whether the rest of the epithelium is thought to be cornifying or dying. With the electron microscope discrete homogeneous eosinophilic units often called Civatte, cytoid, or hyalin bodies can be recognized as dyskeratotic cells in lichen planus and discoid lupus erythematosus and as necrotic cells in phototoxic dermatitis and erythema multiforme. Dyskeratotic cells occur in inflammatory and neoplastic processes.

Necrosis: local death of cells or tissue that occurs within a living organism.

Histologic judgments about necrosis are made on the basis of nuclear changes. These alterations are nuclear fragmentation (karyorrhexis), nuclear ghosts (karyolysis), and nuclear shrinkage with consequent hyperchromasia (pyknosis). Often the cytoplasm of necrotic cells is swollen and eosinophilic. Coagulation necrosis and caseation necrosis are the major types of necrosis in skin. Histologically, in coagulation necrosis cellular outlines are preserved, but cellular detail is lost (e.g., gumma), whereas in caseation necrosis there is complete loss of all structural details, the tissue being replaced by granular material containing nuclear debris (e.g., tuberculoma). Ischemia is the most common cause of necrosis, but toxins (e.g., of Clostridia), enzymes (e.g., pancreatic lipase), and physical and chemical agents (e.g., burns) also produce necrosis. Cells within the dermis, such as fibroblasts and adnexal epithelium, as well as fat cells, can undergo necrosis, just as can epidermal cells. Necrotic keratinocytes are seen in such diverse diseases as erythema multiforme (an inflammation) and basal-cell carcinoma (a neoplasm) (Fig. 3-8C).

Vacuolar alteration (liquefaction degeneration) of the basal-cell layer: minute spaces immediately above and below the basement membrane at the dermoepidermal junction (Fig. 3-10).

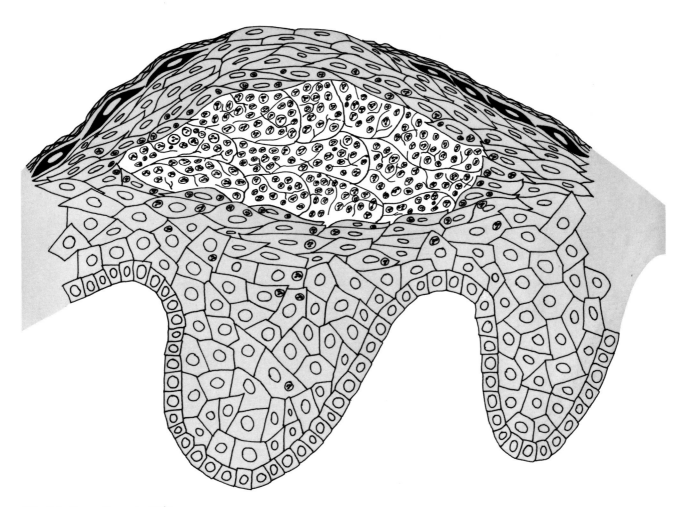

FIG. 3-9. Spongiform pustule.

Confluence of these tiny spaces results in formation of dermoepidermal clefts, which upon receipt of fluid, usually serum, proceed
to subepidermal vesiculation. All diseases with extensive vacuolar
alteration may become bullous (e.g., lichen sclerosus et atrophicus,
lichen planus, erythema multiforme).

Clefts: spaces that do not contain fluid may appear within the
epidermis (Fig. 3-11), (e.g., in keratosis follicularis), below the
epidermis at the dermoepidermal interface (e.g., in lichen planus),
or between epithelial cells and connective tissue (e.g., in basal-cell
carcinoma). These empty spaces result from retraction of tissue
elements during fixation.

Dermal Changes

Histologic changes in the dermis may be seen as cellular infiltrates
or as alterations in the connective tissue itself. The density and
depth of these infiltrates determines whether the clinical lesion
will be a papule, a nodule, or another type of lesion.

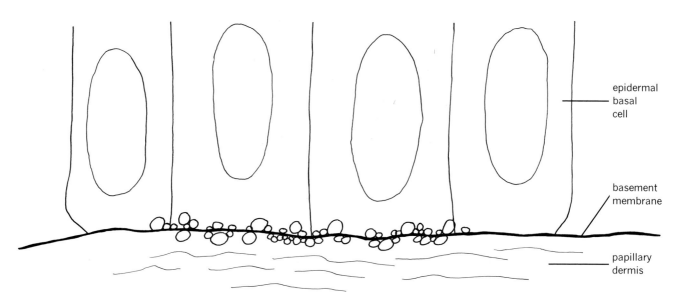

FIG. 3-10. Vacuolar alteration at the dermoepidermal interface.

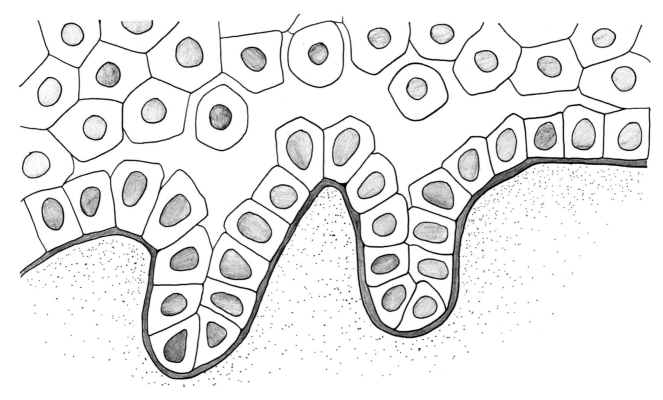

FIG. 3-11. Cleft.

Cellular Infiltrates

Monomorphous: all cells of one type.

Mixed: cells of more than two types.

Lymphohistiocytic: lymphocytes and histiocytes only.

Lichenoid: a bandlike infiltrate of cells, as in lichen planus, that extends across the upper part of the dermis parallel to the epidermis and often obscures the dermoepidermal interface.

The word *lichenoid* is also used clinically for papules that resemble those of lichen planus, i.e., flat-topped.

Nodular (Latin, "small node"): well-circumscribed collections, usually of cells. Like the word *lichenoid, nodular* also has a clinical meaning, namely, a large round elevated lesion.

Leukocytoclastic ("a break-up of leukocytes resulting in nuclear dust"): fragmentation of nuclei, especially of neutrophils. Leukocytoclasis is prominent in leukocytoclastic vasculitis (allergic vasculitis).

Alterations in Connective Tissue

Collagen degeneration: structural and tinctorial changes in collagen. The word *degeneration,* rather than *necrosis,* is applied to collagen because the histologic criteria for necrosis involve nuclei, and collagen is anuclear. Examples of cutaneous collagen degeneration are hyalinization (e.g., in chronic lichen sclerosus et atrophicus and chronic radiodermatitis) and basophilic degeneration (e.g., in acute necrobiosis lipoidica). Basophilic degeneration of collagen should not be confused with the basophilic, spaghettilike connective tissue fibers that are found in the dermis of chronically sun-damaged skin (i.e., elastotic material, solar elastosis).

Hyalinization of collagen (Greek, "made into glass"): confluence and increased eosinophilia of collagen.

Fibrosis (Latin, "condition of thread formation"): increased collagen in altered arrangement, with an increased number of fibroblasts (Fig. 3-12).

Sclerosis: increased collagen in altered arrangement, having a homogeneous, eosinophilic, hyalinized appearance with a decreased number of fibroblasts (Fig. 3-13). Sclerosis sometimes, but not always, represents old fibrosis.

Collagen in vertical streaks: elongated parallel strands of thickened collagen present in a widened papillary dermis and oriented perpendicularly to the surface of the specimen (Fig. 3-14).

This phenomenon occurs in certain thickenings of the papillary dermis, such as in lichen simplex chronicus, and in other lesions that are chronically rubbed, such as in lichen planus, chronic contact dermatitis, and mycosis fungoides.

Lamellated collagen: Coarse collagen in lamellated whorls often forms around increased numbers of melanocytes at the dermoepidermal junction. Thin fibroblasts parallel the whorls of coarse lamellated collagen, which is similar to the coarse collagen in vertical streaks that develops from persistent rubbing in lichen simplex chronicus. This phenomenon of lamellation tends to form

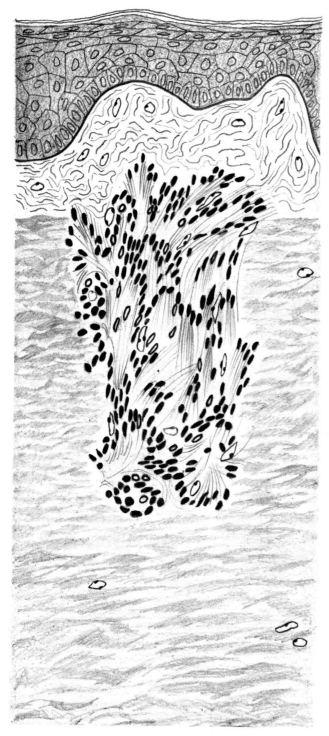

FIG. 3-12. Fibrosis.

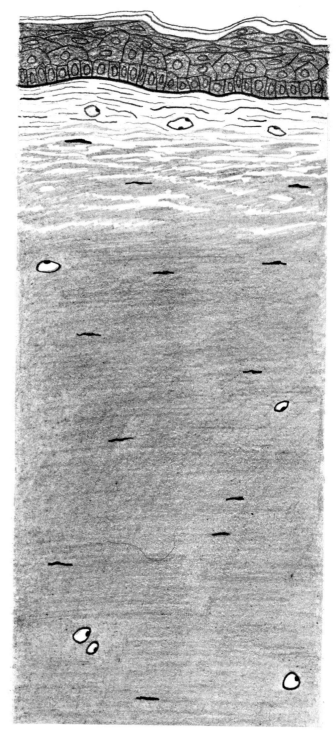

FIG. 3-13. Sclerosis.

episodically in melanocytic hyperplasias, both in those conditions in which melanocytes have normal nuclei (e.g., simple lentigo) and in those characterized by abnormal nuclei (e.g., malignant melanoma in situ).

Papillomatosis: projections of the dermal papillae above the skin surface (e.g., in acanthosis nigricans) (Fig. 3-15).

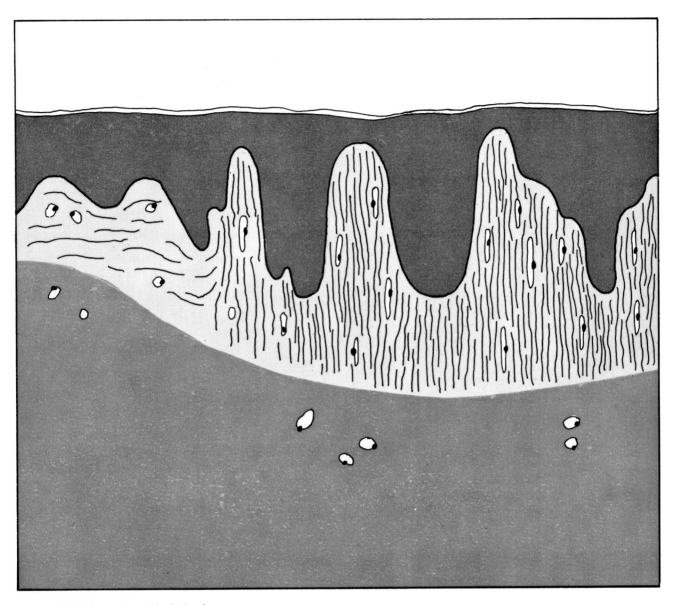

FIG. 3-14. Collagen in vertical streaks.

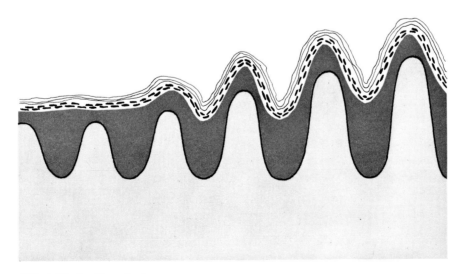

FIG. 3-15. Papillomatosis.

Clinical Terms (Gross Pathologic Skin Lesions)

Even though they are generally considered to be primary (i.e., spontaneous), certain clinical lesions can develop both from internal factors and from wholly external influences. Examples of this principle are the similar-appearing blisters in pemphigus and those induced by cantharidin; the comedones of adolescent acne and those resulting from exposure to hydrocarbons or severe long-standing sun damage ("senile" comedones, better called "solar" comedones); the lichenoid papules of lichen planus and those caused by photographic color developers; hives of a drug eruption and the wheals that follow pressure; purpura of coagulation defects and traumatic ecchymoses; and the scars of atrophic striae induced either by systemic corticosteroids or by topical corticosteroids under occlusion.

Changes such as ulcers, crusts, scales, and scars are generally regarded as secondary skin lesions. They evolve from primary skin lesions or are sometimes artefacts induced by patients.

Primary Clinical Lesions

Macule (Latin, "a spot"): a flat discoloration up to 1 cm in diameter (Fig. 3-16).

A macule can result from pigmentary abnormalities, such as increased epidermal melanin in a freckle or decreased epidermal melanin in confetti-sized lesions of vitiligo. Pinpoint purple macules (petechiae) are caused by extravasated erythrocytes in the papillary dermis and reddish macules, such as in viral exanthems, result from erythrocytes within dilated capillaries. Hemorrhagic spots can be due to trauma as in senile purpura.

Patch: a macular lesion more than 1 cm in diameter (Fig. 3-16).

The causes of patch formation are identical to those of macule production. The café au lait spot of neurofibromatosis (von Recklinghausen's disease) results from increased epidermal melanin. A purple patch, or ecchymosis, is due to extravasation of erythrocytes, and a reddish patch, in a blush or sunburn, results from congestion of erythrocytes within the dilated blood vessels of the superficial dermis.

Papule (Latin, "a small swelling"): a solid, elevated lesion up to 1 cm in diameter (Fig. 3-17).

Papules are usually caused by an infiltrate within the papillary dermis. The infiltrate may be cellular or noncellular. The papule of lichen nitidus results from a dense, primarily histiocytic infiltrate which expands a dermal papilla. Leukemic papules consist of

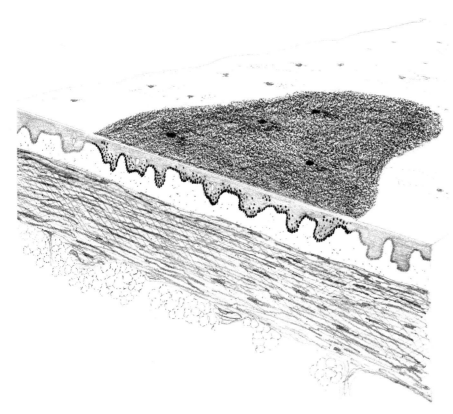

FIG. 3-16. Macule, patch.

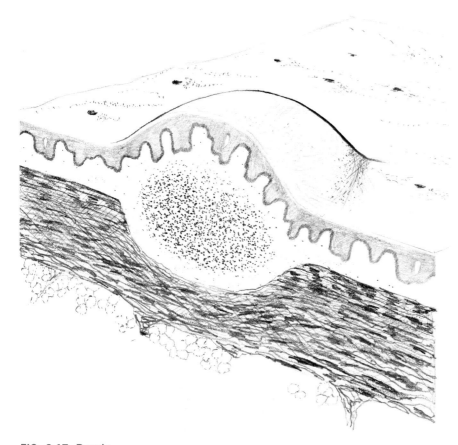

FIG. 3-17. Papule.

dense diffuse dermal infiltrates whose cells are characteristically interposed between collagen bundles. Papules of lichen amyloidosus result from the deposit of amyloid in dermal papillae. Papules associated with hyperkeratosis of the epidermis have traditionally been termed "papulosquamous" lesions, such as in psoriasis, where the papular component is contributed by dermal edema and inflammatory cells and the squamous component by epidermal changes, especially in the cornified layer. Papules can consist mainly of epithelial components, such as the epidermal hyperplasia of a plane wart or the infundibular hyperplasia of molluscum contagiosum. The papules of lichen simplex chronicus are formed by thickening of the epidermis and the papillary dermis, the result of persistent rubbing. *Lichenoid* is descriptive of flat-topped papules like those of lichen planus.

Plaque (Dutch, "a slab of wood"): a flat, solid, elevated lesion more than 1 cm in diameter (Fig. 3-18).

Plaques are formed either by extension or coalescence of papules. Thus, plaques can occur in conditions such as lichen amyloidosus, psoriasis, lichen simplex chronicus, and lichen planus.

Urtica (wheal, hive) (Latin, "nettle"): evanescent pinkish papules and plaques that blanch upon diascopy (viewing of the skin through a firm transparent instrument, such as a glass slide, which is pressed firmly against the lesion) and often have pseudopods at their periphery (Fig. 3-19).

Hives consist of abundant edema and a near absence of inflammatory cells (serous inflammation). A huge hive in distensible sites, such as the lips and eyelids, is called angioedema.

Unlike papules and plaques that are composed of more persistent infiltrates, hives appear and disappear within minutes to hours. Wheal-like, or urticarial, lesions can be differentiated from

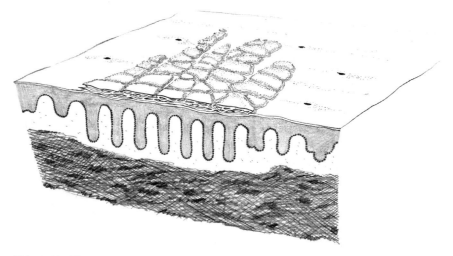

FIG. 3-18. Plaque.

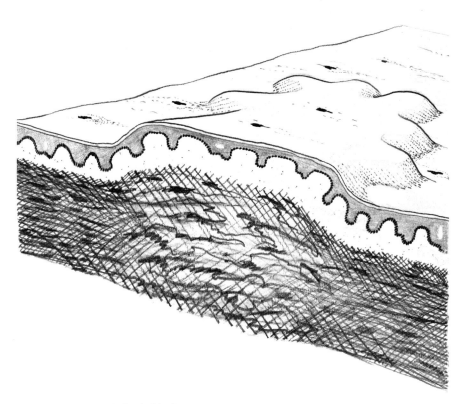

FIG. 3-19. Urtica (wheal, hive).

true wheals despite their morphologic similarities. Urticarial lesions persist for days or weeks and histologically consist of a mixed-cell infiltrate, as well as of noticeable edema. Urticarial clinical lesions occur in some drug eruptions, dermatitis herpetiformis, pemphigoid, herpes gestationis, allergic contact dermatitis, leukocytoclastic vasculitis, and arthropod reactions. Although these lesions have edema of the papillary dermis and a mixed inflammatory-cell infiltrate in common, there are striking histologic differences among them.

Nodule (tumor) (Latin, "small node"): a round elevated lesion greater than 1 cm in diameter (Fig. 3-20).

Nodules usually result from relatively massive infiltrates in the dermis, but they can also arise from large infiltrates in the subcutaneous fat. For example, a dense diffuse dermal infiltrate composed of foamy histiocytes forms the nodule of lepromatous leprosy. Nodules can be produced by dermal infiltrates of atypical cells such as epithelial cells (e.g., malignant melanoma) and mesenchymal cells (e.g., atypical fibroxanthoma). The subcutaneous deposit of fibrin is responsible for the nodules associated with rheumatoid arthritis and the dermal deposit of urate for the nodules of gout. Prurigo nodularis is an exaggerated nodular form of lichen simplex chronicus and consists of a thickened papillary dermis and epidermis.

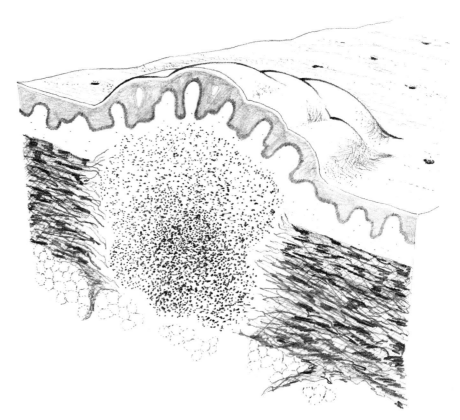

FIG. 3-20. Nodule.

Papilloma (Latin, "nipple"): fingerlike projections above the skin surface due to upward extensions of the dermal papillae (papillomatosis) which are usually covered by hyperplastic epidermis (Fig. 3-21).

The papillary dermis may be thickened, and the overlying epidermis may be normal or even thin in cross sections (e.g., skin tags and acanthosis nigricans). Thickening of the epidermis and the papillary dermis occurs in lesions like seborrheic keratosis. The term *verrucous* is sometimes used synonymously with papillomatous, but the tips of the dermal papillae in verrucous lesions are usually pointed, rather than rounded as in papillomatous ones.

Cyst (Latin, "a sac"): an epithelium-lined cavity containing fluid or solid material (Fig. 3-22).

Cysts in skin are almost always lined by adnexal epithelium (i.e., hair follicles, eccrine, or apocrine). The most common skin cyst involves the superior portion of the hair follicle whose contents are predominantly cornified cells (infundibular cyst). A cyst that contains mostly sebaceous material is the lesion of steatocystoma multiplex whose epithelial lining resembles that of the sebaceous duct. Material that simulates sweat is found in cysts of the sweat ducts (hidrocystomas).

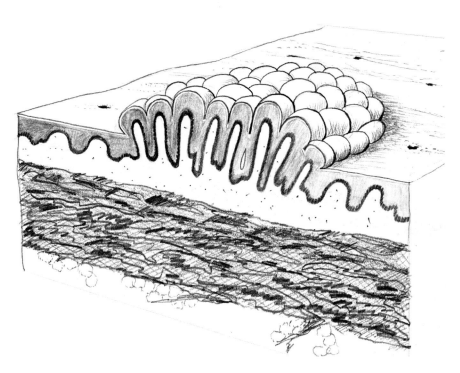

FIG. 3-21. Papilloma.

Some deposits in skin are incorrectly termed "cysts," for example, the "synovial" or myxoid cysts, which are really collections of mucin not enclosed by epithelium. This condition is better named "focal mucinosis."

Vesicle (Latin, a "small blister"): a fluid-filled circumscribed elevated lesion up to 1 cm in diameter (Fig. 3-23).

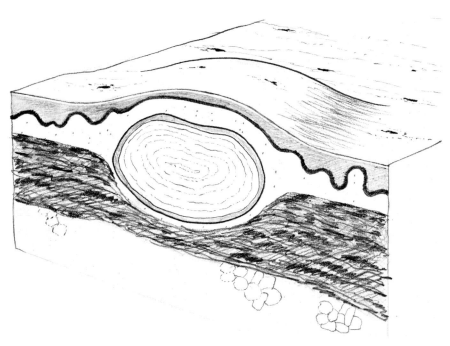

FIG. 3-22. Cyst.

Discrete fluid-filled spaces occur within the epidermis (intraepidermal vesicle). Clinically, it is often impossible to distinguish intraepidermal from subepidermal vesicles. Contrary to the rule that subepidermal vesicles are more distended, intraepidermal vesicles may also be tense (e.g., in chicken pox or herpetic blisters) and subepidermal blisters may be flaccid (e.g., toxic epidermal necrolysis). Of the well-known vesicular skin diseases, intraepidermal vesicles are seen in allergic contact dermatitis, pemphigus vulgaris, and in the viral group of herpes simplex, herpes zoster, and varicella; and subepidermal vesicles are seen in dermatitis herpetiformis, porphyria cutanea tarda, and pemphigoid. Progressive intercellular edema (spongiosis) causes vesiculation in allergic contact dermatitis and increasing intracellular edema contributes to vesiculation caused by herpesvirus. Physical damage, be it chemical, electrical, mechanical, or thermal, can also produce vesicles and bullae.

Bulla (Latin, "blister"): a fluid-filled circumscribed elevated lesion greater than 1 cm in diameter (Fig. 3-23).

Bullae, like vesicles, can also be divided into intraepidermal and subepidermal types. The classic example of the intraepidermal bulla appears in pemphigus vulgaris and of the subepidermal bulla in pemphigoid.

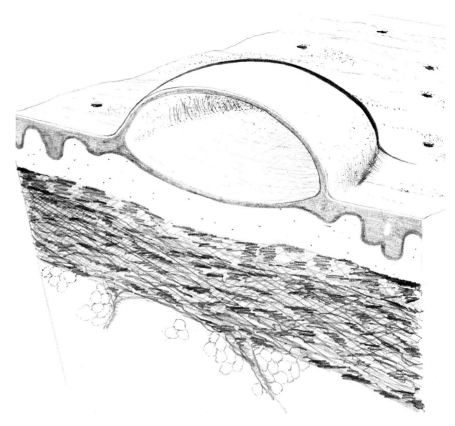

FIG. 3-23. Vesicle, bulla (intraepidermal).

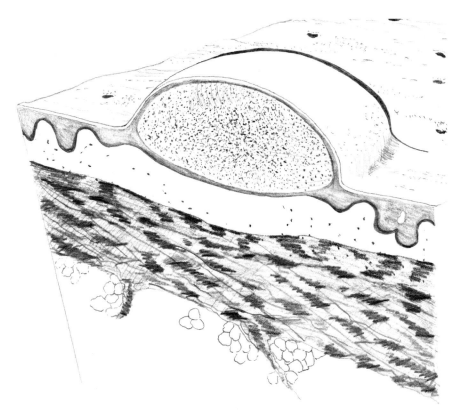

FIG. 3-24. Pustule.

Pustule: a circumscribed collection of pus (neutrophils and necrotic debris) (Fig. 3-24).

Most pustules are intraepidermal in location, but purulent material can accumulate in long-standing or secondarily infected subepidermal vesicles and bullae. Intraepidermal pustules may be intracorneal (e.g., in candidiasis), subcorneal (e.g., in subcorneal pustular dermatosis), or spongiform (e.g., in pustular psoriasis). Follicular pustules occur in acne and other folliculitides. Pustules can be either of infectious or noninfectious cause. Bacterially caused pustules are seen in impetigo and furunculosis. No organisms, however, can be cultured from the pustules of pustular psoriasis or subcorneal pustular dermatosis.

Purpura (Latin, "purple color"): bleeding into the skin (Fig. 3-25).

Petechiae are pinpoint macules much less than 1 cm in diameter, and ecchymoses are patches greater than 1 cm in diameter. A hematoma, a hemorrhagic lesion situated deeper in the dermis or in the subcutis, usually results in a swelling.

Telangiectasia (Greek, "dilated end blood vessel"): dilated capillaries, venules, and arterioles that are visible as tiny blood vessels near the skin surface.

Telangiectases may appear in the absence of an inflammatory reaction, such as in chronically sun-damaged skin. They may also

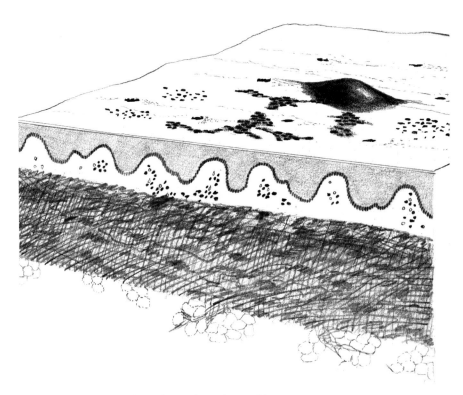

FIG. 3-25. Purpura with ecchymosis and petechiae.

be secondary to inflammatory processes that result in poikiloderma (i.e., telangiectases, atrophy, and hypopigmentation and hyperpigmentation).

Comedo (Latin, "a glutton"): a dilated hair follicle infundibulum filled with cornified cells, sebaceous material, and microorganisms.

Comedones are the primary lesions of acne vulgaris, but they can also be seen secondary to occlusion (such as by machine oils) and to severe long-standing sun damage ("senile" comedones, better called "solar" comedones). Groups of solar-induced comedones surrounded by prominent elastotic material in the skin overlying the zygoma constitute nodular elastoidosis (Favre-Racouchot syndrome). *Steroid acne* refers to comedones induced by systemic or topical corticosteroids.

Secondary Clinical Lesions

Scale: cornified cells that have become visible on the skin surface (Fig. 3-26).

As has been stated, hyperkeratosis (increased thickness of the cornified layer) can be subdivided into parakeratosis (cornification with nuclear retention) and orthokeratosis (cornification without nuclear retention). In some conditions, such as in pityriasis rubra pilaris, both abnormalities are present: parakeratosis alternates,

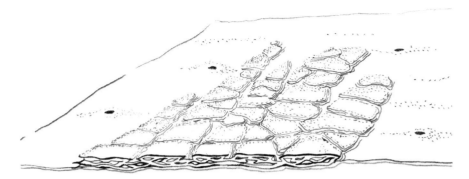

FIG. 3-26. Scale.

vertically and horizontally, with orthokeratosis. Scale is described as micaceous (e.g., the confluent parakeratosis of psoriatic plaques), branny (e.g., the focal scale-crust of seborrheic dermatitis), powdery (e.g., the orthokeratosis of tinea versicolor in which the normal basket-weave pattern of the cornified layer is preserved), adherent (e.g., the confluent compact and laminated orthokeratosis of ichthyosis vulgaris and X-linked ichthyosis), coarse (e.g., the focal vertical parakeratosis of keratosis follicularis and porokeratosis), and greasy (e.g., the delicate, laminated, pigmented orthokeratosis of seborrheic keratosis). Scale can also be follicular as in keratosis pilaris and discoid lupus erythematosus.

Crust: dried exudate composed of serum and cells (Fig. 3-27).

The honey-colored crusts of impetigo consist of serum and leukocytes. A hemorrhagic scab consists of serum, leukocytes, and erythrocytes. *Vegetations* are heaped-up crusts, as seen in pemphigus vegetans and pyoderma vegetans. Necrotic keratinocytes, parakeratotic cells, fibrin, and bacteria may also be found in crusts.

Erosion: defect caused by partial or complete loss of the epidermis (Fig. 3–28).

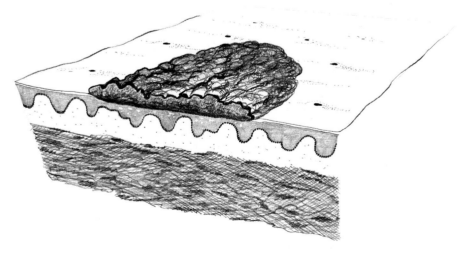

FIG. 3-27. Crust.

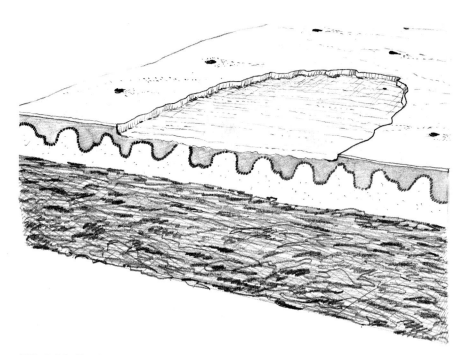

FIG. 3-28. Erosion.

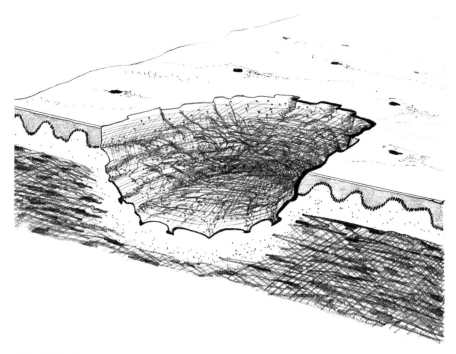

FIG. 3-29. Ulcer.

The prototypic erosion is the denuded lesion of pemphigus vulgaris where the blister has occurred above the basal-cell layer. Erosions, because they do not involve the dermis, heal without scarring unless they become infected.

Ulcer (Latin, "a sore"): a defect caused by complete loss of epidermis and usually part of the underlying dermis (Fig. 3-29). Ulcers can result from diseases such as venous insufficiency (e.g.,

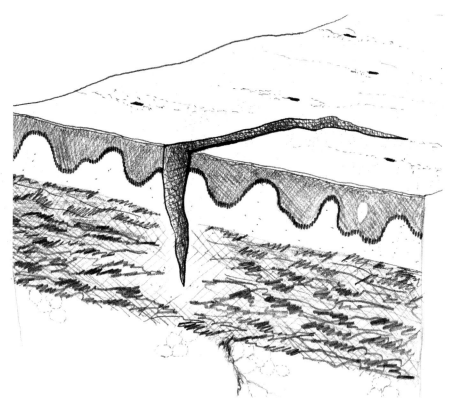

FIG. 3-30. Fissure.

stasis ulcer), vasculitis (e.g., ecthyma gangrenosum in pseudomonas septicemia), chronic infection (e.g., the Chiclero ulcer in leishmaniasis), or from neoplasms (e.g., basal-cell carcinoma). Ulcers can also be factitial, i.e., self-induced by caustics, sharp instruments, or by the patient's own fingernails. Excoriation can produce erosion or ulceration, depending upon how vigorously the fingernails are employed. Ecthyma is an ulcer usually caused by beta hemolytic streptococci. Ulcers, if they destroy the normal collagen pattern in the papillary dermis, inevitably heal with scarring.

Fissure (Latin, "a split"): a linear defect that extends from the skin surface into the dermis (Fig. 3-30).

Fissures are commonly seen over flexural creases in scaly lesions such as in psoriasis that involves the palms, soles, and intergluteal cleft.

Scar: fibrosis that replaces the normal arrangement of collagen (Fig. 3-31).

A scar represents the end stage of an inflammatory process that began with destruction of preexisting tissue and evolved through granulation tissue. Histologically, a scar consists of collagen fibers, oriented parallel to the skin surface, an increased number of fibroblasts and dilated blood vessels oriented perpendicularly to the skin surface. A keloid has thickened, homogeneous, brightly

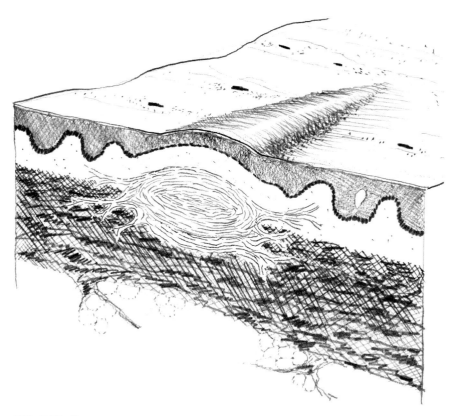

FIG. 3-31. Scar.

eosinophilic, hyalinized randomly arranged collagen bundles associated with an increased number of fibroblasts. The normal skin markings are usually effaced when scars and keloids involve the papillary dermis.

Atrophy: a decrease in the skin substance due usually to decreased thickness of the dermis and less commonly of the subcutaneous fat (Fig. 3-32).

Atrophy can result from thinning of preexisting collagen bundles such as in aging or thinning of the dermis following severe inflammation or ulceration. The clinical characteristics of cutaneous atrophy are shininess, whiteness, loss of the normal skin surface markings, wrinkling, and loss of the cutaneous adnexa, especially hair follicles. Thinness of the skin can be determined clinically, because blood vessels in the atrophic area are easily visualized, whereas those beneath the normal skin are not. When atrophy is accompanied by telangiectasia, hyperpigmentation, and hypopigmentation, the condition is called "poikiloderma."

Sclerosis (Greek, "hardness"): a circumscribed area of diffuse induration of the skin, detectable only by palpation.

The foremost clinical example of sclerosis is scleroderma, but hardening of the skin is also seen in diseases such as scleredema and scleromyxedema. The word *sclerosis* is used histologically to signify hyalinization of collagen bundles, coupled with a decreased number of fibroblasts.

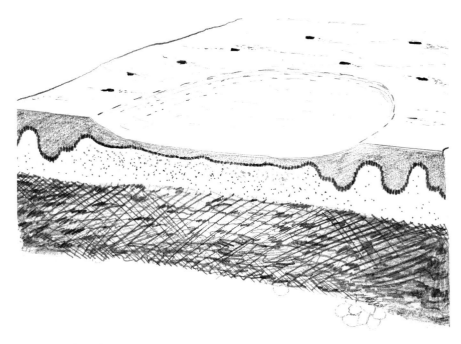

FIG. 3-32. Atrophy.

Lichenification: a papular thickening of the skin associated with accentuation of the normal skin markings, hyperpigmentation, and sometimes scales (Fig. 3-33).

Lichenification results from chronic rubbing of the skin. The classic examples of lichenification are the plaques of lichen simplex chronicus and the nodules of prurigo nodularis. Should prurigo nodularis become eroded or ulcerated from scratching, it

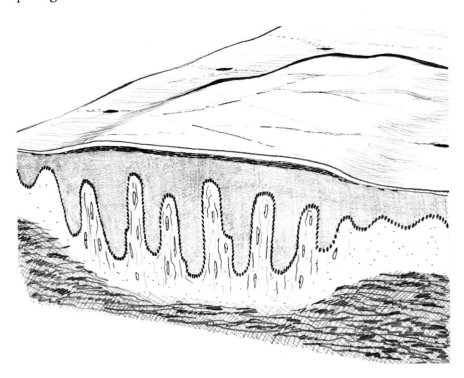

FIG. 3-33. Lichenification.

is termed "picker's nodule." Lichenification can be superimposed upon chronic pruritic dermatitides, such as chronic contact dermatitis and exfoliative erythroderma. Most long-standing lesions of atopic dermatitis are really examples of lichenification due to rubbing and erosions due to scratching. The telltale histologic sign of lichenification is thickening of the papillary dermis by vertically streaked collagen fibers. The thickening of the papillary dermis is usually accompanied by an increased number of plump and stellate fibroblasts, some of which are multinucleated. Epidermal changes in lichenified skin are hyperkeratosis, hypergranulosis, and spinous-cell hyperplasia.

Pigmentation: a coloration caused by a variety of pigments, most commonly melanin.

Melanin is responsible for a variety of colors in skin: black (abundant melanin at all levels of the epidermis, including the cornified layer, as in some junctional melanocytic nevi), blue (melanin within melanocytes and melanophages in the mid and deep dermis of a blue nevus), tan (melanin in the epidermis of a café au lait spot), gray (diffuse dermal melanosis associated with metastatic malignant melanoma), and ashy (melanin within epidermal cells and dermal melanophages of erythema dyschromicum perstans). Differences in coloration among peoples (e.g., black Africans, brown American Negroes, reddish-brown American Indians, and yellow Orientals) are also due to melanin. Loss of epidermal melanin can be seen in vitiligo and in postinflammatory hypopigmentation. Increased epidermal melanin, with melanophages in the papillary dermis, can be seen in postinflammatory hyperpigmentation. Skin colors in tattoos result from pigments other than melanin such as silver (slate-gray), carotene (yellowish-orange), cobalt (blue), cadmium (yellow), mercury (red), carbon (black or blue), and chromium (green). The brownish coloration of hemochromatosis is due primarily to melanin, rather than to hemosiderin.

Burrow: a tunnel, usually in the cornified or spinous layers, fashioned by a parasite or its larva.

The classic burrow is made by the female of the species, Sarcoptes scabiei. The mite deposits her eggs and feces within the burrow and in this location gives rise to intense pruritus. The larva or "creeper" of Ancylostoma braziliense that causes cutaneous larva migrans resides in the lowermost epidermis, where it moves in serpentine tracks.

Sinus tract: an epithelium-lined channel which opens upon the skin surface.

The lesions of the follicular occlusion tetrad (acne conglobata, hidradentitis suppurativa, dissecting cellulitis of the scalp and pilonidal sinus) are examples of sinus tracts in skin. These form as a result of re-epithelization of hair follicle units following rupture and suppuration.

Abscess (Latin, "a departure"): a localized accumulation of pus.

Cutaneous abscesses (suppurative dermatitis or panniculitis) most commonly result from rupture of hair follicle cysts with resultant neutrophilic reaction in response to bacteria, yeasts, cornified cells, and hair. A furuncle is a follicular abscess, usually caused by Staphylococcus aureus. A carbuncle consists of confluent furuncles. The earliest lymphangitic lesions of sporotrichosis are abscesses in the dermis and subcutaneous fat. Microabscesses occur in the epidermis of psoriasis and in the dermis of granuloma inguinale. "Pautrier's abscess" in mycosis fungoides is a misnomer because the cells composing it are mostly mononuclear, rather than neutrophilic polymorphonuclear.

Confusing Terms

Eczema (Greek, "to boil out").

The term *eczema* is indiscriminately invoked and variously defined. Many different kinds of eczema have been described, based upon etiology (e.g., allergic), distribution (e.g., seborrheic), morphology (e.g., asteatotic), occupation (e.g., bakers), anatomy (e.g., folliculorum), age (e.g., rubrum), and season (e.g., winter). These "eczemas" do not all have clinical and histologic features in common. Confusion about the term *eczema* (and eczematoid, eczema-like, eczematous, eczematous dermatitis, eczematization, eczematid, eczematogenic, and eczematosis) abounds.

Therefore, *eczema* is perhaps best discarded altogether in favor of *spongiotic dermatitis* for those papular, papulovesicular, and vesicular diseases that are characterized by spongiosis. There is ample precedent for employing histologic terms for clinical conditions, e.g., granuloma and vasculitis.

Neurodermatitis: inflammation of the skin that in some way is thought to be related to "nerves," either organically or psychologically.

Two types of neurodermatitis have been described: circumscribed (lichen simplex chronicus) and disseminated (atopic dermatitis). There is little agreement among dermatologists about neurodermatitis, clinically, histologically, pathogenetically, or etiologically. The term should be expunged from the vocabulary for skin diseases.

Parapsoriasis (Greek, *para*, "beside," "alongside of," "beyond," "a kind of," "false," "like or resembling," and many more vagaries): in medical contexts, abnormality (e.g., parakeratosis) or resemblance to a presumably true form (e.g., paracoccidioidomycosis).

Parapsoriasis is merely a designation with distinguishing modifiers that has become convenient by usage for several conditions that vaguely resemble psoriasis but that should not be taken literally as relating these conditions to psoriasis or to each other. The term has been given to at least five cutaneous conditions, namely, parapsoriasis en plaques, guttate parapsoriasis, parapsoriasis (pityriasis) lichenoides et varioliformis acuta, parapsoriasis (pityriasis) lichenoides chronica, and parapsoriasis variegata. These diseases, linked only by the name *parapsoriasis* and by that only to suggest vague clinical resemblance, have been uncritically treated as an interrelated group by some authors. Furthermore, other authors who have attempted to differentiate among the diseases dubbed *parapsoriasis* have usually failed to agree about their clinical, histologic, and biologic natures.

In this book, I apply *parapsoriasis en plaques* as a title for a lichenoid or psoriasiform and lichenoid dermatitis that is characterized by reddish-brown, slightly scaly, slightly wrinkled patches. In my opinion, parapsoriasis en plaques is the patch stage of mycosis fungoides and is analogous to the patch stage of multiple idiopathic hemorrhagic sarcoma (Kaposi's sarcoma). This is not to say that every patch must evolve inexorably into a plaque or a nodule of the respective disease nor that plaques and nodules of them must inevitably develop elsewhere in patients who have such patches. In time, however, often decades later, plaques and nodules of mycosis fungoides or multiple idiopathic hemorrhagic sarcoma usually develop in the skin and internal organs of patients who have or have had premonitory patches.

I use *guttate parapsoriasis* to designate a slight spongiotic dermatitis with small mounds of scale-crusts that appears clinically as drop-sized (or somewhat larger) pinkish-tan macules or papules covered by gray waferlike scales. It is notable for chronicity and, as yet, untreatability.

Parapsoriasis (pityriasis) lichenoides et varioliformis acuta (Mucha-Habermann disease) is a superficial and deep perivascular dermatitis with changes of vacuolar alteration and necrotic keratinocytes at the dermoepidermal interface and often intraepidermal vesiculation. Clinically, it consists of erythematous and purpuric macules, papules, and necrotic papulovesicles that sometimes resolve with varioliform scars. *Parapsoriasis (pityriasis) lichenoides chronica* is a lichenoid dermatitis with focal parakeratosis which, I believe, is a scaly, nonvesicular variant of pityriasis lichenoides et varioliformis acuta. It may appear *ab initio* or develop later in the acute form. Because the name *parapsoriasis* has been attached to many different conditions, in order to mitigate confusion the acute and chronic forms of Mucha-Habermann disease are best referred to as *pityriasis* lichenoides et varioliformis acuta and *pityriasis* lichenoides chronica.

Parapsoriasis variegata in its histopathology begins as a psoriasiform dermatitis and ends lichenoid. Clinically, it is highly distinctive, consisting of slightly scaly, slightly atrophic wavy bands that give the skin a zebralike rippled appearance. Whether parapsoriasis variegata is in any way related to mycosis fungoides has yet to be determined. I think that it is.

Dermatosis: any pathologic condition of the skin.

Dermatologists and dermatopathologists sometimes speak of "inflammatory dermatosis" when "dermatitis" is really intended. General pathologists do not refer to "acute appendicosis" or to "ulcerative colosis."

Necrobiosis: a condition of life and death.

The word *necrobiosis* is as confusing histologically as it is etymologically. *Necrobiosis* is applied to connective tissue alterations in certain palisaded granulomatous inflammations of skin such as in granuloma annulare, rheumatoid nodule, and necrobiosis lipoidica. However, the "necrobiotic" alteration is mostly mucin in granuloma annulare, fibrin in rheumatoid nodule, and collagen degeneration and sclerosis in necrobiosis lipoidica. Because of this imprecision, the term *necrobiosis* should not be used except to refer to the disease necrobiosis lipoidica.

Nevus: literally, a "birthmark."

The word *nevus* is used clinically to describe any congenital lesion, such as vascular nevus (e.g., port-wine stain), sebaceous nevus (e.g., nevus sebaceus of Jadassohn), epidermal nevus (e.g., nevus unius lateris), collagenous nevus (e.g., shagreen patch), nevus of fat tissue (e.g., nevus lipomatosus). The term *nevus* is also used histologically for the cells (nevus cells, i.e., melanocytes) that compose the common soft pigmented mole. This usually acquired lesion is also called a "nevus," a "nevus cell nevus," or, more accurately, a "melanocytic nevus." Thus, the word *nevus* is employed (1) clinically to designate birthmarks and acquired soft pigmented moles and (2) histologically for the cells that constitute these moles.

The word *nevus* should never be used alone, but always with a modifier such as melanocytic, epidermal, sebaceous, vascular, collagenous, or fatty.

Active Junctional Nevus: Melanocytes fixed in formalin are no longer active. Cytologically, melanocytes within the epidermis are either typical or atypical. Atypicality of melanocytes does not necessarily imply biologic malignancy as is evident in such lesions as the large spindle- and/or epithelioid-cell nevus (benign juvenile melanoma, Spitz nevus), halo nevus, and recurrent melanocytic nevus following partial surgical excision (pseudomelanoma). Therefore, atypical melanocytes within the epidermis may be a feature of melanocytic nevi, as well as of malignant melanomas. The phrase *active junctional nevus* is often a hedge against committing oneself to a diagnosis of melanocytic nevus or malignant melanoma. In my opinion, the terms *active junctional nevus* and *junctional activity* should not be used.

Leukoplakia (Greek, "white formation").

Clinically, the whiteness of leukoplakia is a manifestation of sodden abnormal cornification (hyperkeratosis) on mucous membranes. The term *leukoplakia* implies that the mucous-membrane lesion is a precursor of squamous-cell carcinoma. Leukoplakia does not apply to other white plaques on mucous membranes, such as keratosis oris, lichen planus, and lichen sclerosus et atrophicus, lesions that in most cases are not premalignant. Histologically, leukoplakia is to mucous membranes what solar keratosis is to skin, an atypical epithelial hyperplasia. The atypical nuclei reside primarily in the lower portion of the epithelium. In time, these mucous-membrane changes may proceed to squamous-cell carcinoma in situ and eventually to "invasive" squamous-cell carcinoma. Because the term *leukoplakia* has different connotations to dermatologists, pathologists, otolaryngologists, gynecologists, and dentists, it is best avoided.

Invasion: The term *invasion* with reference to the skin is generally used in pathology to mean movement of neoplastic cells from the epidermis into the dermis and to imply biological malignancy. For example, squamous-cell carcinoma and malignant melanoma are often referred to as "invasive." Are they any more invasive than a keratoacanthoma or an intradermal melanocytic nevus in which cells have moved from a junctional position in the epidermis into the dermis? To date there are no consistently cogent criteria that define invasion, nor are there well-demarcated boundaries that a neoplasm must reach before it is considered to be "invasive." In my opinion, it is best merely to speak of the depth of extension of a cutaneous neoplasm, whether benign or malignant, into the dermis or subcutaneous fat, rather than of invasion. For example, a squamous-cell carcinoma may extend to the midreticular dermis and beyond, just as may a malignant melanoma. Perhaps the thickness of carcinomas should be measured, just as malignant melanomas are. What has been said of invasion surely applies also to "micro-invasion" in the skin. In my view, both terms are best completely avoided.

Kraurosis vulvae (Latin, "a dry or brittle condition of the vulva").

The term *kraurosis vulvae* has been applied to a number of whitish patches and plaques on the vulva. Most of these lesions are, in actuality, lichen sclerosus et atrophicus; a few are lichen simplex chronicus, and still fewer are carcinoma in situ. Thus, the designation *kraurosis vulvae* is not diagnostically precise, but rather a clinical catchall and should therefore be eliminated in favor of the specific diagnosis.

The Biopsy

The Biopsy

4

It is important to emphasize the value of biopsy in the diagnosis of inflammatory skin diseases. A specific histologic diagnosis can be made in the majority of inflammatory processes in skin, and whenever possible imprecise terms such as "chronic nonspecific dermatitis" should be avoided. In the management of a patient with an inflammatory skin disease, it is often advantageous to perform the biopsy before embarking upon treatment. Frequently, specimens submitted to our laboratory as "eczema" reveal dermatophytic hyphae within epidermal or follicular cornified cells, and many that are submitted as dermatitis herpetiformis show the mite of scabies in the cornified layer.

Biopsy of skin should be considered not merely the mechanical removal of a piece of tissue for histologic interpretation, but rather an important step in a sequence that includes (1) careful selection of one or more lesions, (2) suitable removal of the specimen by the most appropriate surgical method and delicate handling of the specimen, (3) proper fixation of the specimen and preparation of the histologic slide, (4) accurate histologic diagnosis, and (5) thorough review of the histologic sections by the physician who performed the biopsy. The culmination of this cycle, which begins and ends with the clinician, should be the study of each histologic slide by the physician who removed the specimen. Ideally, the dermatopathologist should inspect every skin lesion clinically before a specimen has been removed for biopsy, but such inspection is usually impossible. The lesion itself is a manifestation of a pathologic process; the gross and the light microscopic examinations are but two ways of assessing it. There are also histochemical, electron microscopic, immunofluorescent, and other diagnostic techniques. Close communication between clinician and pathologist is essential for their own greater understanding of the disease process, and for the patient's benefit.

Selection of Site

Many inflammatory diseases of the skin, such as dermatitis herpetiformis, nummular dermatitis, and scabies, are exquisitely pruritic and, as a consequence of scratching, are associated with erosions, ulcerations, and crusts. In general, excoriated lesions, as well as scars and postinflammatory pigmentary changes, should not be chosen as sites for specimens. The surgeon should search for spontaneous early lesions that have not been tampered with in any manner. Such lesions are usually macules, papules, nodules, vesicles, and bullae. Pustules, as in pustular psoriasis, may be the initial lesion and sterile. Some spontaneous macular and papular lesions may be covered by scales. When patients have no underlying skin disease and only various evidences of rubbing and scratching, biopsy can be helpful to verify the absence of a primary cutaneous pathologic process.

In attempting to diagnose specifically vesiculobullous diseases, it is best that the *earliest* lesion be selected for biopsy. In dermatitis herpetiformis, pemphigoid, herpes gestationis, erythema multiforme, and arthropod reactions, the earliest lesion is an edematous papule, *not* a blister. Biopsy of these papular lesions, rather than the sequential vesicles or bullae, is most likely to yield a correct histologic diagnosis. Lesions to be avoided are old blisters, not just because they are often contaminated by bacteria, but because re-epithelization that may have occurred beneath the blister will complicate the histologic picture. In diseases such as pemphigus vulgaris, toxic epidermal necrolysis, and familial benign chronic pemphigus (Hailey-Hailey disease), in which blisters may be the initial lesions, the smallest, clearest vesicle should be selected for biopsy, rather than a crusted, purulent bulla.

Histologic diagnosis of some inflammatory processes is often facilitated by taking more than one biopsy specimen, especially if lesions are in different stages of development, as in pityriasis lichenoides et varioliformis acuta and in leukocytoclastic (allergic) vasculitis. For example, histologic examination of the urticarial, nonpurpuric papules of leukocytoclastic vasculitis may show only neutrophils and nuclear dust around the dermal blood vessels, but neither fibrin nor inflammatory cells within the vessel walls. If purpuric papules or vesicles are both present, biopsy of them often reveals all of the diagnostic histologic features of vasculitis.

Not only the lesions for biopsy, but the method of biopsy must be selected with care. In general, vesicles and bullae should be excised with a scalpel rather than removed by a punch, shave, or saucerization procedure. This rule applies especially to bullae that are flaccid, such as those of pemphigus vulgaris and toxic epidermal necrolysis. In these conditions, the punch shears the epidermal roof from its moorings (Fig. 4-1), and then the pathologist is often presented with a specimen from which the critical epidermal element is missing. Exceptions to the rule of scalpel excision of blisters are tiny tense vesicles such as those of herpes simplex and miliaria crystallina. A 4-mm punch can completely encircle such a small vesicle, which can then be extracted intact for histologic examination.

The punch biopsy is also likely to be inadequate for the diagnosis of panniculitis. Because inflammatory processes involving the fat tend to alter the adhesion of the subcutis to the dermis, a punch biopsy of panniculitis often fails to deliver the fat. Thus, an insufficient specimen consisting only of epidermis and dermis is submitted to the pathologist, who cannot render an opinion about the fat, let alone the precise type of panniculitis. The condition of the large subcutaneous blood vessels is one important differential feature between erythema nodosum and nodular vasculitis. A punch biopsy may miss the critical vessel. Therefore, all biopsies of panniculitis should extend into the deep subcutis and preferably should be performed with a scalpel. The surgeon

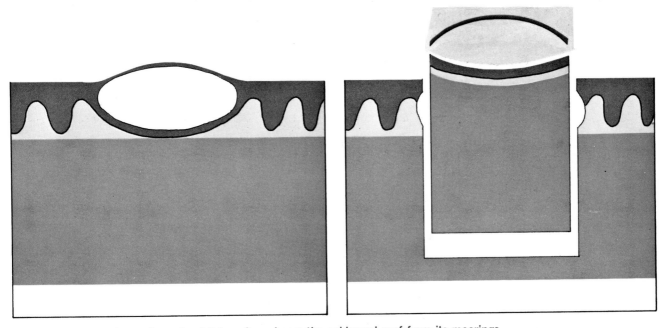

FIG. 4-1. A punch biopsy through a blister often shears the epidermal roof from its moorings.

should routinely examine the specimen to ensure that fat is actually present before submitting it for histologic processing.

What has just been written about adequate biopsy specimens of panniculitides applies equally to those from alopecias from the scalp. The matrical ends of anagen follicles on the scalp, i.e., the bulbs, lie well in the subcutaneous fat. In order to assess accurately hair follicles in the scalp, the biopsy specimen must include a generous amount of subcutaneous fat. Excision by scalpel is preferable, but excision by at least a 5 mm punch in proper alignment parallel to the hair shafts is acceptable. By both methods, sufficient adipose tissue must be provided.

Because a neoplasm such as a keratoacanthoma or a malformation such as a nevus sebaceus cannot always be readily removed in its entirety, only a representative portion need be excised to determine the diagnosis. In the case of keratoacanthoma, the preferred procedure is to use a scalpel to make a fusiform excision enveloping the center of the lesion and extending from normal skin to normal skin and down into the subcutaneous fat. This method is superb because keratoacanthoma can be distinguished histologically from squamous-cell carcinoma by the overall configuration of the lesion rather than by cytologic detail. A less optimal, but sufficient, biopsy of keratoacanthoma is a scalpel excision that extends from the center of the tumor to normal skin and includes the subcutaneous fat. A punch biopsy of a keratoacanthoma does not give any clue to the overall pattern of the lesion and thus is worthless for differentiating keratoacanthoma from squamous-cell carcinoma.

In some instances more than one biopsy specimen is not only desirable, but essential. In a broad patch of Hutchinson's freckle, a determination must be made whether the entire melanocytic process is wholly confined to the epidermis (lentigo maligna) or whether atypical melanocytes are present within the dermis (lentigo maligna melanoma). The size of the lesion and its location may preclude total surgical excision. In such instances, multiple small specimens obtained from several foci within the lesion (preferably the most heavily pigmented, indurated, or elevated) should be obtained. Total, rather than partial, surgical excision of a Hutchinson's freckle, with multiple sections then taken by the pathologist through the entire specimen, is the best method for evaluating the extent of the melanocytic process. More than one biopsy may be necessary when there is a question of hypopigmentation or hyperpigmentation. Either the biopsy specimen must include a portion of the surrounding normal skin or a second biopsy of the normal skin must be taken in order to have a basis for comparing the amounts of epidermal melanin.

In a pigmented lesion suspected of being a superficial spreading malignant melanoma, the most common type of malignant melanoma, it is also advisable to excise the entire lesion by surgical scalpel excision when possible. For a variety of reasons, most commonly because of the size of the lesion or its site, total excision for biopsy is not always advisable. Then the most elevated or firmest portion of the lesion, *i.e.*, the exophytic component, should be removed with a scalpel deep enough to include subcutaneous fat. There is no evidence that cutting into a malignant melanoma enhances the possibility of metastasis. The prognosis and further treatment of malignant melanoma are partly related to the depth of extension of the atypical melanocytes into the dermis and subcutis. In a shave biopsy, atypical melanocytes often extend to the base of the specimen, which in a shave or saucerization procedure may be only the papillary dermis, and therefore the pathologist cannot evaluate the actual depth of tumor extension, and the surgeon cannot recommend for or against lymph-node dissection.

Superficial spreading malignant melanoma arises in association with a benign melanocytic nevus in approximately 50% of the cases. If the procedure is a punch biopsy, which obtains too little tissue, rather than scalpel excision of a significant portion of the tumor, only the benign nevus may be submitted to the pathologist, and the malignant melanoma may remain undiscovered. For a lesion suspected of being malignant melanoma, excision *in toto* without a graft, if possible, is the biopsy procedure of choice.

The shave biopsy has a place in the surgeon's armamentarium, but it is a highly circumscribed one, confined to obviously benign, mostly exophytic hyperplasias, neoplasias, and malformations such as warts, skin tags, seborrheic keratoses, and melanocytic

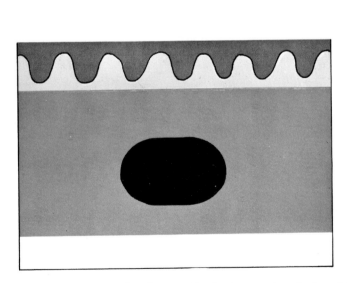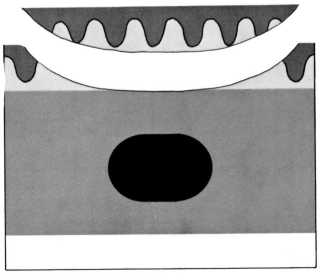

FIG. 4-2. Biopsy by the shave method misses a deep lesion of inflammatory skin disease.

nevi. Such banal lesions can be removed simply and in cosmetically acceptable fashion by simple shave excision, but this method should *not* be utilized for inflammatory diseases (Fig. 4-2), suspected malignant melanoma, or endophytic tumors of undetermined clinical diagnosis. The foregoing applies equally to the scissor biopsy and to curettage. Basal-cell carcinomas, for example, can be diagnosed adequately by shave biopsy or even by curettings.

If the punch technique is used, it should be done correctly. The diameter of the punch (usually not less than 3 mm) should be sufficient to adequately sample the pathologic process, and the specimen should almost always include subcutaneous fat. A common error after punch biopsy is the squeezing of the specimen by forceps as it is lifted by the surgeon. Squeezing causes cellular distortion ("crush" artefact), often rendering the specimen histologically unreadable (Fig. 4-3). Forceps should never touch the specimen. Instead, the syringe needle with which local anesthesia was injected should be used to spear the specimen horizontally and to lift it gently from its socket.

In sum, before proceeding to the biopsy the clinician should always attempt to visualize in his mind's eye the distribution of the pathologic process within the skin, that is, within the epidermis alone, the dermis alone, the subcutaneous fat alone, or within a combination of these. Then he is better led to select the method for surgical removal of the specimen that will permit the pathologist to examine enough of the histologic features to make a specific diagnosis.

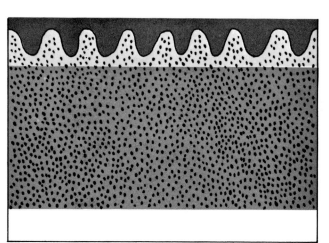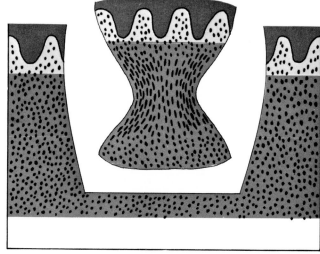

FIG. 4-3. Squeezing of a biopsy specimen by a forceps causes cellular distortion that may render the specimen histologically unreadable.

Fixation of Specimen

Before any type of specimen for biopsy is placed in formalin, it should be flattened on a firm piece of cardboard for proper embedding by the pathologist. The usual fixative for skin specimens is 10% neutral buffered formalin. The amount of formalin should be approximately twenty times that of the specimen by volume. The surgeon should be responsible for ensuring that the specimen is actually placed in the formalin. The cap to the specimen bottle must be firmly tightened. Artificial changes occur rapidly if the specimen is not immediately and continually flooded by formalin. Freezing artefact, which may occur when specimens are accidentally frozen during transport, can be eliminated by the addition of 10% by volume of 95% ethyl alcohol to the formalin.

If electron microscopy is also contemplated as a routine procedure, all skin specimens may be placed in modified Milonig's fixative rather than simply in formalin. Such fixation prepares the specimen for both routine histologic processing and electron microscopy.

Diagnosis by Histopathologic Patterns

Recognition of Major Patterns

 Superficial perivascular dermatitis

 Superficial and deep perivascular dermatitis

 Vasculitis

 Nodular and diffuse dermatitis

 Intraepidermal vesicular and pustular dermatitis

 Subepidermal vesicular dermatitis

 Folliculitis and perifolliculitis

 Fibrosing dermatitis

 Panniculitis

Advantages of Pattern Method

Application of Pattern Method

Diagnosis *by* Histopathologic Patterns

5

THE UNDERSTANDING of disease has traditionally been built upon the triad of diagnosis (what is it?), etiology (what caused it?), and pathogenesis (how did it happen?) Current emphasis in medical education is on the latter two elements, cause and mechanism of disease, rather than on morphology. Yet the etiology of most skin diseases is unknown. Pathogenesis is either understood fragmentarily or not at all. In fact, skin disease has yet to be completely and critically surveyed morphologically. The approach of this book to diagnosing inflammatory skin diseases is rooted firmly in morphology as the direct route to diagnosis and as a springboard for thinking about causes and pathways of pathologic processes. Accurate morphologic diagnosis is a first step toward effective dermatologic therapy and remains important, if only to the patient, who is less concerned about "how did it happen?" than with "how do you treat it?"

To the novice, the split-second accuracy of the experienced ornithologist to identify birds, whether in flight or partially camouflaged, is uncanny. Equally amazing to the beginner in dermatology is the facility of the experienced clinician to make diagnoses, seemingly before the patient has fully exposed the skin lesions. How do the cognoscenti distinguish a particular bird from among thousands or a specific skin disease from among hundreds? The morphologic method requires accurate observation and orderly classification. The morphologist, at a glance, responds reflexly to pattern—shape, form, and structure—on the basis of previous exposures. When experts disagree about identification, of birds or skin lesions, the conflict is resolved by reference to established criteria.

There is currently no orderly approach to the histologic diagnosis of inflammatory skin diseases. Since cause and pathogenesis of most of these entities are unknown, one is justified in grouping them on the basis of common histologic appearances. This book classifies skin diseases by distinctive histopathologic patterns. It is relatively easy to distinguish among the major families of birds by size and shape of beak, body, wing, and tail (Fig. 5-1), but it is more difficult to differentiate between members of the same species. By noting subtle, but characteristic, differences, separations can be made (Fig. 5-2). Using the scanning objective of the light microscope, the histologist can readily classify skin diseases by pattern. Not only can "major families" of skin diseases be distinguished, but "species" differences as well. Examining a histopathologic section under the microscope is like taking an open-book examination: the answers are given; one must only be able to recognize them. Because our ability to recognize accurately is sometimes imperfect, a microscopic diagnosis must on occasion, and of necessity, be tentative. There are times when one simply does not know the answer, even though one is looking at it. At other times, with time, morphologic interpretation will be proven wrong, especially by neoplasms that may refuse to comply with the behavior that the pathologist predicts or ordains.

Recognition of Major Patterns

The method I am espousing utilizes principally the scanning power, because most histologic diagnoses of inflammatory skin diseases can be made using the 2.5 to 4 × objective. Before one can hope to detect pathologic processes in skin, one must be well-schooled in histologic patterns of normal skin. Because the skin has such a remarkably varied terrain, the differences between sites are usually easily identified histologically. An initial reflex in examining a histologic section of skin is to recognize from which part of the body the specimen comes. Certain diseases are limited to certain parts, for example, rosacea to the face, chondrodermatitis nodularis chronica helicis to the ear, and pseudopelade to the

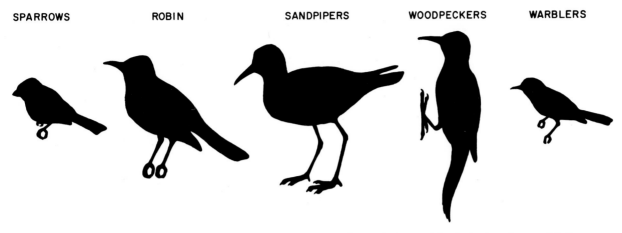

SPARROWS ROBIN SANDPIPERS WOODPECKERS WARBLERS

FIG. 5-1. Patterns of major families of birds. Note variation in size and shape of beak, body, wing, and tail.

scalp. In addition, other diseases favor particular sites, e.g., necrobiosis lipoidica and erythema nodosum, the skin over the anterior tibiae; granuloma faciale and seborrheic dermatitis, the face; and dermatofibroma and nodular fasciitis, the limbs. Thus, by viewing the entire specimen and looking for the telltale topographic markers indicated in Chapter 1, one can make a reasonable judgment about the site from which the biopsy specimen was obtained, which in itself narrows diagnostic possibilities.

Continuing to use the scanning objective, the microscopist should next note the location of the pathologic changes. Are they in the epidermis, dermis, subcutaneous fat, or in a combination of these? When studying a particular histologic section, he must routinely ask himself: "Where is the dominant pathologic change and what is the pathologic pattern?" The histologic expressions of inflammatory skin diseases have been conveniently divided into nine strikingly different major patterns, usually discernible with the scanning objective.

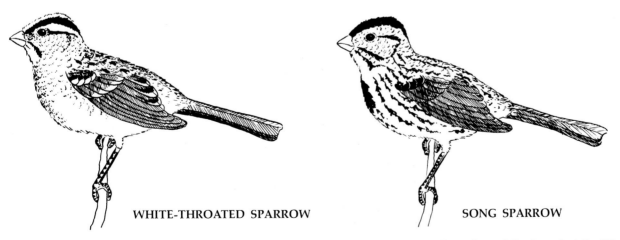

WHITE-THROATED SPARROW   SONG SPARROW

FIG. 5-2. White-throated sparrow and song sparrow, members of the same species. By noting subtle characteristic differences, separation can be made.

The nine major patterns are:

1. Superficial perivascular dermatitis (Fig. 5-3)

2. Superficial and deep perivascular dermatitis (Fig. 5-4)

3. Vasculitis (Fig. 5-5)

4. Nodular and diffuse dermatitis (Fig. 5-6)

5. Intraepidermal vesicular and pustular dermatitis (Fig. 5-7)

6. Subepidermal vesicular dermatitis (Fig. 5-8)

7. Folliculitis and perifolliculitis (Fig. 5-9)

8. Fibrosing dermatitis (Fig. 5-10)

9. Panniculitis (Fig. 5-11)

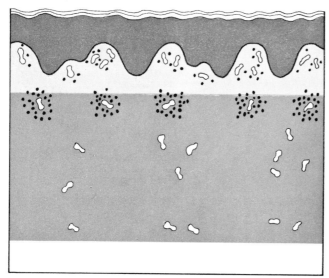

FIG. 5-3. Superficial perivascular dermatitis.

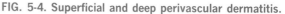

FIG. 5-4. Superficial and deep perivascular dermatitis.

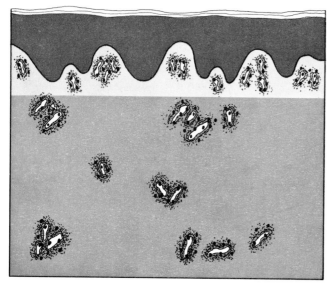

FIG. 5-5. Vasculitis.

Once the major pattern has been identified, the diagnostic possibilities are dramatically reduced. The next step is to home in on the exact diagnosis. For example, cellular infiltrates in the dermis tend to be arranged as (1) superficial perivascular, (2) superficial and deep perivascular, or (3) nodular and diffuse. The most common of these is superficial perivascular dermatitis where the infiltrate is present predominantly around the blood vessels of the superficial plexus. The infiltrate may be lymphohistiocytic (e.g., in gyrate erythema), mixed-cell (e.g., in urticarial allergic eruptions), or monomorphous (e.g., in macular urticaria pigmentosa). The

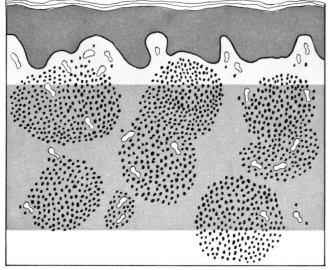

FIG. 5-6. A, Nodular dermatitis.

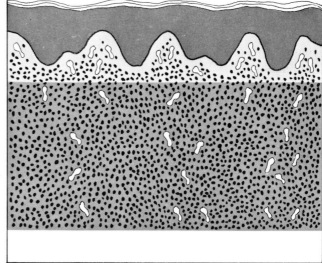

FIG. 5-6. B, Diffuse dermatitis.

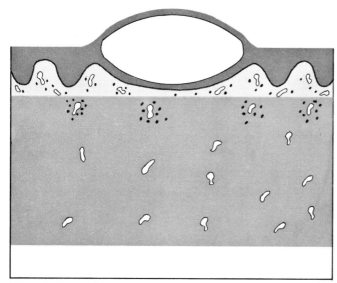

FIG. 5-7. Intraepidermal vesicular and pustular dermatitis

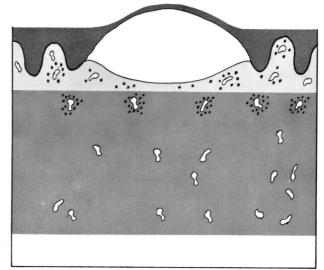

FIG. 5-8. Subepidermal vesicular dermatitis

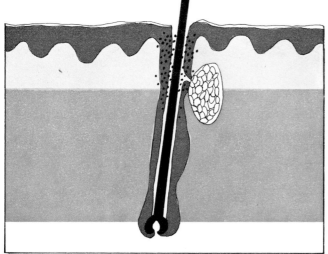

FIG. 5-9. A, Folliculitis.

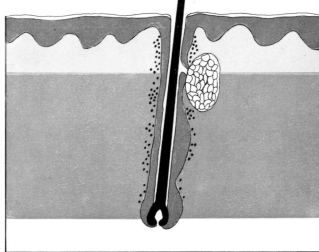

FIG. 5-9. B, Perifolliculitis.

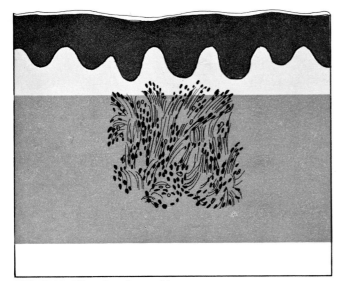

FIG. 5-10. Fibrosing dermatitis.

superficial perivascular pattern can then be subclassified according to associated epidermal alterations: none (perivascular dermatitis, superficial), spongiosis (spongiotic dermatitis), psoriasiform (psoriasiform dermatitis), and abnormalities of the dermoepidermal interface (interface dermatitis). Each of the subdivisions can be further partitioned on the basis of minor variations. An example is spongiotic dermatitis, which includes allergic contact dermatitis, pityriasis rosea, and miliaria rubra among others. Initially, the distinctions among them are detected with difficulty, because they share more similarities than they have differences. I hope that

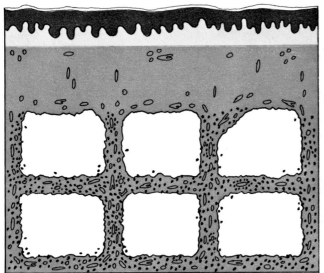

FIG. 5-11. Panniculitis. A, Septal.

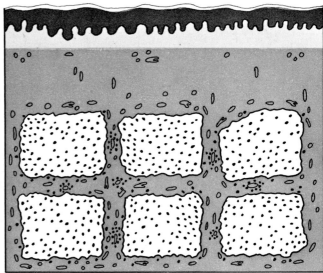

FIG. 5-11. Panniculitis. B, Lobular.

when the reader has completed the section on spongiotic dermatitis in Chapter 6, these subtle, but significant differences will be obvious. If the epidermis shows psoriasiform hyperplasia, as well as spongiosis, the diagnosis is either subacute nummular dermatitis or subacute allergic contact dermatitis (Fig. 5-12). After the major histologic pattern, such as superficial perivascular dermatitis, has been established, it usually is not necessary to subcategorize more than twice. In every instance, higher power is required to verify a tentative scanning power diagnosis, such as the presence of plasma cells in secondary syphilis, neutrophils in dermatitis herpetiformis, nuclear dust in leukocytoclastic vasculitis, or hyphae in dermatophytosis.

By using the pattern method, order can be brought to a group of diseases whose least common denominator is an infiltrate around the blood vessels of the superficial plexus. By subdividing the superficial perivascular dermatitides into diseases that do and do not involve the epidermis, and by further subdividing the former group into spongiotic, psoriasiform, and interface dermatitis, one can vastly simplify diagnosis and more critically consider a remarkably diverse group of diseases that are often dismissed as chronic nonspecific dermatitis. Using this approach, the nonspecific can become specific, and the apparently meaningless can become meaningful.

The foregoing stepwise procedure applies to histologic interpretation of all inflammatory diseases in skin. The morphologic, rather than etiologic, approach to diagnosis is more helpful because the causes of most skin diseases are unknown. Even where etiology has been established such as in viral diseases, the histologic patterns are extraordinarily varied, e.g., (1) erythema infectiosum—perivascular dermatitis, superficial; (2) measles—spongiotic dermatitis; (3) infectious mononucleosis—interface dermatitis; (4) herpesvirus—intraepidermal vesicular dermatitis; (5) verruca plana—epidermal hyperplasia; (6) verruca vulgaris and condyloma acuminatum—papillated epidermal hyperplasia; and (7) molluscum contagiosum—infundibular hyperplasia. With the pattern approach, a unified method for histologic diagnosis is maintained.

These histologic patterns are guidelines to diagnosis as well as to building concepts about pathologic processes in skin. They are not rules to be followed rigidly as if inviolable. Exceptions can be found in every category, and with increasing experience and added knowledge, our thinking about skin diseases should indeed be modified and altered. Just as young birds do not always resemble the adults and human infants do not resemble parents, early skin lesions do not exactly simulate fully developed ones (Fig. 5-13). Just as the seasons influence the color and patterns of birds, so, too, do the site, age, pigment, and extent of exposure to elements, notably the sun, influence the appearance of the skin and its lesions.

Every judgment rendered by the anatomic pathologist is necessarily a subjective one, and the most subjective of all is interpretation. Nonetheless, description of pathologic changes should be reproducibly standardized, comparable to a still life taken by different photographers. The mood may vary according to the artist, but the subject itself does not change. The same principle applies to tissue fixed in formalin. Only the view of it changes. "Describe and diagnose" was the maxim of early histologists. If criteria for diagnosis are clearly established and faithfully followed, diagnosis becomes increasingly objective and thus, reproducible. Histologic diagnosis should *not* be Pirandelloesque: "Right you are, if you think you are."

The significance of the subjective for anatomic pathologists is witnessed by the multiplicity of opinions by different experts in

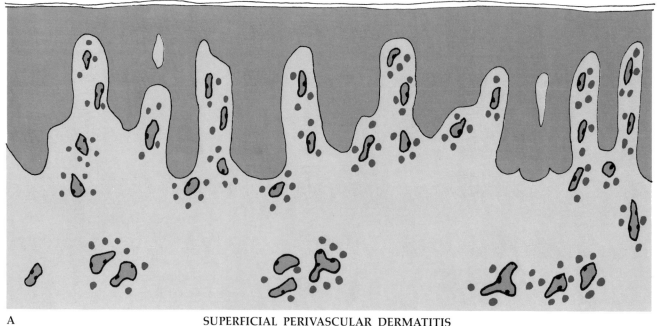

A   SUPERFICIAL PERIVASCULAR DERMATITIS

+

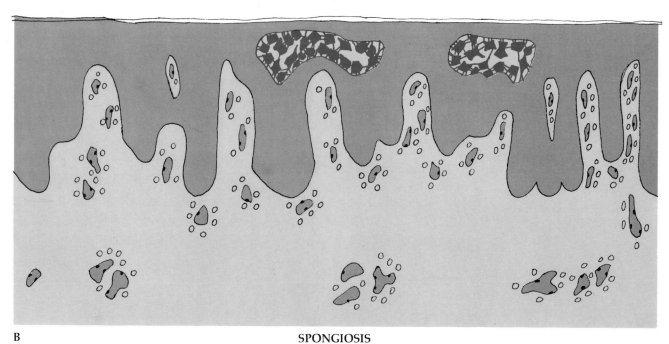

B   SPONGIOSIS

+

FIG. 5-12. Legend on opposite page.

interpretation of the same histologic sections. No approach to skin pathology can possibly avoid the subjective component, nor would it want to, because the subjective is also the creative component. The methodology and philosophy outlined in this text seek to stimulate thinking about skin disease at the same time that they attempt to establish reproducible guidelines for diagnosis.

The pattern method enables the pathologist, once accurate observations have been made, to place every disease process in

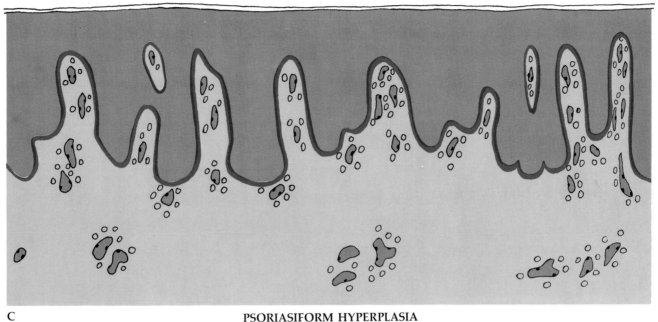

C   PSORIASIFORM HYPERPLASIA

=

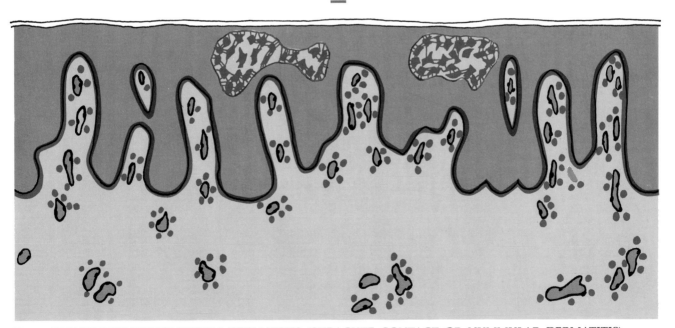

D   SPONGIOTIC PSORIASIFORM DERMATITIS (SUBACUTE CONTACT OR NUMMULAR DERMATITIS)

FIG. 5-12. Diagnosis by histologic pattern. Superficial perivascular dermatitis plus spongiosis and psoriasiform hyperplasia equal spongiotic psoriasiform dermatitis, which is the sole equation for identification of subacute nummular dermatitis or subacute allergic contact dermatitis.

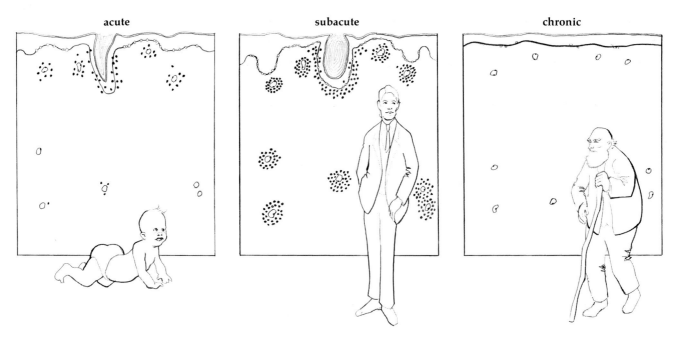

FIG. 5-13. The ages of man and of inflammatory skin diseases (e.g., discoid lupus erythematosus).

every specimen into a well-circumscribed diagnostic category, and to begin to understand the process even if he cannot assign it a proper dermatologic designation. Mastering concepts, rather than names, is our aim. It is this effort to understand a process, not simply to label it, that distinguishes the pathologist from the bird-watcher.

Application of the Pattern Method

Certain generalities about this histologic approach to inflammatory diseases in skin should be mentioned. It is preferable at first to examine sections without reference to the clinician's diagnostic opinion. In this way, the pathologist musters and marshals all of his powers of observation and creativity without the influence of another's bias. If the pathologist can extract the proper meaning from the histologic sections, he will usually do so without assistance from the clinician, and when the pathologist is unable to do so, he can then refer to the clinical data. This approach in no way minimizes the importance of thinking about pathologic processes in both gross and microscopic terms nor does it diminish the importance of close liaison between pathologist and clinician. It is designed to enable the pathologist to maximize his perceptions without prejudice. If the clinical diagnosis differs strikingly from the histologic one, the pathologist should consider obtaining additional sections and consulting directly with the clinician.

One should examine every section on every slide and as many sections of the specimen as possible. Often the critical histologic findings are discretely circumscribed, such as in folliculitis or transient acantholytic dermatosis, and remain embedded in the paraffin block. It is incumbent upon the pathologist to study as much of the specimen by sectioning as is necessary to establish the diagnosis.

After the diagnosis has been reached, the pathologist should search beyond the dominant pathologic process for other abnormalities in the sections. It is helpful to do this by scanning for deviations from normal in an orderly fashion, beginning with the cornified layer, descending through the epidermis into the dermis to include the adnexal structures, and eventually proceeding into the subcutaneous fat. Often these additional abnormalities enhance the pathologist's understanding of skin disease.

Making definitive diagnoses is not always possible. Diseases sometimes evade our attempts to classify them. Therefore, a histologic diagnosis should never exceed more than what the pathologist knows to be completely true and defensible. There is a welcome place for descriptive diagnosis of inflammatory skin diseases. If the process is spongiotic dermatitis and one cannot be more specific than that, the specimen should be diagnosed as spongiotic dermatitis. If the dominant pathologic process is a granulomatous panniculitis and a more specific diagnosis cannot be made, the diagnosis should simply be "granulomatous panniculitis." If one wishes to comment further or to speculate, a note can be appended. In the note, the pathologist may discuss the differential diagnoses and offer his interpretations, but they are clearly conveyed as possibilities or probabilities, rather than as certainties.

If one is uncertain about a histologic diagnosis, representative sections or the tissue block should be sent to a respected colleague for his impression. The consultant's judgment does not necessarily have to be accepted, but it is one way to do fuller justice to the patient and to oneself.

Superficial Perivascular Dermatitis

Perivascular Dermatitis, Superficial

Lymphohistiocytic infiltrate
  Pigmented purpuric dermatitis
  Some viral exanthems
  Gyrate erythema, superficial
  Tinea versicolor
  Erythrasma
  Maculae cerulae
  Postinflammatory pigmentary alteration
  Rocky Mountain spotted fever
Mixed-cell infiltrate
  Urticaria
  Urticarial allergic eruptions, superficial
  Arthropod reactions, superficial
  "Itchy red bump" disease
  Papular eruption of pregnancy
Monomorphous infiltrate
  Urticaria pigmentosa, macular and papular
    lesions

Interface Dermatitis

Vacuolar type
  Erythema multiforme
  Toxic epidermal necrolysis
  Phototoxic dermatitis
  Dermatomyositis
  Discoid lupus erythematosus, acute
  Some morbilliform drug eruptions
  Some morbilliform viral eruptions
  Erythema dyschromicum perstans
  Lichen sclerosus et atrophicus
  Chronic radiodermatitis
  Poikiloderma congenitale
  Pemphigoid, urticarial lesions
Lichenoid type
  Lichen planus
  Lichen-planuslike keratoses
  Lichen-planuslike drug eruptions
  Lichenoid purpura
  Pityriasis lichenoides chronica
  Parapsoriasis en plaques, poikiloderma
    atrophicans vasculare
  Disseminated superficial porokeratosis

Spongiotic Dermatitis

Allergic contact dermatitis, acute
Photoallergic dermatitis, acute
Nummular dermatitis, acute
Id reactions, acute
Dyshidrotic dermatitis, acute
Dermatophytosis, vesicular lesions
Gyrate erythema, superficial
Pityriasis rosea
Guttate parapsoriasis
Acral papular eruption of childhood
Pityriasis alba
Seborrheic dermatitis, acute
Measles
Lichen striatus
Miliaria rubra
Irritant contact dermatitis
Phototoxic contact dermatitis
Stasis dermatitis
Spongiotic simulant of mycosis fungoides
Papular eruption of pregnancy
Eosinophilic spongiosis
  Incontinentia pigmenti
  Allergic contact dermatitis
  Arthropod reactions
  Pemphigoid, urticarial lesions
  Herpes gestationis, urticarial lesions
  Pemphigus vulgaris

Psoriasiform Dermatitis

Psoriasis
Lichen simplex chronicus
Contact dermatitis and nummular dermatitis,
  chronic
Seborrheic dermatitis, chronic
Pityriasis rubra pilaris
Dermatophytosis and candidiasis, scaling le-
  sions
Pellagra
Lamellar ichthyosis
Parapsoriasis variegata
Inflammatory linear verrucous epidermal
  nevus
Incontinentia pigmenti, verrucous lesions
Acrodermatitis enteropathica

Spongiotic Psoriasiform Dermatitis

Nummular dermatitis, subacute
Allergic contact dermatitis, subacute
Seborrheic dermatitis, subacute

Superficial

Perivascular Dermatitis

6

THERE ARE two major vascular plexuses within the dermis: the superficial and the deep (Fig. 1-19). The *superficial vascular plexus* is situated in the upper part of the reticular dermis, immediately beneath the papillary dermis and therefore is also called the subpapillary vascular plexus. The *deep vascular plexus* is located in the lower portion of the reticular dermis.

Most of the common inflammatory diseases of the skin, e.g., seborrheic dermatitis, psoriasis, lichen planus, contact dermatitis, and pityriasis rosea, involve principally the blood vessels of the superficial plexus. There are, however, some inflammatory conditions that involve the blood vessels of both the superficial and the deep plexuses. Inflammatory processes that are limited to the superficial plexus will hereafter be referred to as *superficial perivascular dermatitis* (Fig. 6-1), and those that involve both plexuses as *superficial and deep perivascular dermatitis.* Most of the perivascular infiltrates classified as superficial are confined to the uppermost dermis, but there are some that extend to the level of the mid-reticular dermis. Therefore, for purposes of this classification, an infiltrate around blood vessels anywhere in the upper half of the dermis is considered to be superficial perivascular dermatitis (Fig. 6-2).

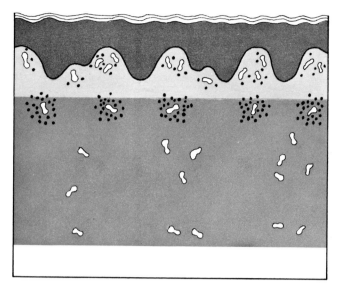

FIG. 6-1. Superficial perivascular dermatitis. Infiltrate is around blood vessels of the superficial plexus.

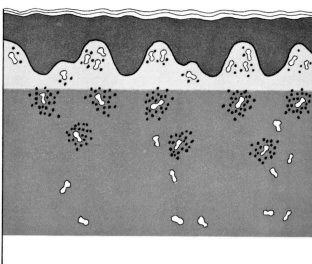

FIG. 6-2. Superficial perivascular dermatitis. Infiltrate is around blood vessels in upper half of dermis.

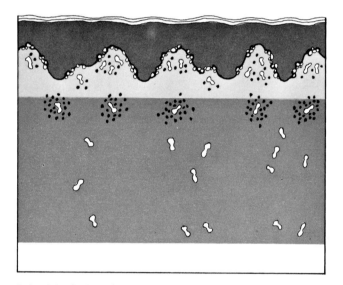

FIG. 6-3. A, Interface dermatitis with vacuolar alteration.

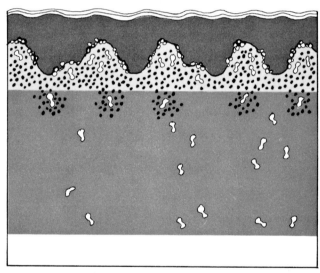

FIG. 6-3. B, Interface dermatitis with lichenoid infiltrate.

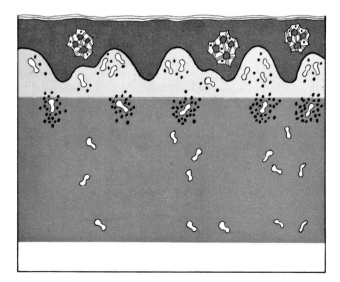

FIG. 6-4. Spongiotic dermatitis.

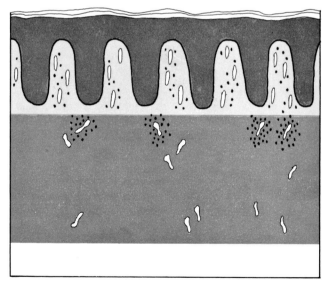

FIG. 6-5. Psoriasiform dermatitis.

The superficial vascular plexus, especially the capillaries in the dermal papillae, the connective tissue of the papillary dermis, and the epidermis constitute a morphologic and biologic unit. Involvement of the blood vessels of the superficial plexus is usually accompanied by alterations in all components of this unit. Only rarely do inflammatory cells surround the superficial blood vessels without any changes being detectable in either the papillary dermis or the epidermis. It is especially important to examine the cornified layer because it contains the historical record of events in the underlying epidermis.

Superficial perivascular dermatitis is subdivided on the basis of whether there are accompanying epidermal changes:

1. Perivascular without epidermal changes (perivascular dermatitis, superficial) (Fig. 6-1)

2. Perivascular with obscuring of the dermoepidermal interface (interface dermatitis) (Fig. 6-3)

3. Perivascular with epidermal spongiosis (spongiotic dermatitis) (Fig. 6-4)

4. Perivascular with epidermal hyperplasia (psoriasiform dermatitis) (Fig. 6-5)

Infiltrates of the superficial perivascular group can be further classified by inflammatory-cell type: lymphohistiocytic, mixed-cell (more than two cell types, usually including eosinophils and/or neutrophils), and monomorphous (usually mast cells).

Perivascular Dermatitis, Superficial (Fig. 6-1)

The inflammatory-cell infiltrate in perivascular dermatitis, superficial, is primarily confined to the region immediately surrounding the vessels of the superficial plexus. Additionally, some cells may be scattered in the papillary dermis, but these remain beneath the dermoepidermal junction so that the epidermis appears unaltered. With the scanning objective, most of the perivascular dermatitides that are wholly superficial without any epidermal involvement resemble one another, and therefore this group of diseases is most often ambiguously diagnosed as "chronic nonspecific dermatitis." When one is familiar with the markers of their individuality, however, specific diagnoses can often be rendered. If, despite careful scrutiny, a specific diagnosis cannot be made, the specimen can be reported descriptively as "perivascular dermatitis, superficial" with the histologic differential diagnosis listed in an appended note. Despite its limitations, the descriptive histologic diagnosis "perivascular dermatitis, superficial" conveys precisely where the inflammatory-cell infiltrate resides.

Lymphohistiocytic Infiltrate

The infiltrate around the superficial vascular plexus consists mainly of lymphocytes and histiocytes in pigmented purpuric dermatitis, superficial gyrate erythema, some viral exanthems, tinea versicolor, erythrasma, maculae cerulae, and postinflammatory pigmentary alteration.

Pigmented Purpuric Dermatitis (Schamberg's Disease) (Fig. 6-6)

—Moderately dense perivascular lymphohistiocytic infiltrate
—Extravasated erythrocytes in the papillary dermis
—Siderophages (macrophages containing hemosiderin) in varying numbers in the papillary dermis
—Early slight edema or later fibrosis of the papillary dermis
—Thick-walled blood vessels with plump endothelial cells in the upper part of the dermis, which is a normal finding for the legs

Pigmented purpuric dermatitis is an idiopathic process that occurs predominantly on the legs as purpuric macules and papules that resemble cayenne pepper. Initially, there are bright red petechiae that, with time, become progressively browner. The purpuric component is seen histologically as numerous extravasated erythrocytes in the papillary dermis. The number of extravasated erythrocytes and siderophages varies, depending on the age of the lesion and the severity of the disease. Although hemosiderin glitters and tends to be more yellow-brown than melanin, it is sometimes impossible to distinguish between the two pigments when they are stained with hematoxylin and eosin. In these instances, a stain for iron, such as Perls' or Prussian blue, is useful.

Clinically, the erythema of Schamberg's disease is usually not discernible because of the predominant purpura. If the lesions are long-standing, there may be mild epidermal hyperplasia and orthokeratosis and/or parakeratosis, reflected clinically in slight scaling. The inflammatory-cell infiltrate and edema of the papillary dermis are largely responsible for the variable sense of firmness of the lesions. Spongiosis occurs rarely. There is no vasculitis.

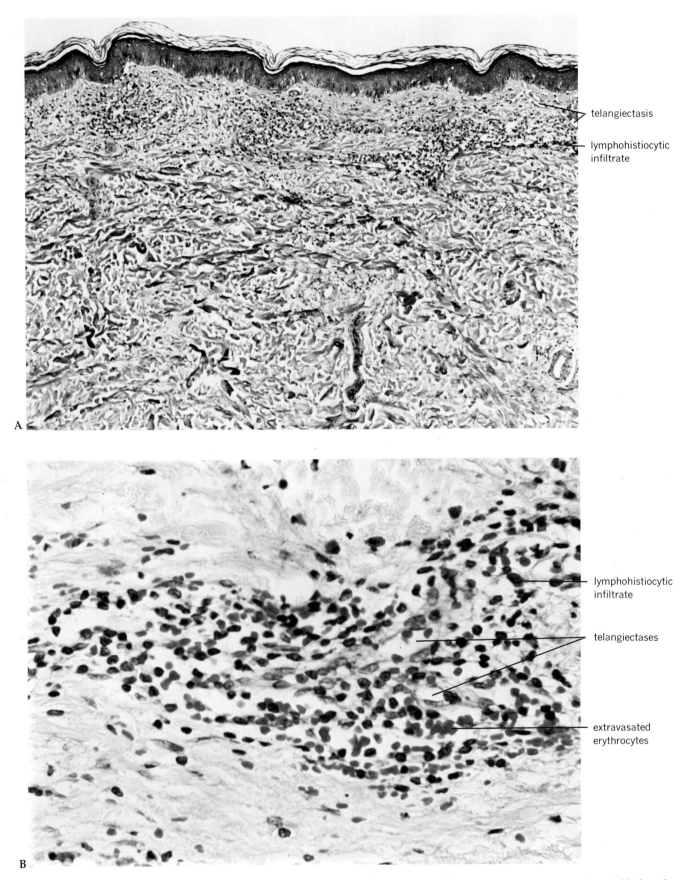

telangiectasis

lymphohistiocytic
infiltrate

lymphohistiocytic
infiltrate

telangiectases

extravasated
erythrocytes

A

B

FIG. 6-6. Pigmented purpuric dermatitis (Schamberg's disease). Characteristics are superficial perivascular lymphohistiocytic infiltrate with extravasated erythrocytes. (A, × 90, B, × 500.)

Some Viral Exanthems

> —Sparse lymphohistiocytic infiltrate around widely dilated blood vessels in the upper and mid dermis
> —Nearly inconspicuous edema of the papillary dermis

The edema and the widely dilated blood vessels are reflected clinically in a blotchy macular and papular eruption characteristic of some viral exanthems, such as erythema infectiosum. The changes are not diagnostic histologically.

Gyrate Erythema, Superficial (Fig. 6-7)

> —Sparse to moderately dense perivascular infiltrate of lymphocytes
> —Mild edema of the papillary dermis

In a biopsy of the advancing edge of the reddish, polycyclic lesions of superficial gyrate erythema, the only pathologic change observed is a superficial perivascular, predominantly lymphocytic, infiltrate that sharply circumscribes the blood vessels. In a biopsy of the circumvallated border of the lesion, focal spongiosis can be seen histologically (see Spongiotic Dermatitis). In a biopsy of the inner scaly edge of the border, foci of parakeratosis are evident, with or without subjacent spongiosis. Finally, only mel-

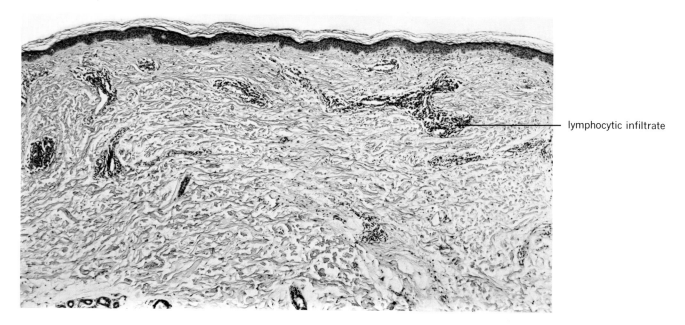

lymphocytic infiltrate

FIG. 6-7. Gyrate erythema, superficial. Advancing edge of erythema annulare centrifugum reveals only predominantly lymphocytic superficial perivascular infiltrate without spongiosis or parakeratosis. (× 50.)

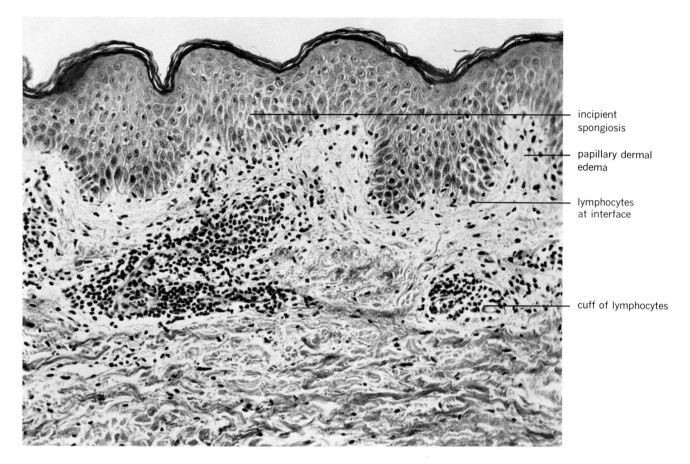

incipient spongiosis

papillary dermal edema

lymphocytes at interface

cuff of lymphocytes

FIG. 6-8. Gyrate erythema, superficial. Little epidermal change is evident in this biopsy specimen from advancing border of erythema annulare centrifugum. Few lymphocytes are seen along dermoepidermal junction, but lymphocytes form cuff around the blood vessels of superficial plexus. (× 193.)

anophages are present in the papillary dermis of the pigmented zone that represents sites previously involved by the advancing erythema. Rarely can incipient spongiosis be detected in biopsy specimens taken from the advancing edge of the lesion (Fig. 6-8).

Tinea Versicolor (Fig. 6-9)

—Sparse perivascular lymphohistiocytic infiltrate
—Abundant hyphae and spores within the cornified layer (Fig. 6-9B)

Within the basket-weavelike pattern of the cornified layer of the lesions of tinea versicolor, there are short, broad hyphae and collections of round spores, a combination that has been dubbed "spaghetti and meatballs" or "frankfurters and beans." The fungal elements of tinea versicolor and of other superficial fungal infections can often be seen in sections stained with hematoxylin and eosin. Therefore, the cornified layer in every skin biopsy slide

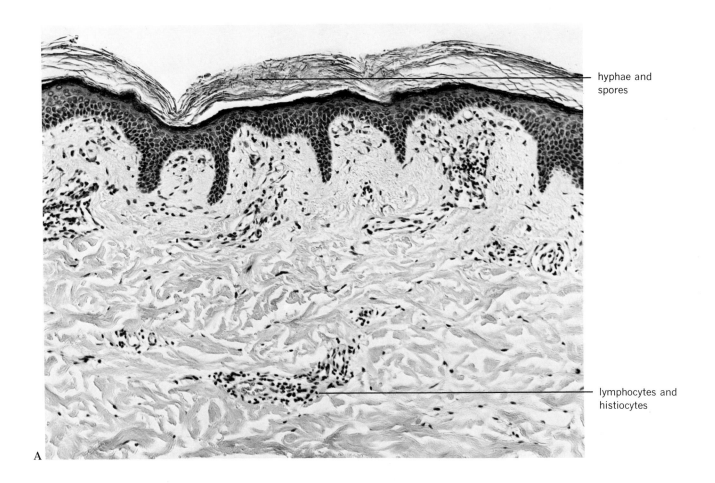

hyphae and
spores

lymphocytes and
histiocytes

A

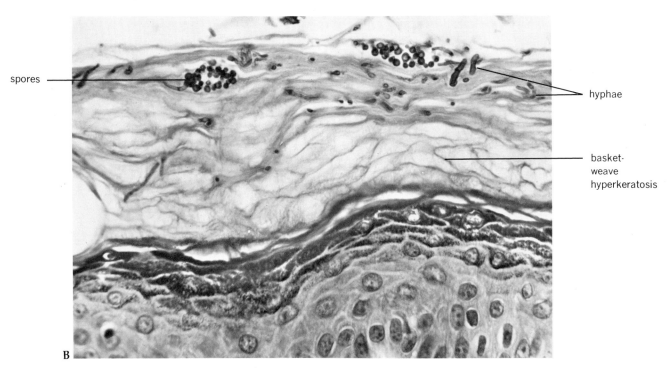

spores

hyphae

basket-
weave
hyperkeratosis

B

FIG. 6-9. Tinea versicolor. A. Even with low power objective, hyphae and spores can be seen in the cornified layer. Note sparse superficial perivascular lymphohistiocytic infiltrate. ($\times$ 141.) B. Ensemble of stubby hyphae and round spores demonstrated in basket-weave patterned hyperkeratotic stratum corneum has been likened to "spaghetti and meat balls" and is diagnostic of tinea versicolor. ($\times$ 565.)

should be studied for the presence of fungi, particularly in those sections in which the cellular infiltrate is sparse, superficial, and perivascular. The PAS or silver methenamine stain aids in confirming the diagnosis. The organism that causes tinea versicolor, Malassezia furfur, can be differentiated from Candida albicans by its shorter, broader hyphae, larger spore size, and septa in budding cells (Plate 2).

Clinically, the lesions of tinea versicolor consist of scales with slight erythema. The scales are composed of orthokeratotic cells. *Versicolor* refers to the apparent change in color of the lesions from light to dark and back again. One theory is that the surrounding normal skin actually changes color as a consequence of sun exposure. Another holds that the hyperpigmented lesions result from large melanosomes well distributed in the epidermis, whereas hypopigmented lesions of tinea versicolor develop when small melanosomes are improperly transferred to the epidermal keratinocytes.

Erythrasma

—Sparse superficial perivascular lymphohistiocytic infiltrate
—Slight hyperkeratosis containing rods and filaments that stain basophilically

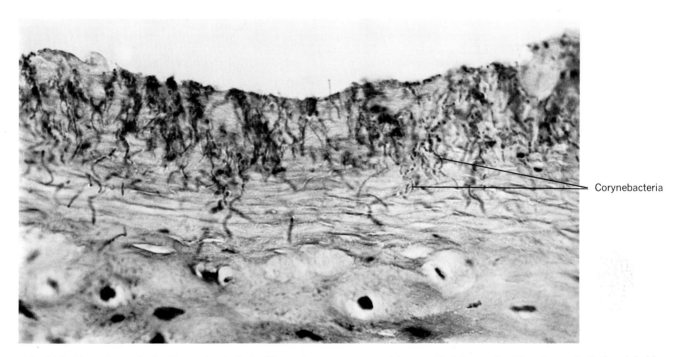

Corynebacteria

FIG. 6-10. Pitted keratolysis. Corynebacteria in filamentous arrangement in cornified layer of epidermis are indistinguishable histologically from those found in cornified layer of erythrasma. (× 710.)

The causative organism of erythrasma, the diphtheroid Corynebacterium minutissimum, is identifiable in sections stained by hematoxylin and eosin as slightly basophilic, delicate rods that form filaments. These bacteria are better visualized with the Gram stain. Similar-appearing diphtheroids cause palmar and plantar lesions known as pitted keratolysis (Fig. 6-10).

Clinically, erythrasma flourishes in intertriginous regions, especially the inguinal, axillary, and inframammary, where it appears as sharply marginated, rust-colored, mildly scaly patches. The lesions of erythrasma fluoresce a magnificient coral red when exposed to long-wave ultraviolet light.

Maculae Cerulae

Maculae cerulae, or sky blue spots, presumably induced by the sucking parts of the crab louse, histologically show a superficial perivascular predominantly lymphocytic infiltrate with associated extravasated erythrocytes.

Postinflammatory Pigmentary Alteration (Fig. 6-11)

> —Lymphohistiocytic infiltrate with melanophages around the superficial vessels and in the dermal papillae
> —Variable thickening of the papillary dermis by fibrosis

In addition to the inflammatory-cell infiltrate containing melanophages, postinflammatory pigmentary alteration often shows fibrotic thickening of the papillary dermis associated with an increased number of plump and stellate fibroblasts. If melanin in the epidermis is decreased, the clinical appearance is that of hypopigmentation. If epidermal melanin is increased, the clinical change is that of hyperpigmentation. Melanophages are present in both postinflammatory hypopigmentation and hyperpigmentation. It is largely the amount of epidermal pigment that actually determines the final color. Histologically, it is impossible to judge the relative amount of epidermal melanin in the lesion unless contiguous normal skin is present. The skin of heavily pigmented people can appear hypopigmented, but histologic study may still reveal more epidermal melanin than there is in lightly pigmented people. The presence of melanophages in the papillary dermis indicates that the inflammatory-cell infiltrate had once involved the dermoepidermal junction, where there was vacuolar alteration, with

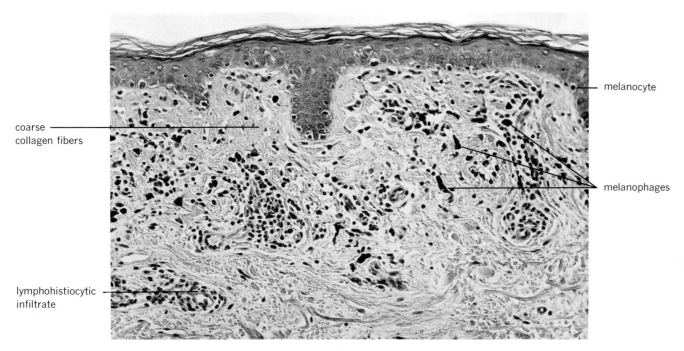

coarse
collagen fibers

melanocyte

melanophages

lymphohistiocytic
infiltrate

FIG. 6-11. Postinflammatory pigmentary alteration. Sparse superficial perivascular lymphohistiocytic infiltrate and numerous melanophages in papillary dermis thickened by coarse collagen fibers signify a previous inflammatory process that encroached upon basal cells and melanocytes of epidermis. Obvious increase in number of epidermal melanocytes indicates that this particular lesion is probably hyperpigmented rather than hypopigmented. (× 220.)

resultant damage to keratinocytes and melanocytes and loss of melanin into the dermis. Coarse collagen in the papillary dermis is the result of a prolonged, rather than an evanescent, inflammatory process. The phrase *postinflammatory pigmentary alteration* describes the end stage of a prior inflammatory process, but provides no clue to the nature of the original dermatitis.

Rocky Mountain Spotted Fever

—Sparse superficial perivascular and interstitial lymphohistiocytic
  infiltrate
—Extravasated erythrocytes in variable numbers within the papillary
  dermis
—Apparent increase in the number of capillaries and venules in the
  upper part of the dermis
—Thrombi occasionally

The eruption of Rocky Mountain spotted fever characteristically begins as reddish macules and papules on the acral parts that soon spreads centrally and becomes purpuric. Fever and headache are nearly constant accompaniments of the eruption in this potentially fatal disease.

The causative organisms of Rocky Mountain spotted fever (Rickettsia rickettsii) are transmitted to humans by the bite of a carrier tick, especially the wood or dog varieties. It may be demonstrated with difficulty in the skin, with Giemsa stain, as small, rod-like structures within endothelial cells of capillaries and venules.

Mixed-cell Infiltrate

A mixed-cell infiltrate is found around the superficial vascular plexus in biopsies from patients with urticaria, urticarial allergic eruptions, and unusually superficial arthropod reactions.

Urticaria (Fig. 6-12)

—Sparse perivascular infiltrate of lymphocytes, histiocytes, mast cells, and occasionally, a few eosinophils
—Severe edema of the reticular dermis
—Dilated blood vessels

When one examines biopsy specimens of urticaria with the scanning objective, the initial impression is one of normal skin. Closer inspection reveals a sparse superficial (and sometimes deep) perivascular inflammatory-cell infiltrate and prominent edema of the reticular dermis. The clue to the diagnosis of urticaria is this extreme paucity of inflammatory cells. Edema can be difficult to detect because the serum in the dermis does not stain. Edema of the papillary dermis is reflected by pallor; edema of the reticular dermis is indicated by slightly widened spaces between the collagen bundles. Thus, edema in the reticular dermis is a more subtle histologic change than is edema in the papillary dermis. The reticular dermis is the major site of edema in urticaria. In the lesions of giant urticaria or angioedema, extravasated erythrocytes can often be found in the upper dermis.

Acute urticaria as a solitary event usually lasts for only a few hours, and the patient has often identified the allergen before arriving at the physician's office. The histologic features of acute urticaria are indistinguishable from those of chronic urticaria, a condition of recurrent acute episodes that persist for weeks, months, or even years and in which a cause is usually not discovered by either patient or physician. The individual lesions of both acute and chronic urticaria are evanescent papules, nodules, or plaques that blanch upon diascopy and are the result of massive edema in the dermis.

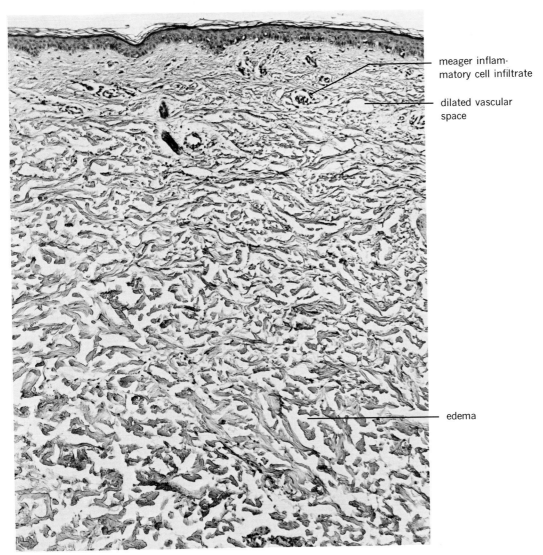

meager inflam-
matory cell infiltrate

dilated vascular
space

edema

FIG. 6-12. Urticaria. Massive edema of reticular dermis, diagnostic of hive or wheal, can be recognized only by noting wide separations of collagen bundles that have been pushed apart by fluid. There are few inflammatory cells. (× 91.)

Urticarial Allergic Eruption, Superficial (Fig. 6-13)

—Moderately dense perivascular and interstitial mixed-cell infiltrate especially of neutrophils, but also of eosinophils, lymphocytes, histiocytes, and mast cells
—Prominent edema of the papillary dermis

Clinically, urticarial allergic eruptions are distinguished from acute and chronic urticaria by the tendency of their individual lesions to persist longer. Although the lesions of true urticaria and urticarial allergic eruptions are similar grossly and have similar causes, their histologic differences are striking. The edematous papules of urticarial allergic eruptions result from edema of the

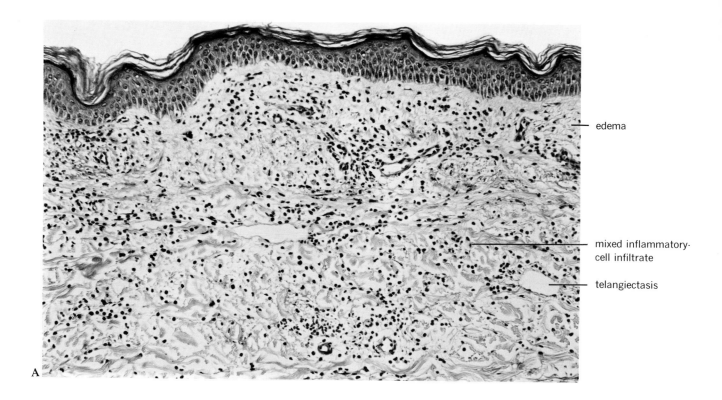

edema

mixed inflammatory-
cell infiltrate

telangiectasis

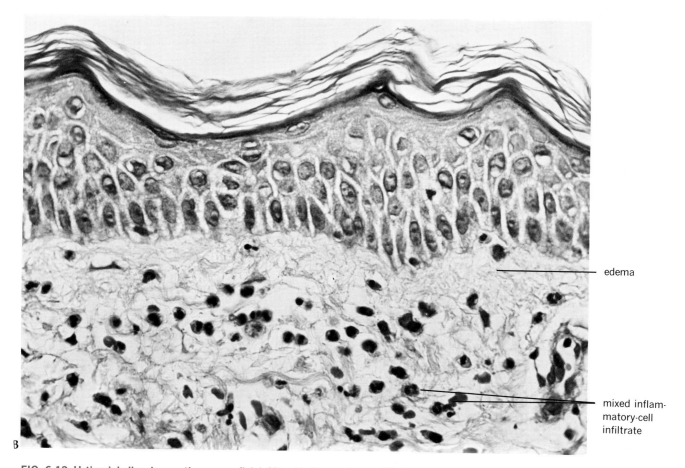

edema

mixed inflam-
matory-cell
infiltrate

FIG. 6-13. Urticarial allergic eruption, superficial. Mixed inflammatory-cell infiltrate of neutrophils, eosinophils, lymphocytes, and histiocytes, arranged perivascularly and interstitially, in an edematous papillary dermis are diagnostic features. Identical changes are seen in chronic urticaria. (A, × 150; B, × 556.)

papillary dermis and a moderately dense mixed-cell infiltrate. By contrast, the lesions of urticaria consist, almost wholly, of edema of the reticular dermis with a dearth of inflammatory cells. In some instances, the mixed inflammatory-cell infiltrate in urticarial allergic reactions is located around the blood vessels of the deep, as well as the superficial, plexus.

Urticarial allergic eruptions are frequently misdiagnosed clinically as erythema multiforme because they often form annular, arcuate, or serpiginous outlines. Unlike erythema multiforme, the lesions of urticarial allergic eruptions do not have "iris" or "target" configurations, are not usually purpuric, and rarely vesiculate. Histologically, urticarial allergic eruptions are readily distinguished from erythema multiforme, which is prototypic of interface dermatitis, vacuolar type, by the absence of both vacuolar alteration and necrotic keratinocytes at the dermoepidermal junction and the presence of neutrophils and eosinophils within dermal infiltrate. Medications, by any route of administration, are the major cause of urticarial allergic eruptions. Other less common causes are allergens, such as inhalants, (e.g., fumes), ingestants (e.g., foods), injectants (e.g., vaccines), and infestations (e.g., gastrointestinal parasites).

Clinically, urticarial lesions may be seen in a variety of diseases other than urticarial allergic eruptions, including dermatitis herpetiformis, pemphigoid, herpes gestationis, early lesions of allergic contact dermatitis, leukocytoclastic vasculitis, and arthropod reactions. Vesicles, and sometimes bullae, often accompany these urticarial lesions, but rarely appear in urticarial allergic eruptions. Biopsy of urticarial lesions will reveal the characteristic histologic changes of the underlying primary disease, i.e., dermatitis herpetiformis, pemphigoid, herpes gestationis, allergic contact dermatitis, leukocytoclastic vasculitis, or arthropod reactions. Thus, the urticarial lesions of different diseases have different histologic appearances and are distinct from the lesions of the urticarial allergic eruption.

Arthropod Reactions, Superficial

Because arthropod reactions usually involve the vessels of both the superficial and deep plexuses, a discussion in depth of this reaction can be found in Chapter 7. Rarely, will arthropod reactions (timid insects) involve only the upper half of the dermis, and they are then seen as lymphohistiocytic infiltrates with eosinophils around the blood vessels and between the collagen bundles. Extravasated erythrocytes and edema are often present in the papillary dermis.

In its literal meaning *arthropod reactions* refers only to inflammatory responses that result from assaults by true arthropods such as mosquitoes, bedbugs, and scabietic mites. However, the same changes in the dermis may also be caused by such dissimilar organisms as the larvae of Ancylostoma braziliense that cause creeping eruption and the cercariae that cause swimmer's itch.

Arthropod reactions are usually accompanied by epidermal changes such as spongiosis or focal necrosis at the actual site of entry of the sucking or biting parts. The clinical and histologic findings are dependent on the type of assaulting arthropod, the depth of the bite, and the duration of the lesion. Clinically, the usual response to an arthropod assault is an urticarial papule, often with a tiny central vesicle. The papular component is accounted for histologically by both edema and a moderately dense mixed inflammatory-cell infiltrate. If a specimen of the periphery of the papule or nodule is examined with the scanning objective, the infiltrate is more often superficial. The central vesicle is situated intraepidermally, but massive subepidermal edema or explosion of a tense intraepidermal vesicle may also eventuate in subepidermal vesiculation.

"Itchy Red Bump" Disease

—Superficial and mid-dermal perivascular and interstitial mixed-cellular infiltrate of lymphocytes, histiocytes, and eosinophils
—Edema of the papillary dermis

This maddeningly pruritic, persistent condition of grouped lesions in middle-aged and older persons consists of widespread edematous papules that are often misinterpreted clinically as dermatitis herpetiformis or transient acantholytic dermatosis. The name *itchy red bump* disease is what patients (and some of their physicians) in Florida have come to call this condition of as yet unknown cause.

Histologically, the changes are similar to those of superficial insect bites, except that the inflammatory-cell infiltrates in the dermis of reactions to arthropod assaults tend to be deeper and wedge-shaped with the V pointing toward the subcutaneous fat. Despite the histologic resemblance of these lesions to arthropod reactions, patients and clinicians who manage these patients insist that the papules are not caused by insects or other arthropods. Whether "itchy red bump" disease is an entity sui generis or a variant of papular urticaria remains to be learned.

—Moderately dense, superficial and mid-dermal infiltrate of lym-
phocytes, histiocytes, and eosinophils
—Slight edema of the papillary dermis
—Slight spongiosis occasionally

This eruptive condition appears toward the termination of pregnancy as pruritic, discrete, edematous papules in patchy distribution on the abdomen. The eruption extends peripherally, especially toward the thighs, and practically never above the breasts. Sometimes a pallid halo appears in the skin immediately surrounding the papules, but vesicles do not develop. The process usually lasts until delivery, or shortly into the postpartum period, and then resolves spontaneously. Immunofluorescent studies have all been negative for suggestion of an immunologic cause.

The clinical differential diagnosis of papular eruption of pregnancy includes herpes gestationis and reactions to arthropod assaults. These conditions differ histologically from papular eruption of pregnancy by having infiltrates that are both superficial and deep, and by their tendency to vesiculation.

Monomorphous (Mast Cell) Infiltrate

A monomorphous infiltrate around the superficial vascular plexus should suggest a diagnosis of the macular or papular forms of urticaria pigmentosa (telangiectasia macularis eruptiva perstans). The mast cell is the dominant cell in the infiltrate, and there are only a few lymphocytes and histiocytes.

Urticaria Pigmentosa, Macular and Papular Lesions (Fig. 6-14)

—Sparse, predominantly perivascular mast-cell infiltrate with some
lymphocytes and histiocytes
—Telangiectases in upper dermis
—Eosinophils, if the lesion was rubbed before biopsy

The histologic common denominator in all forms of urticaria pigmentosa is an infiltrate, usually in the upper half of the dermis, composed mostly of mast cells. One form of the condition has been named telangiectasia macularis eruptiva perstans because the lesions consist of persistent, tan-orange macules (and papules)

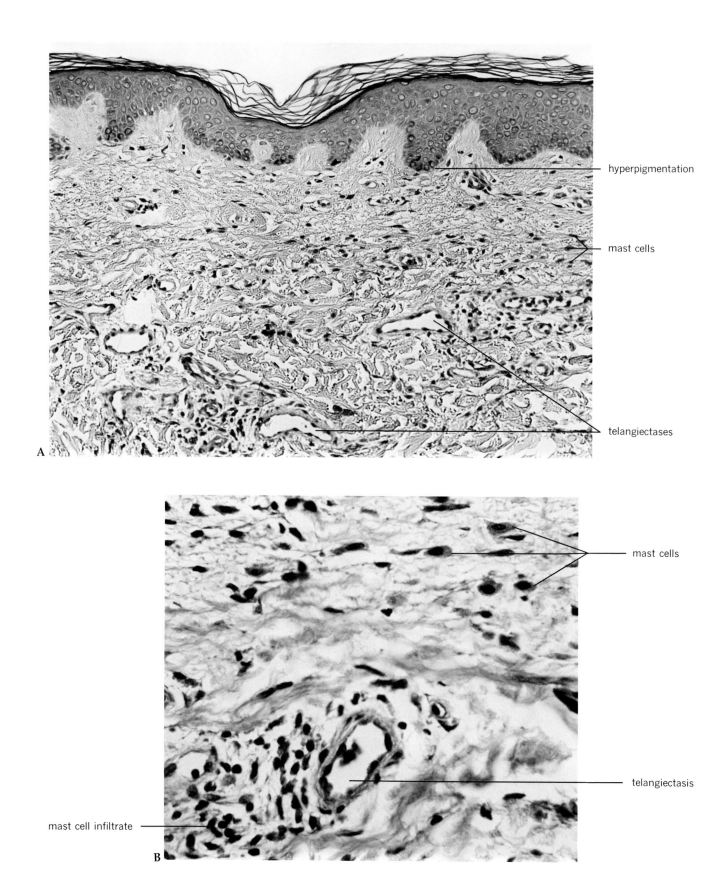

FIG. 6-14. Urticaria pigmentosa, macular and papular lesions. Telangiectases in combination with sparse, but uniform infiltrate of mast cells around widely dilated capillaries and venules and between collagen bundles in upper part of dermis are characteristic of telangiectasia macularis eruptiva perstans. (A, × 168; B, × 600.) The mast cells in this section stained by hematoxylin and eosin can be identified by their dark-staining oval nuclei and pale, finely granular cytoplasm.

interspersed with telangiectases. The macular and papular forms of urticaria pigmentosa are more common in adults, whereas nodular and bullous forms are more frequent in children.

With the scanning objective, the diagnosis of macular or papular urticaria pigmentosa is suggested by a sparse infiltrate around dilated blood vessels of the superficial plexus, and between collagen bundles in the upper dermis. The histologic diagnosis of urticaria pigmentosa can be made on sections stained with hematoxylin and eosin when numerous mast cells are found within the infiltrate. A mast cell has a characteristic cytologic appearance: darkly staining, round to oval nucleus with abundant, pale, pink-purple cytoplasm containing delicate amphophilic granules. When the diagnosis of urticaria pigmentosa is suspected, it should always be confirmed by special stains for mast cells such as the toluidine blue or Giemsa.

Classically, the lesions of macular and papular urticaria pigmentosa become wheals upon rubbing. Biopsy of such artificially provoked wheals will reveal, in addition to mast cells, numerous eosinophils. Some of the mast cells have degranulated.

The lesions of urticaria pigmentosa are tan because there is increased melanin in the epidermis. The telangiectases, which are seen clinically, are a reflection of the widely dilated blood vessels in the upper dermis. Occasionally in nodular lesions of urticaria pigmentosa, massive edema of the papillary dermis, due to histamine release by mast cells, may result in a subepidermal bulla.

Interface Dermatitis

Normally, epidermal rete ridges are so sharply demarcated from dermal papillae that a distinct line can be traced at the dermoepidermal interface. In some superficial perivascular dermatitides this crisp boundary between epidermis and dermis is blurred. Obscuring of the dermoepidermal interface may occur by (1) vacuolar alteration or (2) lichenoid infiltration or both.

When the junction between the epidermis and dermis becomes indistinct as a result of either of these two changes, the histologic picture can be described as superficial perivascular dermatitis with obscuring of the dermoepidermal interface, and the diagnostic category is interface dermatitis. Interface dermatitis can then be subdivided according to whether vacuolar alteration (vacuolar type) or a cellular infiltrate (lichenoid type) is primarily responsible for the blurring of the dermoepidermal interface. Lichenoid infiltrates at the interface are always associated with vacuolar alteration.

Vacuolar Type

In the vacuolar type of interface dermatitis the dermoepidermal interface is obscured by the formation of tiny spaces on either side of the epidermal basement membrane. This histologic pattern is associated with little or no cellular infiltrate at the interface (Fig. 6-3A). Erythema multiforme, with its prominent vacuolar alteration and its meager cellular infiltrate, is the archetype of the vacuolar type.

Erythema Multiforme (including Stevens-Johnson Syndrome) (Fig. 6-15)

—Sparse infiltrate of lymphocytes and histiocytes around the blood vessels of the superficial dermis
—Edema of the papillary dermis
—Extravasated erythrocytes in the papillary dermis
—Vacuolar alteration and a sparse lymphohistiocytic infiltrate along the dermoepidermal interface
—Necrotic keratinocytes at the dermoepidermal junction, throughout the epidermis, and sometimes in the adnexal epithelium
—Slight intracellular epidermal edema (ballooning)
—Slight intercellular epidermal edema (spongiosis)

The features just listed are the earliest histologic changes of erythema multiforme. With time, the infiltrate becomes denser, more extravasated erythrocytes appear in the superficial dermis, the epidermal necrosis becomes more extensive, and the vacuolar alteration can progress to subepidermal separation and eventually to subepidermal vesiculation. Severe ballooning and spongiosis can result in intraepidermal vesiculation. Initially, there are only individually necrotic keratinocytes within the epidermis (Fig. 6-16A). Later, there is confluent epidermal necrosis (Fig. 6-16B). The dermoepidermal junction may be obscured.

The clinical lesions of erythema multiforme are urticarial papules and plaques that become increasingly purpuric and often have an annular configuration. Some lesions, composed of concentric rings, resemble the iris of the eye and the marksman's target. Erythema multiforme usually, but not always, occurs on mucous membranes, especially those of the oral cavity. Intracellular edema and subsequent intraepithelial vesiculation are more prominent in mucous membranes than in skin. The gray color of the blisters in erythema multiforme results from epidermal necrosis; the red indurated rings, from vascular dilatation and dermal edema; and the purpura, from extravasated erythrocytes in the superficial dermis.

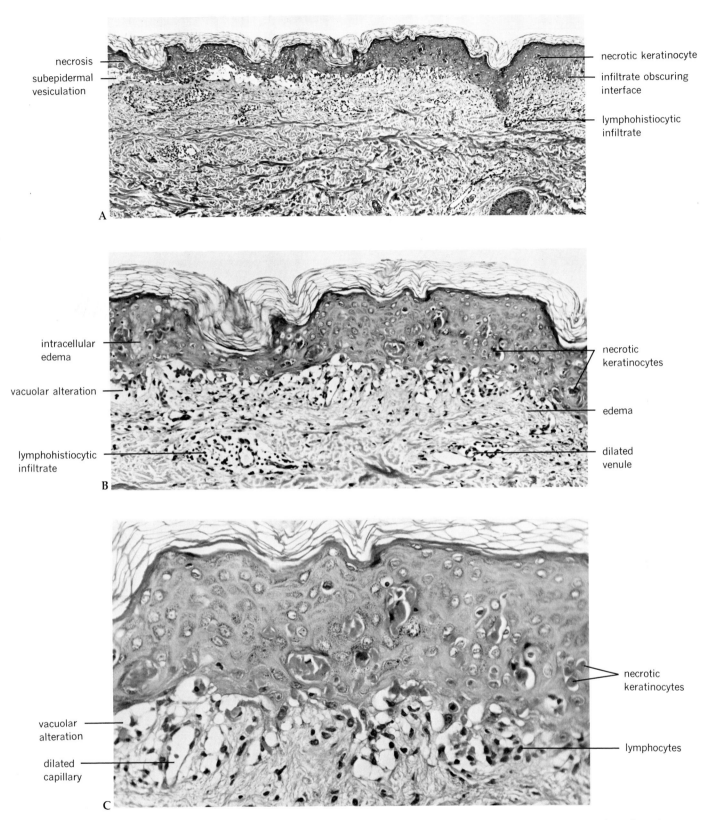

necrosis

subepidermal
vesiculation

necrotic keratinocyte

infiltrate obscuring
interface

lymphohistiocytic
infiltrate

intracellular
edema

vacuolar alteration

lymphohistiocytic
infiltrate

necrotic
keratinocytes

edema

dilated
venule

vacuolar
alteration

dilated
capillary

necrotic
keratinocytes

lymphocytes

FIG. 6-15. Erythema multiforme. A, Even under scanning magnification, the constellation of necrotic epidermal keratinocytes, vacuolar alteration of the dermoepidermal interface, dermoepidermal separation, and sparse superficial perivascular infiltrate of lymphocytes and histiocytes can be seen. (× 68.) B, Early changes of the disease, i.e., individually necrotic keratinocytes, slight ballooning, vacuolar alteration, and sparse superficial infiltrate of lymphocytes and histiocytes, are illustrated. (× 149.) C, The individual necrotic keratinocytes pictured will eventuate in complete epidermal necrosis, and vacuolar alteration will progress to dermoepidermal separation and vesiculation. (× 316.)

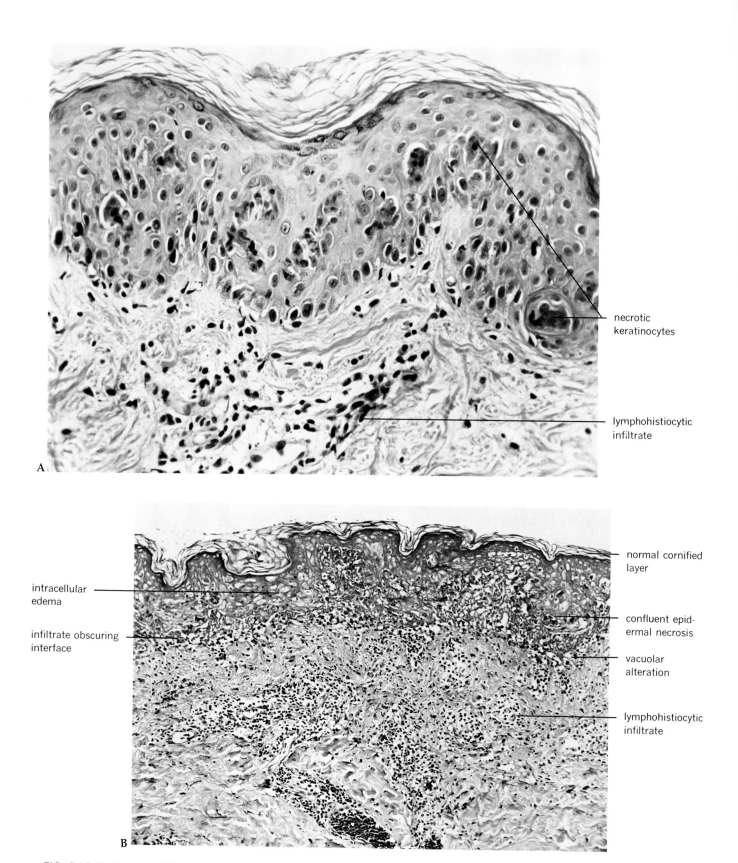

FIG. 6-16. Erythema multiforme. A, Necrotic keratinocytes are scattered throughout epidermis of this section of an early lesion. The patient also had clinical features of toxic epidermal necrolysis in addition to "iris" and "target" lesions. (× 299.) B, In this later lesion, basket-weave pattern of normal cornified layer above complete epidermal necrosis indicates that lesion is still of recent onset, perhaps 24 to 48 hours ago. Mononuclear cells and vacuolar alteration obscure the dermoepidermal junction. (× 140.)

Erythema multiforme has a specific and distinctive histologic pattern. It is a single pathologic process that involves both the dermis and the epidermis. Unfortunately, the clinical diagnosis erythema multiforme is often incorrectly applied to a variety of urticarial eruptions that have annular, arcuate, and serpiginous shapes. Many lesions labeled erythema multiforme clinically are actually urticarial allergic eruptions, usually drug induced, that have a mixed inflammatory-cell infiltrate and are not associated with histologic alterations of the dermoepidermal interface. The urticarial lesions of pemphigoid are also sometimes misdiagnosed, both clinically and histologically, as erythema multiforme. This error is largely left over from that period, before pemphigoid had been specifically recognized, when cases of what are now called pemphigoid were called chronic bullous erythema multiforme. Pemphigoid, unlike erythema multiforme, which usually has no eosinophils, is characterized histologically by the presence of eosinophils. Clinically, pemphigoid lacks iris or target lesions, does not favor acral areas, and usually spares mucous membranes.

The cause of erythema multiforme cannot be ascertained in the majority of cases. Some causal agents are drugs, mycoplasma, herpesvirus, and vaccinia. Regardless of cause, the clinical and histologic lesions of erythema multiforme are characteristic. The histologic differential diagnosis includes toxic epidermal necrolysis and graft-versus-host reactions, from which erythema multiforme cannot always be distinguished. It may well be that these conditions are related and merely different manifestations of the same pathologic process. Epidermal changes indistinguishable from those of erythema multiforme can also be seen in pityriasis lichenoides et varioliformes acuta (Mucha-Habermann disease) and in acute fixed drug eruption.

Toxic Epidermal Necrolysis

Histologically, toxic epidermal necrolysis is often indistinguishable from erythema multiforme. Clinically, toxic epidermal necrolysis consists of flaccid bullae that can easily be peeled off the skin like wet tissue paper. The bullae can be huge and widespread. In some cases of toxic epidermal necrolysis, iris and target lesions characteristic of erythema multiforme are present simultaneously with sheets of flaccid blisters. Because they share histologic and clinical similarities, toxic epidermal necrolysis and erythema multiforme could be different names for the same disease.

Toxic epidermal necrolysis is discussed more fully in Chapter 11. The staphylococcal scalded-skin syndrome is discussed in Chapter 10.

Phototoxic Contact Dermatitis and Phototoxic Dermatitis (Fig. 6-17)

—Sparse superficial perivascular lymphohistiocytic infiltrate
—Vacuolar alteration along the dermoepidermal interface
—Intracellular edema
—Variable epidermal necrosis ranging from individual necrotic keratinocytes to confluent necrosis (Fig. 6-18)

Sunburn is the prototypic example of the phototoxic reaction. Some systemically administered medications, such as the tetracyclines, accentuate the sunburn response (phototoxic dermatitis), as do topically applied materials such as psoralens, tars, and certain dyes (phototoxic contact dermatitis).

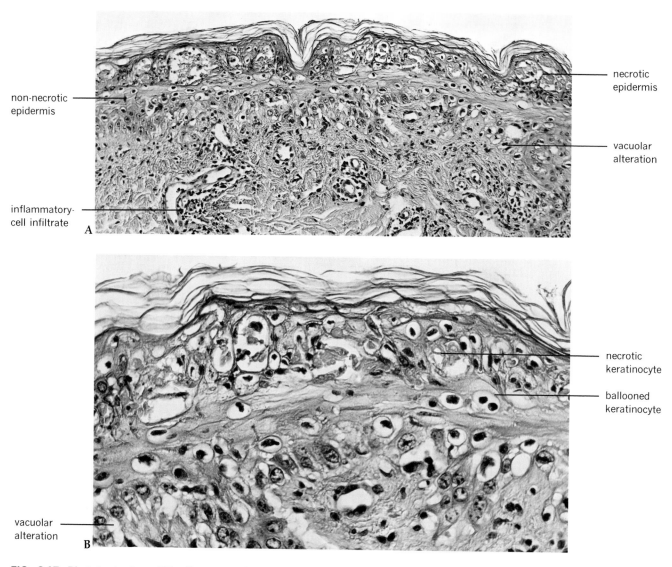

FIG. 6-17. Phototoxic dermatitis. Presence of epidermal necrosis beneath cornified layer with normal basket-weave pattern indicates that injury was sudden and recent. (× 159.) B, Preponderance of necrotic keratinocytes in upper outer portion of epidermis indicates that source of damage to skin was external, as by ultraviolet light. (× 403.)

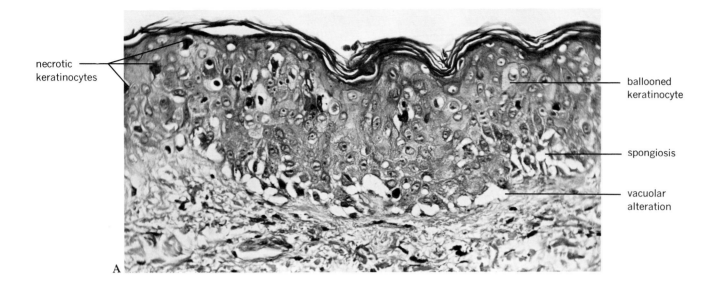

necrotic keratinocytes

ballooned keratinocyte

spongiosis

vacuolar alteration

A

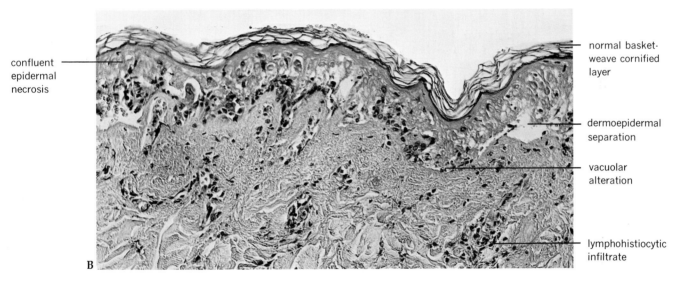

confluent epidermal necrosis

normal basket-weave cornified layer

dermoepidermal separation

vacuolar alteration

lymphohistiocytic infiltrate

B

FIG. 6-18. Phototoxic dermatitis. A, Early stage in patient with sunburn consists of scattered necrotic keratinocytes ("sunburn cells"), vacuolar alteration, and sparse superficial perivascular lymphohistiocytic infiltrate. (× 300.) B, Later stage. Normal basket-weave pattern of cornified layer and necrotic epidermis indicate that precipitating event, damage by ultraviolet radiation, occurred within day or two. (× 227.)

Dermatomyositis (Fig. 6-19)

—Sparse lymphohistiocytic infiltrate both around the vessels of the superficial plexus and scattered throughout the papillary dermis, sometimes with extravasated erythrocytes

—Varying amounts of mucin among collagen bundles in the upper dermis

—Variable edema in the upper dermis

—Vacuolar alteration along the dermoepidermal interface

—Thickened basement membrane in long-standing lesions

—Thin epidermis with a reduced pattern of rete and papillae

The histologic changes of the dermoepidermal interface in dermatomyositis are often indistinguishable from those of discoid lupus erythematosus. In acute discoid lupus erythematosus, however, the dermal infiltrate is usually more dense and may be both superficial and deep, whereas in subacute and chronic discoid lupus erythematosus, the basement membrane and the cornified layer are usually thicker. It may be impossible to distinguish dermatomyositis histologically from the early stages of discoid lupus erythematosus when the infiltrate may be wholly superficial.

Early lesions of dermatomyositis are characterized clinically by violaceous erythema, edema, and telangiectases; later lesions are atrophic with hypopigmentation and hyperpigmentation, as well as telangiectases (poikilodermatomyositis). The widely dilated blood vessels of the superficial plexus are responsible for the telangiectases and contribute to the characteristic heliotrope hue. Periorbital swelling is due to dermal edema. Atrophy results from sclerosis of the papillary dermis.

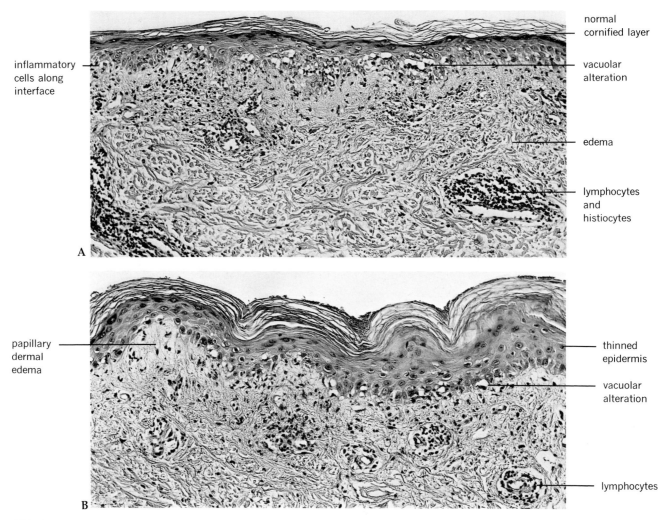

FIG. 6-19. Dermatomyositis, early stage. Thinned epidermis, vacuolar alteration at dermoepidermal interface, edema of papillary dermis, and superficial perivascular predominantly lymphocytic infiltrate are indistinguishable from changes in acute discoid lupus erythematosus. (A, × 133; B, × 136.)

As just noted, early stages of discoid lupus erythematosus may have histologic features that are indistinguishable from those of dermatomyositis. Usually, however, the infiltrate of acute discoid lupus erythematosus is denser and deeper. Abundant mucin may be present in the dermis of both dermatomyositis and discoid lupus erythematosus. Because discoid lupus erythematosus usually involves the deep, as well as the superficial, plexus, it will be discussed in detail in Chapter 7.

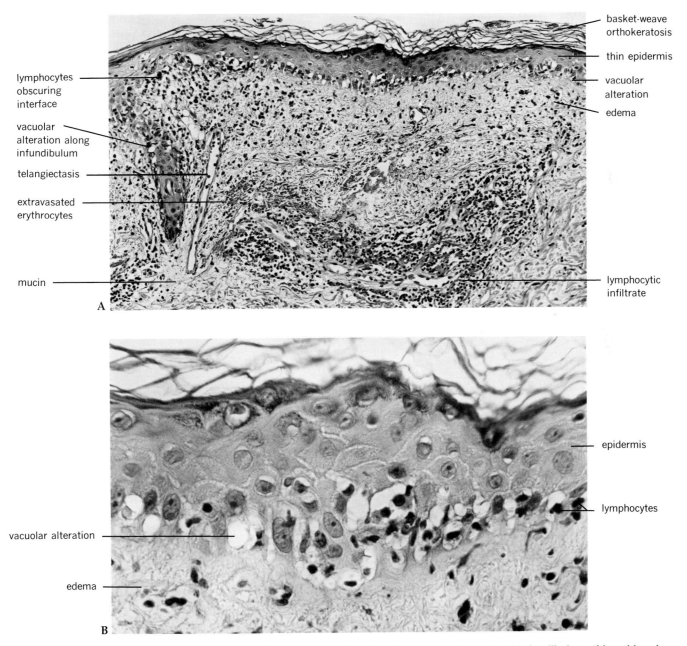

FIG. 6-20. Discoid lupus erythematosus, acute. Prominent vacuolar alteration along epidermis and infundibulum, thin epidermis devoid of rete ridges, lymphocytes obscuring dermoepidermal interface, mucin in upper dermis, and superficial predominantly lymphocytic infiltrate around telangiectatic vessels are features. (A, × 138; B, × 610.)

Some Morbilliform Drug Eruptions (Fig. 6-21)

—Sparse-to-moderately dense infiltrate of lymphocytes and histiocytes around the superficial vascular plexus
—Sparse lymphohistiocytic infiltrate along the dermoepidermal interface
—Slight vacuolar alteration of the dermoepidermal junction
—Occasionally extravasated erythrocytes in the papillary dermis

Among the many histologic patterns produced by drugs is interface dermatitis, vacuolar type. In the past, eruptions with these histologic features were termed toxic erythemas. There is no evidence that toxins in the sense of inherent poisons are involved. In fact, most are morbilliform drug eruptions, to be distinguished from urticarial drug eruptions in which the infiltrate of mixed-inflammatory cells is confined to the dermis and does not involve the dermoepidermal junction.

Drugs, regardless of the route administered, can induce a multiplicity of eruptions simulating almost every inflammatory histologic pattern in skin. For example, drug eruptions can histologically mimic lichen planus, psoriasis, and pityriasis rosea. They can also cause highly specific changes such as the fixed drug

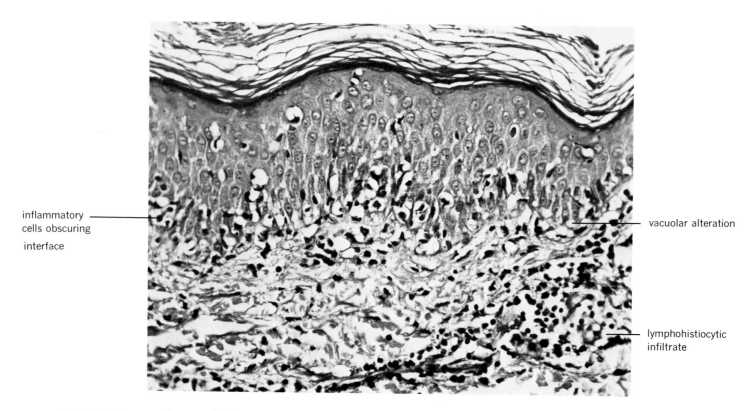

inflammatory cells obscuring interface

vacuolar alteration

lymphohistiocytic infiltrate

FIG. 6-21. Drug eruption, morbilliform type. Histologic changes shown are similar to those of erythema multiforme, but note absence of necrotic keratinocytes. ($\times$ 370.)

eruption. Drugs are among the major causes of erythema multiforme, toxic epidermal necrolysis, erythema nodosum, and urticarial allergic eruptions.

Morbilliform drug eruptions share histologic features in common with erythema multiforme, but differ by the absence of necrotic epidermal keratinocytes in abundance. Morbilliform drug eruptions are distinguishable from older lesions of dermatomyositis and chronic discoid lupus erythematosus by the absence of basement-membrane thickening. Histologic changes similar to those in morbilliform drug eruptions may be seen in some morbilliform viral exanthems.

Some Morbilliform Viral Eruptions

—Sparse lymphohistiocytic infiltrate around the blood vessels of the superficial plexus
—Obscuring of the dermoepidermal interface by the infiltrate in conjunction with vacuolar alteration

The histologic changes in some morbilliform viral eruptions are often identical to those for the morbilliform type of drug eruption. Diseases such as infectious mononucleosis are typical of this group of viral eruptions. In general, these viral exanthems are macular and papular erythemas.

Erythema Dyschromicum Perstans (Fig. 6-22)

—Sparse lymphohistiocytic infiltrate around the vessels of the superficial plexus and, in active lesions, at the dermoepidermal junction
—Melanophages in the papillary dermis
—Vacuolar alteration along the dermoepidermal interface
—Diminished rete-papillae pattern
—Epidermal hyperpigmentation

Early active lesions of erythema dyschromicum perstans may have slightly lichenoid inflammatory-cell infiltrates in the papillary dermis. In older, less active lesions there is only vacuolar alteration, and no inflammatory cells are seen at the dermoepidermal interface.

This disease is named erythema dyschromicum perstans because of its persistent patches of dusky erythema. The ashy color of these patches results in part from the combined influences of

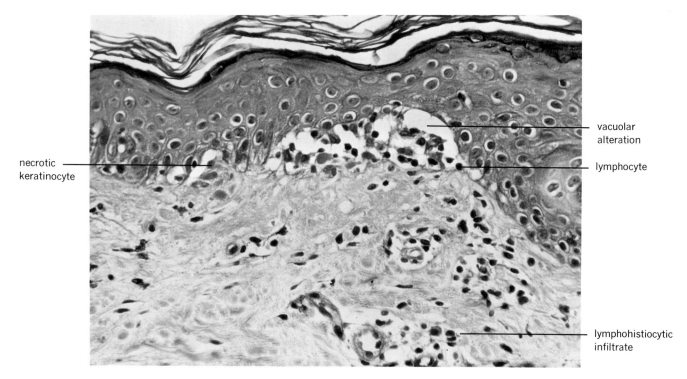

necrotic keratinocyte

vacuolar alteration

lymphocyte

lymphohistiocytic infiltrate

FIG. 6-22. Erythema dyschromicum perstans. Early histologic changes illustrated are especially conspicuous at dermoepidermal interface which is obscured by severe vacuolar alteration, necrotic keratinocytes, and scattered lymphocytes. (×444.)

epidermal hyperpigmentation, melanophages in the papillary dermis, and dilated superficial blood vessels. As the process evolves, there may be simultaneous inflammatory (a lymphohistiocytic infiltrate around dilated blood vessels) and postinflammatory (increased epidermal and dermal melanin) features. The cause of erythema dyschromicum perstans is unknown.

Lichen Sclerosus et Atrophicus (Fig. 6-23)

—Moderately dense predominantly lymphocytic infiltrate with histiocytes and plasma cells around the blood vessels of the depressed superficial plexus
—Prominent edema within thickened papillary dermis and separation of thin collagen fibrils
—Telangiectases throughout the upper half of the dermis
—Vacuolar alteration of the dermoepidermal interface
—Thin epidermis (unless thickened by chronic rubbing)
—Orthokeratosis with infundibular and acrosyringeal plugging

The earliest clinical changes of lichen sclerosus are clearly inflammatory, namely, pink-rose, firm papules and plaques that, in time, proceed to white atrophic patches. During the indurated inflammatory stage, edema of the papillary dermis is prominent (Fig. 6-24A), and the lymphohistiocytic infiltrate is moderately

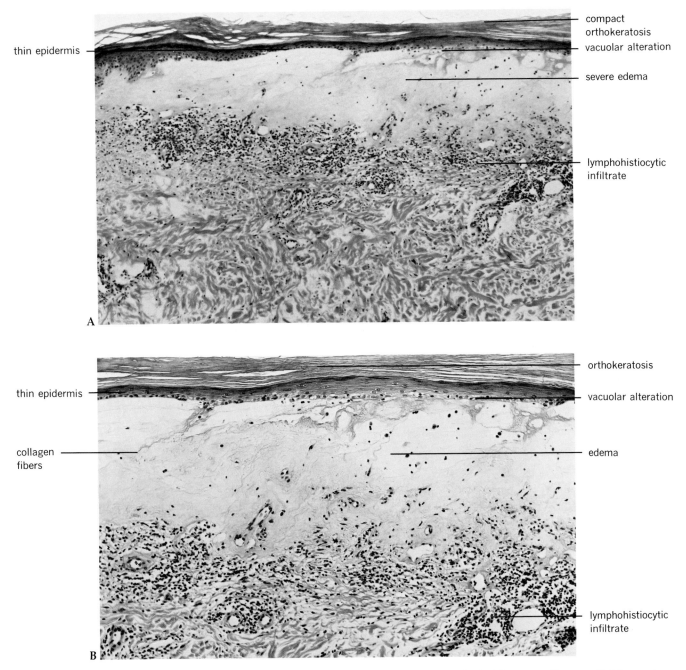

thin epidermis

compact orthokeratosis
vacuolar alteration
severe edema

lymphohistiocytic infiltrate

A

thin epidermis

collagen fibers

orthokeratosis
vacuolar alteration

edema

lymphohistiocytic infiltrate

B

FIG. 6-23. Lichen sclerosus et atrophicus. Note edematous and thickened papillary dermis that depresses the superficial vascular plexus and thus the inflammatory-cell infiltrate. Fine collagen fibers are recognizable in edematous papillary dermis. (A, × 85; B, × 140.)

dense. Acid mucopolysaccharides can be demonstrated in the edematous and thickened papillary dermis. Eventually, the inflammatory-cell infiltrate decreases and the mucinous edema is replaced by sclerotic collagen (Fig. 6-24B). This change is eventually manifested clinically by white atrophic lesions for which the disease is named. Dells within the atrophic areas result from adnexal plugging by cornified cells. Clinical activity can be judged by the presence of erythema at the periphery of the lesions. Some

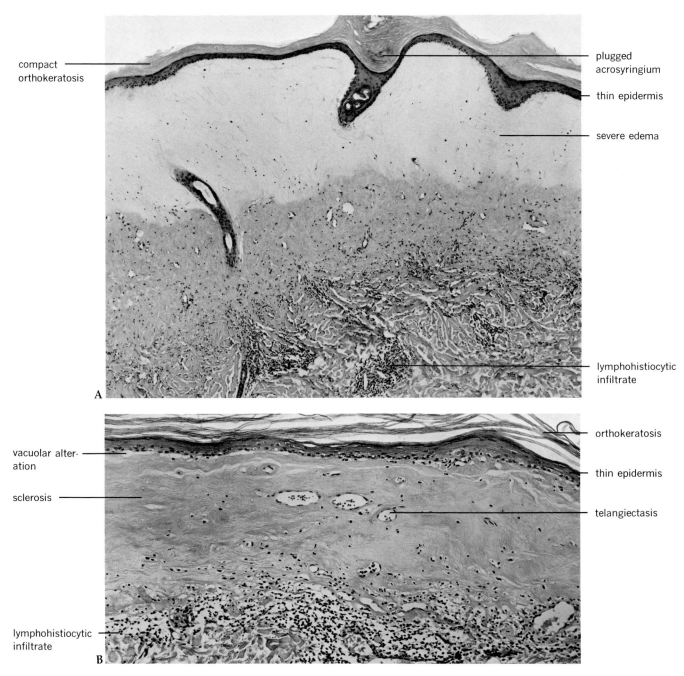

compact orthokeratosis

plugged acrosyringium

thin epidermis

severe edema

lymphohistiocytic infiltrate

A

vacuolar alteration

sclerosis

orthokeratosis

thin epidermis

telangiectasis

lymphohistiocytic infiltrate

B

FIG. 6-24. Lichen sclerosus et atrophicus. A, Relatively early lesion with extensive edema in thickened papillary dermis seated between thin epidermis and moderately dense lymphocytic infiltrate around blood vessels of superficial plexus. Dilated acrosyringium is plugged by cornified cells. (× 60.) B, Older lesion with sclerosis replacing edema in thickened papillary dermis that lies between thin epidermis without rete edges and moderately dense, predominantly lymphocytic infiltrate around blood vessels of superficial plexus. (× 133.)

lesions of lichen sclerosus et atrophicus in children undergo spontaneous and complete involution.

Lichen sclerosus et atrophicus in the anogenital region of women can be distressingly pruritic. When chronically scratched and rubbed, the lesions are altered clinically and histologically by the superimposition of erosions, ulcerations, and features of lichen simplex chronicus.

—Variable infiltrate of lymphocytes, histiocytes and melanophages
—Large bizarre fibroblasts, some multinucleated, within the upper part of the sclerotic dermis
—Absence of adnexal structures
—Some fibrotic blood vessels in the deep dermis and some lumina occluded by intimal thickening and thrombosis
—Subendothelial vacuolar alteration
—Telangiectases throughout the upper part of the dermis
—Fibrillary eosinophilic material (fibrin) at the dermoepidermal interface and around the blood vessels of the superficial plexus
—Prominent vacuolar alteration of the dermoepidermal interface
—Thin epidermis, sometimes hyperkeratotic, eroded, or ulcerated

The presence of bizarre fibroblasts, having large, pleomorphic nuclei, in a sclerotic dermis is diagnostic of radiodermatitis. The clinical expression of chronic radiodermatitis is poikiloderma (hyperpigmentation and hypopigmentation, atrophy, and telangiectasia). Sclerosis of the papillary dermis results in the clinical appearance of atrophy; dilated blood vessels in the papillary dermis cause telangiectases; and an increase or a decrease of epidermal pigment is responsible for the mottled hyperpigmenta-

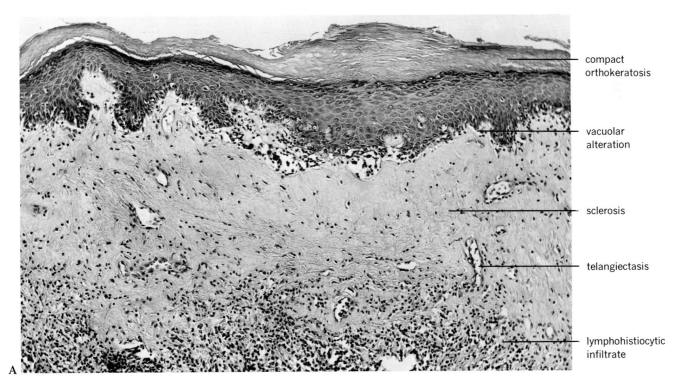

compact orthokeratosis

vacuolar alteration

sclerosis

telangiectasis

lymphohistiocytic infiltrate

A

FIG. 6-25. Radiodermatitis, chronic. A, Histologic changes, i.e., compact orthokeratosis, vacuolar alteration, sclerosis of thickened papillary dermis, and moderately dense infiltrate of lymphocytes and histiocytes around blood vessels of superficial plexus, closely resemble those of lichen sclerosus et atrophicus. (× 120.)

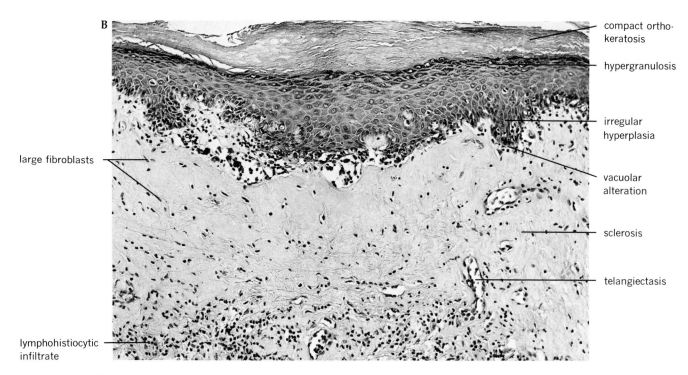

large fibroblasts

lymphohistiocytic infiltrate

compact ortho-keratosis

hypergranulosis

irregular hyperplasia

vacuolar alteration

sclerosis

telangiectasis

FIG. 6-25. B, With higher magnification, large atypical fibroblasts in papillary dermis can be visualized. They help to differentiate chronic radiodermatitis from lichen sclerosus et atrophicus. (× 197.)

tion and hypopigmentation. Ulceration may result from occlusion of dermal blood vessels by intimal thickening or thrombosis.

Keratinocytic and/or melanocytic nuclear atypia may be seen in the epidermis overlying radiation sclerosis. Furthermore, basal-cell carcinomas, squamous-cell carcinomas, keratoses, atypical fibroxanthomas, fibromatoses, sarcomas, and malignant melanomas may develop in areas of chronic radiodermatitis.

Poikiloderma Congenitale (Rothmund-Thomson Syndrome)

—Superficial perivascular lymphohistiocytic infiltrate
—Variable number of melanophages in the papillary dermis
—Telangiectases in the papillary dermis
—Slight fibrosis of the papillary dermis
—Vacuolar alteration at the dermoepidermal junction
—Thin epidermis without the usual configuration of rete and papillae

Poikiloderma congenitale, a recessively inherited inflammatory disease of infancy, begins with widespread erythema that eventually progresses to mottled atrophy, hyperpigmentation, hypopigmentation, and telangiectases. Often there are associated developmental defects such as dwarfism and hypogonadism, as well as cataracts.

—Superficial perivascular lymphohistiocytic infiltrate with numerous eosinophils and rare neutrophils
—Edema of the papillary dermis
—Vacuolar alteration at the dermoepidermal junction
—Few eosinophils within the epidermis

When numerous eosinophils are present within the epidermis, there may be concomitant spongiosis in the urticarial stage of pemphigoid. Slight vacuolar alteration precedes subepidermal vesiculation that is found in the blistering stage of pemphigoid.

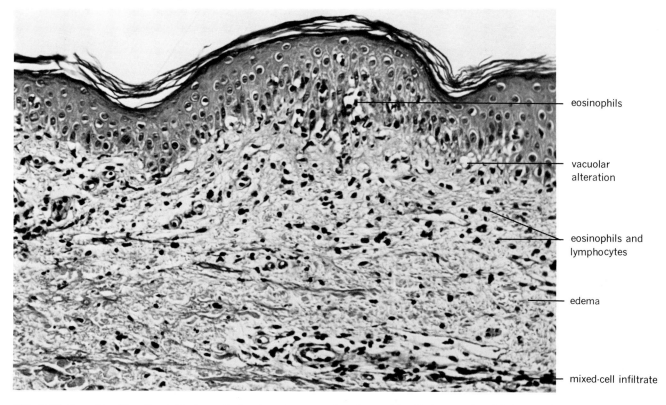

eosinophils

vacuolar alteration

eosinophils and lymphocytes

edema

mixed-cell infiltrate

FIG. 6-26. Pemphigoid, urticarial lesions. Early edematous papules of pemphigoid show eosinophils in dermis, at dermoepidermal interface, and often within epidermis in conjunction with edema of papillary dermis. (× 220.)

Lichenoid Type (Fig. 6-3B)

The second category of infiltrates involving the dermoepidermal interface is characterized by a dense bandlike cellular infiltrate throughout the superficial dermis. With the scanning objective, this dense diffuse superficial infiltrate is seen immediately beneath the epidermis and parallel to it. Some of the cells extend into the epidermis and others obscure the dermoepidermal interface. The archetype of this pattern is lichen planus.

Lichen Planus (Fig. 6-27)

—Dense lymphohistiocytic infiltrate with melanophages around the vessels of the superficial plexus and throughout the papillary dermis, obscuring the dermoepidermal interface
—Coarse collagen bundles in the thickened papillary dermis
—Increased number of dilated, moderately thick-walled blood vessels in the upper dermis
—Vacuolar alteration at the dermoepidermal interface which, when severe, forms subepidermal clefts (Max Joseph spaces) (Fig. 6-28A)
—Homogeneous eosinophilic bodies (Civatte bodies, dyskeratotic cells) in the papillary dermis, at the dermoepidermal interface, and within the epidermis (Fig. 6-28B)
—Irregular epidermal hyperplasia with jagged sawtooth appearance of the rete and a slightly eosinophilic hue (Fig. 6-28A)
—Hypergranulosis, often with V-shaped foci
—Compact orthokeratosis

Each typical, flat-topped, shiny, polygonal papule of lichen planus results from a thickened papillary dermis filled with a dense bandlike infiltrate, as well as from thickening of the epidermis (Fig. 6-29). The characteristic violaceous color probably results from the combined effects of dilated blood vessels, melanophages, the dense superficial inflammatory-cell infiltrate and the thickened papillary dermis.

Atrophic lichen planus differs from the usual type of lichen planus by having a thin epidermis devoid of a rete ridge-dermal papillae pattern and a relatively scant, but bandlike, cellular infiltrate (Fig. 6-30A). Hypertrophic lichen planus differs by having a thickened epidermis with broad, rounded rete and a thickened papillary dermis (Fig. 6-30B). The papillary dermis of hypertrophic lichen planus has features of lichen simplex chronicus, indicating that this form of lichen planus results, in part, from prolonged rubbing. Foci of parakeratosis may indicate that the lesion has also been scratched.

Lichen planus must be distinguished histologically from discoid lupus erythematosus. The major difference is that the infiltrate in lichen planus is confined to the upper part of the dermis, whereas the infiltrate in discoid lupus erythematosus is usually both superficial and deep. In addition, the epidermis in lichen planus is usually thickened, whereas that of lupus erythematosus is usually not associated with hypergranulosis and in time has a prominent basement membrane. Plasma cells are rare in lichen planus but common in discoid lupus erythematosus. Nonetheless, in a particular case, it may be impossible to distinguish lichen planus from discoid lupus erythematosus with certainty.

A reputed variant of lichen planus common to the Middle East occurs only on uncovered parts of the body and is worsened by sunlight. This sun-related form is known, among other names, as lichen planus actinicus.

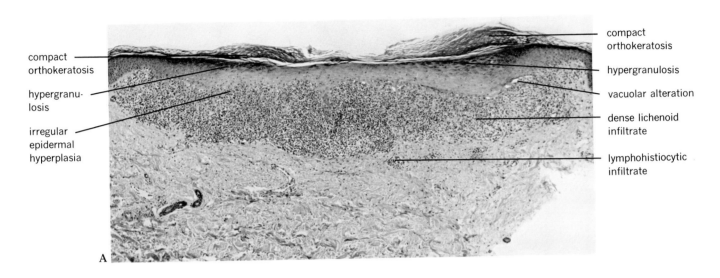

compact orthokeratosis

hypergranu-losis

irregular epidermal hyperplasia

compact orthokeratosis

hypergranulosis

vacuolar alteration

dense lichenoid infiltrate

lymphohistiocytic infiltrate

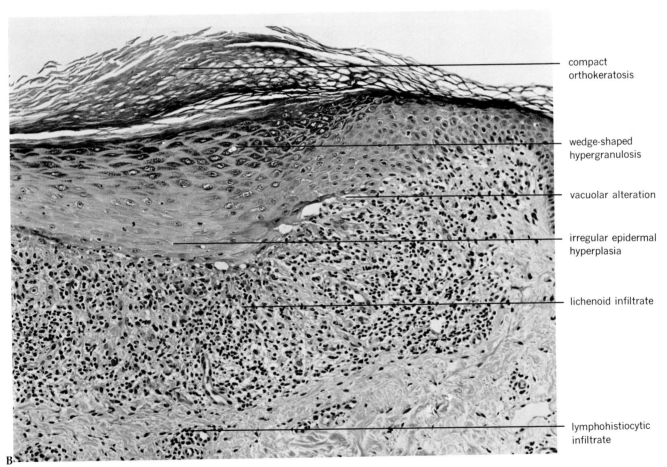

compact orthokeratosis

wedge-shaped hypergranulosis

vacuolar alteration

irregular epidermal hyperplasia

lichenoid infiltrate

lymphohistiocytic infiltrate

FIG. 6-27. Lichen planus. Diagnostic features seen in these photomicrographs include orthokeratosis, focal hypergranulosis, vacuolar alteration, irregular epidermal hyperplasia, and lichenoid infiltrate of lymphocytes and histiocytes that obscures dermoepidermal junction. (A, × 52; B, × 140.)

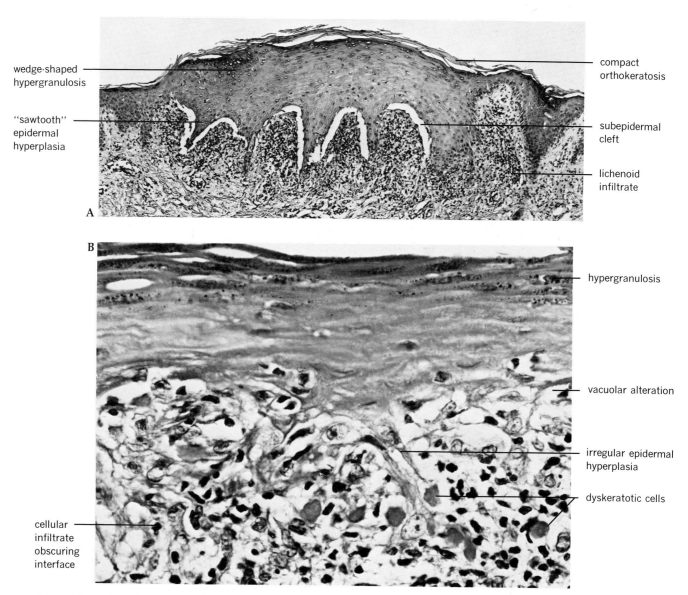

wedge-shaped
hypergranulosis

"sawtooth"
epidermal
hyperplasia

compact
orthokeratosis

subepidermal
cleft

lichenoid
infiltrate

A

B

hypergranulosis

vacuolar alteration

irregular epidermal
hyperplasia

dyskeratotic cells

cellular
infiltrate
obscuring
interface

FIG. 6-28. Lichen planus. A, Note subepidermal clefts formed by coalescence of vacuoles between sawtooth rete ridges and lichenoid infiltrate of lymphocytes and histiocytes. ($\times$ 720.) B, Vacuolar alteration and dyskeratotic cells can be seen. ($\times$ 627.)

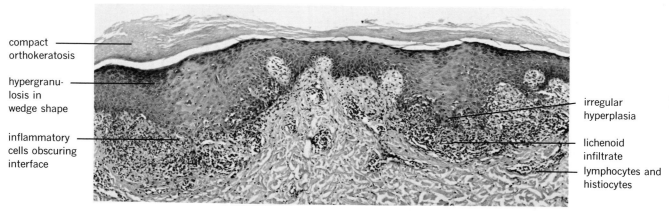

compact
orthokeratosis

hypergranu-
losis in
wedge shape

inflammatory
cells obscuring
interface

irregular
hyperplasia

lichenoid
infiltrate

lymphocytes and
histiocytes

FIG. 6-29. Lichen planus, two early papules. Note two discrete foci of irregular epidermal hyperplasia and lichenoid infiltrate with lymphocytes. Each focus corresponds to a clinical papule. ($\times$ 70.)

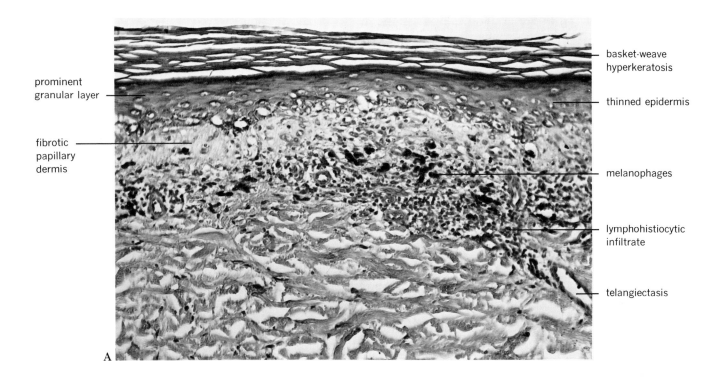

prominent
granular layer

fibrotic
papillary
dermis

basket-weave
hyperkeratosis

thinned epidermis

melanophages

lymphohistiocytic
infiltrate

telangiectasis

A

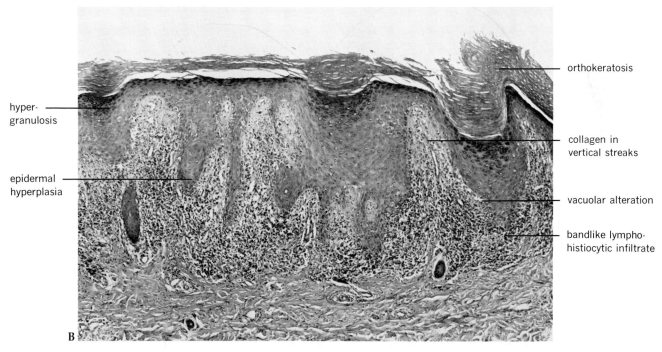

hyper-
granulosis

epidermal
hyperplasia

orthokeratosis

collagen in
vertical streaks

vacuolar alteration

bandlike lympho-
histiocytic infiltrate

B

FIG. 6-30. Lichen planus. A, Atrophic. Atrophic lesions of lichen planus are differentiated histologically from fully developed active lesions of lichen planus by having basket-weave rather than compact orthokeratosis, slightly confluent rather than markedly wedge-shaped hypergranulosis, thinned rather than irregularly hyperplastic epidermis, few rather than many dyskeratotic cells at the dermoepidermal interface, sparse rather than dense bandlike lymphohistiocytic infiltration, and considerable rather than little fibrosis in the papillary dermis. In sum, atrophic lichen planus represents resolving or resolved lichen planus. (× 202.) B, Hypertrophic. The combined features of orthokeratosis, hypergranulosis, irregular epidermal hyperplasia, vacuolar alteration, collagen in vertical streaks within thickened papillary dermis, and bandlike lymphohistiocytic infiltrate in papillary dermis that obscures dermoepidermal interface represent lichen simplex chronicus superimposed upon lichen planus, the result of intense pruritus and persistent rubbing. (× 60.)

Lichen-planuslike Keratoses

Although generally not diagnostic clinically, certain solitary lesions closely resemble those of lichen planus histologically. There are two major variants of keratoses that are lichen-planuslike: one that is virtually indistinguishable histologically from true lichen planus (Fig. 6-31) and the other, a solar keratosis with a dense bandlike cellular infiltrate throughout the papillary dermis that

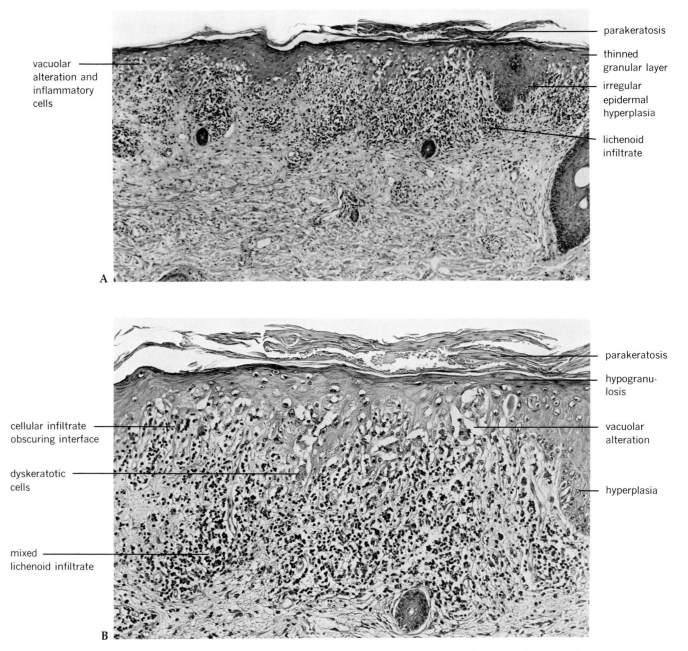

FIG. 6-31. Lichen-planuslike keratosis. Histologic features that may help in differentiating this solitary keratosis from true lichen planus are focal presence of parakeratosis, focal absence or diminution of granular layer, and occasionally plasma cells and eosinophils in the lichenoid infiltrate. (A, × 69; B, × 158.) Note parakeratosis and hypogranulosis, features not usually seen in true lichen planus.

simulates lichen planus (Fig. 6-32). Histologic clues to the detection of keratoses masquerading as lichen planus are the occasional presence of plasma cells and eosinophils within the infiltrate and of focal parakeratosis. An additional clue to the keratosis is the near constancy of elastotic material in the dermis. The lichen-planuslike solar keratosis is distinguished from lichen planus by the presence of atypical keratinocytic nuclei having eosinophilic cytoplasm and by a diminution, rather than thickening, of the granular zone in some lesions.

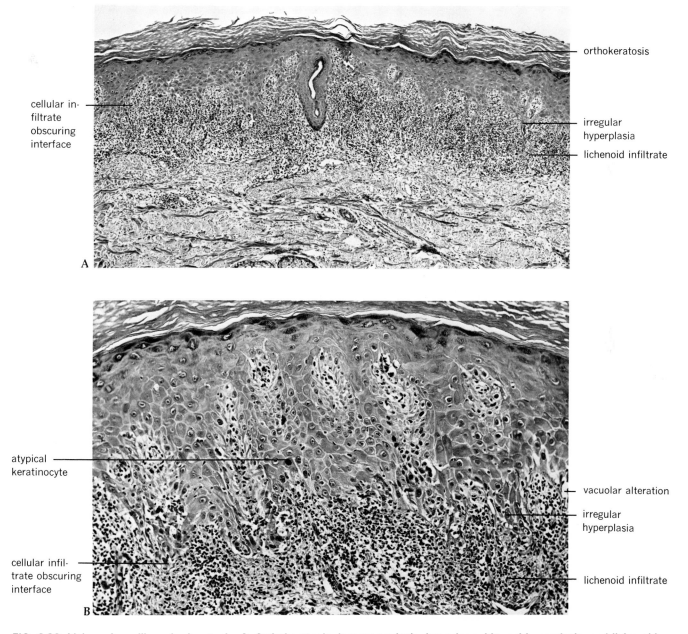

FIG. 6-32. Lichen-planuslike solar keratosis. A, Orthokeratosis, hypergranulosis, irregular epidermal hyperplasia, and lichenoid infiltrate of lymphocytes and histiocytes obscuring the dermoepidermal interface in this specimen are similar to those from a lesion of true lichen planus, (× 60.) B, Atypical epidermal hyperplasia in this solitary lesion indicates it may be an unusual solar keratosis with a lichenoid inflammatory-cell infiltrate. (× 150.)

Lichen-planuslike keratoses occur as solitary lesions predominantly on sun-exposed skin, especially on the chest of older individuals. The presumptive clinical diagnosis is frequently keratosis or basal-cell carcinoma, and only rarely solitary lichen planus or lichen-planuslike keratosis. Lichen-planuslike keratoses are included here because they can be easily confused with lichen planus and lichen-planuslike inflammatory diseases.

Lichen-planuslike Drug Eruptions

The lesions of some drug eruptions are histologically similar to lichen planus. A suggestion of drug etiology is the presence of eosinophils and plasma cells in the infiltrate, rather than just lymphocytes and histiocytes, as is characteristic of lichen planus. In addition, the perivascular infiltrate in lichen-planuslike drug eruptions is often deep, as well as superficial. Focal parakeratosis and a thin epidermis are further evidence that the lesion is an imposter of true lichen planus (Fig. 6-33). These drug-induced lesions also closely simulate lichen planus clinically. Drugs that tend to induce lichen-planuslike eruptions are gold salts, thiazides, and antimalarials.

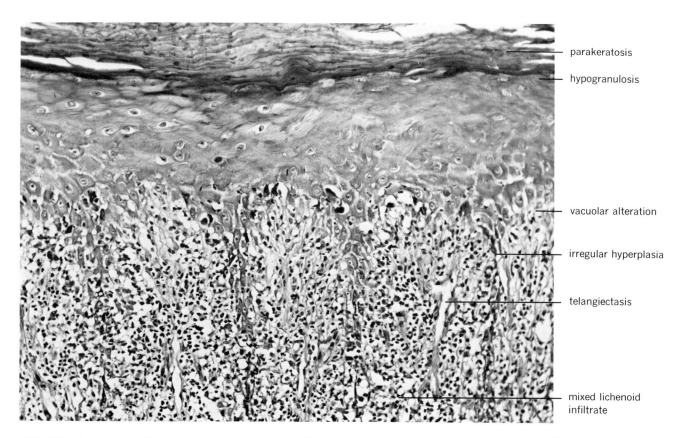

FIG. 6-33. Lichen-planuslike drug eruption from gold. A, Parakeratosis, hypogranulosis, and mixed-cell infiltrate of lymphocytes, histiocytes, and sometimes eosinophils and plasma cells differentiate this dermatitis from true lichen planus. (× 162.)

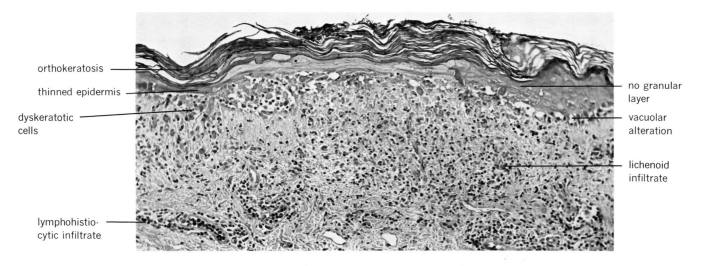

orthokeratosis

thinned epidermis

dyskeratotic cells

lymphohistio-cytic infiltrate

no granular layer

vacuolar alteration

lichenoid infiltrate

FIG. 6-33. B, Note absence of granular layer and thinned epidermis in this lichen-planuslike gold dermatitis. (× 150.)

Lichenoid Purpura (Gougerot-Blum) (Fig. 6-34)

—Dense lymphohistiocytic infiltrate throughout the papillary dermis and obscuring the dermoepidermal interface
—Extravasated erythrocytes in the papillary dermis
—Macrophages containing hemosiderin (siderophages) in the papillary dermis
—Thickening of the papillary dermis by coarse collagen
—Slight epidermal hyperplasia
—Focal parakeratosis

The presence of numerous extravasated erythrocytes, siderophages, and parakeratosis differentiates the lichenoid purpuric eruptions from lichen planus. Clinically, these purpuric papules and plaques of unknown cause, like their macular counterparts in pigmented purpuric dermatitis (Schamberg's disease), occur predominantly on the legs. Lichen aureus is probably a variant of lichenoid purpura, the yellow color largely resulting from the abundant hemosiderin.

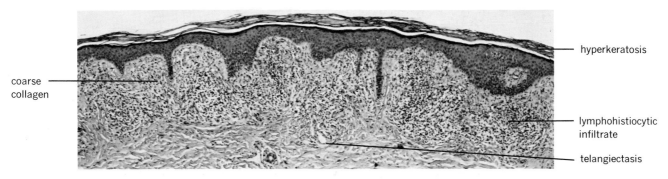

coarse collagen

hyperkeratosis

lymphohistiocytic infiltrate

telangiectasis

FIG. 6-34. Lichenoid purpura (Gougerot-Blum). Dense bandlike infiltrate of lymphocytes, histiocytes, and extravasated erythrocytes that fills papillary dermis thickened by coarse collagen is typical of this variant of persistent pigmented purpuric dermatitides. Siderophages are plentiful in long-standing lesions. Thick-walled capillaries and venules indicate that specimen comes from the leg. (A, × 62; B,× 140.)

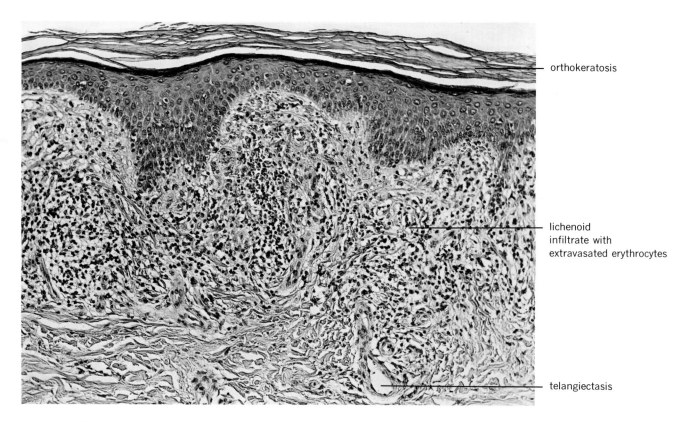

orthokeratosis

lichenoid infiltrate with extravasated erythrocytes

telangiectasis

FIG. 6-34. B.

Pityriasis Lichenoides Chronica (Fig. 6-35)

—Superficial perivascular lymphohistiocytic infiltrate
—Bandlike infiltrate of lymphocytes, histiocytes, melanophages, and extravasated erythrocytes throughout the papillary dermis
—Cellular infiltrate obscures the dermoepidermal junction
—Vacuolar alteration at the dermoepidermal interface
—Relatively thin epidermis with irregular undersurface
—Normal granular zone
—Focal parakeratosis with basket-weave and laminated orthokeratosis

Early lesions of pityriasis lichenoides chronica are characterized by vacuolar, rather than lichenoid, changes at the dermoepidermal interface (Fig. 6-36). The scaly, flat-topped, dull-red papules may occur following pityriasis lichenoides et varioliformis acuta (Mucha-Habermann disease), or they may develop de novo without antecedence of the latter. Pityriasis lichenoides chronica differs clinically from pityriasis lichenoides et varioliformis acuta by the absence of vesicles and scars and histologically by a wholly superficial cellular infiltrate and no intraepidermal edema or vesiculation. Pityriasis lichenoides chronica may well be nothing more than a variant of pityriasis lichenoides et varioliformis acuta.

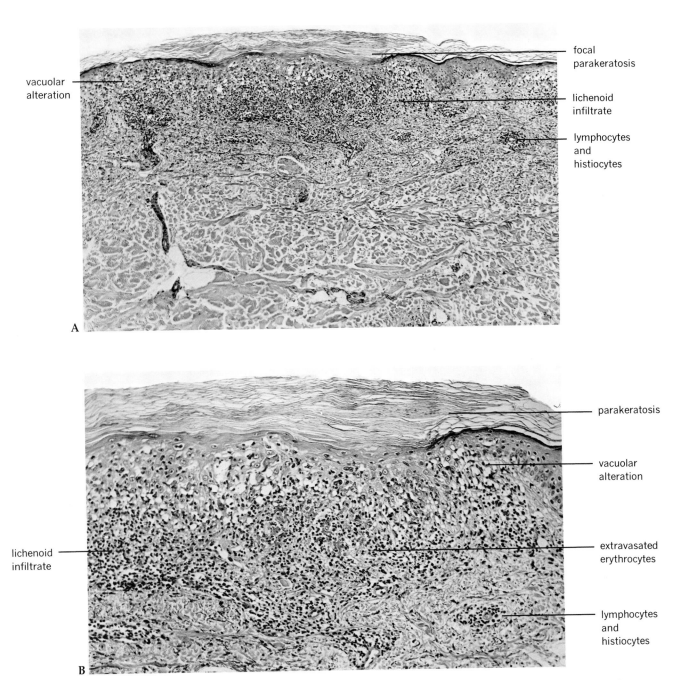

vacuolar alteration

focal parakeratosis

lichenoid infiltrate

lymphocytes and histiocytes

A

parakeratosis

vacuolar alteration

lichenoid infiltrate

extravasated erythrocytes

lymphocytes and histiocytes

B

FIG. 6-35. Pityriasis lichenoides chronica. Focal parakeratosis, lichenoid infiltrate of lymphocytes and histiocytes that obscures dermoepidermal junction, vacuolar alteration, and superficial perivascular infiltrate should suggest the diagnosis. Note how similar the features are to those of pityriasis lichenoides et varioliformis acuta. (A, × 69; B, × 154.)

Some authors have considered pityriasis lichenoides chronica to be synonymous with guttate parapsoriasis, a view with which I do not concur. Clinically, pityriasis lichenoides (et varioliformis) acuta and pityriasis lichenoides chronica seem to be ends of the spectrum of one disease. Histologically, they have many features in common, and both are examples of interface dermatitis. In contrast, guttate parapsoriasis is a spongiotic dermatitis of slight degree.

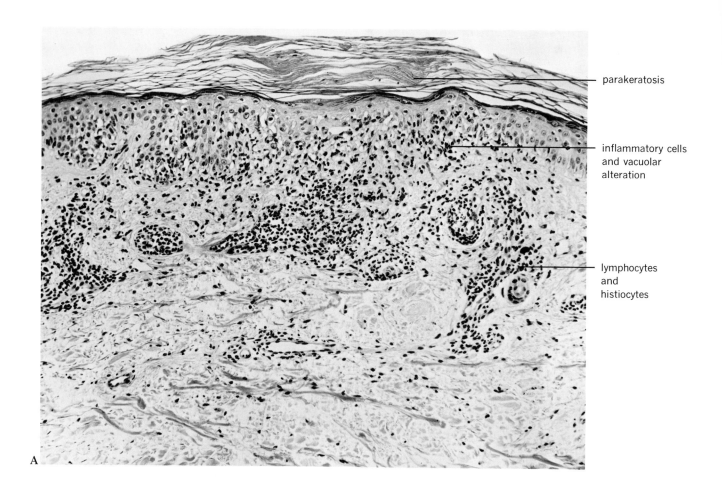

parakeratosis

inflammatory cells and vacuolar alteration

lymphocytes and histiocytes

A

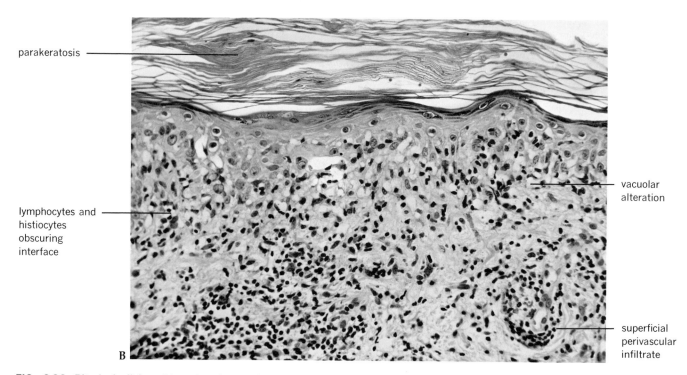

parakeratosis

vacuolar alteration

lymphocytes and histiocytes obscuring interface

superficial perivascular infiltrate

B

FIG. 6-36. Pityriasis lichenoides chronica, early lesion. Vacuolar alteration and sparse, rather than lichenoid, infiltrate of lymphocytes and histiocytes obscure dermoepidermal junction. (A, × 140; B, × 290.)

Parapsoriasis en Plaques (Fig. 6-37); Poikiloderma Atrophicans Vasculare (Fig. 6-38)

—Dense infiltrate of lymphocytes and histiocytes around the dilated
vessels of the superficial plexus and in bandlike array throughout
the thickened papillary dermis
—Mononuclear cells in varying numbers, solitary and in nests, within
the epidermis
—Orthokeratosis, sometimes focal parakeratosis
—Usually diminished rete-papillae pattern

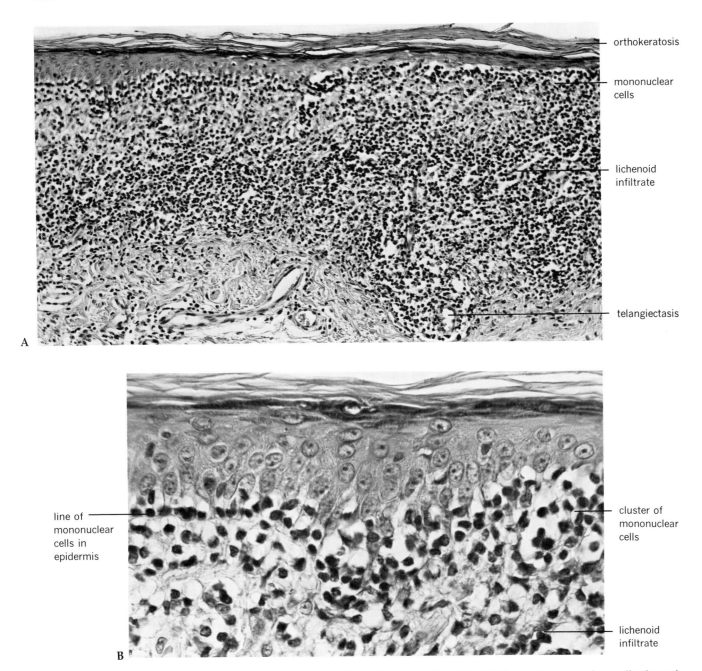

A

B

FIG. 6-37. Parapsoriasis en plaques form of mycosis fungoides. Note dense bandlike infiltrate of mononuclear cells throughout upper part of dermis and within epidermis, both as single cells and as variously sized collections. (A; × 150; B, × 565.)

Parapsoriasis en plaques and poikiloderma vasculare atrophicans, which I regard as patches of mycosis fungoides, are recognized histologically by the density of the cellular infiltrate within the upper part of the dermis and by the presence of mononuclear cells, usually solitary, but sometimes in small collections, within the epidermis. The infiltrate may be present around the deep, as well as the superficial, vascular plexus and within a psoriasiform epidermis (Fig. 6-39). Histologically, the patch stage of mycosis fungoides is differentiated from lichen planus by the absence of significant epidermal changes (orthokeratosis, hypergranulosis, and irregular hyperplasia) characteristic of lichen planus. Furthermore, the mononuclear-cell infiltrate in lichen planus is nearly always confined to the superficial plexus, whereas in patch-stage mycosis fungoides it may involve the deep plexus as well.

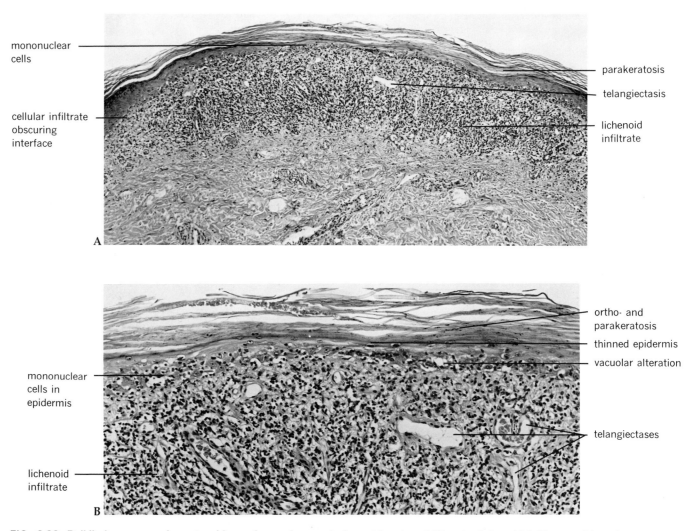

FIG. 6-38. Poikiloderma vasculare atrophicans form of mycosis fungoides. In addition to lichenoid infiltrate of lymphocytes and histiocytes that obscures dermoepidermal interface and mononuclear cells within epidermis, this process is characterized by epidermis without rete ridges and superficial dermis with telangiectases. (A, × 52; B, × 155.)

Clinically, flat lesions of mycosis fungoides may be shiny and telangiectatic with mottled hypopigmentation and hyperpigmentation (poikiloderma vasculare atrophicans) or orange-tan and covered by fine scale (parapsoriasis en plaques). The patches of mycosis fungoides may be present for many years without concomitant or eventual development of plaques or tumors elsewhere, just as patches of Kaposi's sarcoma may be present for years without development of plaques or tumors. Strictly speaking, mycosis fungoides is not an inflammatory disease, but is included in this section because the patch stage can mimic lichenoid dermatitides.

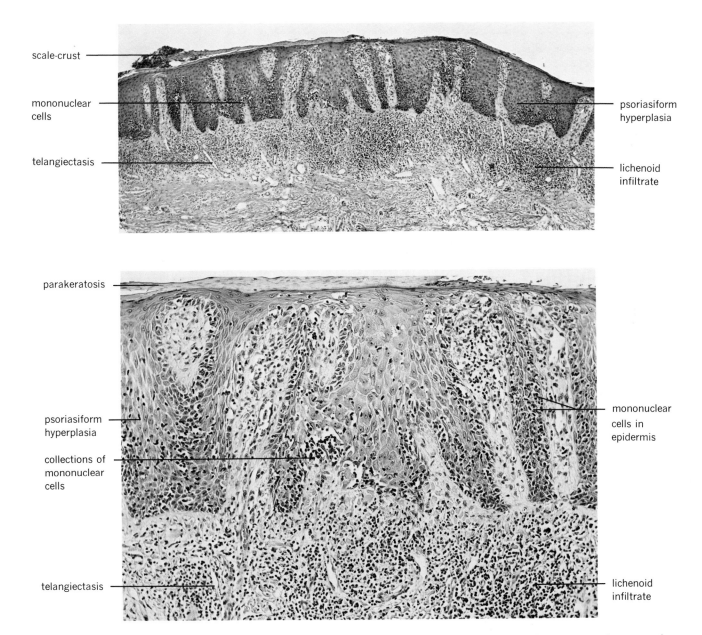

FIG. 6-39. Parapsoriasis en plaques form of mycosis fungoides. An important diagnostic feature is presence of mononuclear cells, both solitary and in small collections, within epidermis of this psoriasiform and lichenoid dermatitis. (A, × 44; B, × 140.)

Disseminated Superficial Porokeratosis (Fig. 6-40)

—Focal or confluent, moderately dense, lymphohistiocytic, lichenoid infiltrate
—Telangiectases in the papillary dermis
—Tall, thin columns of parakeratosis (cornoid lamellae) (Fig. 6-40B)
—Hypogranulosis beneath parakeratotic columns
—Few dyskeratotic and vacuolated cells in the spinous zone beneath the parakeratotic columns

Because the process of disseminated superficial porokeratosis evolves for years, different histologic features are witnessed at different stages of lesions. Common to all forms of porokeratosis (Mibelli, segmental, punctate, and disseminated superficial) is the

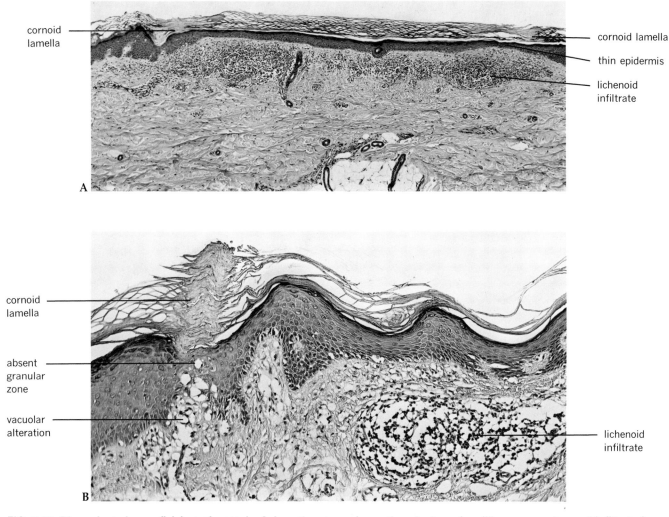

FIG. 6-40. Disseminated superficial porokeratosis. A, In active stage shown there is dense bandlike mononuclear cell infiltrate in upper part of dermis beneath thin epidermis devoid of rete ridges, but dotted by columns of parakeratosis known as cornoid lamellae. (× 33.) B, Lichenoid infiltrate below and to right of cornoid lamella is evidence of active, relatively early stage of disease. (× 142.)

cornoid lamella. In disseminated superficial porokeratosis the parakeratotic column, which is often subtle, leans slightly toward the center of the lesion. The epidermis between the parakeratotic columns is usually thin, sometimes orthokeratotic, but with little of the normal configuration of rete and papillae. In early lesions of disseminated superficial porokeratosis, the lymphohistiocytic infiltrate is present in the papillary dermis immediately beneath the cornoid lamellae. With time, the inflammatory-cell infiltrate becomes more dense and confluent, i.e., lichenoid. Finally, the infiltrate wanes, leaving behind a thickened, fibrotic, telangiectatic papillary dermis containing melanophages.

Clinically, the lesions of disseminated superficial porokeratosis appear on chronically sun-exposed skin, particularly of women, as reddish-brown keratotic papules that gradually extend centrifugally to form round or oval atrophic dells surrounded by slightly raised, sharply defined keratotic ridges. A ridge consists of contiguous parakeratotic columns. The early reddish hue results from telangiectases in the upper dermis, and the late central atrophy is due to a combination of papillary dermal fibrosis, thin, flattened epidermis, and obliteration of the normal epidermal pattern of rete and papillae. Sometimes the cornoid lamella develops from the walls of infundibula and acrosyringia, but does so mostly from intervening epidermis. Rarely will lesions of disseminated superficial porokeratosis involve regions such as the palms and soles that are not chronically exposed to sunlight. Exceptionally, squamous cell carcinomas develop in the atrophic centers of these lesions.

Spongiotic Dermatitis (Fig. 6-4)

Spongiosis is intercellular edema. Because edema appears as clear spaces in preparations stained with hematoxylin and eosin, spongiosis is evinced only by separation of spinous cells from one another. At first the intercellular spines become elongated as fluid accumulates in the intercellular spaces (Figs. 3-14, 6-41A). Eventually a small intraepidermal vesicle forms (Fig. 6-41B). If the fluid accumulation increases, the microscopic intraepidermal vesicle enlarges and becomes evident clinically. A sprinkling of lymphocytes, sometimes of eosinophils, and rarely of neutrophils, is always present within the spongiotic focus. In acantholysis, as in spongiosis, the spinous cells separate completely from their neighbors and in addition also become rounded with homogeneously staining nuclei that are surrounded by perinuclear halos and pe-

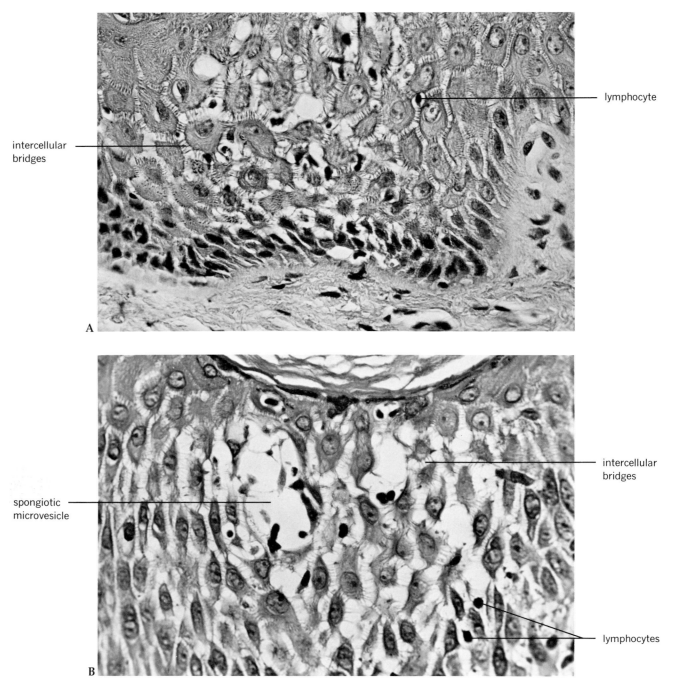

intercellular bridges

lymphocyte

spongiotic microvesicle

intercellular bridges

lymphocytes

A

B

FIG. 6-41. Spongiosis. A, Note stretched intercellular bridges in widened spaces between spinous cells, an early sign of spongiosis. In addition to widened intercellular spaces across which stretch elongated "spines" or bridges, note inflammatory cells in spongiotic loci. (× 592.) B, Spongiosis has evolved into microvesicle. (×656.)

ripheral rims of eosinophilic cytoplasm. Lymphocytes or other inflammatory cells are not necessarily associated with acantholysis.

Certain generalities apply to the evolution of all spongiotic lesions. An infiltrate of inflammatory cells occurs around the dilated blood vessels of the superficial plexus, usually in association with edema of the papillary dermis. The earliest clinical lesions are edematous pink papules.

Spongiosis begins as discrete foci that may increase in size and eventually coalesce with neighboring spongiotic foci. Intracellular edema may be present in addition to intercellular edema. The clinical concomitants are tense vesicles on edematous papular bases. Extreme spongiotic vesiculation may "blow out" the epidermal basal-cell layer, resulting in vesicles that are subepidermal as well as intraepidermal.

The intraepidermal edema inevitably ascends, and when it (homogeneous eosinophilic material) combines with foci of parakeratotic cells on the skin surface, a scale-crust is seen clinically. At this juncture, spongiosis may no longer be seen histologically, but evidence that it was present previously can be inferred from the focal parakeratosis or scale-crust, the scale resulting from increased epidermopoiesis. Clinically, tiny collarettes of scale bear testimony to a prior spongiotic vesicle or intraepidermal pustule.

With time, all spongiotic dermatitides become less spongiotic and more psoriasiform. As the spongiosis diminishes, the psoriasiform hyperplasia increases. Eventually, devoid of spongiosis, these diseases can no longer be recognized as examples of spongiotic dermatitis, but rather of psoriasiform dermatitis (Fig. 6-42).

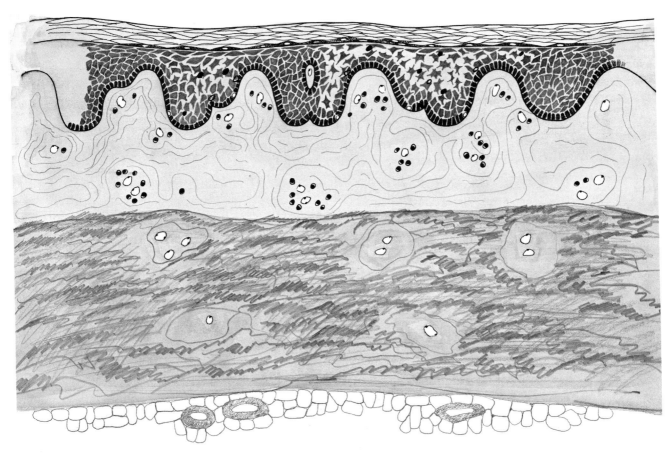

FIG. 6-42. A, Spongiotic dermatitis.

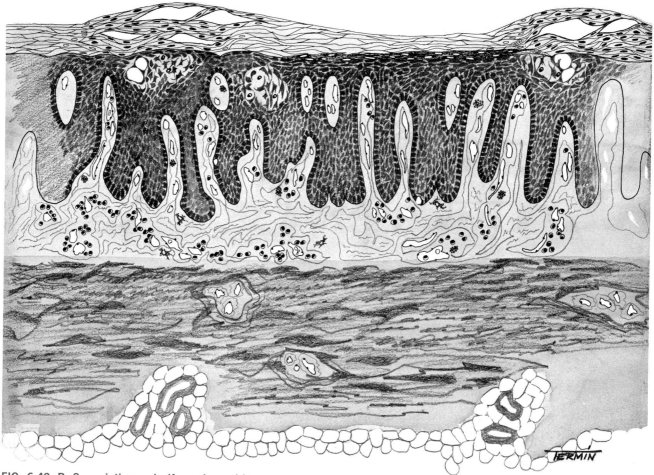

FIG. 6-42. B, Spongiotic psoriasiform dermatitis.

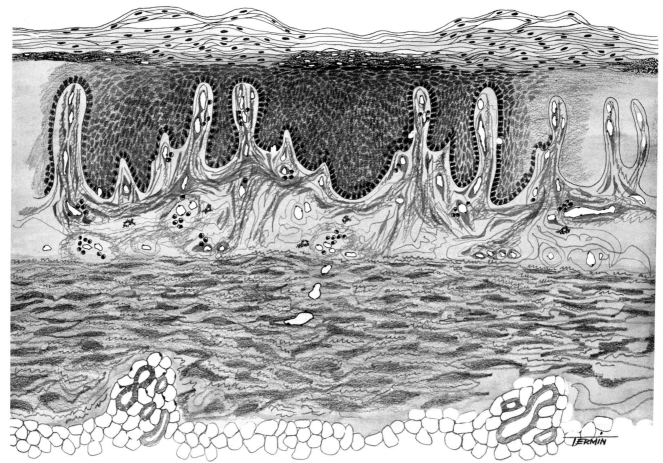

FIG. 6-42. C, Psoriasiform dermatitis.

The prototype of spongiotic dermatitis is allergic contact dermatitis. It will be described in some detail, and the other spongiotic dermatitides will be compared to and differentiated from it. It is sometimes impossible histologically to distinguish one type of acute spongiotic dermatitis from another, e.g., allergic contact dermatitis, nummular dermatitis, dyshidrotic dermatitis, and id reactions. In such instances, an accurate histologic diagnosis can only be spongiotic dermatitis, and a note of histologic differential diagnosis should be added.

Although drugs administered systemically are capable of inducing almost every inflammatory reaction pattern in the skin, they rarely cause a spongiotic dermatitis.

Allergic Contact Dermatitis, Acute (Figs. 6-43, 6-44)

—Superficial perivascular lymphohistiocytic infiltrate with varying numbers of eosinophils ranging from none to numerous
—Edema of the papillary dermis
—Extravasated erythrocytes occasionally present within the papillary dermis
—Focal spongiosis
—Slight intracellular edema

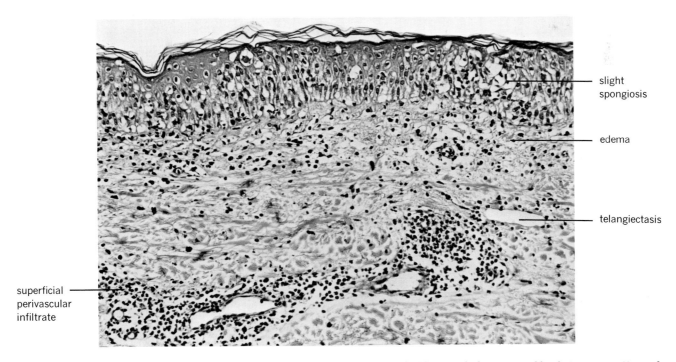

slight spongiosis

edema

telangiectasis

superficial perivascular infiltrate

FIG. 6-43. Allergic contact dermatitis, acute. A, Slightly papular lesion, recognizable as early from normal basket-weave pattern of cornified layer, consists of slight, but diffuse, spongiosis, edema of the papillary dermis, and mixed inflammatory-cell infiltrate containing eosinophils. ($\times$ 220.)

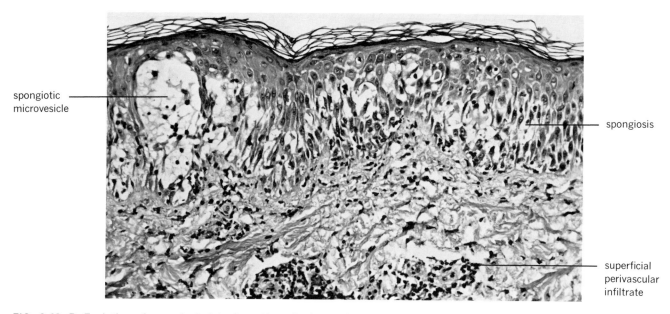

spongiotic
microvesicle

spongiosis

superficial
perivascular
infiltrate

FIG. 6-43. B, Evolution of spongiosis into formation of microvesicle within epidermis is pictured. (× 193.)

By gentle palpation of the surface of early edematous pink papules of allergic contact dermatitis, it is sometimes possible to feel the pinpoint elevations caused by spongiotic vesicles, even when they cannot be seen grossly (Fig. 6-44B). In time, tense vesicles become visible. Bullae of severe allergic contact dermatitis may develop as a result of large, multiloculated intraepidermal

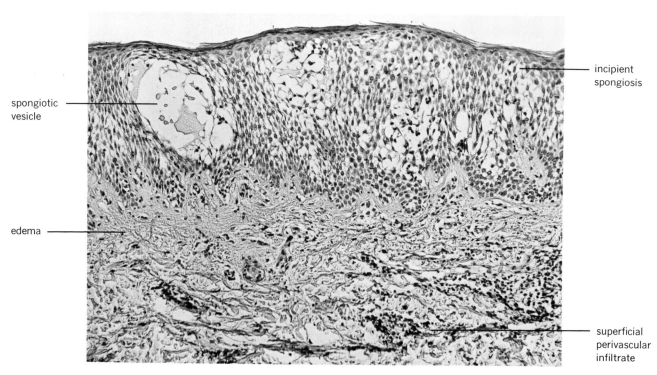

incipient
spongiosis

spongiotic
vesicle

edema

superficial
perivascular
infiltrate

FIG. 6-44. Allergic contact dermatitis, acute. A, Varying degrees of spongiosis, including spongiotic vesicle, are seen in early papulovesicular lesion. (× 138.)

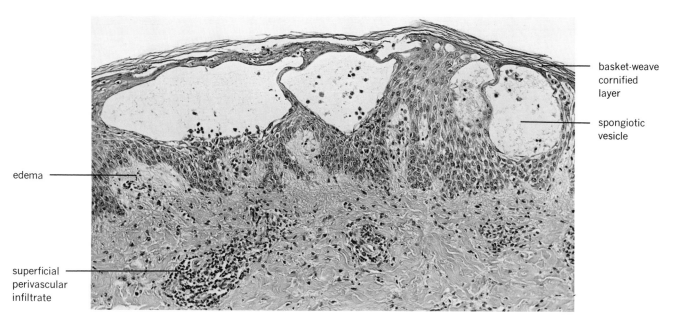

basket-weave
cornified
layer

spongiotic
vesicle

edema

superficial
perivascular
infiltrate

FIG. 6-44. B, Association of several spongiotic vesicles with unaltered basket-weave pattern in cornified layer and edema of papillary dermis indicates that changes pictured are still those of acute type. (× 136.)

vesicles, some of which expand and become subepidermal when the tension within becomes sufficiently great (Fig. 6-45).

Spongiosis is most severe in the acute stage of allergic contact dermatitis. It diminishes in subacute allergic contact dermatitis, in which epidermal hyperplasia and scale-crusts develop. Spongiosis

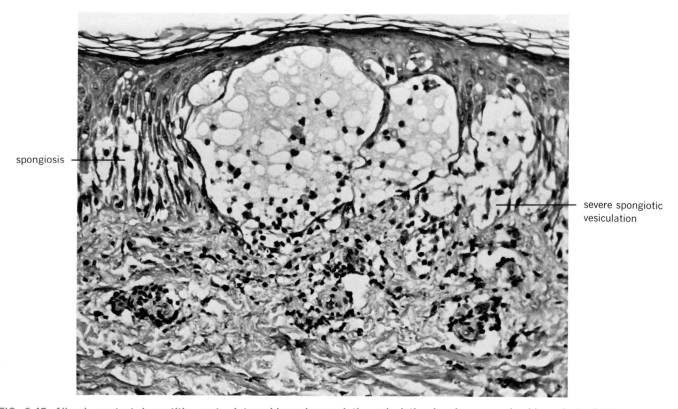

spongiosis

severe spongiotic
vesiculation

FIG. 6-45. Allergic contact dermatitis, acute. Intraepidermal spongiotic vesiculation has become subepidermal. (× 247.)

is virtually absent in chronic allergic contact dermatitis where there is psoriasiform epidermal hyperplasia and parakeratosis.

In some instances of acute allergic contact dermatitis the dermal changes of edema and inflammatory cells overshadow the epidermal spongiosis. These reactions, especially to compounds such as nickel, chromate, and neomycin, have been termed "dermal" contact dermatitis. If serial sections are cut through these specimens, spongiosis will inevitably be found.

The histologic changes of spongiotic dermatitis may be indistinguishable in allergic contact dermatitis, id reactions, dyshidrotic dermatitis, nummular dermatitis, and dermatophytic vesicles.

Photoallergic Contact Dermatitis and Photoallergic Dermatitis

The histologic changes in the epidermis of photoallergic contact dermatitis are indistinguishable from those of allergic contact dermatitis. In contrast to allergic contact dermatitis, however, the inflammatory-cell infiltrate in photoallergic contact dermatitis may be both deep and superficial. Morphologically, the clinical lesions of photoallergic contact dermatitis are identical to those of allergic contact dermatitis. The distribution of photoallergic contact dermatitis, however, is usually limited to the sun-exposed areas, ordinarily sparing the shaded areas immediately below the eyebrows, nose and mandible. Photoallergic contact dermatitis can be induced by topical application of certain chemicals, such as the halogenated salicylanimides, which are used in antiseptics in some toilet soaps.

Photoallergic dermatitis, unlike photoallergic contact dermatitis, results from the combination of systemic administration of a drug such as chlorpromazine to a previously sensitized person and exposure to ultraviolet light. Histologically, like photoallergic contact dermatitis, photoallergic dermatitis shows spongiosis, edema of the papillary dermis, and a moderately dense predominantly lymphocytic infiltrate around the blood vessels of the superficial plexus and sometimes of the deep one too. Clinically, photoallergic dermatitis differs from photoallergic contact dermatitis by being a monomorphous eruption of myriad tiny papules and papulovesicles on light-exposed sites.

In order to emphasize an analogy that exists between the two types of photoallergic reactions (induced by light in the range of 330 to 380 nm) and phototoxic reactions (induced by light in the range of 290 to 390 nm), I have termed those reactions in which topically applied materials combine with light to cause inflammatory changes either *photoallergic contact dermatitis* or *phototoxic contact dermatitis*. Those reactions in which systemically administered agents plus light cause eruptions are either photoallergic dermatitis or phototoxic dermatitis.

Nummular Dermatitis, Acute

The early changes in the epidermis and dermis of nummular dermatitis are indistinguishable histologically from those of acute allergic contact dermatitis. In both conditions there are foci of spongiosis, edema of the papillary dermis, and a superficial perivascular infiltrate of lymphocytes, histiocytes, and sometimes eosinophils. Clinically, acute nummular dermatitis consists of tense vesicles grouped in coin-shaped clusters of various sizes. The accompanying pruritus is so intense that the roofs of the vesicles are quickly scratched away, leaving behind erosions, ulcerations, and often hemorrhagic crusts.

Id Reaction, Acute

Classically, tense vesicles occur in the id reaction, especially on the hands, secondary to inflammatory dermatophytic infections that are situated on the feet. Widespread id reactions can also be secondary to other florid cutaneous inflammations such as allergic contact dermatitis from sensitization to materials in shoes. These generalized id reactions (commonly termed "autosensitization" eruptions) mimic allergic contact dermatitis, clinically and histologically. The mechanism whereby id reactions develop is not fully understood, but they are thought to represent a reaction to an allergen initially applied at one skin site and subsequently hematogenously disseminated.

Dyshidrotic Dermatitis, Acute (Fig. 6-46)

Dyshidrotic dermatitis is a type of spongiotic dermatitis that occurs on the hands and feet, especially on the palmar and plantar surfaces and along the sides of the digits. Dyshidrotic dermatitis is indistinguishable histologically from allergic contact dermatitis, nummular dermatitis, id reactions, some vesicular dermatophytic infections, and from id reactions, all of which may also involve acral volar skin.

Clinically, the tiny vesicles of dyshidrotic dermatitis simulate tapioca, sago, or small bubbles lodged immediately beneath the skin surface. They are intensely pruritic.

The term *dyshidrotic* is a misnomer. There is as yet no absolute evidence that this idiopathic dermatitis is related to an aberration of structure or function of the sweat ducts.

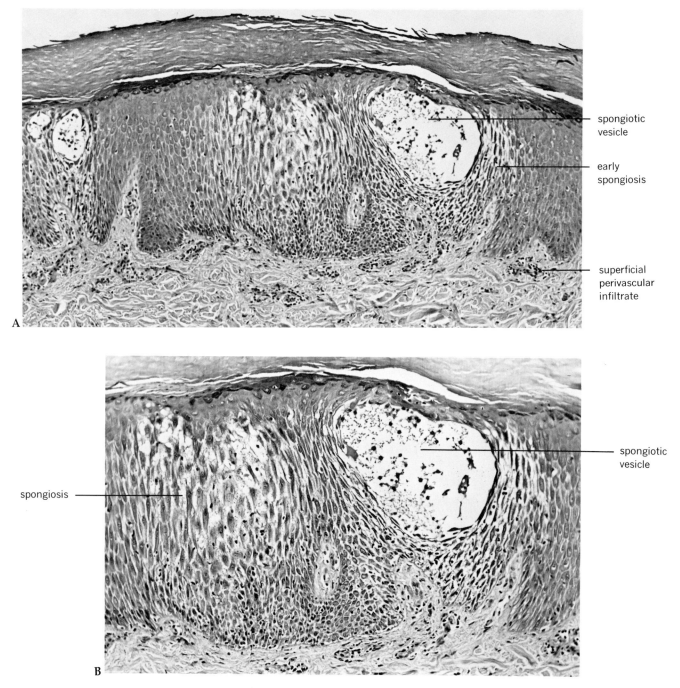

FIG. 6-46. Dyshidrotic dermatitis, acute. Histologic changes in biopsy specimen from palm of patient with clinical features of dyshidrotic dermatitis are indistinguishable from those in acute allergic contact dermatitis, nummular dermatitis, id reactions, and some vesicular dermatophytic infections. (A, × 96; B, × 162.) Note progression from intercellular edema at left of picture to spongiotic vesiculation at right.

—Superficial perivascular infiltrate of lymphocytes, histiocytes, neutrophils, and, rarely, eosinophils
—Edema of the papillary dermis
—Focal spongiosis, sometimes spongiotic intraepidermal vesiculation
—Neutrophils often present within the epidermis and within spongiotic foci
—Hyphae, especially within the orthokeratotic portions of the cornified layer.

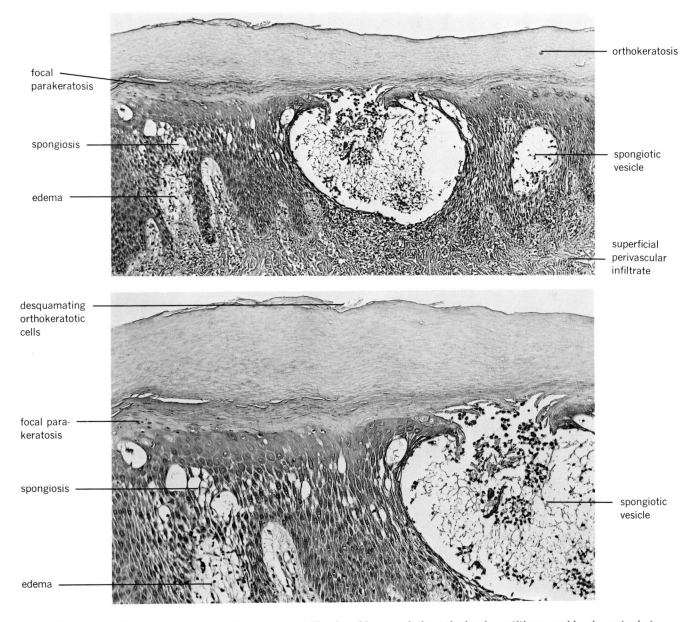

FIG. 6-47. Dermatophytosis, vesicular. A, With low magnification this spongiotic vesicular dermatitis caused by dermatophytes cannot be differentiated from allergic contact dermatitis, nummular dermatitis, dyshidrotic dermatitis, or id reaction. (× 106.) B, With higher magnification evolution from spongiosis to spongiotic vesiculation can be seen. Note that hyphae are not always discernible by hematoxylin and eosin stain at this magnification. (× 175.)

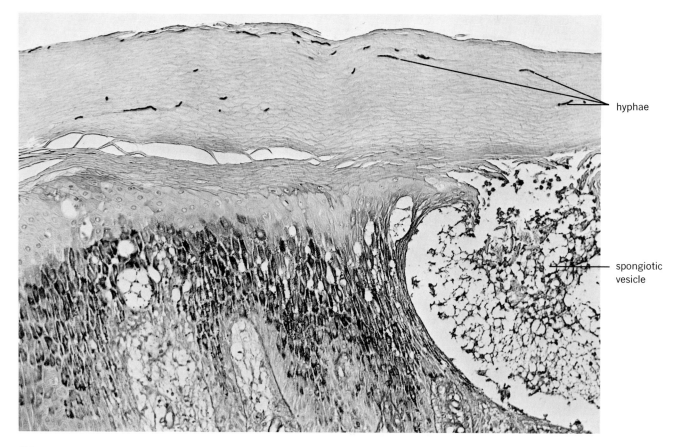

hyphae

spongiotic vesicle

FIG. 6-48. Dermatophytosis, vesicular. Numerous hyphae can be seen in orthokeratotic portion of cornified layer in PAS-stained section of biopsy specimen in Fig. 6-47. (× 140.)

Superficial fungal infections, such as "ringworm" in children and "athlete's foot" in adults, are manifested clinically as vesicles and scales. Sometimes the two types may coexist. Dermatophytic vesicular lesions are a form of spongiotic dermatitis, whereas dermatophytic scaly lesions are a type of psoriasiform dermatitis. Common causes of vesicular dermatophytic eruptions are Microsporum canis and Trichophyton mentagrophytes. Rarely, Trichophyton rubrum can also cause vesiculation. The periodic acid-Schiff (PAS) stain should be ordered for all spongiotic dermatitides of the palms and soles (Fig. 6-49), those having neutrophils within the epidermis, and for undiagnosed pustular dermatitides. The finding of neutrophils within the epidermis is a clue to the possible presence of fungal elements within the cornified layer.

The dermatophytoses are but one illustration of the many morphologic expressions that infectious agents may evoke. Vesicles and scales are the most common lesions of dermatophytoses, but some fungi that cause superficial infections are also capable of causing pustules, suppurative and suppurative-granulomatous folliculitis (Majocchi's granuloma), onychomycosis, and scarring and nonscarring alopecias.

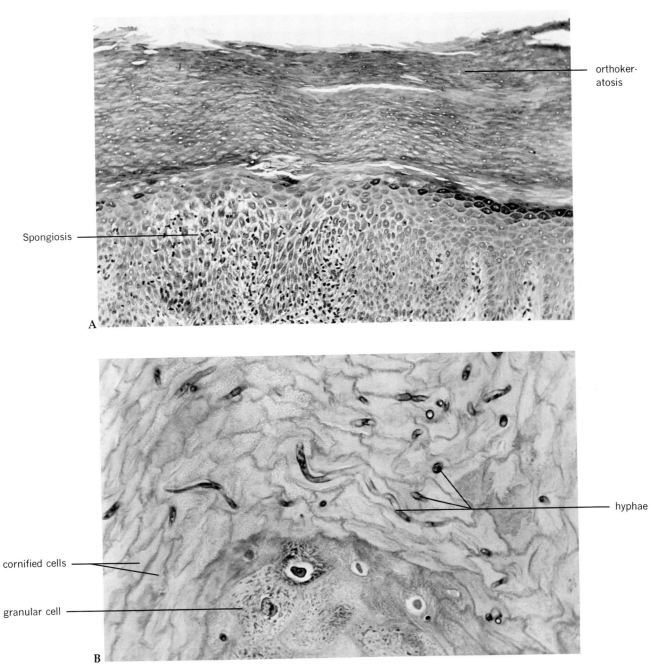

FIG. 6-49. Dermatophytosis, vesicular. A, Spongiotic dermatitis in biopsy specimen from palm should always prompt search for hyphae. ($\times$ 149.) B, PAS stain uncovers hyphae that may not be easily discerned with hematoxylin and eosin stain. ($\times$ 678.)

Gyrate Erythema, Superficial (Fig. 6-50)

—Moderately dense superficial perivascular infiltrate of lymphocytes and some histiocytes, and, rarely, eosinophils
—Slight edema of the papillary dermis
—Focal spongiosis
—Focal parakeratosis occasionally

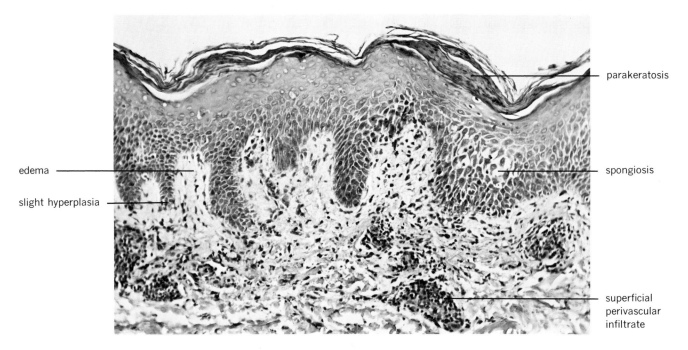

parakeratosis

edema

slight hyperplasia

spongiosis

superficial
perivascular
infiltrate

FIG. 6-50. Gyrate erythema, superficial. Focal parakeratosis, spongiosis, slight epidermal hyperplasia, edema of papillary dermis, and superficial perivascular infiltrate of lymphocytes and histiocytes are features common to erythema annulare centrifugum and to pityriasis rosea. (× 192.)

Clinically, the lesions of superficial gyrate erythema are known by a variety of names, the most familiar of which is erythema annulare centrifugum. The gyrate erythemas may be polycyclic, serpiginous, arcuate, or annular. The clinical hallmarks of this condition are firm, reddish, variably complete ringed lesions with delicate scales on the inner margins of their rims. The firmness results primarily from edema of the papillary dermis. The delicate scale is a clinical consequence of focal parakeratosis, beneath which there is usually spongiosis. Sometimes multiple sections must be scanned before spongiotic foci are found, but spongiosis will inevitably be present if the biopsy is taken from the firmest portion of the rim. Sometimes the biopsy of a superficial gyrate erythema will show only a superficial perivascular dermatitis without any significant epidermal change (Fig. 6-7). Rarely will eosinophils appear in addition to lymphocytes and histiocytes within the infiltrate. In other instances there may be parakeratosis without spongiosis. These are simply histologic reflections of one pathologic process at different moments in its evolution and at different loci in its centrifugal spread. Superficial fungal infections of skin may also have an annular configuration like that of the gyrate erythemas, but their scale contains hyphae and is at the outermost advancing border of the periphery, rather than at the inner rim. Both gyrate erythemas and dermatophytoses leave hyperpigmentation in the wake of their outward advance.

Not all gyrate erythemas are of the superficial type. In lesions of the deep type of gyrate erythema (e.g., erythema gyratum repens), the blood vessels of the deep plexus are also involved. In this deep type there is no spongiosis or parakeratosis and, hence, no scale. Because of the additional involvement of the deep plexus, the lesions tend to be more indurated than those of erythema annulare centrifugum. Annular lesions can occur in a variety of skin diseases besides erythema annulare centrifugum, namely, granuloma annulare, erythema multiforme, sarcoidosis, lichen planus, secondary syphilis, and dermatophytosis. For unknown reasons, annular lesions of syphilis, sarcoidosis, and lichen planus are much more common in dark-skinned peoples. The histologic differential diagnosis of superficial gyrate erythema is pityriasis rosea from which it may be indistinguishable.

Pityriasis Rosea (Fig. 6-51)

—Superficial perivascular infiltrate of lymphocytes and histiocytes
—Eosinophils, in variable numbers, occasionally
—Edema of the papillary dermis
—A few or many extravasated erythrocytes within the papillae (Fig. 6-52)
—Focal spongiosis
—Slight epidermal hyperplasia
—Focal parakeratosis in mounds

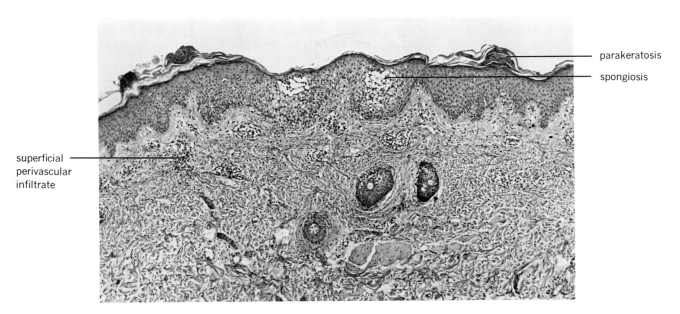

FIG. 6-51. Pityriasis rosea. Foci of parakeratosis and spongiosis associated with superficial perivascular infiltrate of lymphocytes and histiocytes are features of pityriasis rosea and erythema annulare centrifugum. (× 67.)

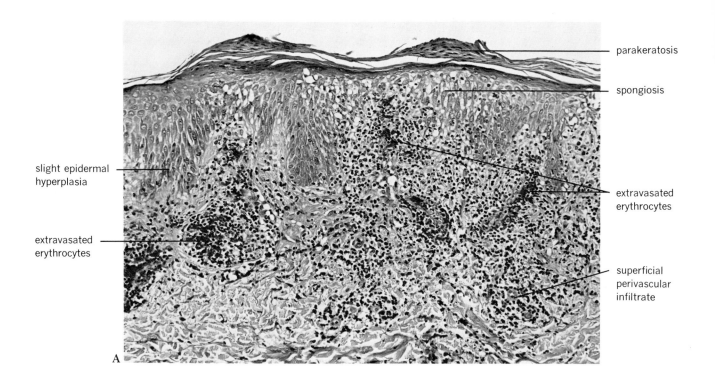

slight epidermal
hyperplasia

extravasated
erythrocytes

parakeratosis

spongiosis

extravasated
erythrocytes

superficial
perivascular
infiltrate

A

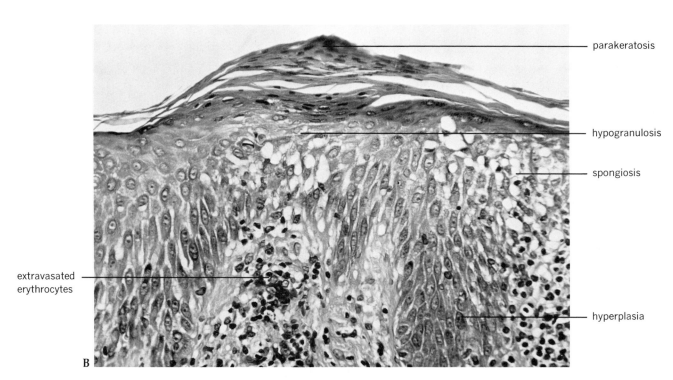

extravasated
erythrocytes

parakeratosis

hypogranulosis

spongiosis

hyperplasia

B

FIG. 6-52. Pityriasis rosea. Typical histologic features, requiring differentiation only from erythema annulare centrifugum, are focal parakeratosis, spongiosis, slight epidermal hyperplasia, edema of papillary dermis, and superficial perivascular lympho-histiocytic infiltrate with varying numbers of extravasated erythrocytes. (A, × 167; B, × 345.)

An interesting, and exceptional, finding in the epidermis of pityriasis rosea is multinucleated epithelial cells (Fig. 6-53).

Pityriasis rosea typically involves the body from the neck to the knees with salmon-pink oval lesions that have wrinkled centers and delicate collarettes of scale at their peripheries. The long axes of these oval lesions tend to be aligned parallel to the ribs, creating a Christmas-tree pattern. Clinically, vesicles are exceedingly rare. The eruption is often portended by a lesion ("herald" or "mother" patch) that, with time, becomes the largest and most psoriasiform. Biopsy of this oldest lesion shows histologic changes similar to those already described, but the perivascular infiltrate is often both superficial and deep, and there are less spongiosis, greater epidermal hyperplasia, and a gentle undulation to the surface. Pityriasis rosea persists for several weeks before disappearing spontaneously.

The histologic features of pityriasis rosea may be indistinguishable from those of superficial gyrate erythema (erythema annulare centrifugum). Guttate parapsoriasis may usually be differentiated histologically from pityriasis rosea by crusts in addition to scales, less spongiosis, and fewer inflammatory cells in the infiltrate.

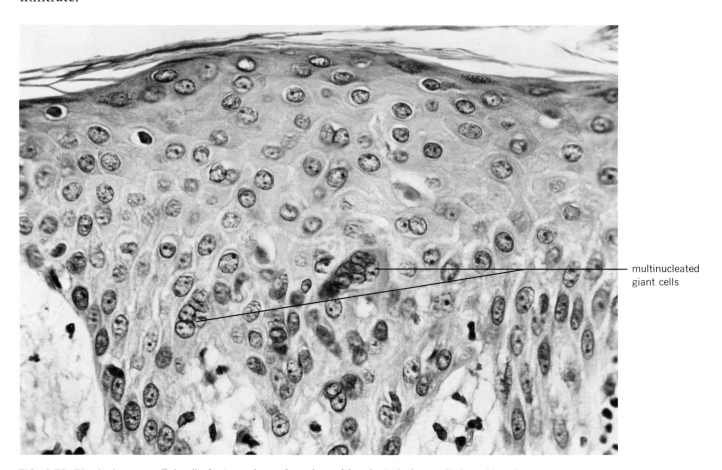

multinucleated giant cells

FIG. 6-53. Pityriasis rosea. Episodic feature shown here is multinucleated giant cells in epidermis. ($\times$ 608.)

Guttate Parapsoriasis (Fig. 6-54)

—Sparse superficial perivascular lymphohistiocytic infiltrate
—Slight epidermal hyperplasia
—Slight focal spongiosis
—Scale-crusts

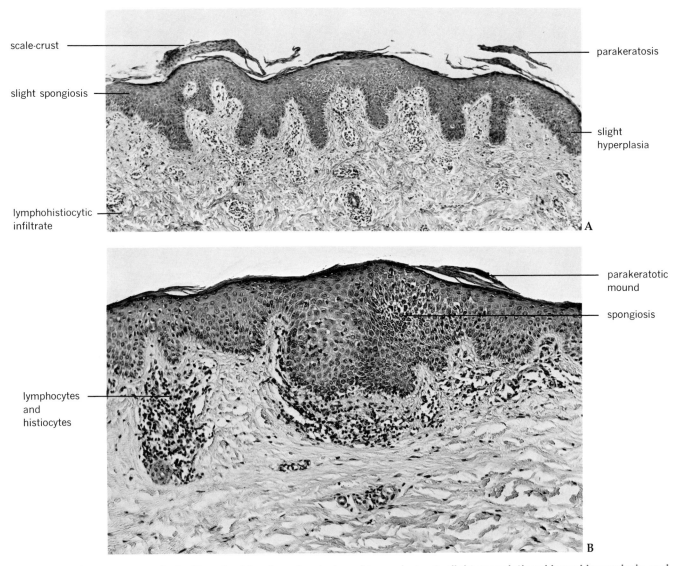

scale-crust

parakeratosis

slight spongiosis

slight hyperplasia

lymphohistiocytic infiltrate

A

parakeratotic mound

spongiosis

lymphocytes and histiocytes

B

FIG. 6-54. Guttate parapsoriasis. Mounds of focal parakeratosis and/or scale-crust, slight spongiotic epidermal hyperplasia, and sparse superficial perivascular lymphohistiocytic infiltrate are typical features. Digitate dermatosis shows histologic features indistinguishable from those of guttate parapsoriasis. (A, × 67; B, × 134.)

Because the spongiosis in guttate parapsoriasis is so slight, often not detectable, it may not always be possible to classify guttate parapsoriasis as a type of spongiotic dermatitis (Fig. 6-55). The presence of a crust in the absence of erosion or ulceration implies preceding spongiosis.

Guttate parapsoriasis may be difficult to distinguish histologically from pityriasis rosea. In guttate parapsoriasis, however, there is usually more serum in parakeratotic foci, less spongiosis, fewer or no extravasated erythrocytes, and a sparser inflammatory-cell infiltrate. Clinically, guttate parapsoriasis consists of drop-sized, pinkish-orangy-tan papules covered by a waferlike scale. The disease is notoriously refractory to all therapy.

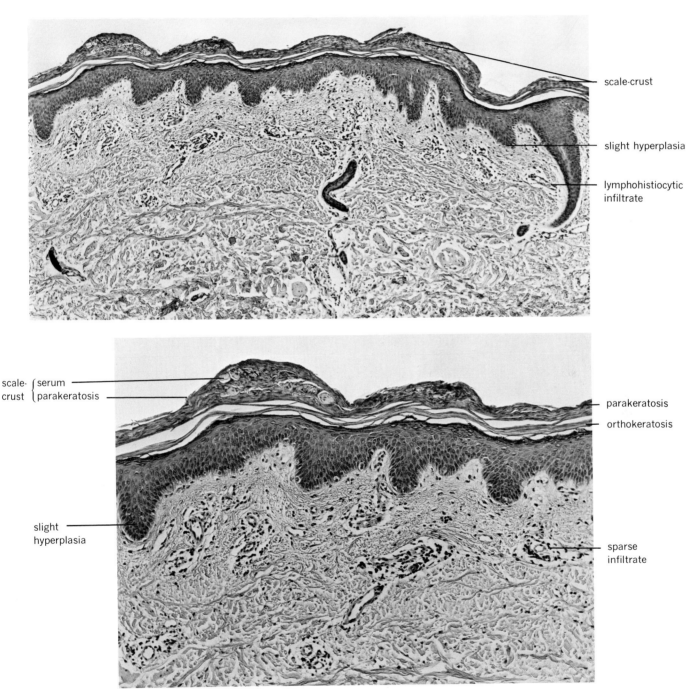

FIG. 6-55. Guttate parapsoriasis. Mounds of parakeratosis or scale-crust, slight epidermal hyperplasia, and slight or no spongiosis with sparse superficial perivascular lymphohistiocytic infiltrate are characteristic features. Serum in scale-crust indicates that spongiosis was formerly present in epidermis. Episodic nature can be inferred from confluent orthokeratosis beneath largely confluent parakeratosis. (A, × 60; B, × 140.)

Acral Papular Eruption of Childhood (Gianotti-Crosti Syndrome) (Fig. 6-56)

—Sparse superficial perivascular lymphohistiocytic infiltrate
—Edema of the papillary dermis
—Variable numbers of extravasated erythrocytes
—Focal spongiosis
—Focal scale-crust

The erythematous, edematous papules of acral papular eruption of childhood are found mostly on the extremities, buttocks, and face. The "juicy" character of the papules results from edema in the papillary dermis and from spongiosis. Depending upon the number of extravasated erythrocytes, the papules may or may not be slightly purpuric. Some lesions of Gianotti-Crosti syndrome have atypical mononuclear cells within the spongiotic foci and must be differentiated histologically from mycosis fungoides and histiocytosis X.

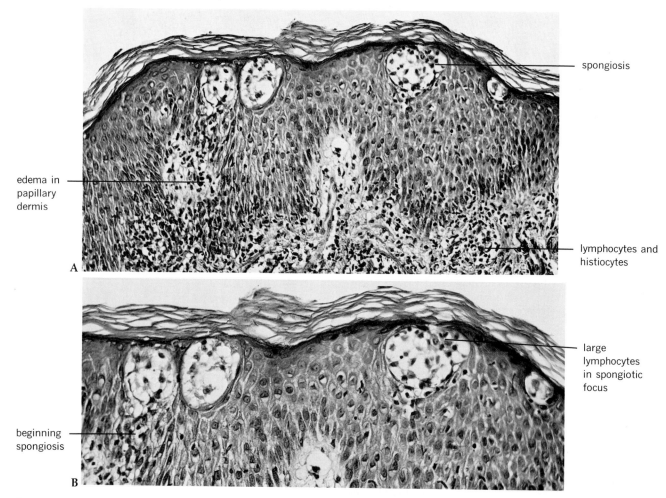

FIG. 6-56. Gianotti-Crosti syndrome. Spongiotic foci within epidermis may contain some atypical lymphocytes as shown. Spongiosis in lesions helps distinguish them from mycosis fungoides in which Pautrier's microabscesses are present. (A, × 199; B, × 272.)

—Sparse superficial perivascular lymphohistiocytic infiltrate
—Slight focal spongiosis
—Slight focal parakeratosis

Clinically, pityriasis alba consists of round, hypopigmented patches that are covered by fine, powdery scales. These asymptomatic lesions occur predominantly on the face of young children.

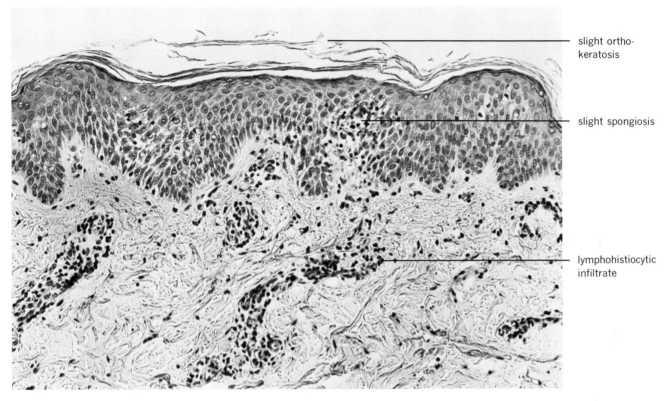

slight ortho-
keratosis

slight spongiosis

lymphohistiocytic
infiltrate

FIG. 6-57. Pityriasis alba. Slight orthokeratosis and spongiosis, in combination with sparse superficial perivascular lymphohistiocytic infiltrate, are features shown. (× 182.)

Seborrheic Dermatitis, Acute (Fig. 6-58)

—Sparse superficial perivascular lymphohistiocytic infiltrate with few
   neutrophils
—Widely dilated blood vessels of the superficial plexus
—Edema of the papillary dermis
—Slight focal spongiosis
—Scale-crust containing neutrophils, especially at the margins of the
   follicular ostia

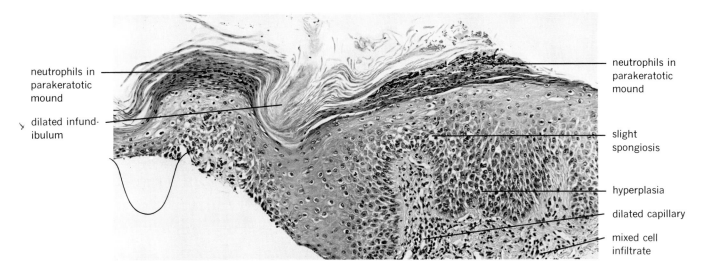

neutrophils in parakeratotic mound

dilated infund- ibulum

neutrophils in parakeratotic mound

slight spongiosis

hyperplasia

dilated capillary

mixed cell infiltrate

FIG. 6-58. Seborrheic dermatitis, acute. Characteristics are mounds of scale-crusts containing neutrophils adjacent to infundib- ular ostia that are plugged by orthokeratotic cells, slight spongiosis and epidermal hyperplasia, and dilated capillaries surrounded by sparse infiltrate of lymphocytes histiocytes, and neutrophils. (× 139.)

Seborrheic dermatitis begins as pinpoint pink papules that soon coalesce to form reddish, slightly elevated plaques covered by branny grey-yellow scale-crusts. The clinical diagnosis is usu- ally made by distribution, rather than by the vague morphologic features of the condition. Seborrheic dermatitis tends to involve the center of the face, including the forehead, eyebrows, paranasal and nasolabial folds, and the malar and postauricular regions. The prominent histologic feature of dilated blood vessels is responsible for the dominant clinical feature of erythema. The scale-crusts are especially situated at the perimeters of follicular ostia. In short, the histologic changes in seborrheic dermatitis are surprisingly few. Long-standing lesions of seborrheic dermatitis are psoriasi- form. By contrast to seborrheic dermatitis, dandruff is neither inflammatory nor spongiotic, but consists only of orthokeratotic clumps with minute parakeratotic foci.

Measles (Plate 4)

—Sparse lymphohistiocytic infiltrate around the blood vessels of the superficial plexus
—Slight focal epidermal hyperplasia
—Focal intracellular edema
—Focal spongiosis
—Multinucleated epithelial cells in the foci of intracellular and inter- cellular edema
—Occasional necrotic keratinocytes
—Focal parakeratosis

The histologic changes in Koplik's spots are similar to those in the skin lesions of measles. The electron microscope has revealed the presence of the measles virus within the epidermal multinucleated cells. Clinically, the reddish papules of measles result primarily from the focal epidermal edema and the dermal vasodilatation.

Lichen Striatus (Fig. 6-59)

—Superficial perivascular lymphohistiocytic infiltrate
—Focal collections of histiocytes, some multinucleated, within the papillary dermis
—Vacuolar alteration at the dermoepidermal junction, sometimes with subepidermal clefts, above the histiocytic collections in the dermal papillae
—Dyskeratotic cells within the epidermis, at the dermoepidermal junction, and in the papillary dermis
—Slight parakeratosis above spongiotic foci

Lichen striatus consists of linearly arranged tiny papules, some flat-topped and smooth, others scaly, usually on an extremity of a child. The lesions erupt, persist for months, and disappear spontaneously.

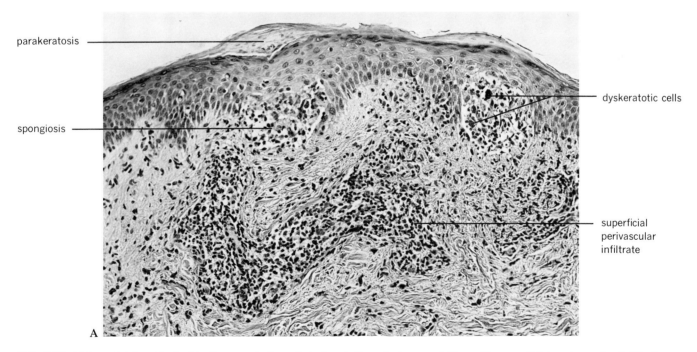

FIG. 6-59. Lichen striatus. Foci of both spongiosis and dyskeratotic cells in association with superficial perivascular infiltrate containing numerous histiocytes with some lymphocytes are diagnostic findings. Higher magnification shows combination of spongiosis and dyskeratotic cells. (A, × 149; B, × 510.)

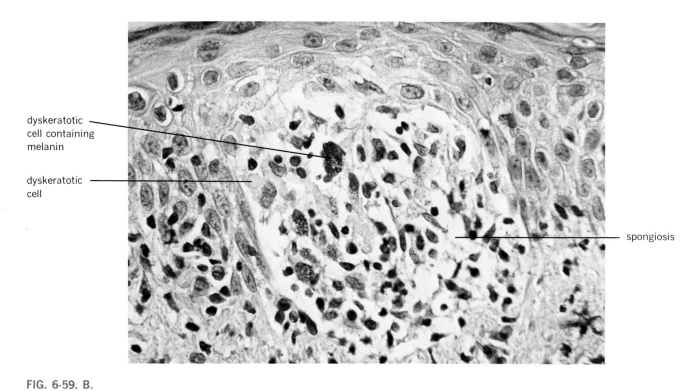

dyskeratotic cell containing melanin

dyskeratotic cell

spongiosis

FIG. 6-59. B.

Miliaria Rubra (Fig. 6-60)

—Superficial perivascular infiltrate of lymphocytes, histiocytes, and, often, neutrophils
—Focal spongiosis involving the intraepidermal portion of the eccrine sweat duct (acrosyringium)

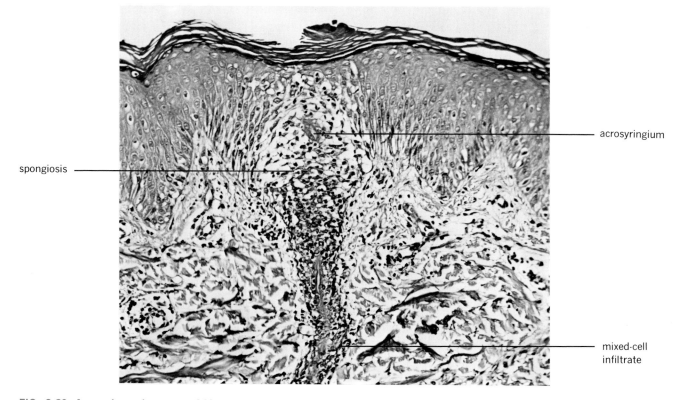

acrosyringium

spongiosis

mixed-cell infiltrate

FIG. 6-60. A, see legend on page 243.

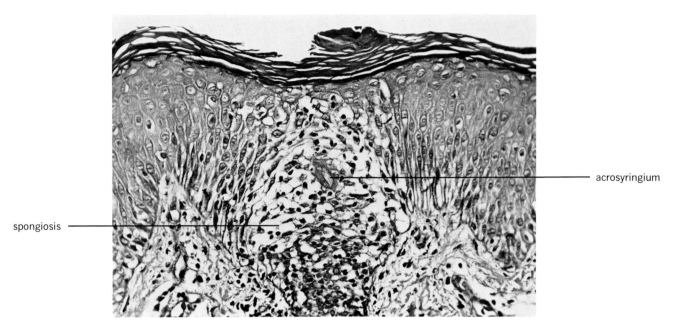

spongiosis

acrosyringium

FIG. 6-60. Miliaria rubra. Diagnostic features are spongiosis around intraepidermal portion of eccrine duct and sparse mixed inflammatory-cell infiltrate around straight dermal portion of eccrine duct. (A, × 176; B, × 265.)

Clinically, miliaria rubra (heat rash, prickly heat) consists of multiple, minute, discrete reddish papules that rarely vesiculate. Each pinpoint papule represents a spongiotic focus in and around an acrosyringium. Patients with milaria rubra are unable to sweat in the affected areas because the acrosyringia are occluded in the inflammatory process.

Irritant Contact Dermatitis (Fig. 6-61)

—Superficial perivascular infiltrate of neutrophils, lymphocytes, and and histiocytes
—Extensive ballooning
—Slight spongiosis
—Varying degrees of epidermal necrosis
—Scale-crust, depending on the age of the lesion
—Erosion or ulceration, depending on the severity of the process

Irritant contact dermatitis is distinguished histologically from allergic contact dermatitis by having neutrophils (rather than eosinophils), prominent intracellular edema (rather than intercellular edema), and epidermal necrosis. Unlike allergic contact dermatitis, which results from cutaneous hypersensitivity and is mediated by lymphocytes, irritant contact dermatitis, as its name denotes, is nonallergic. The inflammatory skin changes of irritant contact dermatitis vary from mild redness and scaling, as from overexposure to detergents, to severe blistering and ulceration, as from acid or alkali burns.

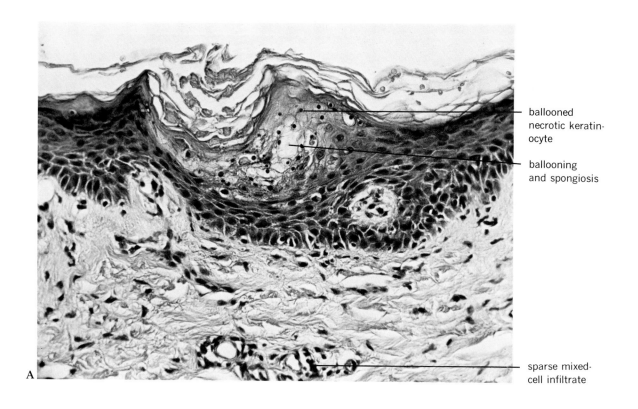

ballooned
necrotic keratin-
ocyte

ballooning
and spongiosis

sparse mixed-
cell infiltrate

A

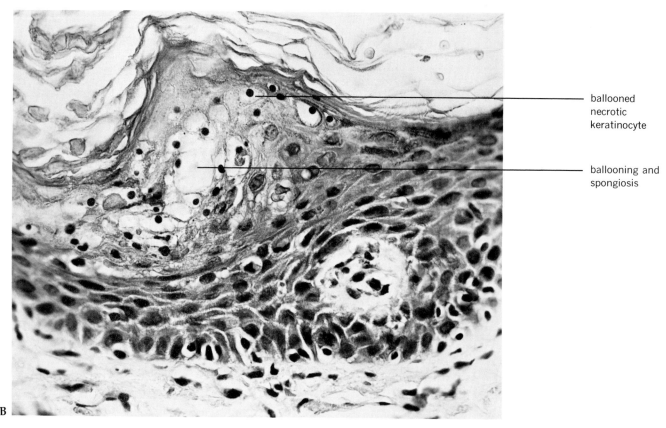

ballooned
necrotic
keratinocyte

ballooning and
spongiosis

B

FIG. 6-61. Irritant contact dermatitis, early changes. Note slight spongiosis, ballooning, and necrosis of keratinocytes in discrete foci. (A, × 291; B, × 620.)

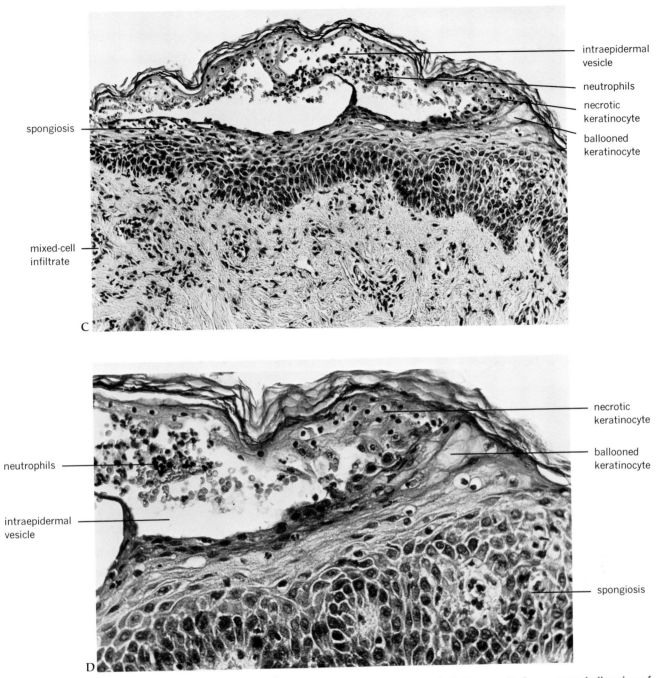

intraepidermal
vesicle

neutrophils

necrotic
keratinocyte

ballooned
keratinocyte

spongiosis

mixed-cell
infiltrate

C

necrotic
keratinocyte

ballooned
keratinocyte

neutrophils

intraepidermal
vesicle

spongiosis

D

FIG. 6-61. (continued). Irritant contact dermatitis, late changes. C, Intraepidermal vesiculation results from severe ballooning of keratinocytes. ($\times$ 168.) D, Ballooned and necrotic keratinocytes seen within epidermal blister are also features of phototoxic dermatitis but are not as sharply circumscribed in the latter. ($\times$ 336.)

Phototoxic Contact Dermatitis

The histologic changes of phototoxic contact dermatitis are similar to those of irritant contact dermatitis. The prime clinical example of phototoxic contact dermatitis is berloque dermatitis due to perfumes that contain 5-methoxypsoralen. Phototoxic contact dermatitis must be distinguished from systemic phototoxic dermatitis such as that induced by demeclocycline (Declomycin). Phototoxic dermatitides, irrespective of whether the photosensitizing agent is applied topically or given systemically, have similar histologic features.

The inflammatory-cell infiltrates in photodermatitides tend to surround the blood vessels of the deep, as well as the superficial, plexus, although they may be wholly limited to the superficial plexus. The deep plexus is almost always affected in polymorphous light eruptions and in photo-induced lesions of discoid lupus erythematosus and is affected less often in photoallergic and phototoxic dermatitides.

Stasis Dermatitis

—Superficial perivascular lymphohistiocytic infiltrate with a few neutrophils around thick-walled capillaries and venules
—Siderophages and often extravasated erythrocytes
—Slight epidermal hyperplasia
—Focal spongiosis
—Focal scale-crust

In severe, long-standing stasis dermatitis, the epidermis may be eroded or ulcerated. The diagnostic hints of this type of dermatitis are spongiotic changes in concert with features of chronic stasis: increased numbers of thick-walled superficial blood vessels and numerous siderophages. Clinically, mottled, tan-brown pigmentation represents persistent leakage of red blood cells from the superficial dermal blood vessels, and petechiae indicate recent extravasation of erythrocytes. The tiny papules in stasis dermatitis result primarily from spongiotic epidermal hyperplasia.

It may be that spongiotic changes in areas of stasis actually represent a contact dermatitis superimposed upon skin already compromised by stasis. Patients often apply numerous nostrums in these locations.

Papular Eruption of Pregnancy

The pruritic condition of the waning days of pregnancy, known as papular eruption of pregnancy, has been discussed earlier in the chapter because it usually consists histologically of a superficial perivascular and interstitial infiltrate of lymphocytes, histiocytes, and eosinophils. Sometimes there may be slight spongiosis.

The lymphocytes in the spongiotic foci of the spongiotic dermatitides seldom have atypical nuclei, but when they do, histologic
findings may be misinterpreted as those of the Pautrier abscesses

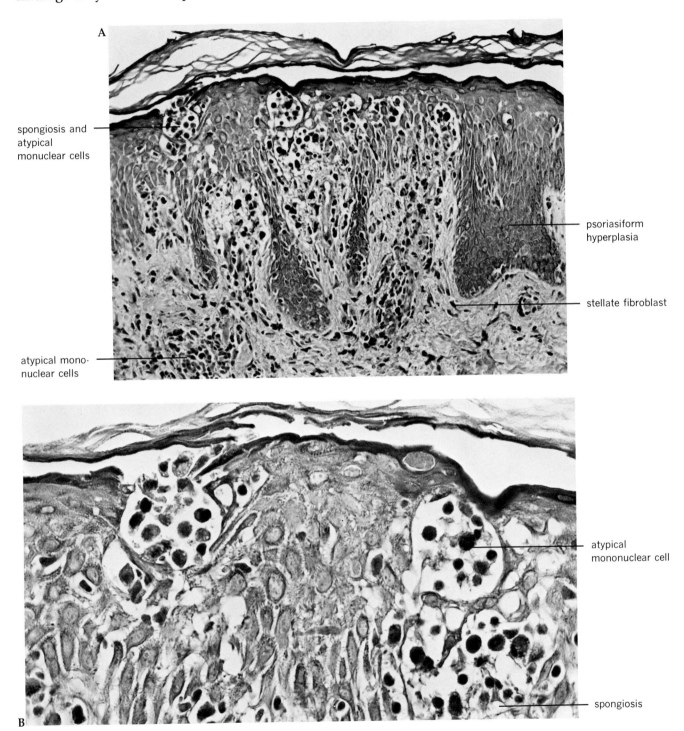

FIG. 6-62. Spongiotic simulation of mycosis fungoides in subacute allergic contact dermatitis. In rare cases, as in this photomicrograph, atypical mononuclear cells in spongiotic foci can be confused with those in mycosis fungoides. The differentiating
feature is absence of spongiosis in mycosis fungoides. Atypical mononuclear cells, presumably T-lymphocytes activated by
responsible contact allergen, can be seen associated with intercellular edema. (A, × 187; B, × 456.)

of mycosis fungoides. The simulant is differentiated from authentic mycosis fungoides by the presence of spongiosis, the absence of many cells having cerebriform nuclei (Fig. 6-63), and relatively sparse dermal infiltrate. Examples of spongiotic simulators are some lesions of acute allergic contact dermatitis and of Gianotti-Crosti syndrome.

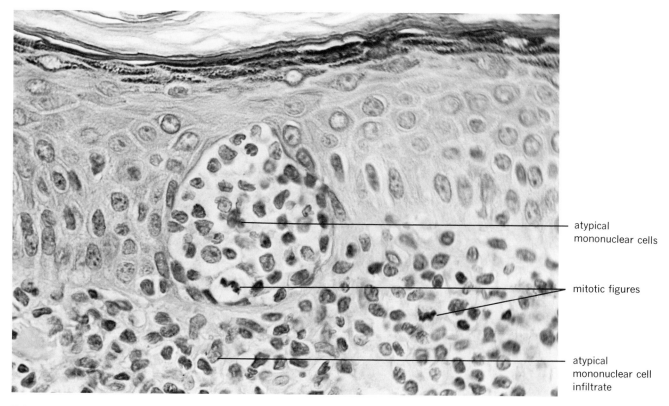

atypical
mononuclear cells

mitotic figures

atypical
mononuclear cell
infiltrate

FIG. 6-63. Mycosis fungoides. Note cytologic similarity between atypical cells within dermis and epidermis. Some nuclei have convoluted, cerebriform shape, and some are in mitosis. There is no spongiosis. ($\times$ 610.)

Eosinophilic Spongiosis (Fig. 6-64)

Eosinophilic spongiosis is distinctive because of the numerous eosinophils within the spongiotic foci and around the blood vessels of the superficial plexus. This type of spongiotic dermatitis occurs as a cardinal feature of incontinentia pigmenti (vesicular stage), an occasional finding in allergic contact dermatitis and arthropod reactions, infrequently in the urticarial lesions of pemphigoid and herpes gestationis, and exceptionally in pemphigus vulgaris.

Incontinentia pigmenti, a multisystem disease that usually is present at birth, clinically proceeds through several skin stages: vesicular, warty-crusted, whorly-pigmented, and, rarely, atrophic. The vesicular stage is characterized histologically by eosinophilic spongiosis.

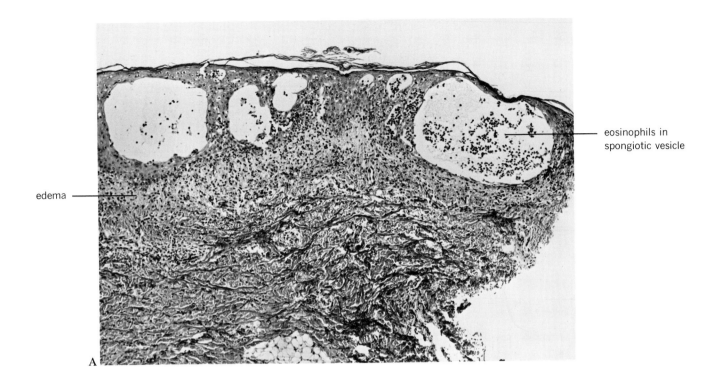

eosinophils in
spongiotic vesicle

edema

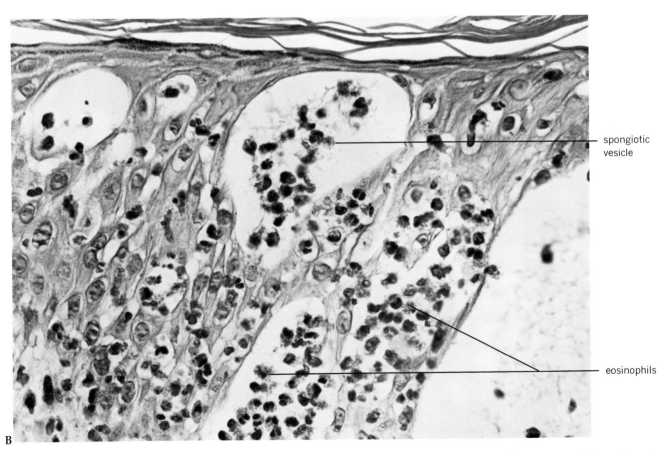

spongiotic
vesicle

eosinophils

FIG. 6-64. Eosinophilic spongiosis: incontinentia pigmenti. Numerous eosinophils in spongiotic vesicles are seen within epidermis of this lesion in early vesicular stage. (A, × 88; B, × 508.)

Acute allergic contact dermatitis is characterized by a spongiotic dermatitis in which eosinophils may or may not be present. In unusual instances, when large numbers of eosinophils occur in the superficial dermis, spongiosis with eosinophils may be seen within the epidermis.

Arthropod reactions, including those of scabies, usually consist of a superficial and deep perivascular dermatitis in which eosinophils are a prominent feature. The vesicle of an arthropod bite is spongiotic and, in some cases, contains numerous eosinophils.

Pemphigoid is a subepidermal vesicular dermatitis with a superficial dermal infiltrate containing eosinophils, lymphocytes, histiocytes, and, occasionally, neutrophils. Sometimes, within the epidermis at the sides of the subepidermal blister, small foci of eosinophilic spongiosis can be seen. More commonly, eosinophils are scattered singly throughout the epidermis of the early urticarial lesions of pemphigoid. What has just been written for pemphigoid applies also to herpes gestationis.

Typical pemphigus vulgaris is diagnosed histologically by intraepidermal vesiculation with the blister forming above the basal-cell zone. Acantholytic cells are present in the suprabasalar cleft and beneath the mostly intact epidermis. Rarely will patients with pemphigus vulgaris also have lesions that reveal eosinophilic spongiosis when a biopsy is done.

Psoriasiform Dermatitis (Fig. 6-5)

Psoriasiform refers to a particular pattern of epidermal hyperplasia, namely, elongation of the rete ridges that accentuates the undulations seen in ordinary cross sections between the epidermal rete and the dermal papillae. This elongation may be subtle, as in early guttate lesions of psoriasis, or extensive, as in long-standing psoriatic plaques. When the psoriasiform pattern is recognized in conjunction with an infiltrate around the blood vessels of the superficial plexus, the question should immediately be posed, "Psoriasis or not psoriasis?" To answer this query properly requires familiarity with the varied histologic presentations of psoriasis and the features that distinguish psoriasis from the other psoriasiform dermatitides.

The classic histologic picture of psoriasis applies to only one presentation of the disease, a lesion of weeks' or months' duration. A papule of eruptive guttate psoriasis, clinically only days old, has a much different histologic appearance and, paradoxically, is not even psoriasiform.

—Sparse lymphohistiocytic infiltrate around the blood vessels of the superficial plexus (rare eosinophils or plasma cells may be found)
—Dilated tortuous capillaries in the papillary dermis
—Thin dermal papillae
—Prominent psoriasiform epidermal hyperplasia with thin but club-shaped rete ridges of approximately equal length
—Increased numbers of mitotic figures in keratinocytes of the lower epidermis
—Thin suprapapillary plate
—Hypogranulosis or absence of the granular layer
—Confluent parakeratosis with small orthokeratotic foci

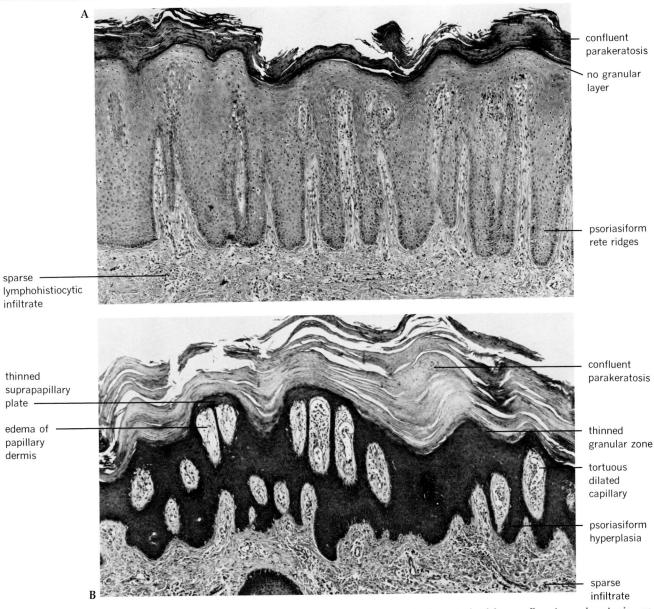

FIG. 6-65. Psoriasis, long-standing plaque. A, Fully developed lesion shown is characterized by confluent parakeratosis, no granular layer, elongated rete ridges of approximately equal length, and sparse inflammatory-cell infiltrate devoid of neutrophils in both dermis and epidermis. (× 73.) B, Confluence of bulbous ends of club-shaped rete ridges is common in specimens from plaques of psoriasis and results from slightly tangential sectioning. (× 80.)

Psoriasis, Early Guttate Lesions (Fig. 6-66)

—Sparse mixed inflammatory-cell infiltrate of lymphocytes, histiocytes, and neutrophils; extravasated erythrocytes common
—Dilated, slightly tortuous capillaries in the papillae
—Slight edema of the papillary dermis
—Slight psoriasiform epidermal hyperplasia
—Small collections of neutrophils within the epidermis, especially within the spinous and granular layers (spongiform pustules), beneath the cornified layer (subcorneal pustules), and within mounds of parakeratosis (pustular scale-crusts)
—Granular layer largely preserved
—Orthokeratosis above regions of intact granular layer and between pustular scale-crusts

During the progression from early papules to chronic plaques there is a series of pathologic changes in psoriasis.

Perhaps the most important consistent sign of psoriasis is the illusion of an increased number of capillaries that spiral upward in the dermal papillae to almost touch the epidermis. The illusory appearance is created by the sectioning through corkscrew-shaped vessels in histologic processing. The tortuous capillaries are surrounded by a few neutrophils and extravasated erythrocytes in evolving lesions and by lymphocytes and histiocytes in those resolving.

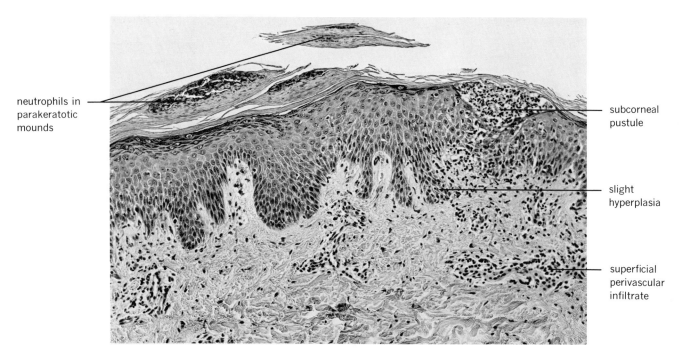

neutrophils in parakeratotic mounds

subcorneal pustule

slight hyperplasia

superficial perivascular infiltrate

FIG. 6-66. Psoriasis, early guttate lesion. Neutrophils within epidermis in spongiform and subcorneal pustules, as well as within parakeratotic foci, are important diagnostic features of early stage. (× 136.)

—Sparse lymphohistiocytic infiltrate with neutrophils around the blood vessels of the superficial plexus
—An apparent increase in number of dilated blood vessels in the papillae (tortuous blood vessels cut in cross section give the impression of an actual increase in the number of blood vessels)
—Extravasated erythrocytes within the papillae
—Extensive edema of the papillary dermis
—Slight to moderate epidermal hyperplasia, usually psoriasiform
—Increased mitotic figures in and above the basal layer
—Neutrophils scattered throughout the epidermis (spongiform pustules)
—Focal parakeratosis, often admixed with neutrophils

When plaques of psoriasis begin to resolve, they show more orthokeratosis than parakeratosis, a well-defined granular zone, and no neutrophils. Among the last features to disappear is the tortuosity of the capillaries.

The clinical features of psoriasis can be reconstructed from the histologic alterations. The clinical counterpart of confluent parakeratosis is gray-white, silvery scales, dilated blood-filled vessels produce redness, edema in the papillary dermis combined with epidermal hyperplasia contributes a sense of firmness to the lesion, and the thin suprapapillary plate allows bleeding when scale

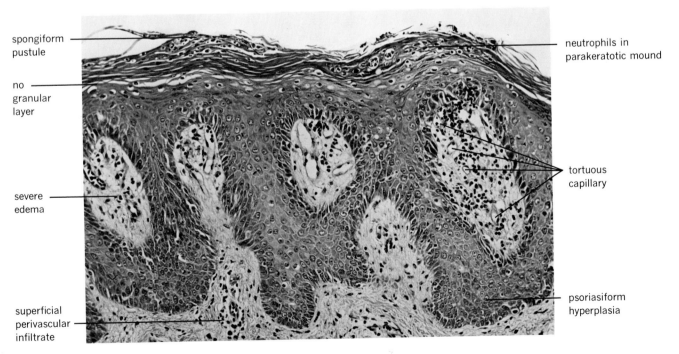

FIG. 6-67. Psoriasis, guttate lesion. A, Tiers of neutrophils within mounds of parakeratosis, spongiform pustules, slight psoriasiform hyperplasia, tortuous capillaries in edematous papillary dermis, and sparse mixed inflammatory-cell infiltrate containing neutrophils are diagnostic of early eruptive psoriasis. (× 164.)

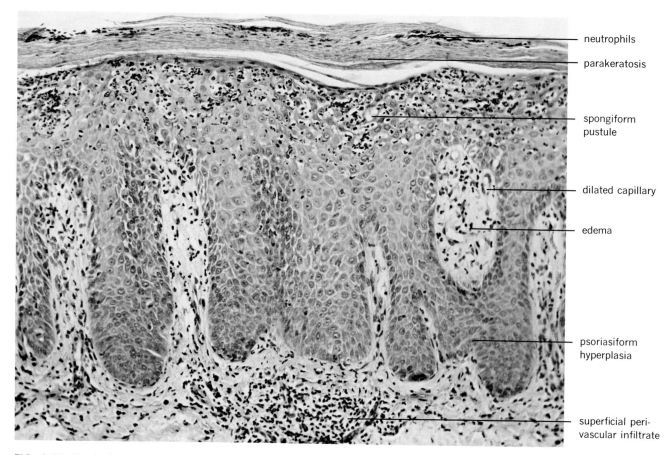

neutrophils

parakeratosis

spongiform
pustule

dilated capillary

edema

psoriasiform
hyperplasia

superficial peri-
vascular infiltrate

FIG. 6-67. Psoriasis, guttate lesion. B, Slightly older active lesion. (× 205.)

is abruptly ripped from the lesion (Auspitz sign). Guttate psoriatic lesions have similar clinical features, but they are less pronounced. In psoriatic erythroderma the histologic character of psoriasis is usually preserved. As a rule, erythrodermas due to different diseases are more easily differentiated from one another histologically than clinically.

Acceleration and exaggeration of the psoriatic process may result in the production of macroabscesses (i.e., pustular psoriasis). Neutrophils emerge from the dilated capillaries in the dermal papillae and ascend into the epidermis where they accumulate in the spinous, granular, and even cornified layers. Histologically, the spongelike appearance results from innumerable neutrophils framed by trabeculations formed by residual keratinocytic membranes. The movement of neutrophils from the papillary dermis into the epidermis often occurs so rapidly that the epidermis does not have time to become hyperplastic. Thus, spongioform pustules may or may not be associated with psoriasiform epidermal hyperplasia. Small pustules (Munro) and spongiform pustules (Kogoj) may also occur in guttate lesions that are not pustular clinically. Scattered neutrophils, rather than collections of them, within the epidermis are significant to diagnose evolving psoriasis.

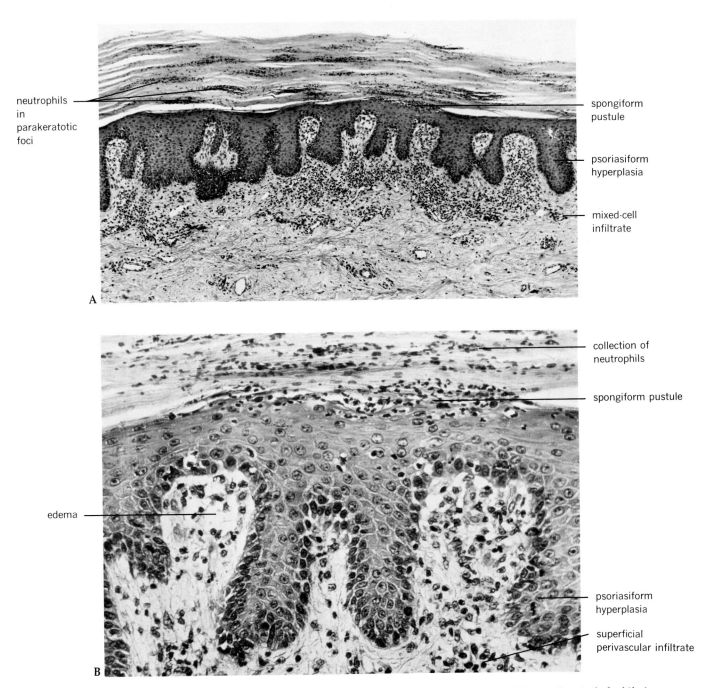

neutrophils in parakeratotic foci

spongiform pustule

psoriasiform hyperplasia

mixed-cell infiltrate

collection of neutrophils

spongiform pustule

edema

psoriasiform hyperplasia

superficial perivascular infiltrate

FIG. 6-68. Psoriasis, periphery of small plaque. Neutrophils at all levels of epidermis, especially within parakeratotic foci that are staggered throughout thickened cornified layer, are characteristic of active lesions. Other features are edematous papillary dermis, slightly psoriasiform epidermis, and spongiform pustules. The greatest activity occurs at periphery of plaque. (A, × 92; B, × 408.)

Sometimes a biopsy obtained from a rapidly developed small pustule of pustular psoriasis reveals a subcorneal pustule, histologically indistinguishable from that of subcorneal pustular dermatosis (Sneddon-Wilkinson syndrome) or impetigo. The neutrophils stream upward to the subcorneal region with such celerity that none are left to form a sponge among the subjacent cells. Similarly, the epidermis may not have time to become psoriasiform or parakeratotic. Simultaneously sampled pustules in the same patient with pustular psoriasis will often reveal both spongiform pustules and subcorneal pustules, depending upon the moment at which their evolution has been interrupted by biopsy.

Spongiform pustules are seen in a variety of clinical diseases, most of which are probably variants of the psoriatic process, for example, pustular psoriasis, acrodermatitis continua, keratoderma blenorrhagicum (Reiter's disease) and impetigo herpetiformis. Occasionally, spongiform pustules are seen in other diseases, namely, secondary syphilis (especially the rupial type), nonlipid reticuloendotheliosis (Letterer-Siwe disease), halogenodermas, pyoderma gangrenosum, and pustular drug eruptions. Theoretically, spongiform pustules can occur in any subcorneal pustular dermatitis because, in order for neutrophils to reach a subcorneal position, they must migrate through the spinous layer. The clinical counterparts of large spongiform pustules are tiny, discrete pustules that form purulent lakes upon coalescence. The pustules resolve with crusts and sheets of delicate scales. Collarettes of scale-crusts are clinical signs of former pustules.

Pustular psoriasis may develop in preexisting psoriatic plaques, appear as an explosive generalized eruption (von Zumbusch type), or be limited to the palms and/or soles (Barber type). However, not all pustular eruptions of the palms and soles represent psoriasis.

Lichen Simplex Chronicus (Figs. 3-14, 6-69)

—Lymphohistiocytic infiltrate with melanophages and occasionally plasma cells, primarily around dilated blood vessels with slightly thickened walls in the superficial dermis
—Thickened papillary dermis composed of laminated coarse collagen bundles oriented parallel to the rete and perpendicular to the surface of the specimen (collagen in vertical streaks)
—Dilated blood vessels in the papillary dermis parallel the coarse collagen in vertical streaks
—Plump, stellate, and multinucleated fibroblasts in the thickened papillary dermis
—Psoriasiform epidermal hyperplasia with rete ridges of unequal length and breadth
—Hypergranulosis
—Compact orthokeratosis with focal parakeratosis

Lichen simplex chronicus is the term applied to thickened skin lesions that result from long-standing rubbing. Persistent rubbing thickens both the epidermis and the papillary dermis, especially

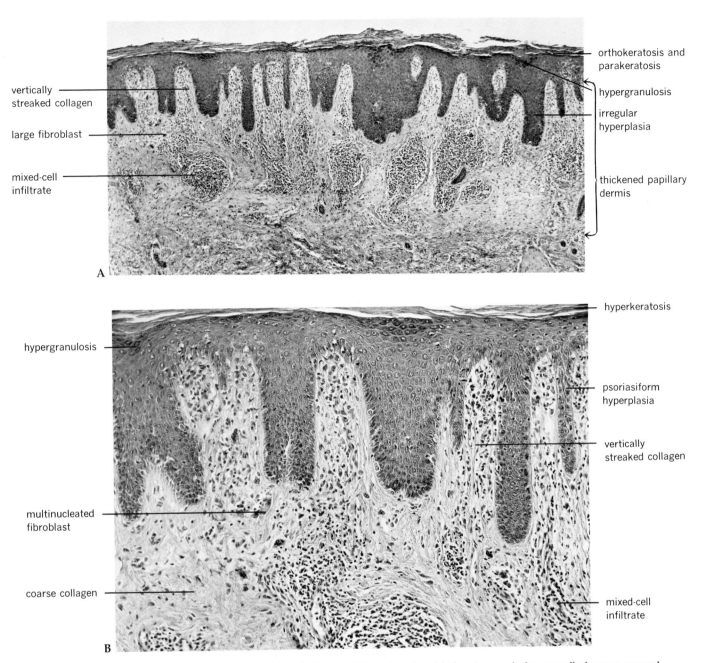

vertically streaked collagen

large fibroblast

mixed-cell infiltrate

orthokeratosis and parakeratosis

hypergranulosis

irregular hyperplasia

thickened papillary dermis

A

hyperkeratosis

hypergranulosis

psoriasiform hyperplasia

vertically streaked collagen

multinucleated fibroblast

coarse collagen

mixed-cell infiltrate

B

FIG. 6-69. Lichen simplex chronicus. Moderately dense infiltrate of lymphocytes, histiocytes, and plasma cells is seen around blood vessels of superficial plexus. A, Between arrows note vast thickening of papillary dermis. (× 50.) B, Note collagen in vertical streaks and increased number of plump, stellate, and multinucleated fibroblasts within thickened papillary dermis. (× 144.)

the latter. In severely rubbed skin, the papillary dermis may be 20 times its normal thickness. Crucial to the diagnosis of lichen simplex chronicus is thickening of the papillary dermis by vertically streaked lamellae of coarse collagen (Figs. 3-14, 6-70). If scratching dominates, there may be prominent parakeratosis, erosion, and even ulceration. The clinical lesion is lichenified because of the thickened papillary dermis and epidermis. The normal skin markings are accentuated because the rete-papillae

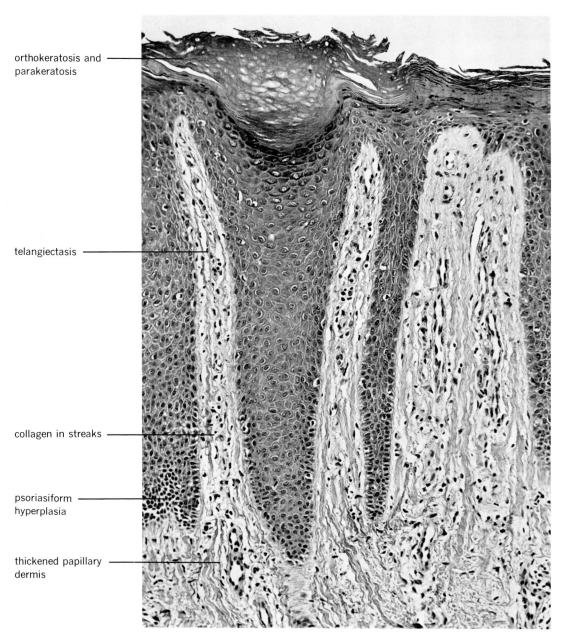

orthokeratosis and
parakeratosis

telangiectasis

collagen in streaks

psoriasiform
hyperplasia

thickened papillary
dermis

FIG. 6-70. Lichen simplex chronicus. Note telangiectases and collagen in vertical streaks oriented parallel to hyperplastic rete ridges and perpendicular to skin surface. Collagen in vertical streaks is diagnostic histologic sign of prolonged rubbing of skin. Thickening of papillary dermis is also evident. (× 187.)

pattern is exaggerated. Increased epidermal melanin plus melanophages is responsible for hyperpigmentation, and the compact confluent orthokeratosis produces an adherent scale. The condition of nodular lesions that results from persistent rubbing of discrete foci is called "prurigo nodularis." The lesions merely represent dome-shaped caricatures of the lesions of lichen simplex chronicus (Fig. 6-71). Eroded or ulcerated nodular lesions, in consequence of having been both rubbed and picked, are termed "picker's nodule" (Fig. 6-72). *Granuloma fissuratum* is a misnomer for lesions of prurigo nodularis that develop secondary to long-standing focal irritations, such as caused by poorly fitting prostheses (e.g., eyeglass frames).

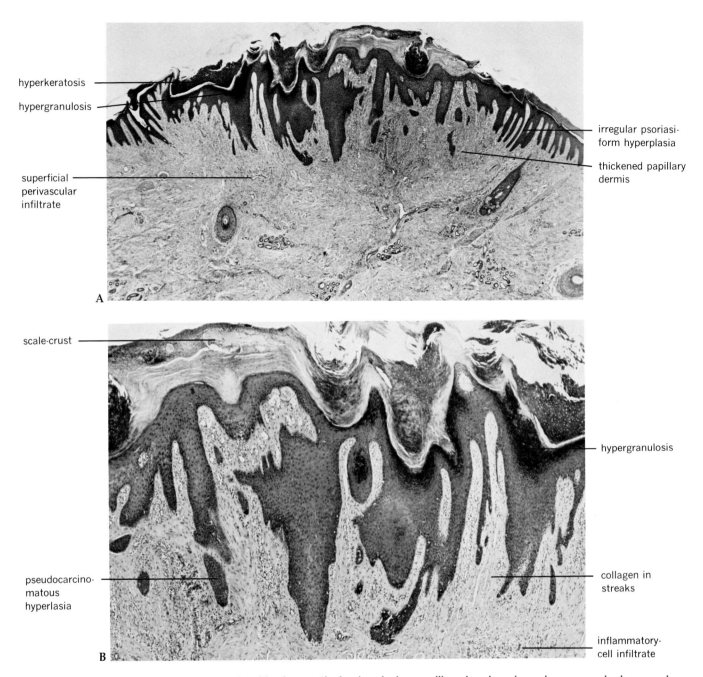

hyperkeratosis

hypergranulosis

superficial
perivascular
infiltrate

irregular psoriasi-
form hyperplasia

thickened papillary
dermis

A

scale-crust

hypergranulosis

pseudocarcino-
matous
hyperlasia

collagen in
streaks

inflammatory-
cell infiltrate

B

FIG. 6-71. Prurigo nodularis. Note that entire skin above reticular dermis, i.e., papillary dermis, spinous layer, granular layer, and cornified layer, is thickened. A, Dome-shaped lesion such as this results from persistent rubbing of well-circumscribed spot and is nothing more than nodular variant of lichen simplex chronicus. ($\times$ 20.) B, Collagen in vertical streaks is seen in thickened papillary dermis. ($\times$ 48.)

Atopic dermatitis is also largely caused by rubbing and scratching. If the fingers of a patient with atopic dermatitis could be restrained, the skin lesions would virtually disappear, although the itching would doubtless persist.

Because itching and resultant rubbing are practiced on diverse pruritic skin lesions, the histologic features of lichen simplex chronicus may be superimposed upon many underlying pathologic processes. For example, repeated rubbing of lichen planus,

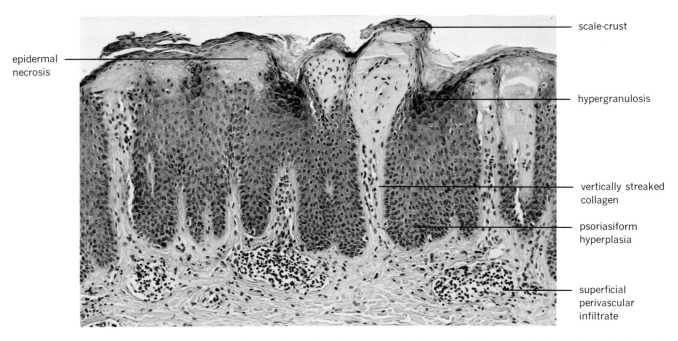

epidermal necrosis

scale-crust

hypergranulosis

vertically streaked collagen

psoriasiform hyperplasia

superficial perivascular infiltrate

FIG. 6-72. Picker's nodule. Foci of epidermal necrosis and scale-crusts result from scratching; psoriasiform hyperplasia and collagen in vertical streaks result from persistent rubbing. (× 142.)

especially lesions on the legs, produces hypertrophic lichen planus. Other lesions that commonly provoke a rubbing response, and consequently are associated with superimposed clinical and histologic features of lichen simplex chronicus, are chronic contact dermatitis, chronic photodermatitis (actinic reticuloid), and mycosis fungoides. Lichen simplex chronicus itself results from the rubbing of what was previously clinically normal skin.

Collagen similar to the coarse, laminated type that occurs in lichen simplex chronicus and its variants (prurigo nodularis and picker's nodule), may also be found in the angiofibromas common to fibrous papule of the face, adenoma sebaceum, and acral fibrokeratomas. The altered collagen in these conditions, just as in lichen simplex chronicus, is produced by plump, stellate, and striking multinucleated fibroblasts.

Contact Dermatitis and Nummular Dermatitis, Chronic (Fig. 6-73)

—Moderately dense lymphohistiocytic infiltrate with melanophages around the vessels of the superficial plexus
—Varying thickening of the papillary dermis by coarse collagen fibers in vertical streaks
—Psoriasiform epidermal hyperplasia
—Focal parakeratosis above hypogranulosis, alternating with orthokeratosis

Eosinophils are occasionally present in chronic allergic contact dermatitis, and a few neutrophils may be seen in chronic irritant contact dermatitis. Eosinophils in a psoriasiform dermatitis are a clue to the diagnosis of chronic allergic contact dermatitis. Spongiosis is usually absent, but when it is present, the diagnostic considerations are subacute allergic contact dermatitis and nummular dermatitis. Chronic nummular dermatitis is indistinguishable histologically from chronic contact dermatitis. Both pruritic conditions are almost always subjected to vigorous rubbing by patients so that there are concurrent histologic signs of lichen simplex chronicus.

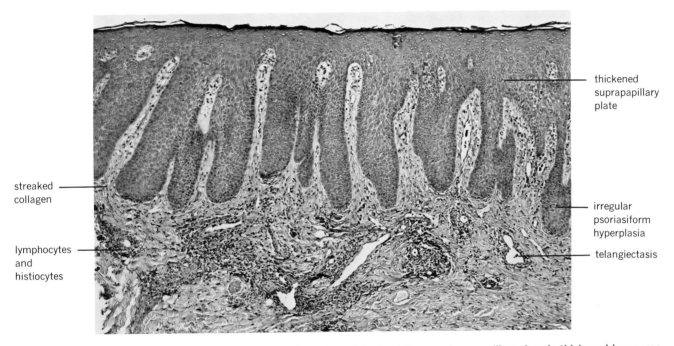

FIG. 6-73. Allergic contact dermatitis, chronic. Some sign of persistent rubbing, such as papillary dermis thickened by coarse collagen fibers arranged in vertical streaks, is usually superimposed upon nonspongiotic psoriasiform dermatitis. ($\times$ 78.)

Some patients are exposed for extended periods to contactants that cause allergic or irritant dermatitis. Common examples of responsible allergens are chromium in cement, nickel in rings and earrings, and plastics in eyeglass frames. Long-standing irritant contact dermatitis can be incited by such chemicals as detergents, turpentine, and gasoline. Clinically, chronic contact dermatitis is characterized by patches and plaques composed of scales (orthokeratosis and parakeratosis) with varying shades of erythema (dilated, blood-filled vessels). Uncommonly, chronic contact dermatitis becomes so widespread that an exfoliative erythroderma results. Clinical and histologic features of lichen simplex chronicus are frequently superimposed upon the erythroderma of chronic contact dermatitis.

Seborrheic Dermatitis, Chronic (Fig. 6-74)

—Sparse superficial perivascular lymphohistiocytic infiltrate
—Widely dilated capillaries and venules in the superficial plexus
—Psoriasiform epidermal hyperplasia
—Parakeratotic follicular plugs
—Focal parakeratosis, especially at the lips of adnexal ostia

Unlike the lesions of acute and subacute seborrheic dermatitis, those of chronic seborrheic dermatitis show neither spongiosis nor neutrophils within the papillary dermis and epidermis. There are striking telangiectases and few inflammatory cells. Clinically, the lesions of chronic seborrheic dermatitis are psoriasiform and covered by scales, rather than scale-crusts.

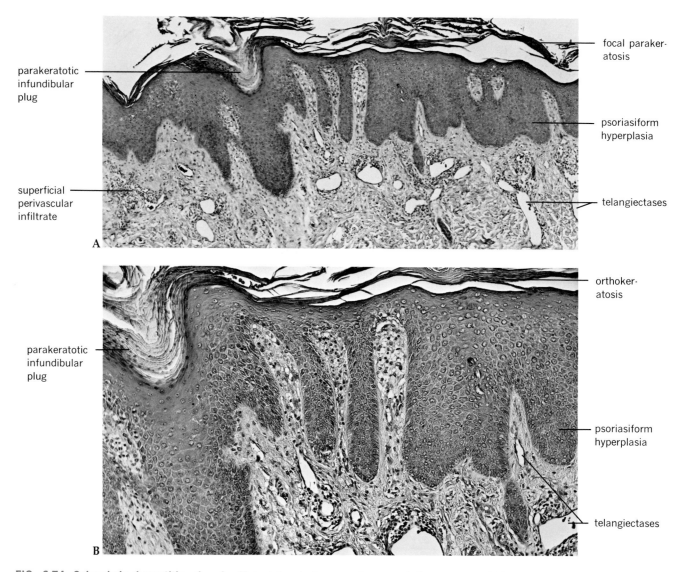

FIG. 6-74. Seborrheic dermatitis, chronic. Note telangiectases and sparse inflammatory-cell infiltrate beneath psoriasiform epidermis, parakeratotic infundibular plug, and alternating orthokeratosis and parakeratosis. (A, × 62; B, × 136.)

—Sparse lymphohistiocytic infiltrate around the dilated blood vessels of the superficial plexus and around infundibular blood vessels
—Psoriasiform epidermal hyperplasia, ranging from slight to extensive
—Dilated follicular infundibula filled with cornified cells
—Alternating orthokeratosis and parakeratosis, both vertically and horizontally

The histologic changes of pityriasis rubra pilaris are present in lesions that, clinically, are strikingly follicular; i.e., keratotic plugs emanate from hair-follicle ostia. Follicular keratoses in pityriasis rubra pilaris may be prominent, extend considerably above the skin surface, and be associated with a dense perifollicular lymphohistiocytic infiltrate. Similar histologic changes in and around follicles can be seen in keratosis pilaris and in lichen spinulosus.

The discrete follicular keratotic papules of pityriasis rubra pilaris are best seen on the dorsa of the hands, but they also occur on the trunk and extremities. Other clinical concomitants are salmon-colored, psoriasiform plaques, erythrodermas within which are small islands of normal skin, severe keratoderma of the palms and soles, and profuse scaling of the face and scalp.

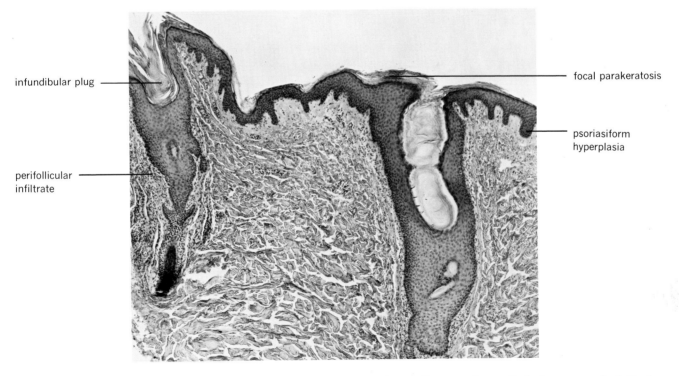

infundibular plug

perifollicular infiltrate

focal parakeratosis

psoriasiform hyperplasia

FIG. 6-75. Pityriasis rubra pilaris. Photomicrographs of two biopsy specimens illustrate diagnostic features, namely, follicular keratotic plugs in association with slight psoriasiform dermatitis and alternating orthokeratosis and parakeratosis. However, follicular plugs are not present in every specimen of pityriasis rubra pilaris. (A, × 57; B, × 84.)

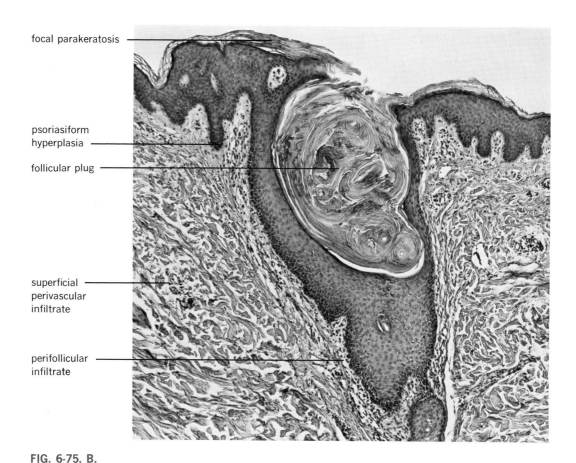

focal parakeratosis

psoriasiform
hyperplasia

follicular plug

superficial
perivascular
infiltrate

perifollicular
infiltrate

FIG. 6-75. B.

Pityriasis Rubra Pilaris without Follicular Involvement (Fig. 6-76)

—Sparse lymphohistiocytic infiltrate around dilated blood vessels of
the superficial plexus
—Epidermal hyperplasia, ranging from slight to psoriasiform
—Focal orthokeratosis and parakeratosis, vertically and horizontally

In the absence of follicular plugging, it is not possible to make
an unequivocal histologic diagnosis of pityriasis rubra pilaris. As
in all skin lesions, microscopic definition will be dependent upon
the site from which the biopsy is obtained. This is of special
importance in pityriasis rubra pilaris because some lesions are
clinically follicular and others are not. The diagnosis of pityriasis
rubra pilaris can be only suggested from the nonfollicular, scaly,
pinkish-orange lesions by the presence of alternating orthokeratosis and parakeratosis, both vertically and horizontally, in association with slight epidermal hyperplasia and sparse superficial
perivascular dermatitis. Unlike the situation in psoriasis, where
there may also be alternating orthokeratosis and parakeratosis, no
neutrophils are present in the parakeratotic foci of pityriasis rubra
pilaris (Fig. 6-77), and the parakeratosis is not in mounds.

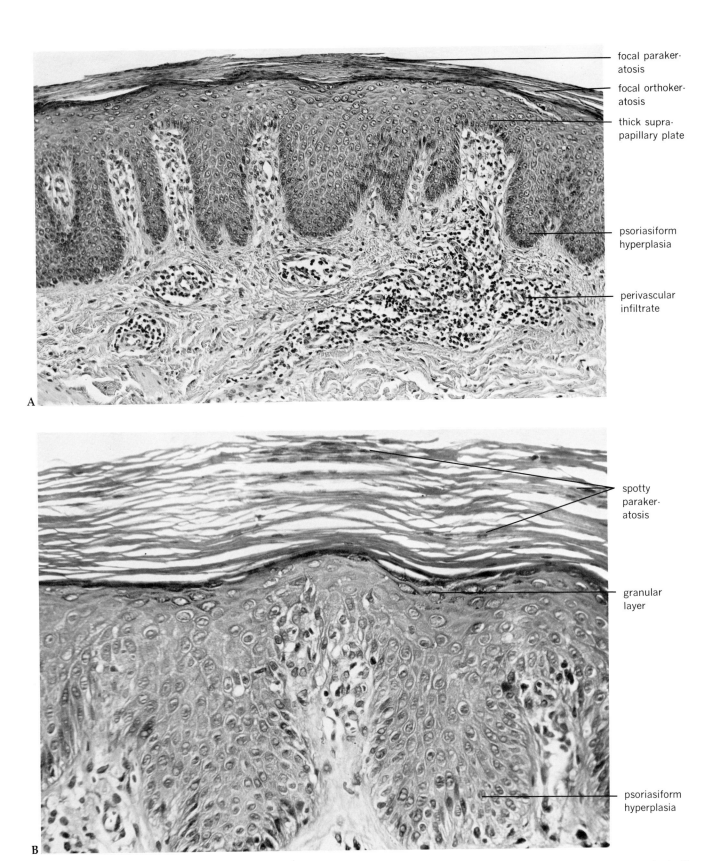

focal paraker-
atosis

focal orthoker-
atosis

thick supra-
papillary plate

psoriasiform
hyperplasia

perivascular
infiltrate

spotty
paraker-
atosis

granular
layer

psoriasiform
hyperplasia

A

B

FIG. 6-76. Pityriasis rubra pilaris without follicular keratotic plugs. A, Parakeratosis that alternates with orthokeratosis, both vertically and horizontally, psoriasiform dermatitis, and absence of neutrophils within epidermis (unlike psoriasis) are characteristic features. (× 136.) B, Diagnosis can be made by noting spotty parakeratosis that alternates with orthokeratosis in both vertical and horizontal directions, an intact granular zone, psoriasiform hyperplasia, no neutrophils within epidermis, and sparse superficial perivascular lymphohistiocytic infiltrate. (× 244.)

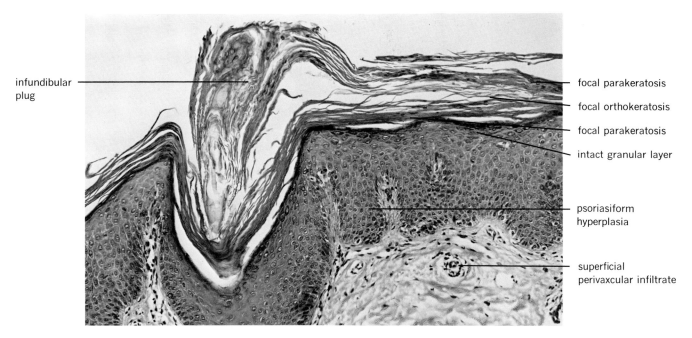

FIG. 6-77. Pityriasis rubra pilaris. Note alternating orthokeratosis and parakeratosis, prominent follicular plug, psoriasiform hyperplasia with intact granular zone, sparse superficial perivascular cellular infiltrate, and absence of neutrophils with epidermis. (× 128.)

Dermatophytosis (Fig. 6-78) and Candidiasis (Fig. 6-79)—Scaling Lesions (Plate 2)

—Sparse lymphohistiocytic infiltrate, occasionally with neutrophils, around the dilated blood vessels of the superficial plexus
—Slight psoriasiform epidermal hyperplasia
—Orthokeratosis occasionally with focal parakeratosis
—Hyphae within the orthokeratotic areas

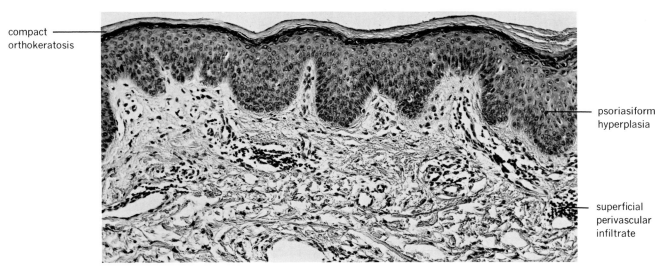

FIG. 6-78. Dermatophytosis, scaly lesion. Example of slightly psoriasiform dermatitis associated with compact orthokeratosis that should prompt a search for fungi in cornified layer. (× 140.)

The critical diagnostic finding in dermatophytosis and candidiasis with scaling lesions is hyphal elements within the cornified layer. These can be identified by careful search of sections routinely stained with hematoxylin and eosin, but they are better visualized by staining with periodic acid-Schiff (PAS) or silver methenamine. To avoid missing the microscopic diagnosis of dermatophytosis and candidiasis, the pathologist should regularly scan the cornified layer (especially if compact orthokeratotic) of every specimen with superficial perivascular dermatitis, looking for opalescent hyphal and/or budding forms. Fungal elements are much more easily discerned in basket-weave rather than compact

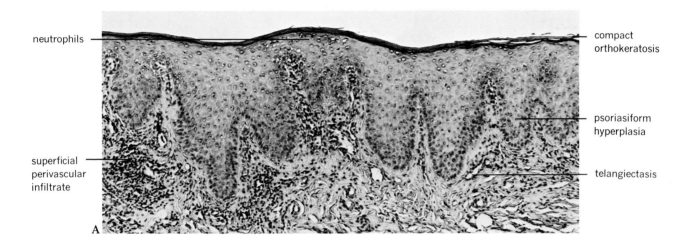

neutrophils — compact orthokeratosis

psoriasiform hyperplasia

superficial perivascular infiltrate — telangiectasis

A

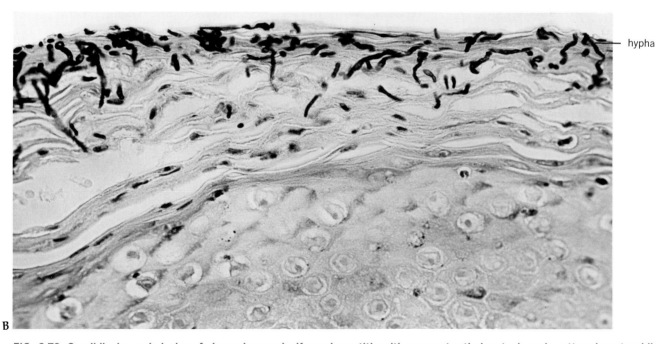

hypha

B

FIG. 6-79. Candidiasis, scaly lesion. A, Irregular psoriasiform dermatitis with compact orthokeratosis and scattered neutrophils within epidermis should strongly suggest diagnosis of candidiasis or dermatophytosis. (× 199.) B, Note the hyphal elements, characteristic of candidiasis, lodged high in the cornified layer. (PAS stain; × 524.)

hyperkeratosis (Fig. 6-80). A helpful aid in identifying hyphae in compact orthokeratosis of sections stained by hematoxylin and eosin is to cut down the light by lowering the condenser of the microscope. The refractility of the fungi is thereby enhanced. Neutrophils in the papillary dermis or epidermis should alert one to the possibility of a superficial fungus infection (Plate 1).

Two fundamental types of pathologic change are induced by dermatophytic infection of skin: (1) vesicles and (2) scales. The fine scale of superficial fungal infections results from orthokeratosis, and the mild erythema results from dilated blood vessels in the superficial plexus. Clinically, candidiasis can present a pustular eruption or scaly plaques.

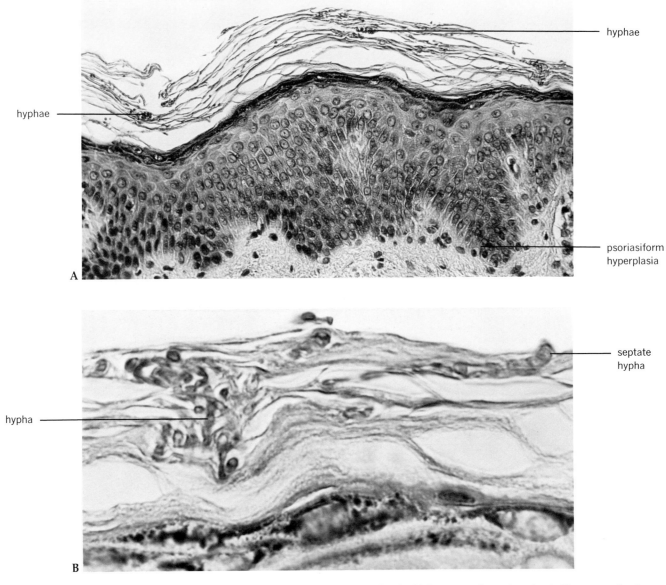

FIG. 6-80. Dermatophytosis, scaly lesion. Photomicrographs of section stained with hematoxylin and eosin. A, Numerous hyphae are seen in basket-weave patterned orthokeratotic stratum corneum. (× 308.) B, Note hyphae oriented longitudinally and in cross section. Dermatophytes are usually found in orthokeratotic horn that is compact rather than basket-weave. (× 835.)

—Sparse superficial perivascular lymphohistiocytic infiltrate
—Varying numbers of extravasated erythrocytes
—Increased number of dilated capillaries in the papillary dermis
—Slight psoriasiform epidermal hyperplasia
—Abundant pale cytoplasm of cells in the superficial epidermis
—Confluent parakeratosis, usually surmounted by basket-weave cornified cells

The lipocytes in the subcutis of patients with pellagra are often shrunken, an evidence of malnutrition and weight loss that usually accompany the disease.

Pellagra, which results from a deficiency of nicotinic acid, is characterized, when clinically classic, by the tetrad of dermatitis, diarrhea, dementia, and, if untreated, death. The redness (owing to dilatation of the vessels of the superficial capillary-venular plexus) and scaling (the result of confluent parakeratosis) occur mostly on areas exposed to sunlight and to friction. If the patient responds to treatment, the dermatitis resolves with hyperpigmentation. Blisters may develop in pellagra as a result of severe intracellular edema in spinous cells. Histologic changes similar to those in pellagra occur in acrodermatitis enteropathica and necrolytic migratory erythema, both also deficiency diseases.

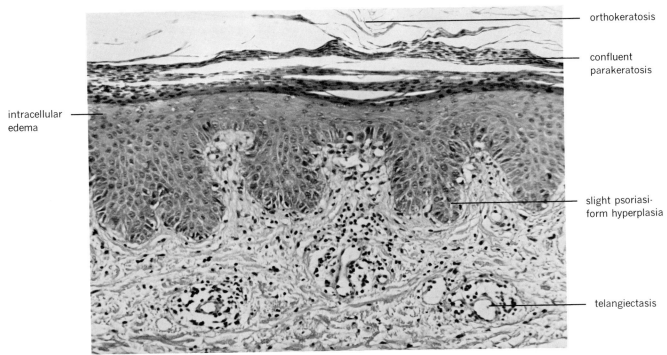

FIG. 6-81. Pellagra. Scaly lesions of this disease are characterized by basket-weave pattern of orthokeratosis in original cornified layer, confluent parakeratosis, slight psoriasiform epidermal hyperplasia, and few inflammatory cells around widely dilated blood vessels of superficial plexus. (× 190.)

Lamellar Ichthyosis (Nonbullous Congenital Ichthyosiform Erythroderma) (Fig. 6-82)

—Sparse lymphohistiocytic infiltrate around the dilated blood vessels of the superficial plexus
—Psoriasiform epidermal hyperplasia
—Normal or thickened granular zone
—Compact laminated orthokeratosis

Lamellar ichthyosis, a congenital disease, is truly an ichthyosis (unlike bullous congenital ichthyosiform erythroderma [epidermolytic hyperkeratosis] which actually is an epidermal nevus) because it consists of fishlike scales. Clinically, these scales differ from those of ichthyosis vulgaris and of X-linked ichthyosis by being much broader and being associated with underlying erythema. Histologically, the epidermis of lamellar ichthyosis is more hyperplastic than that of either ichthyosis vulgaris or X-linked ichthyosis and, unlike ichthyosis vulgaris, has a normal or thickened granular zone. The scale is caused by prominent compact laminated orthokeratosis, and the redness by dilated superficial blood vessels.

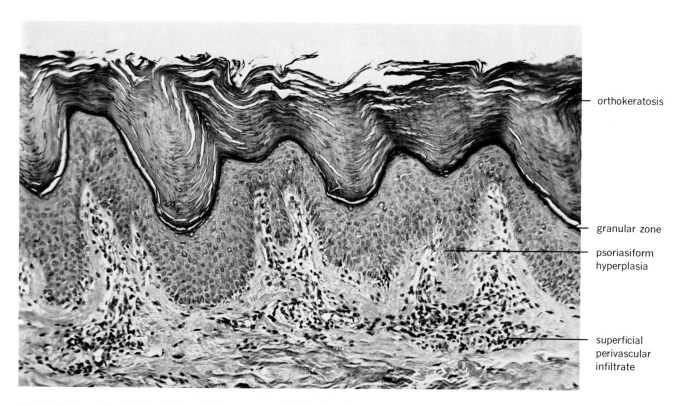

FIG. 6-82. Lamellar ichthyosis (nonbullous congenital ichthyosiform erythroderma). Note inflammatory-cell infiltrate around blood vessels of superficial plexus, as well as psoriasiform epidermis with intact granular zone and compact and laminated orthokeratosis. ($\times$ 133.)

—Superficial perivascular lymphohistiocytic infiltrate
—Psoriasiform epidermal hyperplasia
—Some mononuclear cells within the hyperplastic epidermis
—Focal parakeratosis

Parapsoriasis variegata is more distinctive clinically than it is histologically, consisting of reddish, slightly scaly, longitudinally oriented, gently wavy bands that interweave to form a reticulated pattern. The lesions are persistent and refractory to therapy. They resolve with slight atrophy. Whether parapsoriasis variegata is related to mycosis fungoides has not yet been clarified.

Inflammatory Linear Verrucous Epidermal Nevus (Fig. 6-83)

—Sparse lymphohistiocytic infiltrate around the dilated blood vessels of the superficial plexus
—Slightly papillated psoriasiform epidermal hyperplasia
—Multiple foci of hypogranulosis
—Relatively short, broad zones of parakeratosis, sharply demarcated from orthokeratosis, overlying regions of hypogranulosis

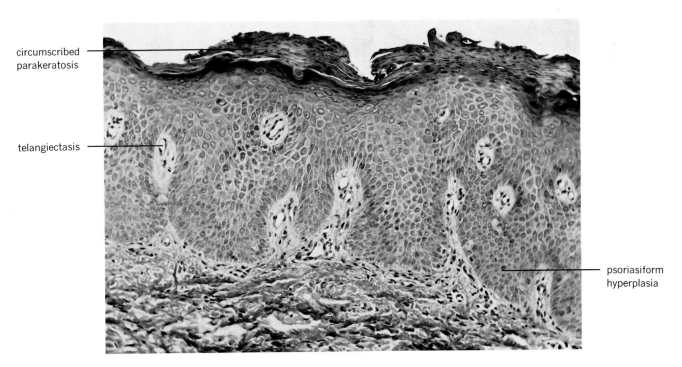

circumscribed parakeratosis

telangiectasis

psoriasiform hyperplasia

FIG. 6-83. Inflammatory linear verrucous epidermal nevus. Presence of well-circumscribed zones of parakeratosis above psoriasiform epidermis should suggest diagnosis. (× 167.)

Inflammatory linear verrucous epidermal nevus, one of the various epidermal nevi, is characterized clinically by discrete, reddish-brown, scaly, slightly verrucous papules that tend to coalesce and form a linear streak. This nevus occurs especially on the left leg, thigh, or buttock of girls, at birth or in early childhood.

The histologic differential diagnosis of inflammatory linear verrucous epidermal nevus is linear porokeratosis that usually has thinner zones of parakeratosis, less epidermal hyperplasia, and little inflammatory-cell infiltrate, but their histologic similarities suggest that the two conditions may be related. In rare instances, slight spongiosis or neutrophils are present in the epidermis of the inflammatory linear verrucous epidermal nevus.

There are several different morphologic expressions of epidermal nevi in addition to the inflammatory linear verrucous epidermal nevus and linear porokeratosis, such as nevus verrucosus and ichthyosis hystrix. In my opinion, bullous congenital ichthyosiform erythroderma is a widespread epidermal nevus and not a type of ichythyosis. I also contend that acanthosis nigricans is not an epidermal nevus, but a kind of papillomatosis in which the epidermis is usually thinned rather than thickened.

Incontinentia Pigmenti, Verrucous Lesions (Fig. 6-84)

—Sparse superficial perivascular lymphohistiocytic infiltrate
—Melanophages scattered throughout the dermis
—Telangiectases in the papillary dermis
—Irregular and extreme psoriasiform hyperplasia
—Numerous large dyskeratotic cells, some calcified, throughout the hyperplastic epidermis
—Increased number of mitotic figures in the lower portion of the epidermis
—Orthokeratosis and parakeratosis

The histologic features in the verrucous lesions of incontinentia pigmenti are absolutely distinctive and diagnostic. The many large dyskeratotic cells scattered throughout the psoriasiform epidermis are not found in any other inflammatory process.

Incontinentia pigmenti is a hereditary systemic disease of females. The skin lesions are usually present at birth and proceed through vesicular, verrucous, and pigmented stages. The vesicular lesions show eosinophilic spongiosis, the verrucous lesions large dyskeratotic cells, and the pigmented lesions melanophages in the dermis. In addition to the cutaneous changes, there may also be skeletal, dental, ocular, and neurologic developmental defects.

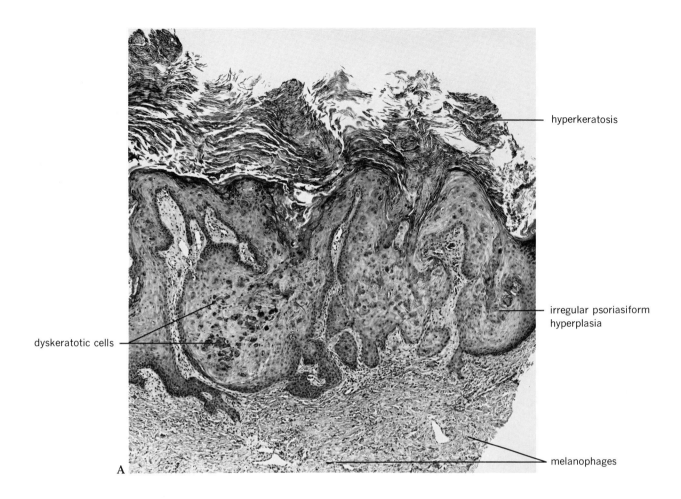

hyperkeratosis

irregular psoriasiform
hyperplasia

dyskeratotic cells

melanophages

A

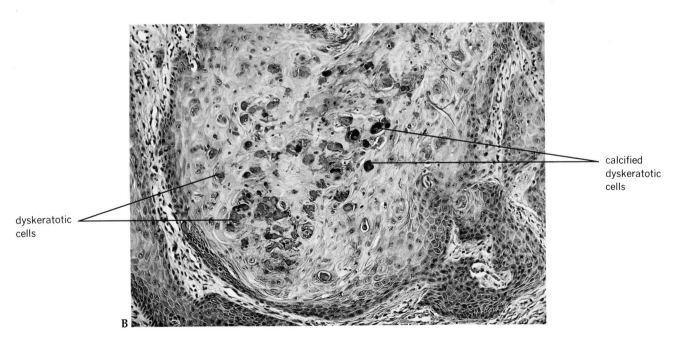

dyskeratotic
cells

calcified
dyskeratotic
cells

B

FIG. 6-84. Verrucous stage of incontinentia pigmenti. A, Numerous dyskeratotic cells in hyperplastic epidermis that is also hyperkeratotic and many melanophages throughout dermis enable an unequivocal diagnosis to be made, (× 53.) B, Note dyskeratotic cells that are apparently calcified. (× 121.)

Acrodermatitis Enteropathica (Fig. 6-85)

—Sparse superficial perivascular lymphohistiocytic infiltrate
—Tortuous capillaries in the papillary dermis
—Psoriasiform hyperplasia
—Few scattered dyskeratotic cells
—Prominent parakeratosis

The psoriasiform lesions of acrodermatitis enteropathica, a disease that begins in infancy, must be differentiated from those of psoriasis, clinically and histologically. In the psoriasiform epidermis of acrodermatitis enteropathica, unlike in psoriasis, there are often dyskeratotic cells and no neutrophils. The psoriasiform lesions of acrodermatitis enteropathica occur especially around the orifices, as well as on the elbows, knees, and paronychial regions and in the intergluteal fold. Vesiculopustular and vesiculobullous lesions may precede the psoriasiform plaques. Alopecia and diarrhea are other features of this disease.

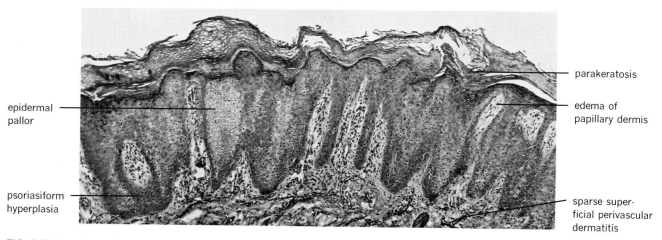

FIG. 6-85. Acrodermatitis enteropathica. Plaque, clinically psoriasiform, shows characteristic histologic features of a psoriasiform dermatitis. Hyperplastic epidermis is covered by parakeratosis and contains dyskeratotic and pale cells. (× 77.)

Spongiotic Psoriasiform Dermatitis (Fig. 6-86)

Spongiotic psoriasiform describes an epidermal pattern of elongated rete ridges with spongiosis. Any spongiotic process that persists may become spongiotic and psoriasiform. However, for practical purposes, there are only two common dermatitides that are spongiotic psoriasiform, namely, subacute allergic contact dermatitis and subacute nummular dermatitis. Both of these diseases, unlike seborrheic dermatitis which has only slight spongiosis and epidermal hyperplasia, may be attended by vesicles.

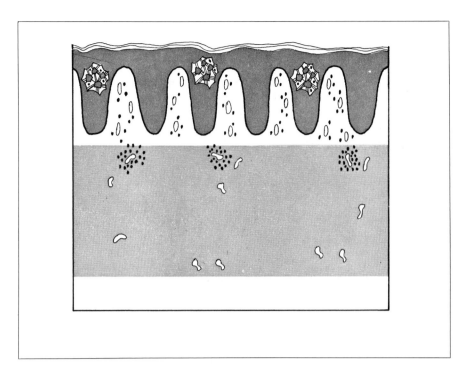

FIG. 6-86. Spongiotic psoriasiform dermatitis.

Nummular Dermatitis, Subacute

Allergic Contact Dermatitis, Subacute (Fig. 6-87)

—Moderately dense mixed-cell infiltrate composed of lymphocytes, histiocytes, occasional plasma cells, and varying numbers of eosinophils (often numerous) around the blood vessels of the superficial plexus
—Edema of the papillary dermis
—Psoriasiform epidermal hyperplasia
—Focal spongiosis
—Focal parakeratosis with homogeneous eosinophilic material containing inflammatory cells (scale-crust)

Subacute nummular dermatitis cannot be distinguished histologically from subacute allergic contact dermatitis. Both are characterized by spongiotic psoriasiform dermatitis, and eosinophils are often found in the dermal infiltrate. Long-standing lesions are less spongiotic and more psoriasiform (Fig. 6-88).

Nummular dermatitis received its name because of the coinlike configuration of the clinical lesions. Clinically, nummular dermatitis consists of well-circumscribed, closely set, tense spongiotic vesicles. When the serum from these intraepidermal vesicles

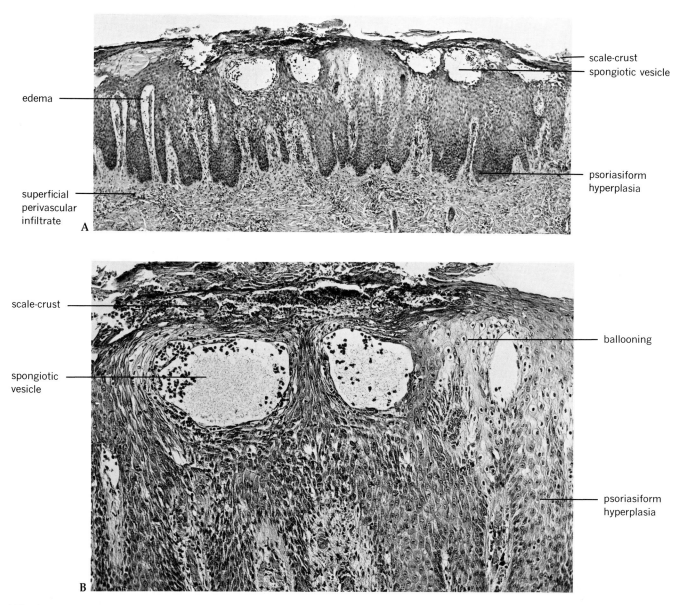

edema —

superficial
perivascular
infiltrate   A

scale-crust
spongiotic vesicle

psoriasiform
hyperplasia

scale-crust —

spongiotic
vesicle

balloning

psoriasiform
hyperplasia

B

FIG. 6-87. Nummular dermatitis, subacute. A, Spongiotic psoriasiform dermatitis, as pictured here, is almost pathognomonic of either subacute nummular dermatitis or subacute allergic contact dermatitis. (× 50.) B, Scale-crusts, as seen in this higher magnification, commonly surmount spongiotic lesions of nummular dermatitis. The numerous neutrophils within the epidermis are signs of impetiginization secondary to scratching. (× 135.)

ascends to the skin surface, crusts form in association with scale. The fierce scratching that accompanies the intense pruritus of nummular dermatitis quickly replaces the vesicles with erosions. Induration results from the thickened epidermis and edematous papillary dermis. In long-standing lesions, coarse collagen in vertical streaks, the telltale sign of rubbing (lichen simplex chronicus), is present in the papillary dermis of both subacute nummular dermatitis and subacute allergic contact dermatitis (Fig. 6-89).

The distinctive exudative discoid and lichenoid chronic dermatosis (Sulzberger-Garbe disease) is probably a variant of nummular dermatitis.

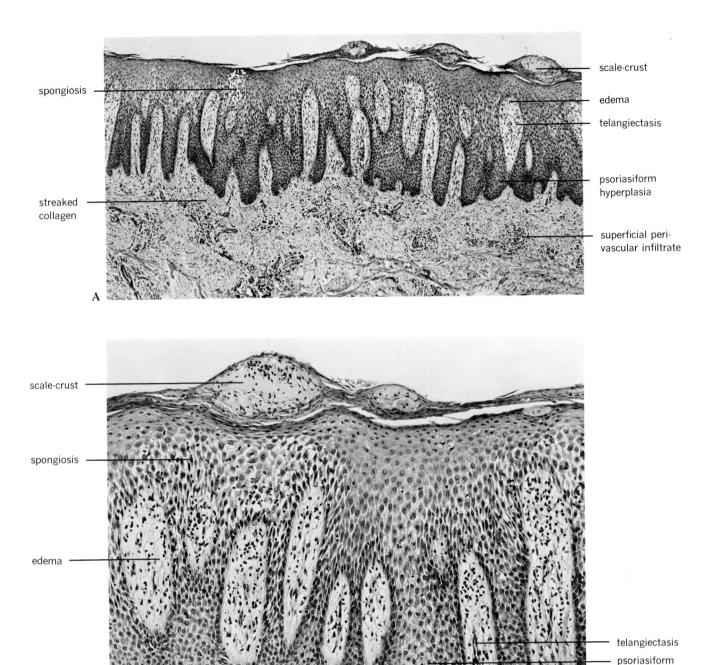

spongiosis

streaked collagen

scale-crust

edema

telangiectasis

psoriasiform hyperplasia

superficial perivascular infiltrate

scale-crust

spongiosis

edema

telangiectasis

psoriasiform hyperplasia

FIG. 6-88. Nummular dermatitis, subacute. A, Multiple scale-crusts, spongiotic psoriasiform hyperplasia, and mixed inflammatory-cell infiltrate are features of either subacute nummular dermatitis or subacute allergic contact dermatitis. Older lesions of nummular dermatitis are marked by pronounced psoriasiform hyperplasia and relatively little spongiosis (A, × 54; B, × 140.)

Just as the acute forms of allergic contact dermatitis, nummular dermatitis, dyshidrotic dermatitis, id reactions, and vesicular dermatophytoses may be indistinguishable from one another histologically, so too may the subacute forms of these conditions be spongiotic psoriasiform dermatitides. Each may also show evidences of lichen simplex chronicus as a result of persistent rubbing.

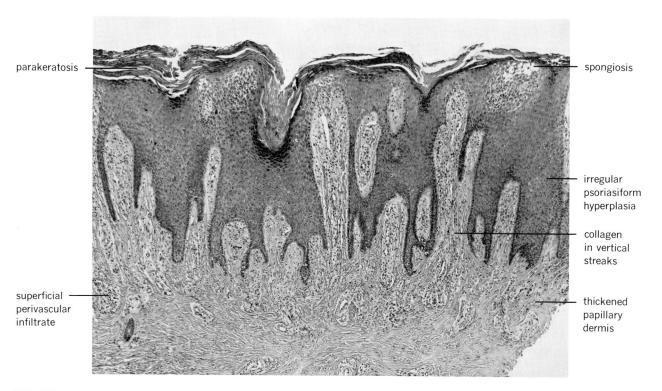

parakeratosis

spongiosis

irregular
psoriasiform
hyperplasia

collagen
in vertical
streaks

superficial
perivascular
infiltrate

thickened
papillary
dermis

FIG. 6-89. Subacute contact or nummular dermatitis, persistently rubbed. Papillary dermis thickened by collagen in vertical streaks sandwiched between spongiotic psoriasiform hyperplasia and lymphohistiocytic infiltrate around dilated blood vessels of superficial plexus are diagnostic features of lichen simplex chronicus superimposed upon subacute contact or nummular dermatitis. ($\times$ 53.)

Seborrheic Dermatitis, Subacute (Fig. 6-90)

—Sparse superficial perivascular infiltrate of lymphocytes and histiocytes
—Prominent telangiectases
—Slight spongiosis
—Slight psoriasiform hyperplasia
—Follicular plugging by orthokeratosis and parakeratosis
—Scale-crusts containing neutrophils at the lips of the follicular ostia

Subacute seborrheic dermatitis has spongiosis in common with acute seborrheic dermatitis, as well as psoriasiform hyperplasia in common with chronic seborrheic dermatitis. In the subacute stage spongiosis and hyperplasia are less prominent.

At most stages in its evolution, important diagnostic signs of seborrheic dermatitis are mounds of scale-crusts containing neutrophils at the lips of dilated horn-filled follicular infundibula. It may be that the acrosyringia, as well as the acrotrichia, are plugged by cornified cells in seborrheic dermatitis, because sweating is significantly diminished within the lesions.

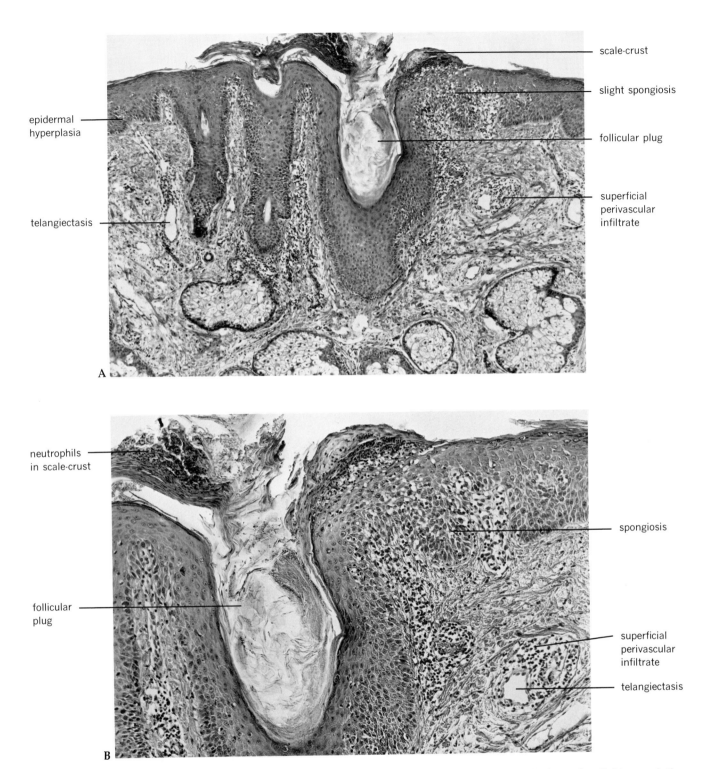

scale-crust

slight spongiosis

follicular plug

superficial perivascular infiltrate

epidermal hyperplasia

telangiectasis

A

neutrophils in scale-crust

spongiosis

follicular plug

superficial perivascular infiltrate

telangiectasis

B

FIG. 6-90. Seborrheic dermatitis, subacute. Note follicular plugs, scale-crusts at margins of infundibular ostia, slight spongiotic epidermal hyperplasia, and sparse inflammatory-cell infiltrate around telangiectasias. Note neutrophils at periphery of infundibular orifice. (A, × 92; B, × 189.)

Superficial and Deep Perivascular Dermatitis

Primarily Perivascular

Lymphohistiocytic infiltrate

Lymphocytic infiltration (Jessner)

Gyrate erythema, deep

Scleroderma, inflammatory stage

Indeterminate leprosy

Polymorphous light eruption

Mixed-cell infiltrate, neutrophils prominent

Cellulitis (including erysipelas)

Acute febrile neutrophilic dermatosis
(Sweet's syndrome)

Erythropoietic protoporphyria

Tick bite

Fleabite

Mixed-cell infiltrate, eosinophils prominent

Most reactions to arthropods, creeping eruption, cercarial dermatitis, caterpillar dermatitis, coral dermatitis, and "itchy red bump" disease

Herpes gestationis, urticarial lesions

Pemphigoid, urticarial lesions

Mixed-cell infiltrate with neutrophils and eosinophils prominent

Urticarial allergic eruptions, deep type

Interface Dermatitis

Lymphohistiocytic infiltrate

Discoid lupus erythematosus, acute

Discoid lupus erythematosus, chronic

Discoid lupus erythematosus, subacute

Pityriasis lichenoides et varioliformis acuta

Lymphomatoid papulosis

Lichenoid photodermatitis

Mixed-cell infiltrate

Fixed drug eruption

Syphilis, secondary stage

Spongiotic Dermatitis

Photocontact dermatitis

Reactions to arthropods, creeping eruption, cercarial dermatitis

Fixed drug eruption

Dermatophytosis, vesicular lesions

Cellulitis

Psoriasiform Dermatitis

Scabies, keratotic-crusted lesions

Syphilis, secondary stage

Actinic reticuloid

Pityriasis rosea, herald patch

Superficial *and* Deep Perivascular Dermatitis

A CELLULAR infiltrate that surrounds the blood vessels of the superficial and deep plexuses denotes superficial and deep perivascular dermatitis (Fig. 1-19). The cellular composition of the infiltrate may be either lymphohistiocytic or mixed. As with superficial perivascular dermatitis, superficial and deep perivascular dermatitis may be wholly dermal, or there may be associated epidermal alteration at the interface or in the form of spongiotic or psoriasiform changes. Superficial perivascular dermatitides tend to be skin diseases that have no accompanying systemic manifestations. By contrast, superficial and deep perivascular dermatitides occasionally have concomitant involvement of internal organs.

Some of the diseases that I have classified as superficial and deep perivascular dermatitides, for example, pityriasis lichenoides et varioliformis acuta and arthropod reactions, may at times be marked by superficial perivascular dermatitis only.

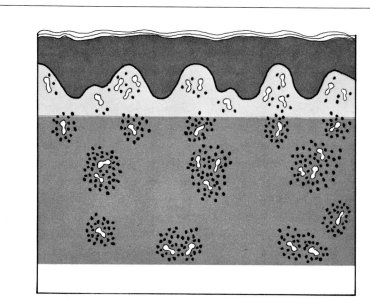

FIG. 7-1. Superficial and deep perivascular dermatitis.

Primarily Perivascular (Fig. 7-1)

Superficial and deep perivascular dermatitis that is wholly dermal and mostly perivascular may be characterized by infiltration of lymphocytes and histiocytes, as in deep gyrate erythema, or by a mixture of cells, as in cellulitis where neutrophils are prominent, in most reactions to arthropods where eosinophils are numerous, and in deep urticarial allergic eruptions where there are both neutrophils and eosinophils.

Lymphohistiocytic Infiltrate

Lymphocytic infiltrates in the dermis are almost always those of inflammatory diseases. Only rarely will a lymphocytic infiltrate around the blood vessels of both plexuses be that of chronic lymphocytic leukemia.

Lymphocytic Infiltration (Jessner) (Fig. 7-2)

—Moderately dense lymphohistiocytic infiltrate around the vessels of the superficial and deep plexuses
—Mucin often between collagen bundles of the reticular dermis

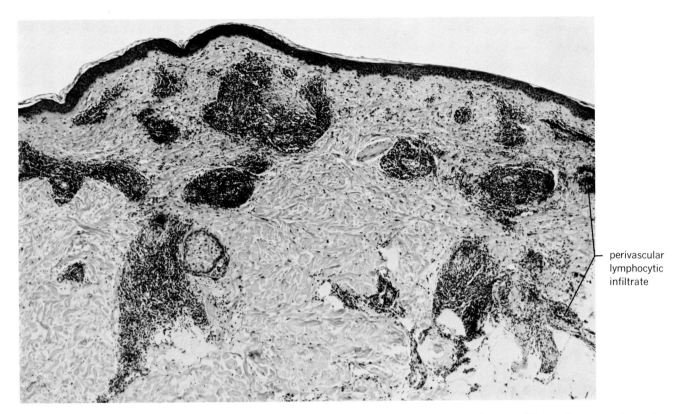

perivascular
lymphocytic
infiltrate

FIG. 7-2. Lymphocytic infiltration (Jessner). As in discoid lupus erythematosus there is superficial and deep perivascular predominantly lymphocytic infiltrate, but vacuolar alteration and thickening of basement membrane are absent. (× 51.)

The diagnosis "lymphocytic infiltration" is not specific, but rather descriptive of certain histologic findings of which the exact nosologic position is uncertain. Lymphocytic infiltration can usually be distinguished histologically from polymorphous light eruption by the near absence of edema in the papillary dermis and from discoid lupus erythematosus by the absence of alterations at the dermoepidermal interface. Clinically, the lesions of lymphocytic infiltration are firm, pink to red-brown, smooth-surfaced papules and plaques, usually on the face, the result of both the cellular infiltrate and mucin deposition. Some plaques are annular because of central clearing.

A noninflammatory disease that also consists of a monomorphous infiltrate of lymphocytes around the blood vessels of both plexuses is lymphocytic leukemia. That condition must therefore be considered in the differential diagnosis of lymphocytic infiltration (Jessner) and its look-alikes, the deep form of gyrate erythema and nonedematous lesions of polymorphous light eruption.

The early inflammatory stage of scleroderma may also be confused with lymphocytic infiltration. Clues to scleroderma in earliest development are occasional presence of plasma cells and a septal panniculitis, assuming a deep enough biopsy specimen is examined.

Gyrate Erythema, Deep (Fig. 7-3)

—Moderately dense lymphohistiocytic infiltrate around the blood vessels of the superficial and deep plexuses
—Slight edema of the papillary dermis

Gyrate erythemas are of two types: (1) superficial and (2) deep. Deep lesions, unlike the superficial ones, show neither focal epidermal spongiosis nor parakeratosis. Clinically, the lesions of the deep type are firmer than those of the superficial type, and they lack peripheral scales. The reddish, firm lesions may be annular, arcuate, polycyclic, or serpentine. No cause is usually discoverable for the persistent gyrate erythemas of either the superficial or the deep types, but one of the deep types (erythema gyratum repens) is found in association with internal malignant tumors often enough to suggest causal relationship. Another variant (erythema chronicum migrans) may follow an insect or tick bite. The deep form of gyrate erythema rarely occurs in female carriers of chronic granulomatous disease.

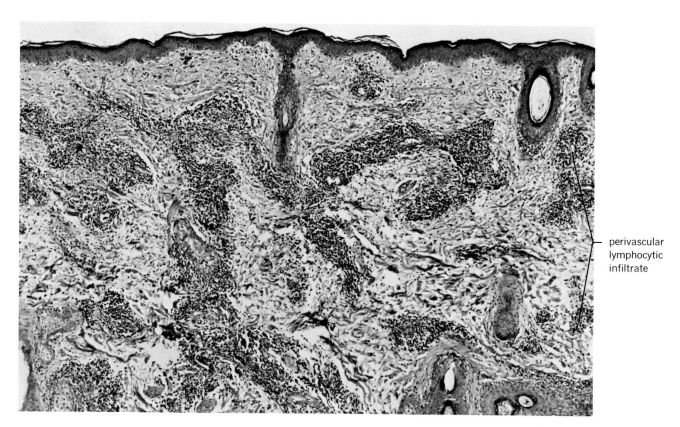

perivascular lymphocytic infiltrate

FIG. 7-3. Gyrate erythema, deep. Histologic changes pictured are indistinguishable from those of lymphocytic infiltration (Jessner) and of nonedematous lesions of polymorphous light eruption. They are easily distinguishable from those of superficial gyrate erythema (erythema annulare centrifigum) in which the infiltrate is wholly superficial and there are focal spongiosis and parakeratosis. (× 51.)

—Moderately dense lymphohistiocytic infiltrate, sometimes with plasma cells and eosinophils, around the vessels of the superficial and deep plexuses
—Varying degrees of sclerosis within the reticular dermis

In addition to the superficial and deep perivascular dermatitis, a neutrophilic vasculitis in the subcutis (Chapter 8) and a panniculitis in which lymphocytes, histiocytes, eosinophils, and plasma cells abound, may be seen in early stages of scleroderma (Chap-

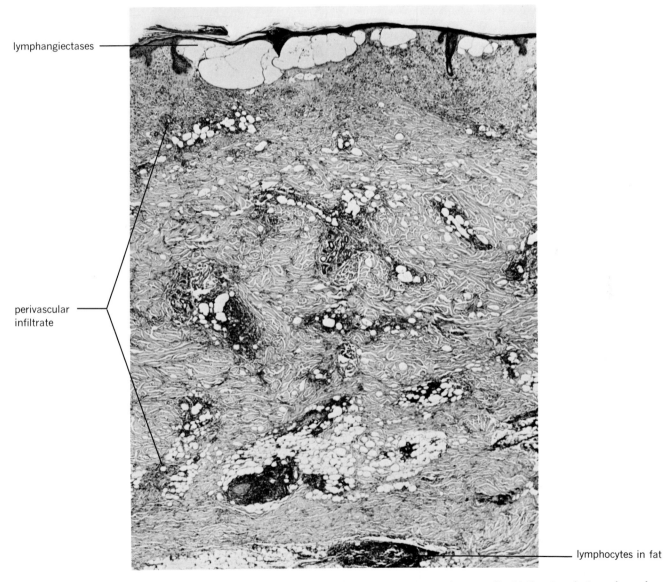

lymphangiectases

perivascular infiltrate

lymphocytes in fat

FIG. 7-4. Scleroderma. Superficial and deep perivascular infiltrate of lymphocytes, plasma cells, histiocytes, but rarely eosinophils, is characteristic of early inflammatory stage. A, Concomitant panniculitis results in destruction of subcutaneous fat and its subsequent replacement by fibrosis. Lymphangiectases, as pictured, rarely develop. ($\times$ 39.)

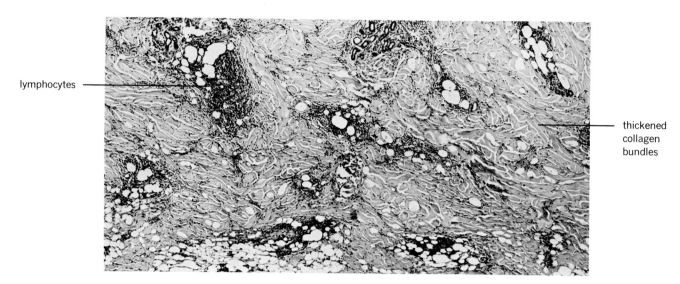

lymphocytes

thickened collagen bundles

FIG. 7-4. B, Thickening of collagen bundles throughout dermis follows appearance of inflammatory-cell infiltrate in this higher magnification of A (× 50.)

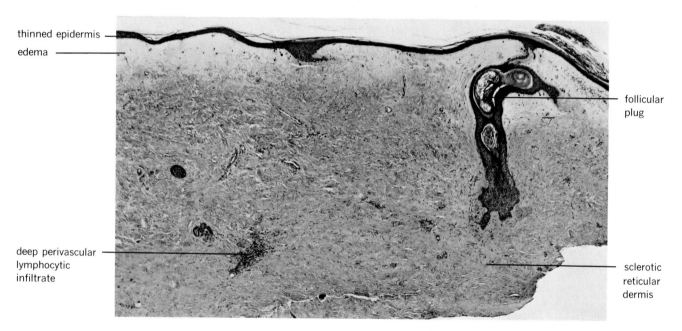

thinned epidermis

edema

follicular plug

deep perivascular lymphocytic infiltrate

sclerotic reticular dermis

FIG. 7-4. C, Morphea and lichen sclerosus et atrophicus in same lesion, a rare occurrence. Thinned epidermis, plug of corni-fied cells in dilated infundibulum, and thickened edematous papillary dermis are features of lichen sclerosus et atrophicus. Deep perivascular lymphocytic infiltrate in sclerotic reticular dermis is feature of scleroderma. (× 31.)

ter 14). At this early point there may be slight or no thickening of the collagen bundles. Adnexa are usually still intact, and fibro-blasts are normal in number. The superficial and deep perivascular infiltrate precedes the sclerotic changes. An uncommon finding in scleroderma is lymphangiectases in the superficial dermis. Except for minor variations, these comments apply to all forms of sclero-derma, to wit, the localized, widespread, and acral. Localized lesions of scleroderma can be subdivided into the following types: guttate, plaque (morphea), and linear (one variant of which is "en coup de sabre" and another is facial hemiatrophy). The guttate

and plaque lesions may also be widespread. Idiopathic atrophoderma of Pasini and Pierini probably is widespread "burned-out"
atrophic hyperpigmented patches of morphea. Progressive systemic sclerosis is often associated with acrosclerotic skin lesions.

Sclerodermoid skin lesions may occur in some patients with
porphyria cutanea tarda and with chronic forms of graft-versus-
host reactions. Fasciitis with eosinophilia seems to me to be a
variant of scleroderma.

Rarely, lesions of localized scleroderma, especially morphea,
and of lichen sclerosus et atrophicus may occur in the same
patient, and even more exceptionally, both processes may be
present in the same lesion (Fig. 7-4C).

The early inflammatory lesions of localized scleroderma often
are lilac-colored, especially at their borders. Later, they are white
and hard centrally. The inflammatory-cell infiltrate is most dense
in the lilac rim, whereas sclerosis predominates centrally. The
early clinical changes in acrosclerosis are better appreciated by
palpation of a sense of doughiness than by inspection.

Indeterminate Leprosy (Fig. 7-5)

—Sparse lymphohistiocytic infiltrate around the blood vessels of the
 superficial and deep plexuses
—Occasional inflammatory cells around and within cutaneous nerves
 (Fig. 7-5B)

As one would expect from the meagerness of the dermal
infiltrate, the lesions of indeterminate leprosy are macules and
patches that are not firm to touch. They are often hypoesthetic
secondary to involvement of nerves and hypopigmented secondary to diminution of epidermal melanin. Indeterminate leprosy is
usually an incipient form of the disease not yet clinically, histologically, or immunologically directed to a lepromatous or tuberculoid course.

A suggestive, but not unequivocal, diagnosis of leprosy in any
form may be made from sections stained with hematoxylin and
eosin. Acid-fast stains, such as the Fite, must be done in an
attempt to demonstrate the lepra bacillus. In indeterminate leprosy, which has neither clinical nor histologic features of lepromatous or tuberculoid leprosy, it is usual to find only a few
organisms within the histiocytes. Sometimes no lepra bacilli can
be found in lesions of indeterminate leprosy.

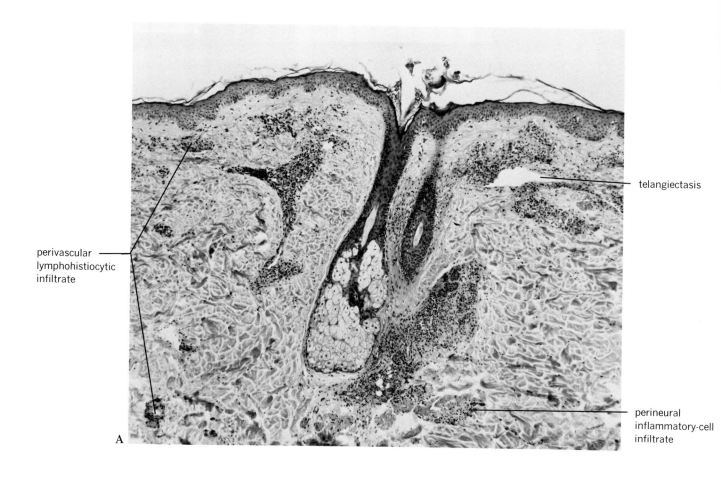

perivascular
lymphohistiocytic
infiltrate

telangiectasis

perineural
inflammatory-cell
infiltrate

A

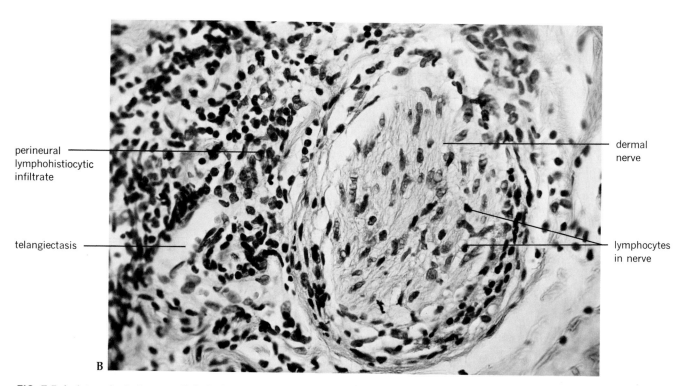

perineural
lymphohistiocytic
infiltrate

telangiectasis

dermal
nerve

lymphocytes
in nerve

B

FIG. 7-5. Indeterminate leprosy. Relatively sparse superficial and deep perivascular and perineural inflammatory-cell infiltrate of histiocytes and lymphocytes should suggest diagnosis. Fite stain may enable confirmation of diagnosis by demonstrating acid-fast bacilli within some histiocytes. (A, × 86; B, × 475.)

—Moderately dense lymphohistiocytic infiltrate around the blood vessels of the superficial and deep plexuses

—Edema of the papillary dermis in varying degree and, if severe, subepidermal vesiculation

—Extravasated erythrocytes in the superficial dermis

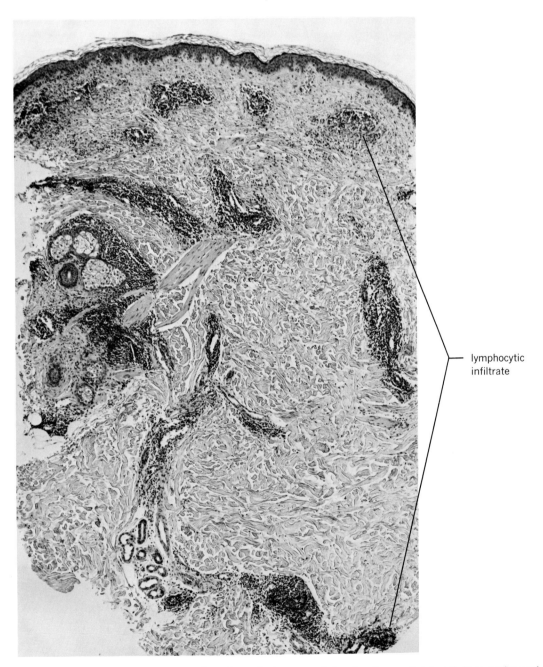

lymphocytic
infiltrate

FIG. 7-6. Polymorphous light eruption. Some lesions consist only of superficial and deep perivascular lymphocytic infiltrate, indistinguishable from lymphocytic infiltration (Jessner) and gyrate erythema, deep type. (× 62.)

A superficial and deep perivascular lymphohistiocytic infiltrate with edema of the papillary dermis is practically diagnostic of polymorphous light eruption. The collagen fibers of the papillary dermis still cling to the epidermis until they are completely separated from it by edema. When edema is massive, a subepidermal blister forms. A similar pattern can be seen with the scanning

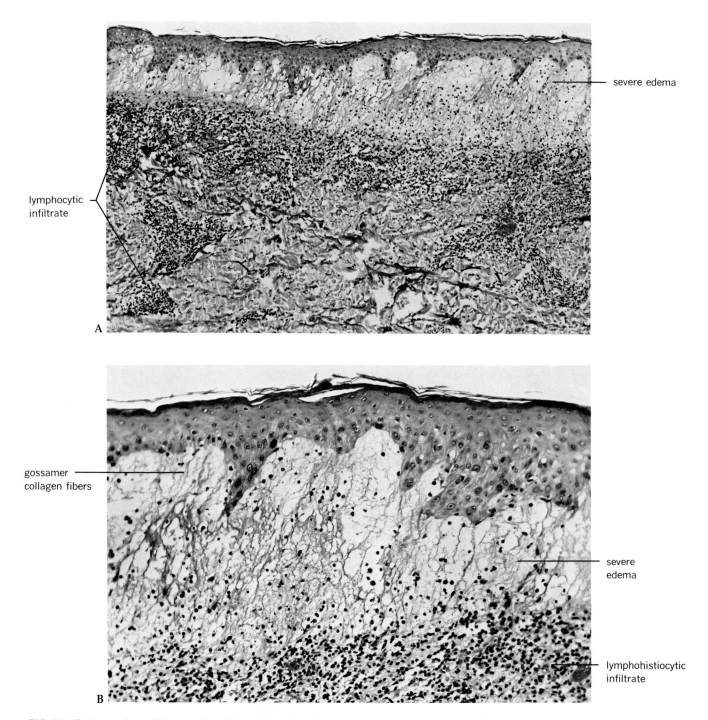

FIG. 7-7. Polymorphous light eruption. Biopsy of a "juicy" papule or plaque reveals superficial and deep perivascular lymphohistiocytic infiltrate with massive edema of papillary dermis. Gossamer collagen fibers still attached to epidermis, despite severe edema. (A, × 68; B, × 166.)

objective in some arthropod reactions, but they are almost always associated with many eosinophils, not only around blood vessels, but between the collagen bundles as well. Massive edema that may dislodge the epidermis can also be found in erysipelas, which is a cellulitis with a sparse superficial and deep dermal mixed-cell infiltrate. Early lesions of lichen sclerosus et atrophicus also show striking edema in the papillary dermis, but the lymphohistiocytic infiltrate is confined to the upper half of the dermis.

Absence of vacuolar alteration at the dermoepidermal junction and lack of basement-membrane thickening in polymorphous light eruption usually allow differentiation from discoid lupus erythematosus. Additionally, in polymorphous light eruption, the follicular infundibula are usually not dilated by cornified cells as they frequently are in discoid lupus erythematosus. Lesions of polymorphous light eruption which lack prominent edema in the papillary dermis may be indistinguishable histologically from lymphocytic infiltration (Jessner) (Fig. 7-6). A helpful clue in differentiation of such cases is the presence of mucin in the reticular dermis in some lesions of lymphocytic infiltration (Jessner).

The primary clinical lesions of polymorphous light eruptions are edematous papules that may evolve into plaques or vesicles. The papules and plaques are secondary to both the edema in the papillary dermis and the superficial and deep perivascular lymphohistiocytic infiltrate. Vesicles form when the superficial edema separates the epidermis from the dermis. Because the lesions of polymorphous light eruption occur predominantly in sun-exposed sites, elastotic material is frequently and incidentally found.

Mixed-Cell Infiltrate with Neutrophils Prominent (phlegmonous dermatitis)

Cellulitis (including Erysipelas)

—Sparse infiltrate mostly of neutrophils, but also of lymphocytes, histiocytes, and mast cells (rarely plasma cells and eosinophils) around the blood vessels of the superficial and deep plexuses
—Inflammatory cells scattered diffusely among collagen bundles
—Widely dilated blood vessels and lymphatics in the superficial dermis
—Extravasated erythrocytes throughout the superficial dermis
—Edema of the papillary dermis
—Occasional subepidermal vesiculation secondary to massive papillary dermal edema

Edema and neutrophils predominate during the early, erythematous, and plaque stages of erysipelas. As the process progresses, lymphocytes and histiocytes increase in number and may eventually outnumber the neutrophils. Edema in the papillary dermis may become so severe that subepidermal vesiculation results, presenting itself clinically as tense vesicles and bullae. The intensity of purpura varies with the number of extravasated erythrocytes. These histologic changes described for erysipelas apply to all cellulitides, regardless of causation.

Acute Febrile Neutrophilic Dermatosis (Sweet's Syndrome)

—Dense infiltrate of neutrophils, nuclear dust, lymphocytes, and histiocytes around the vessels of the superficial and deep plexuses.
—Neutrophils among collagen bundles
—Edema, especially of the superficial dermis
—Widely dilated vascular spaces
—Often extravasated erythrocytes

Clinically, in acute febrile neutrophilic dermatosis painful plaques and nodules occur primarily on the faces and acral areas of middle-aged women who have recently experienced an upper respiratory infection. The eruption, with its associated fever and malaise, tends to recur. The relationship of acute febrile neutrophilic dermatosis to leukocytoclastic vasculitis, if any, is yet unresolved. Occasionally early urticarial lesions of leukocytoclastic vasculitis have no fibrin within the walls of small blood vessels; only a perivascular and interstitial predominantly neutrophilic infiltrate with nuclear dust is present. In some patients, Sweet's syndrome has occurred in concert with leukemia.

Acute febrile neutrophilic dermatosis can be differentiated histologically from cellulitis by the much greater density of its neutrophilic infiltrate and from urticarial allergic eruptions by its greater tendency to subepidermal vesiculation. (See Chapter 9).

Erythropoietic Protoporphyria (Fig. 7-8)

—Sparse superficial and deep perivascular infiltrate predominantly of neutrophils and nuclear "dust" or debris, but also of lymphocytes, histiocytes, and eosinophils
—Thick rim of homogeneous pink material around the capillaries and venules of the superficial plexus

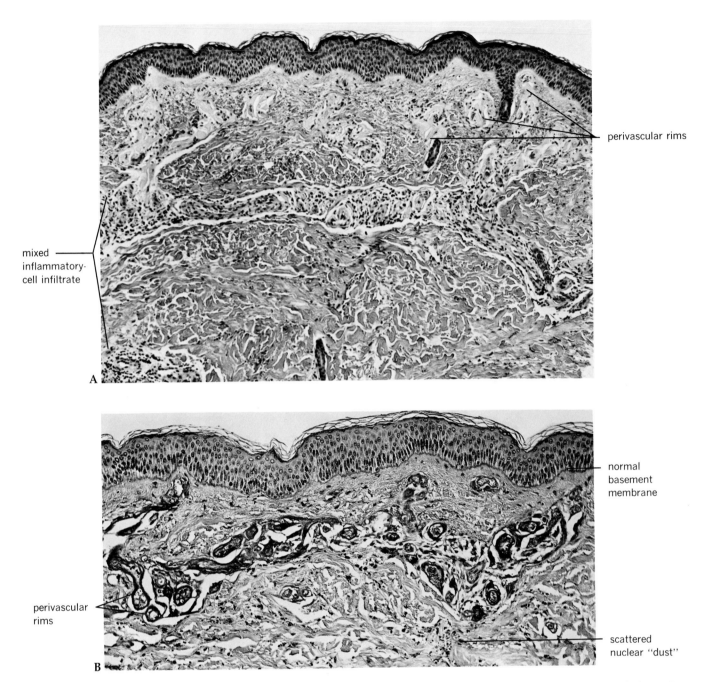

mixed inflammatory-cell infiltrate

perivascular rims

normal basement membrane

perivascular rims

scattered nuclear "dust"

A

B

FIG. 7-8. Erythropoietic protoporphyria. Rims of homogeneous eosinophilic material around blood vessels in upper half of dermis in combination with mixed inflammatory-cell infiltrate containing neutrophils are diagnostic findings. PAS stain accentuated these perivascular rims. (A, × 95; B, × 140.)

The most common lesions of erythropoietic protoporphyria are urticarial papules. Rarely, there are subepidermal vesicles. These lesions develop after exposure to sunlight, even through window glass.

The crucial diagnostic histologic feature is a homogeneous rim of eosinophilic material around the blood vessels of the superficial plexus. This material is PAS-positive, diastase resistant. Similar appearing material is seen in lipoid proteinosis. The histologic changes in erythropoietic protoporphyria can be confused with those of leukocytoclastic vasculitis because of the combination of neutrophils and nuclear "dust" with perivascular homogeneous eosinophilic material. In leukocytoclastic vasculitis, however, the eosinophilic material is fibrillary (fibrin) and is located within and around the blood vessel walls.

The porphyrin abnormality in erythropoietic protoporphyria is the excessive production of protoporphyrin in the bone marrow and the liver. Elevated protoporphyrin levels are found in erythrocytes and in feces, but not in the urine.

Tick Bite

> —Dense superficial and deep infiltrate composed predominantly of neutrophils with varying numbers of lymphocytes, histiocytes, and eosinophils
> —Many neutrophils interposed between collagen bundles throughout the dermis, often extending into the subcutaneous fat
> —Tick often visible on the surface of the specimen, the mouth parts embedded in the superficial dermis

Unlike many reactions to arthropods—such as those caused by mosquitoes, bedbugs, and scabies—tick bites induce a largely neutrophilic, rather than eosinophilic, inflammatory cell response. Flea bites are also associated with a dermal infiltrate consisting mostly of neutrophils rather than of eosinophils, but the infiltrate is much less dense than that evoked by tick bites.

Fleabite

> —Sparse to moderately dense perivascular and interstitial infiltrate of neutrophils and some lymphocytes and histiocytes
> —Dermal edema

Unlike most reactions to arthropods in which eosinophils are plentiful, fleabite reactions contain many neutrophils.

Mixed-cell Infiltrate with Eosinophils Prominent

In addition to arthropod reactions and urticarial lesions of herpes gestationis, the urticarial lesions of pemphigoid and "itchy red bump" disease may sometimes have this pattern.

Most Reactions to Arthropods (e.g., mosquitos, bedbugs, and scabies mite), Creeping Eruption, and Cercarial Dermatitis (Fig. 7-9)

—Moderately dense wedge-shaped infiltrate of eosinophils, lympho-cytes, and histiocytes around the blood vessels of the superficial and deep plexuses
—Inflammatory cells sometimes in blood vessel walls
—Eosinophils, especially among collagen bundles
—Edema of the papillary dermis with occasional subepidermal ve-siculation
—Varying numbers of extravasated erythrocytes
—Scale-crust on the surface and neutrophils in the superficial dermis of eroded lesions

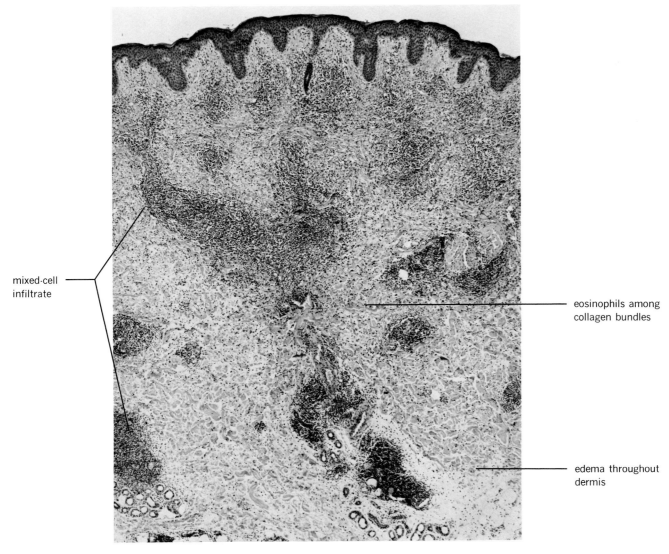

mixed-cell infiltrate

eosinophils among collagen bundles

edema throughout dermis

FIG. 7-9. Reaction to arthropod. Superficial and deep mixed inflammatory-cell infiltrate with eosinophils scattered among collagen bundles in edematous dermis are characteristic changes. (A, × 47; B, × 340.)

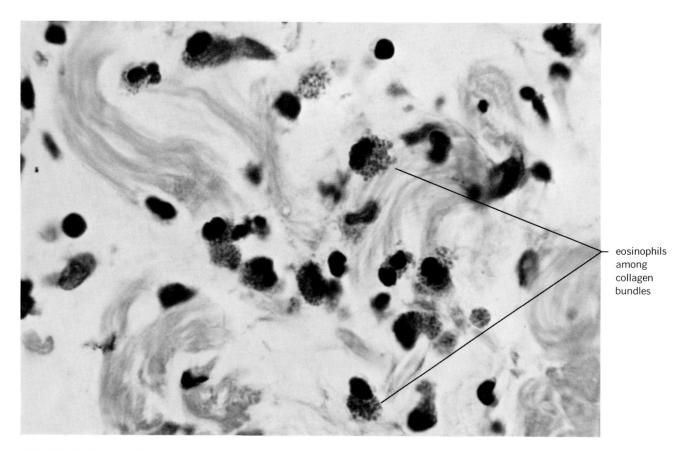

eosinophils among collagen bundles

FIG. 7-9. B, Giemsa stain.

Reactions to arthropods vary enormously in their histologic appearance, depending upon the offending arthropod, the capacity of the host to react, the age of the lesion, and the site of the biopsy (vesicular center or urticarial periphery). In the initial papular stage, there may be an infiltrate of eosinophils, lymphocytes, and histiocytes around only the vessels of the superficial and deep plexuses. Rarely, the infiltrate may be wholly superficial. Sometimes the inflammatory cells are in blood vessel walls, as well as around them. As the lesion evolves toward clinical vesiculation, subepidermal edema and intraepidermal (ballooning and spongiotic) edema increase. The vesicle usually results primarily from intraepidermal edema, but in severe reactions a subepidermal vesicle can also occur. Papular urticaria (lichen urticatus) results from insect bites and shows the same histologic features.

It is important to be aware that eosinophils may not always be present in insect reactions. In these rare instances, there may be only lymphocytes and histiocytes, and in reactions to fleas, neutrophils may be the dominant cell.

Reactions to arthropods may also be granulomas and/or pseudomalignant lymphomas. Such reactions develop when an insect, such as a bee or tick, leaves a stinger or mouth part within the dermis, which then induces a foreign-body reaction. Lesions of these types can last months or years, and atypical histiocytes and lymphocytes suggestive of malignant lymphoma often appear in the cellular infiltrate.

The usual acute reaction to an insect consists of urticarial lesions with central vesiculation in which eosinophils are numerous. Acute insect bite reactions in which neutrophils predominate are less common, and chronic granulomatous reactions, which may resemble malignant lymphoma, are unusual.

Scabies is caused by the mite, Sarcoptes scabiei. One must scrutinize the cornified layer in search of mites or their eggs in all superficial and deep perivascular dermatitides that contain eosinophils (Fig. 7-10). Serial sections may be required to demonstrate organisms or ova. Frequently neither are found, especially in small biopsy specimens. The lesions of scabies can be differentiated histologically from those of insect bites and creeping eruption only by the finding of the female mite or her ova within the cornified layer (Plate 2).

The characteristic clinical lesion of scabies is the burrow (Fig. 7-11), which often has a tiny intraepidermal vesicle at the far end. The female mite lodges in the cornified layer at the distal end of

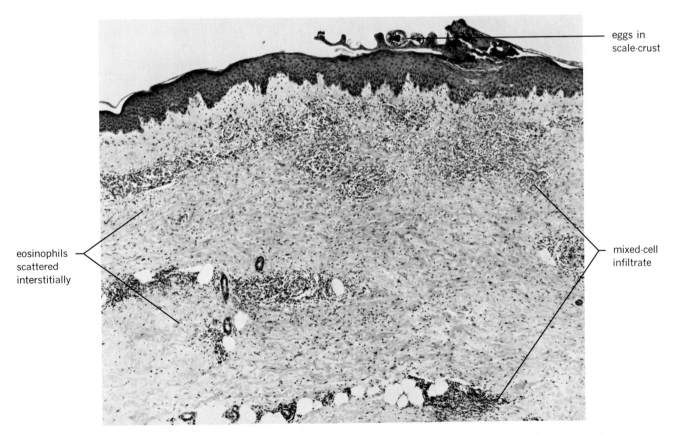

eggs in
scale-crust

eosinophils
scattered
interstitially

mixed-cell
infiltrate

FIG. 7-10. Scabies, papular lesion. As in reactions to arthropods there is interstitial infiltrate of lymphocytes, histiocytes, and eosinophils. Finding a scabietic mite, its parts, or its excreta confirms diagnosis. (A, × 58.)

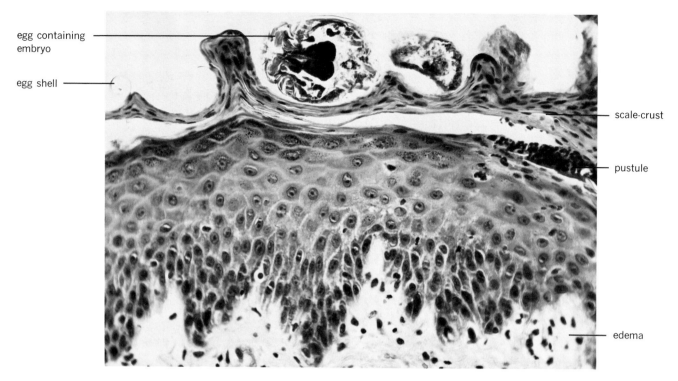

egg containing embryo

egg shell

scale-crust

pustule

edema

FIG. 7-10. Scabies, papular lesion. B, × 306.

the burrow (Fig. 7-11). Sometimes, for various reasons, one may see merely an empty gallery. Because pruritus in scabies is intense, vesicles may be destroyed by scratching and be replaced by erosions and ulcerations. Neutrophils are then seen within scale-crusts on the surface of the specimen and in the superficial dermis.

Sometimes the papules of scabies become as large as nodules and hard. Nodular scabies occurs primarily in the pubic area in males, especially on the penis and scrotum. The nodules result from an extremely dense mixed inflammatory-cell infiltrate around the blood vessels at all levels of the dermis and sometimes around those in the subcutaneous fat. The mononuclear cells within the infiltrate often have large hyperchromatic and pleomorphic nuclei, some in mitosis. Eosinophils may be numerous. The histologic features of nodular scabies are an exaggeration of the usual arthropod reaction and often mimic a malignant lymphoma. It is important to be alert to this phenomemon so as to avoid interpreting nodular scabies as malignant lymphoma. Collagen in vertical streaks is frequently present in the thickened papillary dermis of nodular scabies, indicating that some of the clinical nodularity is secondary to rubbing. The mite of scabies is almost never found in nodular lesions.

Keratotic-crusted scabies, a psoriasiform dermatitis, sometimes pejoratively referred to as Norwegian scabies, is an extreme form of the disease in which thousands of mites invade the skin. As in other forms of scabies, a dense mixed inflammatory-cell infiltrate

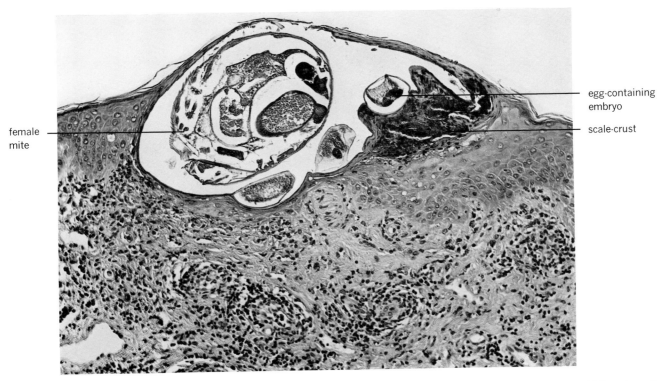

female
mite

egg-containing
embryo

scale-crust

FIG. 7-11. Scabietic burrow. Typical internal structure of scabietic gallery situated intracorneally consists of gravid female and extruded ova in linear arrangement behind her. (× 142.)

is present in the superficial and deep dermis. Both the mites and the scratching they induce cause the epidermis to become hyperplastic and topped by prominent scale-crust. The innumerable mites are easily visualized microscopically within tiers of the thickened cornified layer (Fig. 7-12), in contrast to ordinary scabies in which the mite is discovered with difficulty. Clinically, the patient is diffusely covered by foul-smelling scales and crusts and is highly contagious because the scale-crusts teem with mites.

Biopsy specimens from lesions of scabies are often submitted with a clinical diagnosis of dermatitis herpetiformis because of the pruritic papules and papulovesicles on the sacrum, buttocks, and extensor surfaces of the limbs. Dermatitis herpetiformis, unlike scabies, often involves the scalp, and scabies, unlike dermatitis herpetiformis, favors the interdigital webs. Biopsy specimens of what is clinically taken to be scabies often turn out to be those of suppurative folliculitis.

Creeping eruption is caused by hookworm larvae (Ancylostoma species). Histologically, the lesions of creeping eruption are indistinguishable from insect bite reactions and from scabies. All have a superficial and deep perivascular, as well as an interstitial, lymphohistiocytic infiltrate with eosinophils. All may have edema of the papillary dermis, focal intraepidermal vesiculation, erosions, ulcers, or scale-crusts.

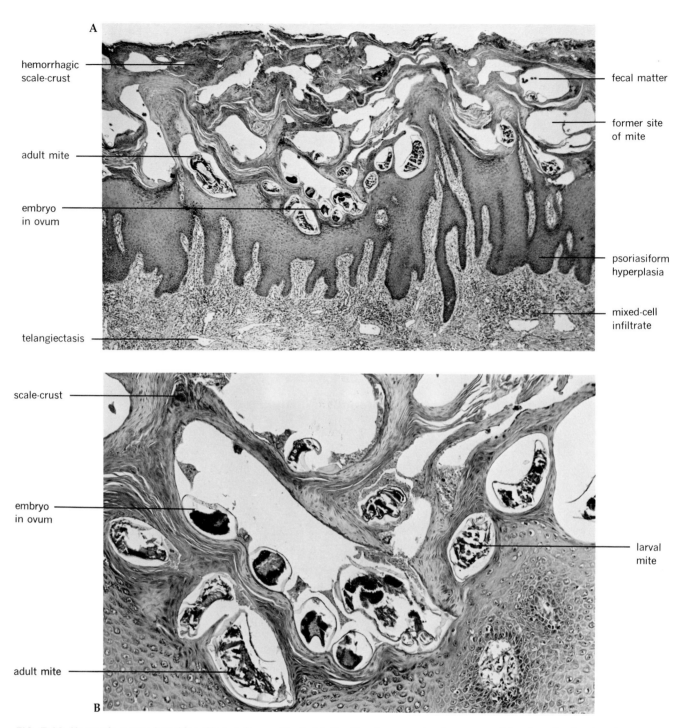

FIG. 7-12. Keratotic-crusted scabies (Norwegian scabies). Adult mites, larvae, nymphs, ova, and fecal matter in abundance are lodged within compartments of hyperkeratotic and crusted cornified layer. (A, × 46; B, × 149.)

On occasion, scabies is diagnosed histologically with certainty, inasmuch as the mite is identified within the cornified layer (Fig. 7-13). Creeping eruption, however, is practically never definitively diagnosed histologically, since the clinician is unable to determine the exact location of the larva for biopsy because of its erratic, zigzag migration through the skin. When the larva is captured, it is situated at the base of the epidermis (Fig. 7-14; Plate 2).

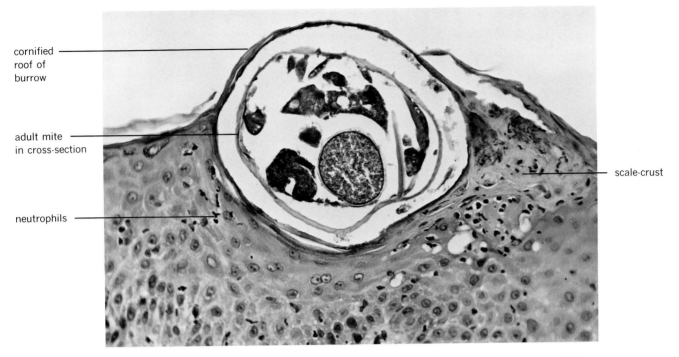

cornified roof of burrow

adult mite in cross-section

neutrophils

scale-crust

FIG. 7-13. Scabies. The mite of scabies is usually lodged in burrow within epidermal cornified layer. ($\times$ 306.)

Clinically, the lesions of creeping eruption are serpentine, sometimes vesicular, tracks. The vesicle is intraepidermal, and the induration is secondary to the subepidermal edema and the inflammatory cell infiltrate.

Cercarial dermatitis, also known as "swimmer's itch," results from superficial penetration of skin by the cercariae of avian schistosomes. The exquisitely pruritic macules, papules, and papulovesicles of the condition occur on uncovered parts of the body that are exposed to infested waters. In histologic sections, cercariae can sometimes be found within intraepidermal spongiotic vesicles (Fig. 7-15). The superficial and deep perivascular and interstitial infiltrates of lymphocytes, histiocytes, and eosinophils are indistinguishable from those of arthropod bites and creeping eruption (Plate 2).

The bristly hairs or spines of caterpillars, particularly of the puss caterpillar, and moths, especially the brown-tail moth, contain an irritating substance. When these hairs or spines pierce the skin, urticarial and papulovesicular lesions are induced. These have histologic features like those of insect bites, creeping eruption, and cercarial dermatitis.

The dermatitis that results from injury to the skin by coral may be indistinguishable from that caused by arthropod assaults. "Itchy red bump" disease also shows histologic changes similar to those of arthropod reactions, although the infiltrate is more often superficial only.

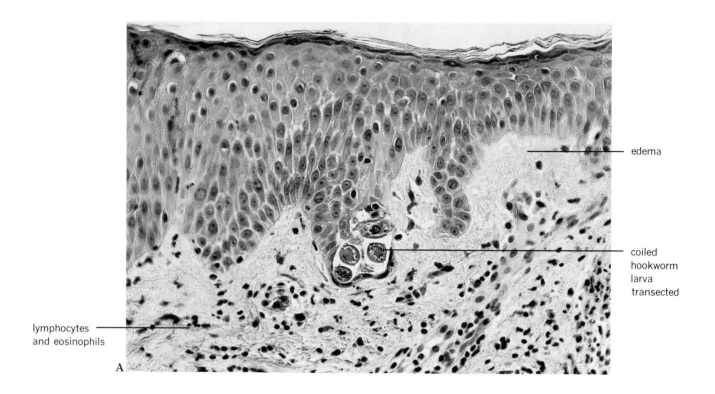

edema

coiled
hookworm
larva
transected

lymphocytes
and eosinophils

A

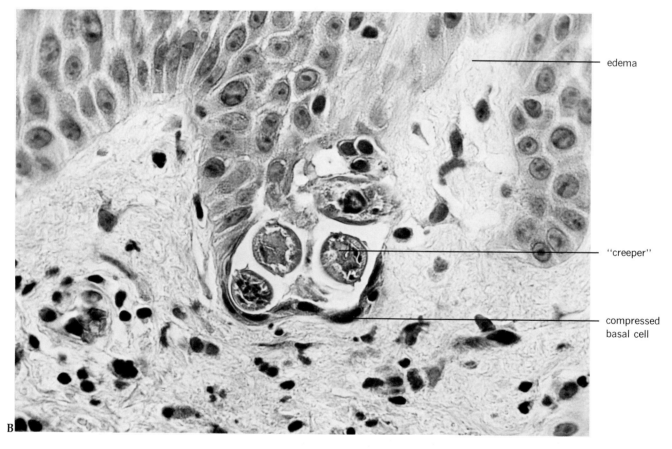

edema

"creeper"

compressed
basal cell

B

FIG. 7-14. Creeping eruption. Pattern and composition of inflammatory-cell infiltrate are just like those of insect bites, scabies, and cercarial dermatitis. In scabies the mite resides in cornified layer of epidermis, whereas in creeping eruption the creeper lies immediately above basal-cell layer. (A, × 306; B, × 578.)

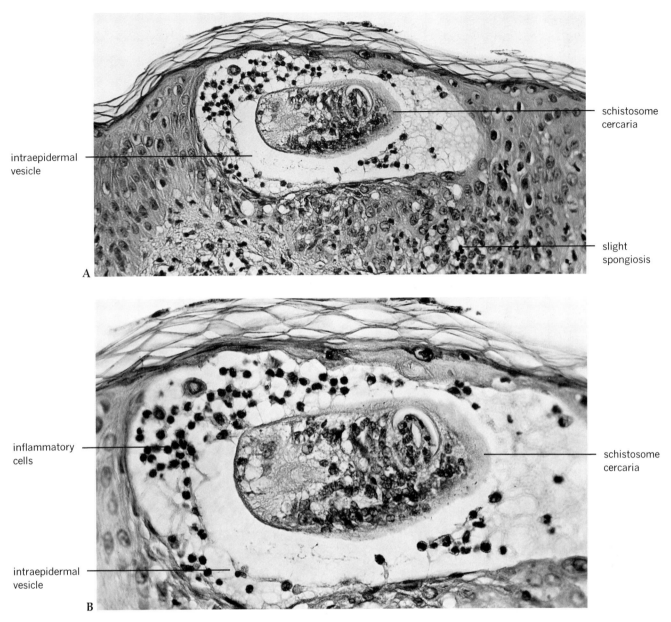

intraepidermal vesicle

schistosome cercaria

slight spongiosis

A

inflammatory cells

schistosome cercaria

intraepidermal vesicle

B

FIG. 7-15. Cercarial dermatitis. Finding cercaria of avian schistosomes in spongiotic vesicle is critical to diagnosis. (A, × 288; B, × 501.)

Herpes Gestationis, Urticarial Lesions (Fig. 7-16)

The early edematous papular lesions of herpes gestationis consist of a superficial and deep perivascular infiltrate of lymphocytes, histiocytes, and numerous eosinophils. Some eosinophils may be scattered among the collagen bundles. The papillary dermis is usually extremely edematous. With time, subepidermal vesicles develop. A more complete exegesis of histologic and clinical features of herpes gestationis is found in Chapter 11. What has been written about herpes gestationis applies also to some urticarial lesions of pemphigoid.

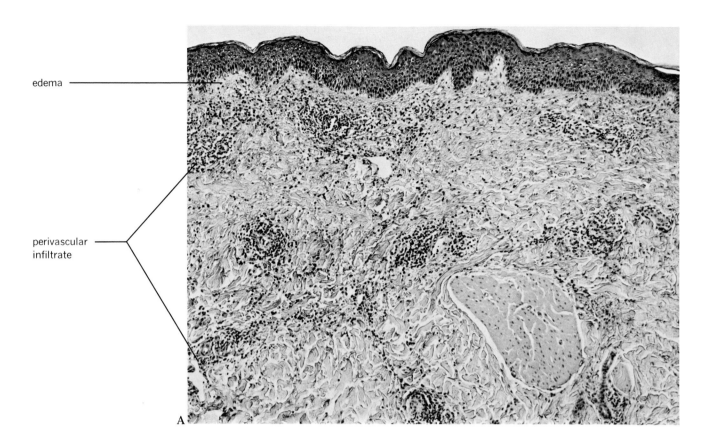

edema ———

perivascular
infiltrate ———

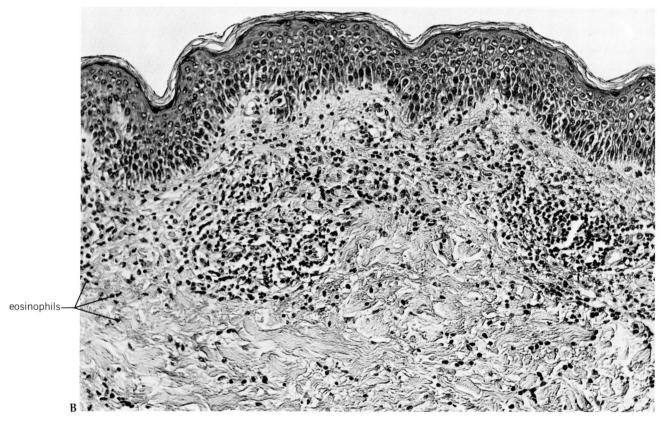

eosinophils ———

FIG. 7-16. Herpes gestationis, urticarial lesion. Pattern and composition of inflammatory-cell infiltrate in early edematous papular lesions are similar to those in reactions to arthropods. Eosinophils are present perivascularly and interstitially. (A, × 83; B, × 160.)

Mixed-cell Infiltrate with Neutrophils and Eosinophils Prominent

Urticarial Allergic Eruptions, Deep Type (Fig. 7-17)

Among the most common eruptions due to drug ingestion or injection is a superficial and deep perivascular dermatitis in which there is abundant edema and a predominance of eosinophils and neutrophils. Urticarial drug eruptions are differentiated from arthropod reactions by the usual presence of neutrophils.

Clinically, urticarial allergic drug eruptions are edematous papules, nodules, and plaques. Similar-appearing clinical lesions can also be produced by a wholly superficial perivascular dermatitis in which neutrophils predominate and are associated with eosinophils, lymphocytes, and histiocytes, as well as severe edema in the papillary dermis. Other chemical allergens, ingestants, injectants, inhalants, or infectants can also cause such cutaneous reactions.

As in all inflammatory diseases of the skin, the most active zones in urticarial allergic eruptions are at the peripheries of the lesions. This is readily apparent clinically and histologically in diseases such as gyrate erythemas and urticarial allergic eruptions, whose lesions have advancing borders, but is equally true for papules of lichen planus and plaques of psoriasis.

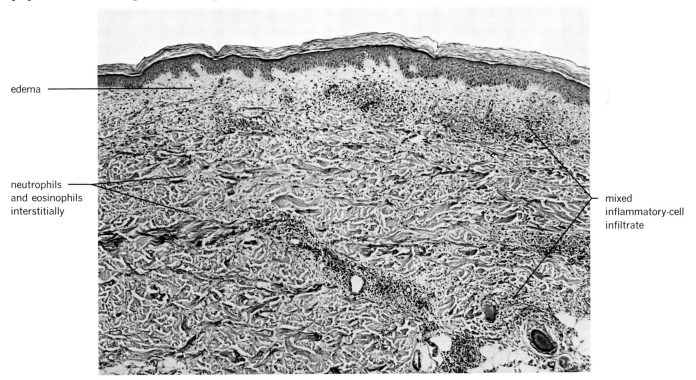

FIG. 7-17. Urticarial allergic eruption, deep type. Perivascular and interstitial mixed inflammatory-cell infiltrate of neutrophils, eosinophils, lymphocytes, and histiocytes in an edematous dermis is seen. Superficial plexus alone or both plexuses may be involved. (× 75.)

Interface Dermatitis (Fig. 7-18)

In interface dermatitis, another type of superficial and deep perivascular dermatitis, lymphocytes and histiocytes or a mixture of inflammatory cells may ascend into the epidermis and in so doing obscure the dermoepidermal interface where there is vacuolar alteration or a lichenoid infiltrate.

Lymphohistiocytic Infiltrate

Discoid Lupus Erythematosus

Discoid lupus erythematosus is one of the interface dermatitides in which a primarily lymphohistiocytic infiltrate obscures the interface. It presents several types of clinical lesions. Early there are erythema, scaling (including "carpet-tack" follicular scales), and induration; later, hyperpigmentation and hypopigmentation, scarring, which may be atrophic, and telangiectasia. The histologic findings reflect the clinical appearance. These pathologic changes can be roughly divided into active or acute discoid lupus erythematosus (the spectrum of erythema through induration) and resolving or chronic discoid lupus erythematosus (permanent changes that often follow induration). Subacute discoid lupus erythematosus has some features of both. The active stages, however, may persist for months or years, and not every active lesion progresses irrevocably through all subsequent stages. Some lesions resolve spontaneously before permanent changes supervene.

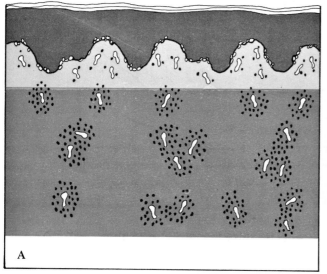 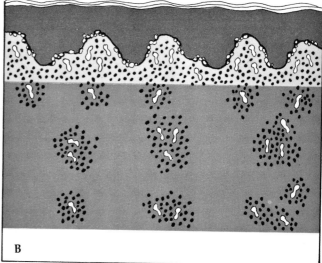

FIG. 7-18. Superficial and deep perivascular dermatitis. A, With vacuolar alteration. B, With lichenoid infiltrate.

—Varyingly dense lymphohistiocytic infiltrate around the blood ves-
sels of the superficial and deep plexuses
—Infiltrate often around adnexal blood vessels
—Rarely, numerous plasma cells
—Melanophages in the papillary dermis
—Edema of the papillary dermis with widely dilated vascular spaces
—Mucin in varying amount among collagen bundles, especially in the
upper half of the dermis
—Variable numbers of extravasated erythrocytes in the superficial
dermis
—Increased number of plump and stellate fibroblasts, some multi-
nucleated, in the superficial dermis
—Vacuolar alteration at the dermoepidermal interface; sometimes
necrotic keratinocytes and even confluent epidermal necrosis in
early lesions
—Epidermal atrophy; sometimes focal epidermal hyperplasia
—Orthokeratosis

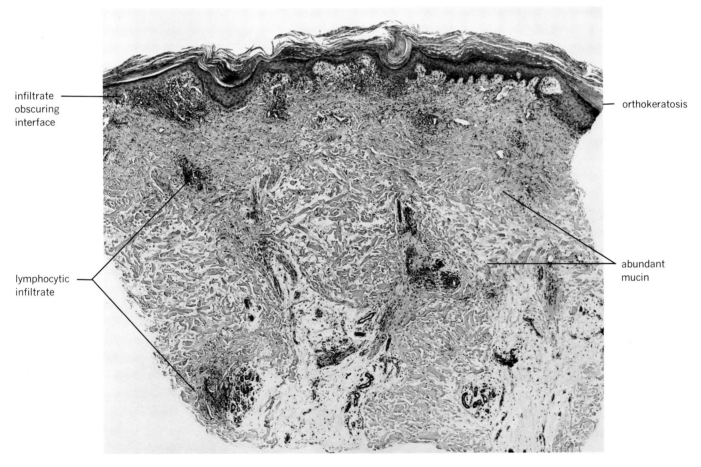

FIG. 7-19. Acute discoid lupus erythematosus. Vacuolar alteration at dermoepidermal junction is sign of acute form. Another feature shown is abundant mucin within reticular dermis. Acute dermatomyositis cannot always be differentiated histologically from acute discoid lupus erythematosus. (A, × 39; B, × 166.)

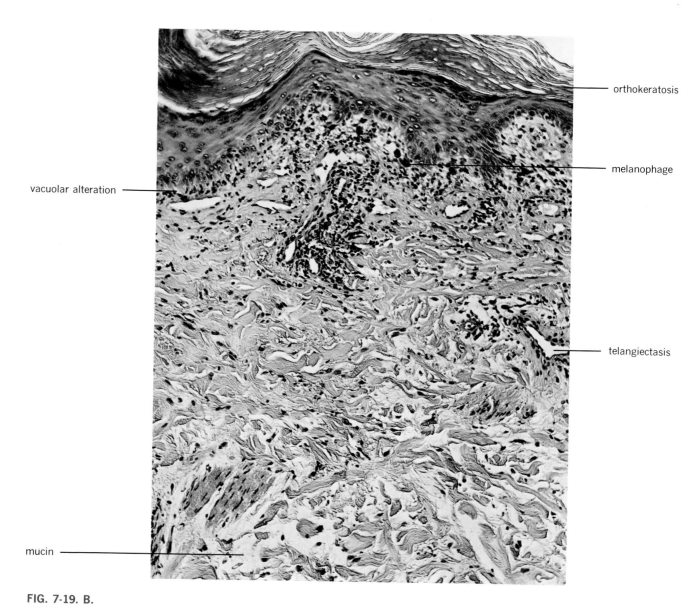

orthokeratosis

melanophage

vacuolar alteration

telangiectasis

mucin

FIG. 7-19. B.

Discoid Lupus Erythematosus, Chronic (Fig. 7-20)

—Varyingly dense lymphohistiocytic infiltrate around the vessels of the superficial and deep plexuses, or no infiltrate
—Sclerotic superficial dermis with stellate fibroblasts
—Widely dilated blood vessels in the superficial dermis, some surrounded by homogeneous eosinophilc material (Fig. 7-21)
—Melanophages in the superficial dermis
—Vacuolar alteration at the dermoepidermal interface
—Thickened basement membrane (Fig. 7-22)
—Epidermal and adnexal atrophy
—Widened follicular infundibula plugged by orthokeratotic cells (follicular plugs)
—Orthokeratosis

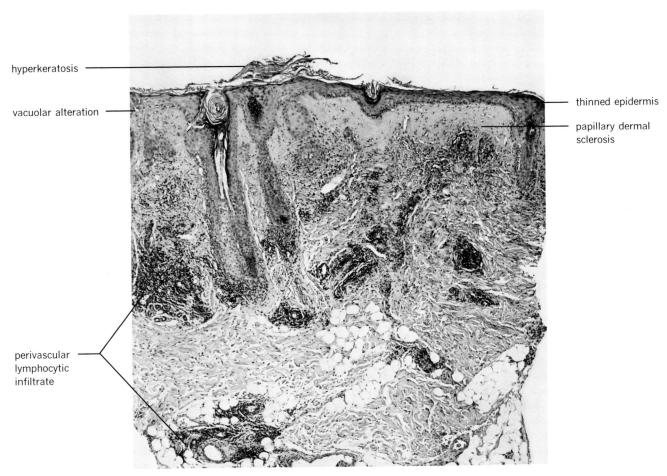

hyperkeratosis

vacuolar alteration

thinned epidermis

papillary dermal
sclerosis

perivascular
lymphocytic
infiltrate

FIG. 7-20. Chronic discoid lupus erythematosus. Fibrosis in upper part of dermis, together with thickened basement membrane, is unequivocal sign of chronicity. (× 50.)

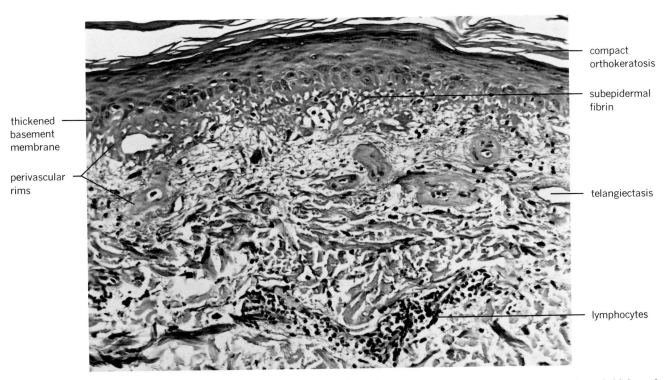

compact
orthokeratosis

subepidermal
fibrin

thickened
basement
membrane

perivascular
rims

telangiectasis

lymphocytes

FIG. 7-21. Chronic discoid lupus erythematosus. Homogeneous eosinophilic material, similar in appearance to that of thickened basement membrane, sometimes rims superficial blood vessels of chronic lesions. (× 162.)

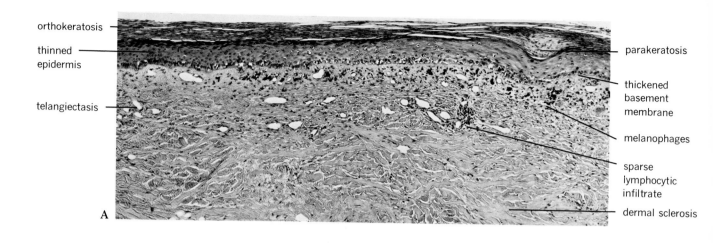

orthokeratosis

thinned epidermis

telangiectasis

parakeratosis

thickened basement membrane

melanophages

sparse lymphocytic infiltrate

dermal sclerosis

A

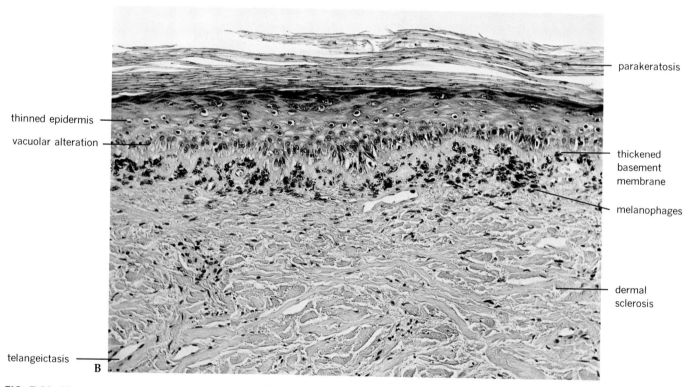

thinned epidermis

vacuolar alteration

parakeratosis

thickened basement membrane

melanophages

dermal sclerosis

telangeictasis

B

FIG. 7-22. Chronic discoid lupus erythematosus. Hyperkeratosis, thinned epidermis devoid of rete ridges, thickened basement membrane, numerous melanophages, telangiectases, and sclerosis in upper part of dermis are classic features. The single most important diagnostic feature is thickened basement membrane. (A, × 63; B, × 147.)

Subacute discoid lupus erythematosus describes that intermediate stage between acute and chronic discoid lupus erythematosus where histologically vacuolar alteration and thickening of the basement membrane zone are both evident at the dermoepidermal interface, widened infundibula are often plugged by compact orthokeratotic cells, (Fig. 7-23) a moderately dense predominantly lymphocytic perivascular infiltrate persists throughout the dermis and there is little or no fibrosis (Fig. 7-24).

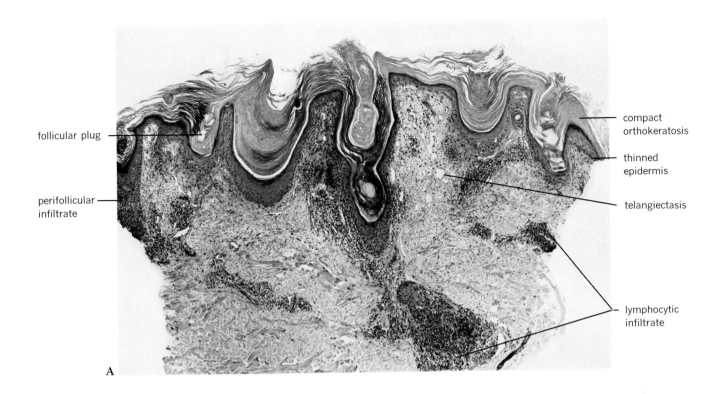

follicular plug

perifollicular infiltrate

compact orthokeratosis

thinned epidermis

telangiectasis

lymphocytic infiltrate

A

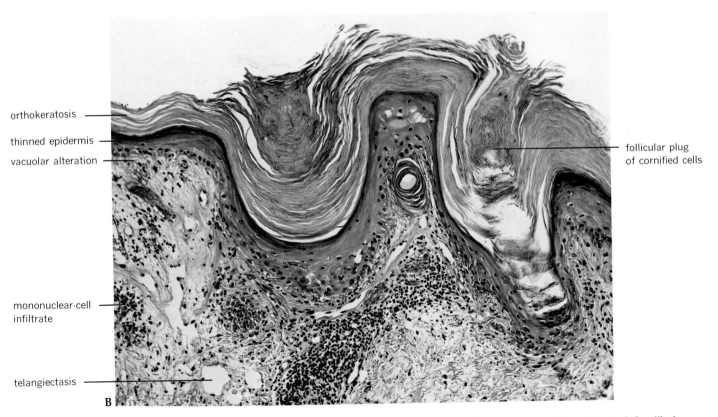

orthokeratosis

thinned epidermis

vacuolar alteration

follicular plug of cornified cells

mononuclear-cell infiltrate

telangiectasis

B

FIG. 7-23. Subacute discoid lupus erythematosus. A, Plugs of cornified cells in adnexal ostia, especially in follicular infundibula, are characteristic features of lesions of subacute and chronic forms. (× 50.) B, Higher magnification to show widely dilated follicular infundibula are plugged by cornified cells. Note that inflammatory-cell infiltrate obscures interface between infundibula and dermis, as well as that between epidermis and dermis. (× 170.)

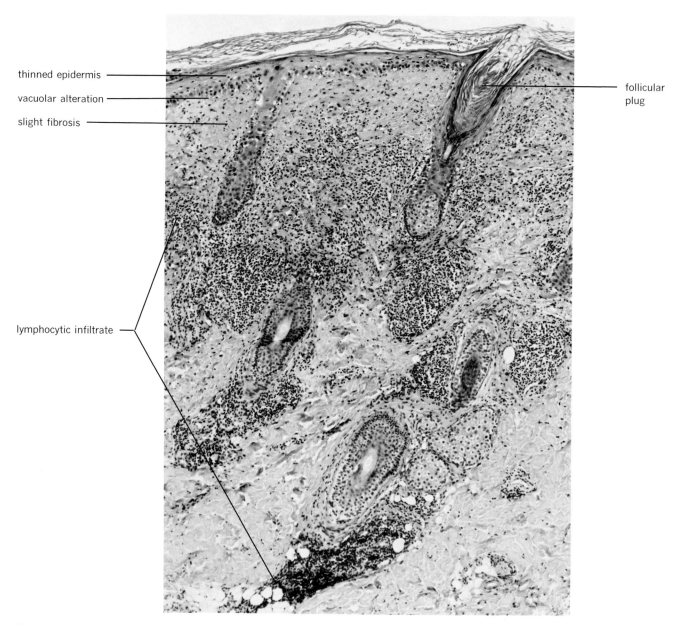

thinned epidermis

vacuolar alteration

slight fibrosis

follicular plug

lymphocytic infiltrate

FIG. 7-24. Subacute chronic discoid lupus erythematosus. Combination of dense inflammatory-cell infiltrate and fibrosis makes this the picture of transition between subacute and chronic forms. (A, × 88; B, × 365.)

The critical diagnostic features in discoid lupus erythematosus are at the dermoepidermal interface in the form of vacuolar alteration in acute lesions and both vacuolar alteration and basement-membrane thickening in chronic lesions (Fig. 7-25). These changes may be found at the junction of the follicular epithelium and the dermis (Figs. 7-23, 7-25). Without these changes at the dermoepidermal interface, discoid lupus erythematosus cannot be unequivocally distinguished from lymphocytic infiltration (Jessner), polymorphous light eruption, or the deep type of gyrate erythema. Rarely, early acute discoid lupus erythematosus may not have interface changes, but later biopsy specimens will likely display diagnostic features.

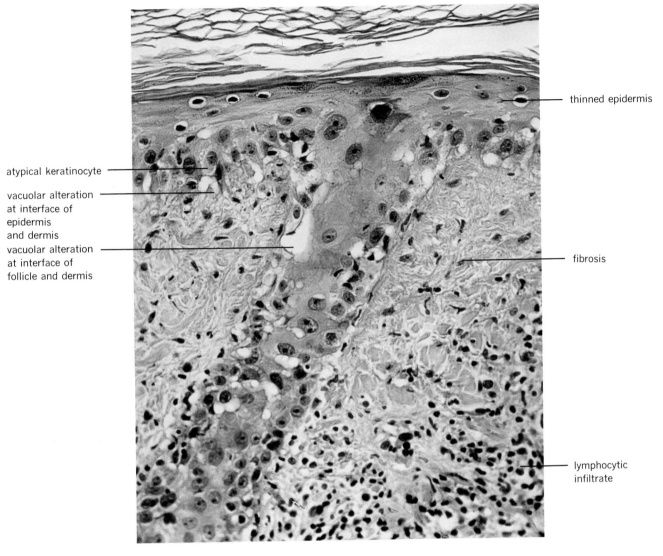

atypical keratinocyte

vacuolar alteration
at interface of
epidermis
and dermis

vacuolar alteration
at interface of
follicle and dermis

thinned epidermis

fibrosis

lymphocytic
infiltrate

FIG. 7-24. B.

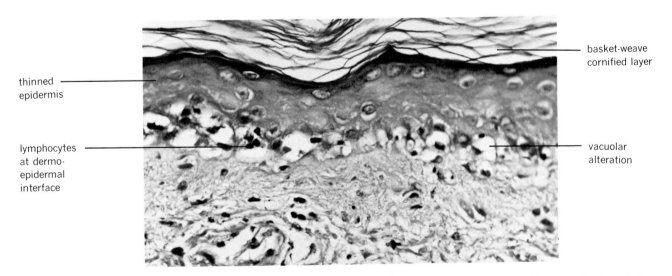

thinned
epidermis

lymphocytes
at dermo-
epidermal
interface

basket-weave
cornified layer

vacuolar
alteration

FIG. 7-25. Acute discoid lupus erythematosus. A, Note prominent vacuolar alteration at dermoepidermal interface, but no thickening of basement membrane as in subacute and chronic forms. Normal basket-weave configuration of cornified layer is evidence that lesion is of recent onset. (× 670.)

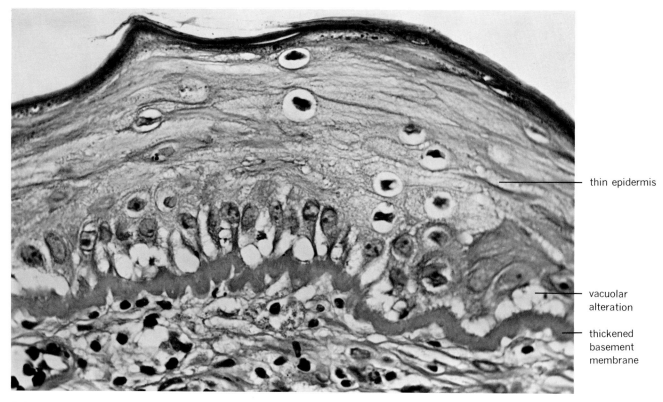

FIG. 7-25. Chronic discoid lupus erythematosus. B, Thickened basement membrane, as pictured in specimen stained by PAS, is particularly diagnostic. Note epidermis devoid of normal pattern of rete ridges and dermal papillae. (× 535.)

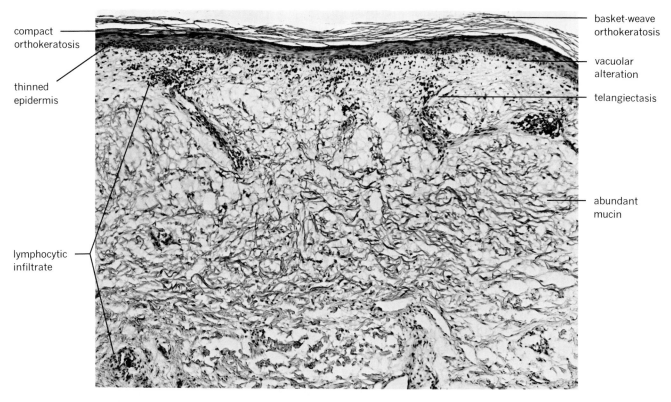

FIG. 7-26. Acute discoid lupus erythematosus, tumid type. Common feature of acute lesions is abundance of acid mucopolysaccharide within dermis. Differentiating features from mucinoses are vacuolar alteration at dermoepidermal interface and lymphocytes around dermal blood vessels. Sometimes these features are very subtle. (× 69.)

Another rarity is the tumid form of discoid lupus erythematosus in which clinically there are indurated reddish plaques with no scales or follicular plugs and histologically there are few changes at the dermoepidermal interface or in the epidermis, but abundant mucin, as well as typical inflammatory cell changes, is found within the dermis (Fig. 7-26). Interface changes similar to those of discoid lupus erythematosus may be seen in dermatomyositis, but there the lymphohistiocytic infiltrate is usually not so dense or deep. Both diseases may have abundant mucin in the dermis. Rarely, the infiltrate of discoid lupus erythematosus may be lichenoid (Fig. 7-27) whereupon it must be differentiated from lichen planus, a disease that involves the superficial plexus rather than both plexuses and does not have a thickened basement membrane (Plate 1).

Dilated follicular infundibula filled with cornified cells are frequent, but not constant, features of discoid lupus erythematosus, especially of the subacute and chronic stages. The prominent periadnexal arrangement of the inflammatory-cell infiltrate in discoid lupus erythematosus is secondary to involvement of the periadnexal blood vessels. In both early and late lesions of discoid lupus erythematosus, the inflammatory-cell infiltrate may be sparse and restricted to the superficial dermis. Plasma cells may be a major component of the infiltrate. Because the lesions of discoid lupus erythematosus commonly occur on skin chronically exposed to sunlight, elastotic material is often found in the dermis.

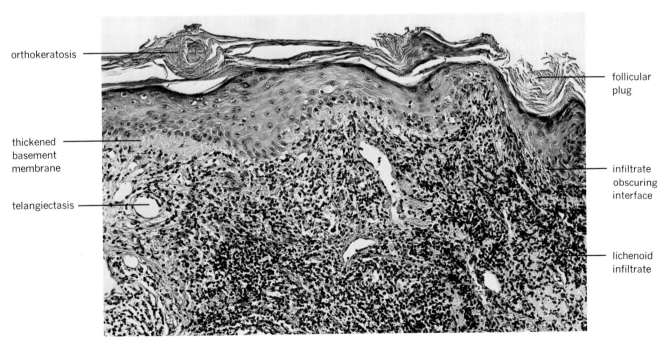

FIG. 7-27. Discoid lupus erythematosus, lichenoid type. Thickened basement membrane distinguishes lichenoid infiltrate from that of other diseases, especially lichen planus. ($\times$ 147.)

Discoid lupus erythematosus may or may not be associated with systemic lupus erythematosus. The former has characteristic clinical and histologic features which when present are pathognomonic, although no judgment can be rendered from the biopsy about the association of internal organ disease.

Discoid lupus erythematosus is the major cutaneous manifestation of systemic lupus erythematosus, but leukocytoclastic vasculitis, livedo reticularis, leg ulcers, digital gangrene, Raynaud's phenomenon, purpuric and bullous lesions, "butterfly blush," periungual telangiectases, and alopecias are other cutaneous signs. Many patients who never show evidence of systemic lupus erythematosus do harbor, sometimes for decades, typical skin lesions of discoid lupus erythematosus. The evanescent butterfly blush of systemic lupus erythematosus consists histologically of telangiectasis surrounded by a superficial sparse infiltrate.

Discoid lupus erythematosus is to systemic lupus erythematosus what psoriasis is to psoriatic arthritis: the lesions are clinically and histologically the same. Most patients with discoid lupus erythematosus do not have systemic lupus erythematosus, just as most patients with psoriasis do not have arthritis. No clinician can diagnose either psoriatic arthritis or systemic lupus erythematosus by studying only the skin lesions. Likewise, no histologist can predict psoriatic arthritis or systemic lupus erythematosus by scrutinizing a biopsy specimen only from the skin.

Drugs, such as procainamide, hydralazine, and diphenylhydantoin (Dilantin), can induce lesions that are indistinguishable clinically and histologically from the lesions of discoid lupus erythematosus.

Pityriasis Lichenoides et Varioliformis Acuta (Mucha-Habermann Disease) (Fig. 7-28)

—Moderately dense lymphohistiocytic infiltrate arranged in a V-shape around the blood vessels of the superficial and deep plexuses
—Atypical mononuclear cells in varying numbers, from none to many
—Extravasated erythrocytes, sometimes numerous, in the papillary dermis and within the epidermis
—Lymphohistiocytic infiltrate obscuring the dermoepidermal interface and within the epidermis
—Vacuolar alteration at the dermoepidermal interface; rarely, subepidermal vesicles
—Necrotic keratinocytes initially at the dermoepidermal interface and eventually throughout the epidermis (Fig. 7-29)
—Intracellular and intercellular edema; frequently intraepidermal vesicles
—Focal parakeratosis and/or scale-crusts, often with neutrophils

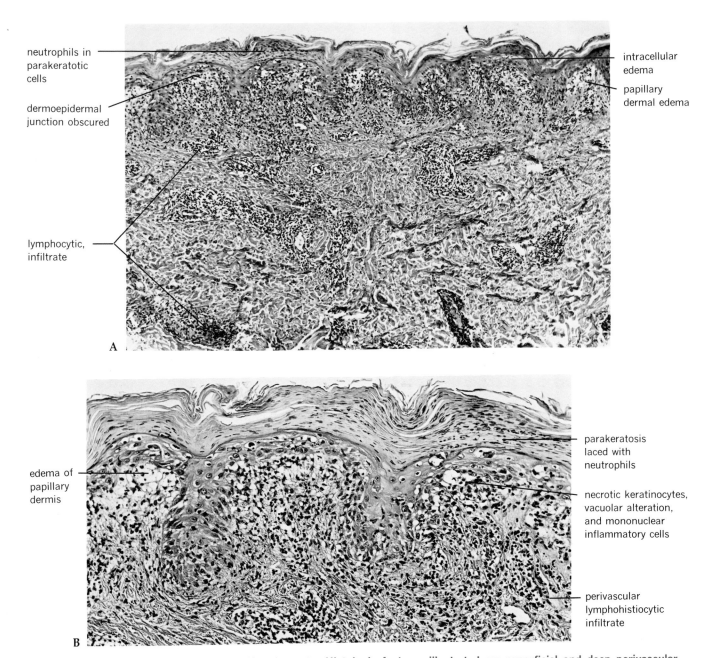

neutrophils in parakeratotic cells

dermoepidermal junction obscured

lymphocytic, infiltrate

intracellular edema

papillary dermal edema

edema of papillary dermis

parakeratosis laced with neutrophils

necrotic keratinocytes, vacuolar alteration, and mononuclear inflammatory cells

perivascular lymphohistiocytic infiltrate

A

B

FIG. 7-28. Pityriasis lichenoides et varioliformis acuta. Histologic features illustrated are superficial and deep perivascular lymphohistiocytic infiltrate that obscures dermoepidermal interface where there are also vacuolar alteration and necrotic keratinocytes. These changes can be differentiated from those of discoid lupus erythematosus in which there is no significant parakeratosis, but commonly there is thickening of basement membrane. (A, × 63; B, × 158.)

Sometimes, the inflammatory-cell infiltrate in pityriasis lichenoides et varioliformis acuta is present around the blood vessels of the superficial plexus only, rather than around both plexuses. When both plexuses are involved, the infiltrate often has a wedge shape with the point toward the subcutis. In *exceptional* cases of this disease lymphocytes may be present within blood vessel walls in conjunction with fibrin. These vasculitic changes are an inconstant feature of the disease.

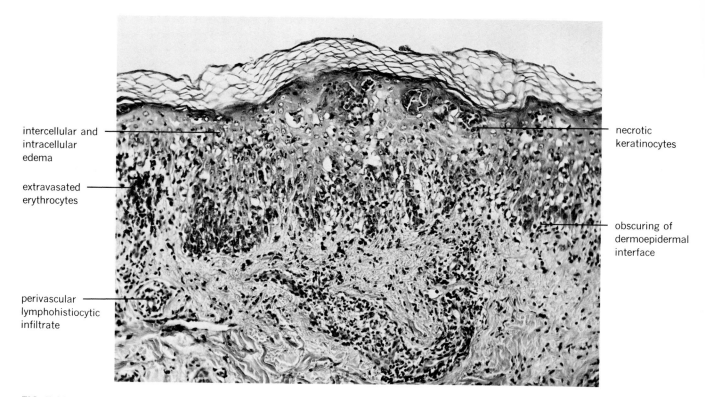

intercellular and intracellular edema

extravasated erythrocytes

perivascular lymphohistiocytic infiltrate

necrotic keratinocytes

obscuring of dermoepidermal interface

FIG. 7-29. Pityriasis lichenoides et varioliformis acuta. Cornified layer in normal basket-weave pattern devoid of parakeratosis or scale-crust indicates that these changes are of recent development. Epidermal changes pictured closely resemble those of erythema multiforme, but dermal changes are different, the infiltrate being deep as well as superficial. (× 162.)

Pityriasis lichenoides et varioliformis acuta is characterized clinically by a polymorphous eruption of widespread small lesions, namely, papules with scales (pityriasis), pink papules that are flat-topped (lichenoides), purpuric and necrotic papules, vesicles, ulcers, and characteristic scars (varioliformis). All these lesions, except the scars, show histologically a superficial and deep perivascular dermatitis with vacuolar alteration of the dermoepidermal interface and extravasated erythrocytes. The disease affects children as well as adults.

Some long-standing cases of pityriasis lichenoides et varioliformis acuta may be attended by scaly papules that differ histologically from earlier lesions by an infiltrate that is wholly superficial and by absence of intraepidermal edema. Such lesions are called pityriasis lichenoides chronica. Rarely, the scaly papules of pityriasis lichenoides chronica can develop without being preceded by the polymorphous lesions of pityriasis lichenoides et varioliformis acuta.

Epidermal necrosis surmounting vesicles is commonly found in pityriasis lichenoides et varioliformis acuta, erythema multiforme, leukocytoclastic vasculitis, fixed drug eruption, septic vasculitis, purpura fulminans, and burns. The necrotic epidermis imparts a grayish hue to the vesicle.

Pityriasis lichenoides et varioliformis acuta is distinguished from discoid lupus erythematosus by the presence of intracellular and intercellular edema and numerous necrotic keratinocytes, as well as by the absence of a periadnexal inflammatory-cell infiltrate and a thickened basement membrane.

Lymphomatoid papulosis (Fig. 7-30)

—Moderately dense superficial and deep perivascular predominantly lymphohistiocytic infiltrate with atypical mononuclear cells
—Infiltrate obscures the dermoepidermal interface
—Vacuolar alteration at the dermoepidermal interface
—Atypical mononuclear cells within the usually hyperplastic epidermis (Fig. 7-31)

Occasionally, atypical mononuclear cells dominate the infiltrate in pityriasis lichenoides et varioliformis acuta. The lesions then histologically resemble those of malignant lymphomas. Many of the cases termed "lymphomatoid papulosis" are undoubtedly instances of pityriasis lichenides et varioliformis acuta in which, for unknown reasons, the cells in the infiltrate show significant atypicality. Other cases of lymphomatoid papulosis differ histo-

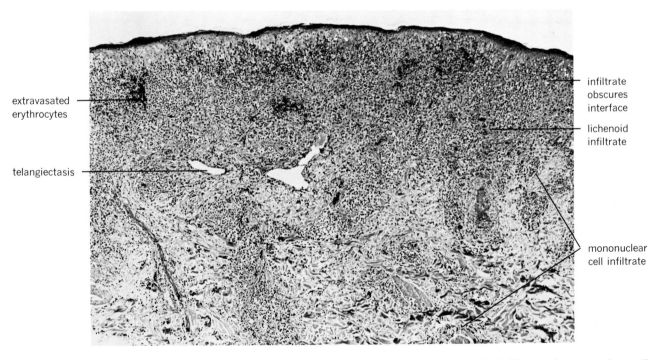

FIG. 7-30. Lymphomatoid papulosis. Changes illustrated are superficial and deep perivascular infiltrate of mononuclear cells, many of which are atypical, in lichenoid arrangement in upper part of dermis where they obscure dermoepidermal interface and from whence they migrate into epidermis. (A, × 57; B, × 173.)

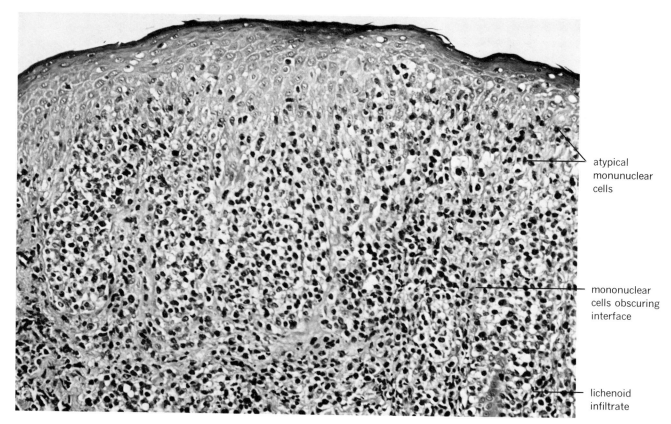

atypical
mononuclear
cells

mononuclear
cells obscuring
interface

lichenoid
infiltrate

FIG. 7-30. B.

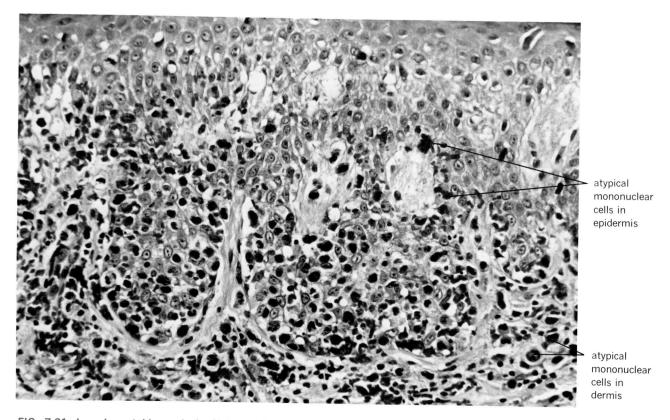

atypical
mononuclear
cells in
epidermis

atypical
mononuclear
cells in
dermis

FIG. 7-31. Lymphomatoid papulosis. Note atypical mononuclear cells scattered throughout epidermis with no tendency to conglomeration as in mycosis fungoides. (× 302.)

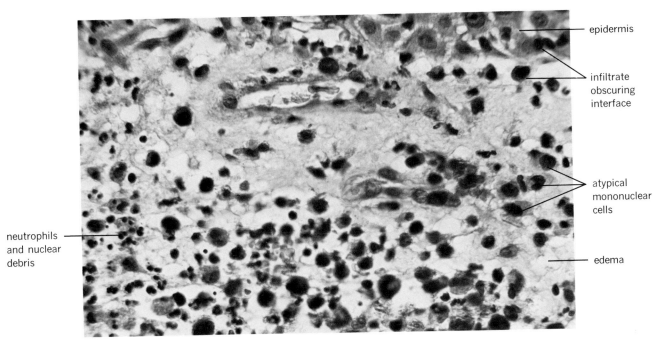

FIG. 7-32. Lymphomatoid papulosis. Dermal infiltrate is sometimes mixed, consisting of neutrophils, plasma cells, and occasionally eosinophils, in addition to atypical mononuclear cells. Edema usually signifies inflammatory disease. (× 520.)

logically from pityriasis lichenoides et varioliformis acuta by the presence of numerous neutrophils, eosinophils, and plasma cells, in addition to atypical mononuclear cells within the infiltrate (Fig. 7-32) and sometimes by the absence of epidermal changes. Clinically, lymphomatoid papulosis is often indistinguishable from pityriasis lichenoides et varioliformis acuta, but unlike pityriasis, the lesions of lymphomatoid papulosis tend to be more persistent, often lasting for years, and to affect adults overwhelmingly.

Lichenoid Photodermatitis (Fig. 7-33)

—Superficial and deep perivascular predominantly lymphocytic infiltrate
—Dense bandlike lymphocytic infiltrate across the upper part of the dermis, obscuring the dermoepidermal interface
—Vacuolar alteration at the junction of the dermis and the epidermis
—Dyskeratotic cells in variable numbers (from none to many) within the epidermis
—Focal parakeratosis or scale-crust occasionally

Lichenoid photodermatitis is precipitated most often by photosensitizing systemic medications such as the chlorthiazides. Clinically, erythematous edematous papules are confined to parts of the body that have been exposed to sunlight.

focal parakeratosis

lichenoid infiltrate

superficial and
deep perivascular
infiltrate

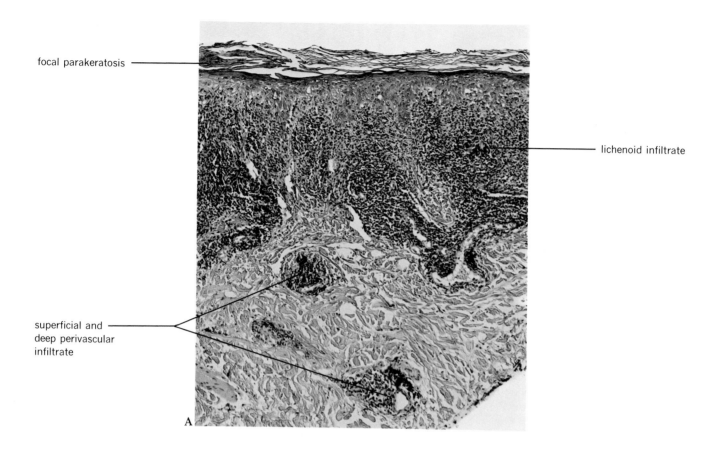

A

infiltrate obscuring
interface

vacuolar
alteration

lichenoid
infiltrate

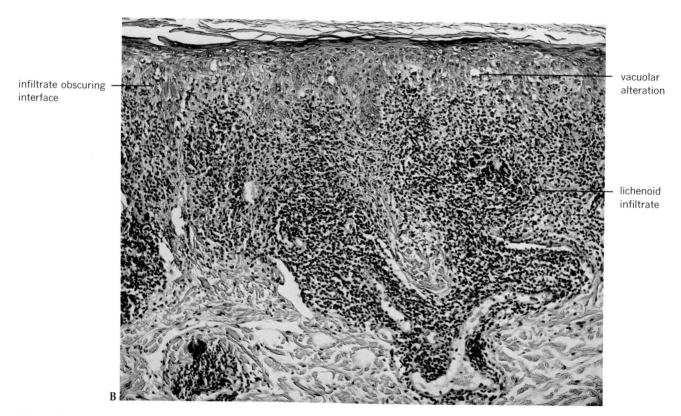

B

FIG. 7-33. Photodermatitis, lichenoid type. Lichenoid infiltrate resembles that of lichen planus, but depth of infiltrate, basket-weave pattern of cornified layer, and absence of hypergranulosis are distinguishing features. (A, × 82; B, × 147.)

—Moderately dense mixed-cell infiltrate of neutrophils, eosinophils, lymphocytes, and histiocytes around the blood vessels of the superficial and deep plexuses
—Extensive edema of the papillary dermis
—Variable numbers of extravasated erythrocytes
—Vacuolar alteration at the dermoepidermal interface, subepidermal clefts, and subepidermal vesiculation
—Necrotic keratinocytes along the dermoepidermal interface and throughout the epidermis; sometimes confluent epidermal necrosis
—Intracellular and intercellular edema, occasionally intraepidermal vesiculation.

The histologic changes apply to the early stage of fixed drug eruption. At this stage, the epidermal features of fixed drug eruption and erythema multiforme cannot always be distinguished. The differentiation between them can only be accomplished by scrutinizing the dermis. In fixed drug eruption, there is a superficial and deep mixed inflammatory-cell infiltrate; in erythema multiforme, there is a superficial lymphohistiocytic infiltrate.

In a fixed drug eruption, the lesions recur in precisely the same site with each administration of the offending chemical. The early clinical lesion is a reddish-purple indurated plaque upon which a bulla with a gray top may develop. The partially necrotic blister has both intraepidermal and subepidermal components, the intraepidermal blister resulting from intracellular and intercellular edema and the subepidermal blister from edema in the papillary dermis. (These changes are pictured in Chapter 10.)

The late lesion of fixed drug eruption, a pigmented patch, shows only a sparse lymphohistiocytic infiltrate and numerous melanophages in the thickened papillary dermis. Depending upon the stage at which the lesion is examined microscopically, the histologist will see the florid changes of early plaques and vesicles, residual hyperpigmentation, or a mixture of these features.

In histologic interpretation, the term *drug eruption* is inadequate because drugs can induce many patterns of inflammation in the skin. It is impossible to look at a particular biopsy specimen of erythema multiforme or erythema nodosum and conclude that a drug rather than any other noxa is the cause. Such is not the case with fixed drug eruption that is specifically related to taking a drug. The exact drug, whether barbiturate, phenolphthalein, or other, cannot be surmised from study of histologic sections.

Syphilis, Secondary Stage (Fig. 7-34)

—Mixed inflammatory-cell infiltrate, usually of histiocytes, lympho-cytes, and plasma cells around the vessels of the superficial and deep plexuses and often bandlike across the papillary dermis
—Increased number of plump endothelial cells lining the dilated blood vessels of the superficial dermis
—Cellular infiltrate at the dermoepidermal interface
—Vacuolar alteration at the dermoepidermal interface
—Thickened papillary dermis, initially by edema, later by fibrosis
—Neutrophils occasionally in the papillary dermis and within the epidermis
—Rarely, intraepidermal neutrophilic abscesses (spongiform pus-tules)
—Irregular or psoriasiform epidermal hyperplasia
—Epidermal pallor, often
—Scale-crusts, often

The skin lesions of secondary syphilis are remarkably protean, both clinically and histologically. The constellation of histologic changes just described is prototypic of secondary syphilis, but there are many variations: absence of plasma cells; presence of eosinophils: granulomatous infiltrate with histiocytic giant cells; vasculitis; superficial, rather than superficial and deep, inflamma-tory-cell infiltrate; and thin, rather than hyperplastic, epidermis. The most common histologic presentation of secondary syphilis is a superficial and deep perivascular infiltrate containing plasma cells that obscures the dermoepidermal junction of a hyperplastic epidermis. The thickened blood vessels are lined by a seemingly increased number of plump endothelial cells. This presentation of secondary syphilis is differentiated from mycosis fungoides by the absence of atypical mononuclear cells and the presence of vascular changes.

The clinical lesions of secondary syphilis are as varied as the histologic features. There may be flat-topped papules like those of lichen planus, scaly papules like those of pityriasis rosea, annular lesions like those of granuloma annulare, acuminate papules like those of sarcoidosis, scaly plaques like those of psoriasis, purulent crusts like those of halogenodermas, and nodules like those of mycosis fungoides. In adults, the lesions of syphilis are never vesicular.

These clinical variations of secondary syphilis reflect the un-derlying histologic changes. Histologically, nodular secondary syphilis is granulomatous. The crusted lesions of rupial syphilis show spongiform pustules. Early condylomata lata also have spongiform pustules, and later papillomatous lesions are often

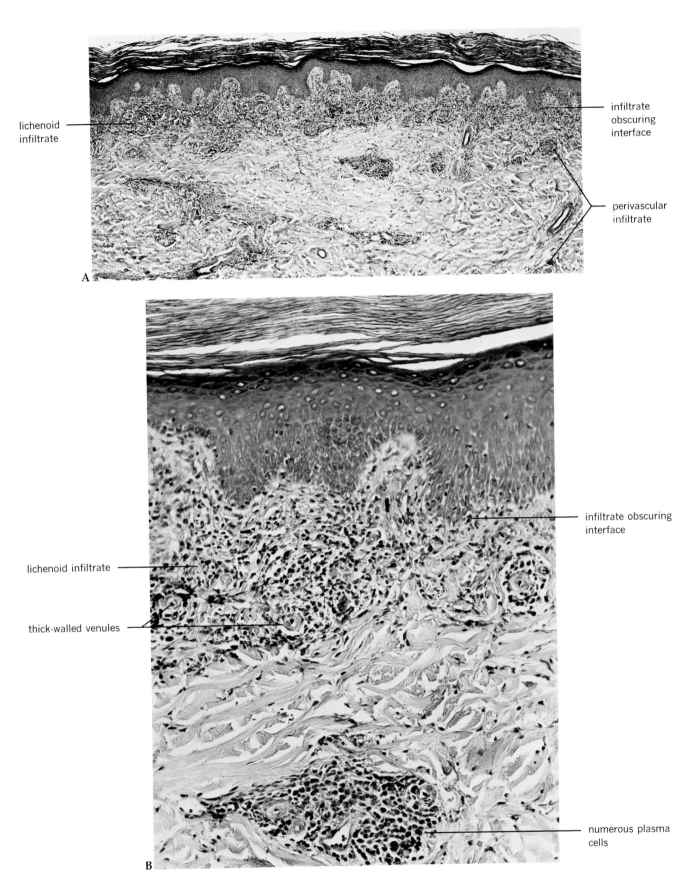

lichenoid infiltrate

infiltrate obscuring interface

perivascular infiltrate

A

infiltrate obscuring interface

lichenoid infiltrate

thick-walled venules

numerous plasma cells

B

FIG. 7-34. Secondary syphilis, lichenoid lesion. The fact that the infiltrate is superficial and deep rather than wholly superficial and contains plasma cells and that the epidermis has rounded, not jagged, rete ridges favors diagnosis of lichenoid secondary syphilis rather than lichen planus. (A, × 53; B, × 209.)

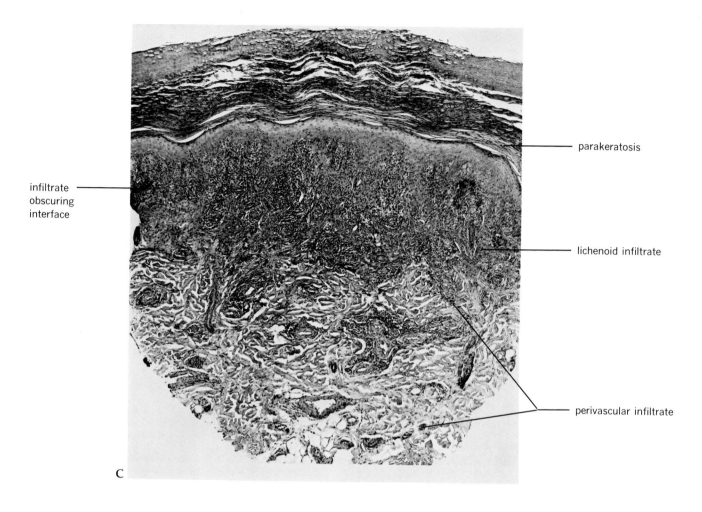

parakeratosis

infiltrate
obscuring
interface

lichenoid infiltrate

perivascular infiltrate

C

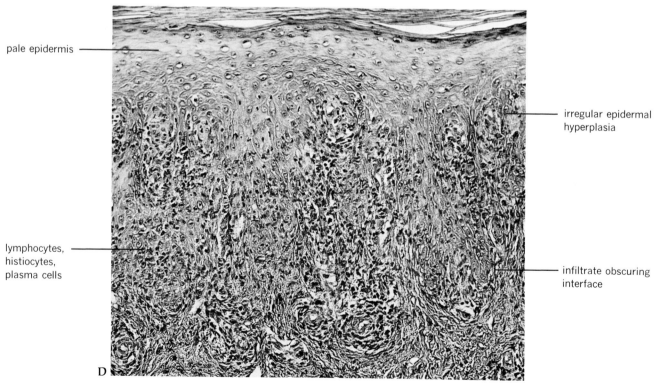

pale epidermis

irregular epidermal
hyperplasia

lymphocytes,
histiocytes,
plasma cells

infiltrate obscuring
interface

D

FIG. 7-34 (continued). (C, × 47; D, × 166.)

eroded or ulcerated. Lichen-planuslike secondary syphilis demonstrates the epidermal and superficial dermal pattern of true lichen planus, but the syphilic infiltrate is deep, as well as superficial, and it usually contains plasma cells. Such histiologic correlations can be made with each of the many clinical manifestations of secondary syphilis.

Secondary syphilis can occasionally be confirmed histologically by silver stains such as the Warthin-Starry or Steiner, which reveals spirochetes, if present, most often within the epidermis and less frequently around blood vessels in the dermal papillae. Ultimate confirmation is by darkfield examination showing spirochetes and by fluorescent antibody test (Plate 1).

Spongiotic Dermatitis (Fig. 7-35)

In photocontact dermatitis, including persistent light reactions; reactions to insect bites, scabies, creeping eruption, and cercarial dermatitis; fixed drug eruption; and cellulitis, including erysipelas, the infiltrate is both superficial and deep perivascular, but in some instances, it is wholly superficial. Each may be associated with both intraepidermal vesiculation, primarily due to spongiosis, and subepidermal vesiculation, primarily due to edema of the papillary dermis. These conditions have been discussed either in Chapter 6 or previously in this chapter. Persistent light reactions are a type of photoallergic contact dermatitis.

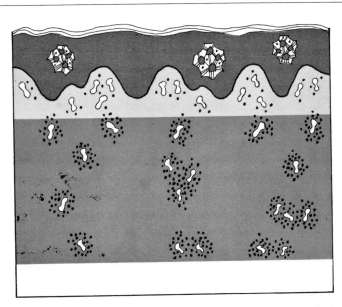

FIG. 7-35. Superficial and deep perivascular dermatitis with spongiosis.

Psoriasiform Dermatitis (Fig. 7-36)

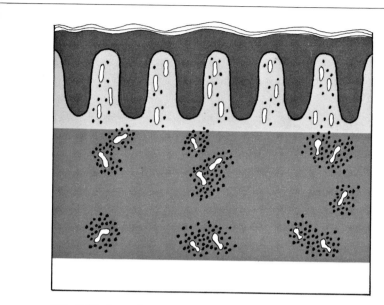

FIG. 7-36. Superficial and deep perivascular dermatitis with psoriasiform hyperplasia.

Most of the features of keratotic-crusted scabies (Norwegian scabies) and the secondary stage of syphilis have already been discussed. The psoriasiform lichenoid pattern is the most common of the many histiologic presentations of secondary syphilis.

Keratotic-crusted Scabies (Fig. 7-37)

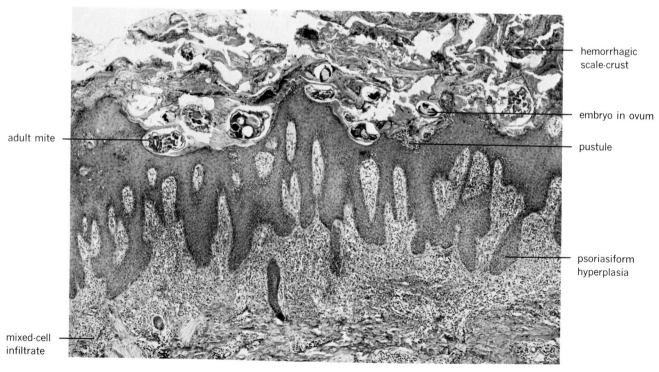

FIG. 7-37. Keratotic-crusted scabies (Norwegian scabies). This psoriasiform dermatitis is distinctive because of numerous mites in all stages of development in hyperkeratotic and crusted cornified layer. (× 56.)

Syphilis, Secondary Stages (Fig. 7-38)

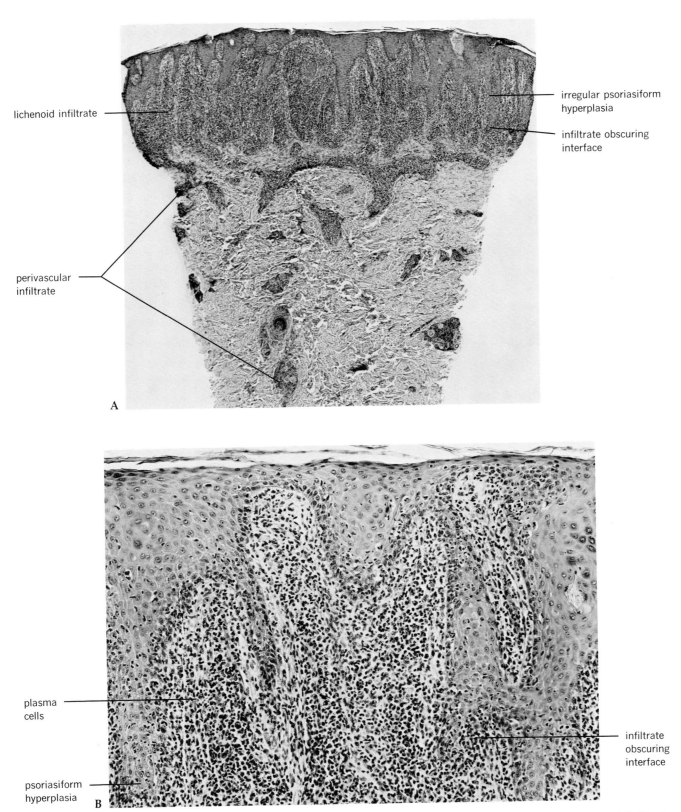

lichenoid infiltrate

irregular psoriasiform hyperplasia

infiltrate obscuring interface

perivascular infiltrate

A

plasma cells

infiltrate obscuring interface

psoriasiform hyperplasia

B

FIG. 7-38. Secondary syphilis, psoriasiform lichenoid lesion. Superficial and deep perivascular mononuclear cell infiltrate containing plasma cells and obscuring dermoepidermal interface of irregularly psoriasiform epidermis is virtually diagnostic of this disease. (A, × 30; B, × 163.)

Actinic Reticuloid (Fig. 7-39)

—Moderately dense superficial and deep mixed inflammatory-cell infiltrate of lymphocytes, histiocytes, plasma cells, eosinophils, and atypical mononuclear cells
—Papillary dermis thickened by collagen in vertical streaks
—Plump, stellate, and multinucleated fibroblasts in the thickened papillary dermis
—Epidermal hyperplasia, sometimes psoriasiform
—Slight orthokeratosis and parakeratosis

The clinical lesions of actinic reticuloid are scaly, indurated, hyperpigmented plaques, mostly on sun-exposed sites. The induration is largely the result of a thickened papillary dermis caused by long-standing rubbing.

Although the exact nosologic status of actinic reticuloid is not really known, most patients with this condition have a persistent photoallergic dermatitis with superimposed lichen simplex chronicus. Some patients who actually have mycosis fungoides are occasionally misdiagnosed histologically as actinic reticuloid, and the reverse also occurs. The ultimate diagnostic procedure is phototesting for evidences of persistent light reaction. Unlike actinic reticuloid, mycosis fungoides in the patch and plaque stages is characterized histologically by the presence of mononu-

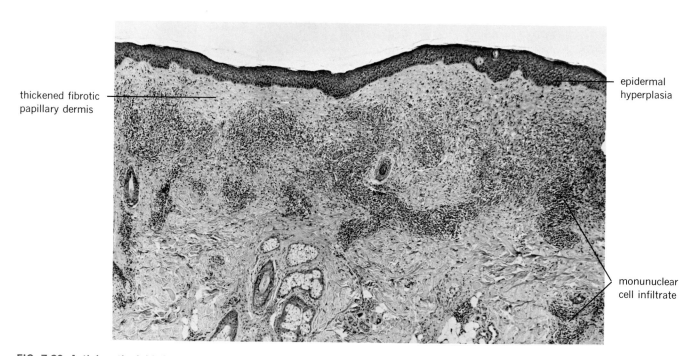

thickened fibrotic papillary dermis

epidermal hyperplasia

monunuclear cell infiltrate

FIG. 7-39. Actinic reticuloid. Superficial and deep perivascular mononuclear cell infiltrate is one sign of photodermatitis. Coarse collagen fibers and multinucleated fibroblasts are indications of persistent rubbing. The disorder results from lichen simplex chronicus superimposed upon a photoallergic contact dermatitis. (A, × 40; B, × 160.)

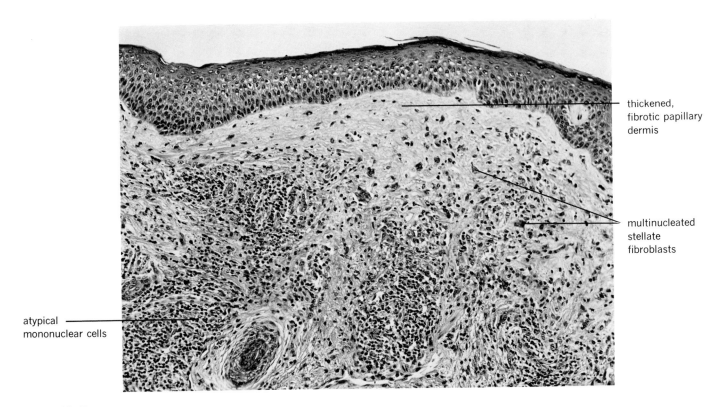

thickened, fibrotic papillary dermis

multinucleated stellate fibroblasts

atypical mononuclear cells

FIG. 7-39. B.

clear cells (not necessarily atypical ones), singly and in conglomerations within the epidermis.

Pityriasis Rosea, Herald Patch

Unlike the eruptive lesions of pityriasis rosea that show spongiosis and a superficial perivascular lymphohistiocytic infiltrate, the original herald or mother patch usually shows psoriasiform epidermal hyperplasia with parakeratosis and a superficial and deep perivascular lymphohistiocytic infiltrate. Sometimes slight spongiosis is present in the herald patch, especially in an early lesion.

Vasculitis

Neutrophilic Vasculitis

Leukocytoclastic vasculitis
  Small vessel involvement, capillary-venule
    Henoch-Schönlein syndrome
    Systemic lupus erythematosus
    Rheumatoid arthritis
    Erythema elevatum diutinum
    Polyarteritis nodosa
    Allergic granulomatosis
    Wegener's granulomatosis
    Cryoglobulinemia
    Hyperglobulinemic purpura of Walden-
      ström
    Reactions to drugs
    Leprosy in reaction
      Lucio's phenomenon
      Erythema nodosum leprosum
    Granuloma faciale
    Herpesvirus infections
    Granuloma annulare
    Necrobiosis lipoidica
  Large vessel involvement, arterial
    Polyarteritis nodosa
    Subcutaneous polyarteritis nodosa
Nonleukocytoclastic vasculitis
  Small vessel involvement, capillary-venule
    Gonococcemia
    Meningococcemia
    Pseudomonas vasculitis
    Staphylococcal septicemia
    Spirochetal (syphilitic) vasculitis
  Large vessel involvement, venous
    Migratory thrombophlebitis
    Varicose thrombophlebitis
    Mondor's disease

Large vessel involvement, arterial
  Nodular vasculitis
  Scleroderma

Lymphocytic Vasculitis

Small vessel involvement, capillary-venule
  Pityriasis lichenoides et varioliformis
    acuta
  Lymphomatoid papulosis

Histiocytic Vasculitis (Granulomatous Vasculitis)

Small vessel involvement, capillary-venule
  Necrobiosis lipoidica
Large vessel involvement, arterial
  Allergic granulomatosis
  Wegener's granulomatosis
  Lethal midline granuloma
  Giant-cell arteritis

Miscellaneous Vasculitides

Small vessel involvement
  Malignant atrophic papulosis
  Livedo vasculitis and atrophie blanche
  Lymphomatoid granulomatosis
  Hyperparathyroidism with vascular calci-
    fication

Thromboses without Vasculitis

Small vessel involvement, capillary-venule
  Disseminated intravascular coagulation
  Waldenström's macroglobulinemia
  Paroxysmal nocturnal hemoglobinuria
  Coumarin-induced necrosis
  Atheroemboli
Large vessel involvement, venous
  Phlebothromboses

Vasculitis

8

VASCULITIS denotes an inflammatory process in which inflammatory cells are within and around the walls of blood vessels and in which there are concomitant signs of damage to blood vessels, such as deposits of fibrin, degeneration of collagen, and necrosis of endothelial and muscle cells (Fig. 8-1).

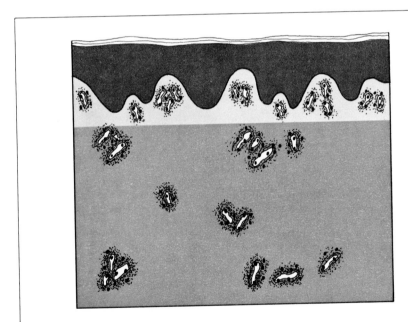

FIG. 8-1. Leukocytoclastic vasculitis.

Cutaneous blood vessels of all sizes, from the smallest capillaries in the papillary dermis to the large arteries in the subcutis, may be affected by vasculitis (Figs. 8-2–8-6). The essential microscopic findings of vasculitis are inflammatory cells within blood

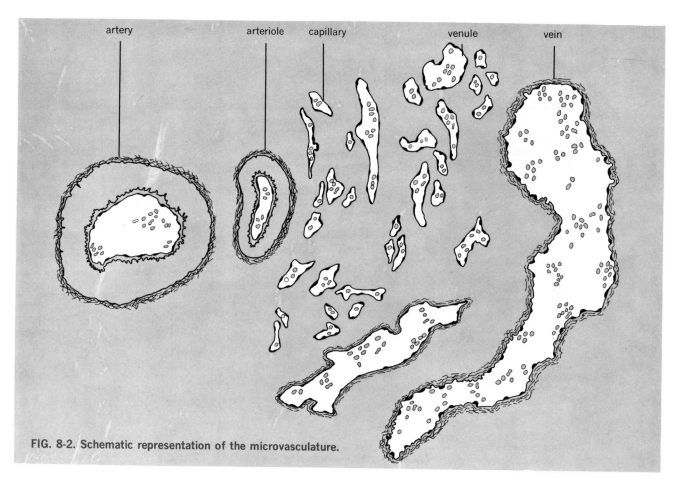

artery   arteriole   capillary   venule   vein

FIG. 8-2. Schematic representation of the microvasculature.

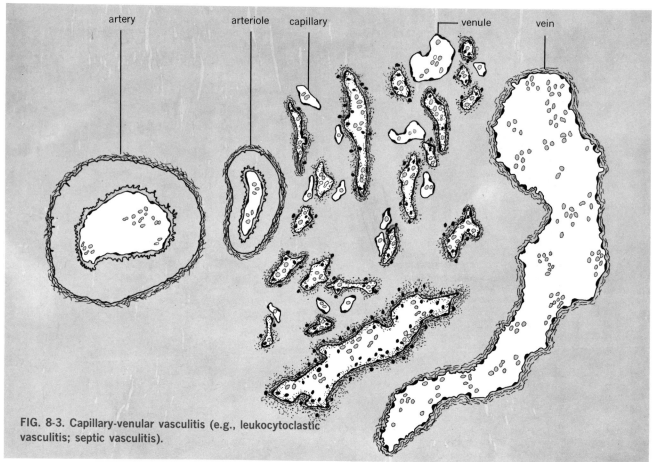

artery   arteriole   capillary   venule   vein

FIG. 8-3. Capillary-venular vasculitis (e.g., leukocytoclastic vasculitis; septic vasculitis).

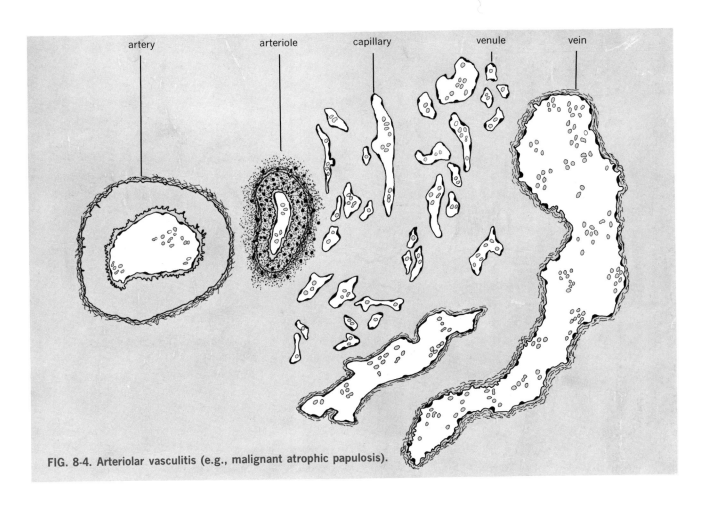

FIG. 8-4. Arteriolar vasculitis (e.g., malignant atrophic papulosis).

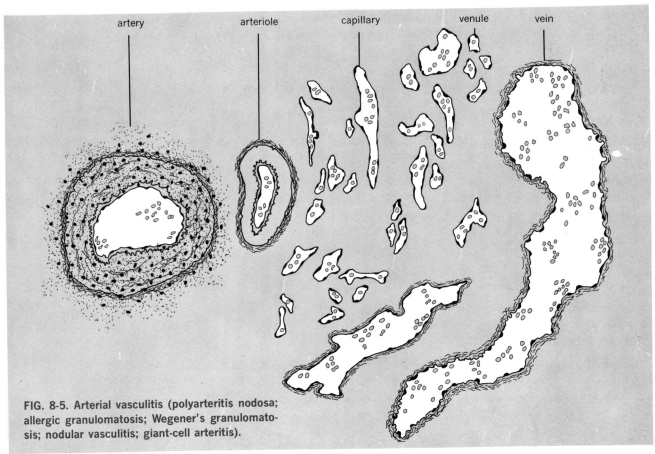

FIG. 8-5. Arterial vasculitis (polyarteritis nodosa; allergic granulomatosis; Wegener's granulomatosis; nodular vasculitis; giant-cell arteritis).

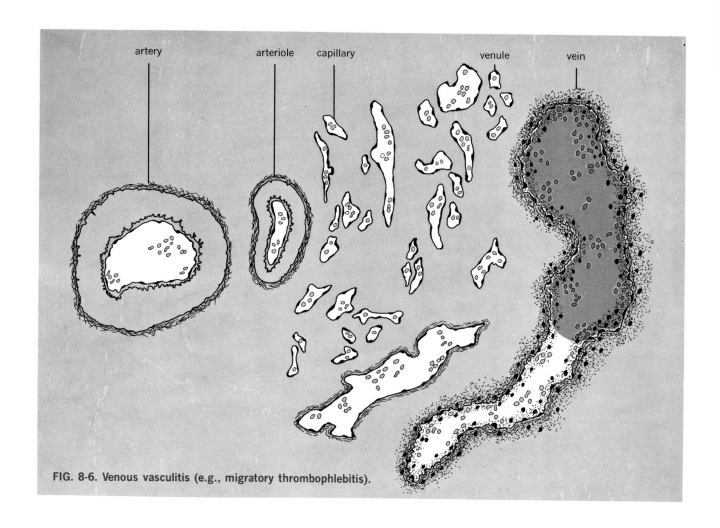

FIG. 8-6. Venous vasculitis (e.g., migratory thrombophlebitis).

artery   arteriole   capillary   venule   vein

vessel walls in association with either fibrillary, homogeneous, or granular eosinophilic material (fibrin*) and/or degenerative and necrotic changes in the blood vessel walls. Thrombi may be present. These changes distinguish vasculitis from perivascular infiltration with inflammatory cells. Both are inflammatory processes, but in vasculitis the major changes occur in the blood vessel walls, rather than around them. The inflammatory cells in vasculitis may be predominantly neutrophils (neutrophilic vasculitis), lymphocytes (lymphocytic vasculitis), or histiocytes (granulomatous vasculitis).

The descriptions of vasculitis in this classification are based upon (1) the dominant type of inflammatory cell (neutrophil, lymphocyte, or histiocyte) within vessel walls and (2) the size of the involved cutaneous blood vessels. The localization of the process, either in the skin alone (cutaneous) or in both skin and other organs (cutaneous and systemic) is also considered.

* The fibrillary, homogeneous, or granular eosinophilic material that is seen with the light microscope and called *fibrinoid* has been shown by electron microscopy to be fibrin. Associated with the fibrin there may be various proteins, such as immunoglobulins and complement, as well as platelets.

The reader must be alert to the fact that in each type of vasculitis, namely, neutrophilic, lymphocytic, and histiocytic, the inflammatory-cell infiltrate is *not* monomorphous, but rather is mixed. For example, in leukocytoclastic vasculitis, eosinophils are often present in addition to neutrophils. Furthermore, the dominant cell type may vary at different stages in the progression of the vasculitis. A case in point is allergic granulomatosis in which eosinophils and neutrophils predominate in early lesions; in later lesions histiocytes are most numerous. Thus, the vasculitides, like all inflammatory conditions in the skin, should be viewed as dynamic processes that have different clinical and histologic features at different times in their evolution.

Neutrophilic Vasculitis

Neutrophilic vasculitis can be subdivided into one type that is associated with fragmented nuclei of neutrophils, also called nuclear "dust" (leukocytoclastic vasculitis), and another in which there is practically no nuclear dust (nonleukocytoclastic vasculitis).

Leukocytoclastic Vasculitis

Many clinicians and pathologists of different nationalities and of different medical specialties, employing different histologic and clinical criteria, have written about leukocytoclastic vasculitis under different titles. Thus, one finds designations like allergic cutaneous arteriolitis, Gougerot-Ruiter syndrome, allergic angiitis, necrotizing angiitis, anaphylactoid purpura, microscopic polyarteritis nodosa, hypersensitivity angiitis, arteriolitis allergica, nodular dermal allergids, hemorrhagic microbids, monosymptom, bisymptom, trisymptom, and pentasymptom complexes, dermatitis nodularis necrotica, purpura rheumatica, and urticarial vasculitis. It would seem wise to settle for a single designation—leukocytoclastic vasculitis.

Leukocytoclastic vasculitis is thought to result, in most instances, from circulating antigen-antibody complexes that are deposited within and around the blood vessel walls. At this target site, the immune complexes activate the complement system that then attracts neutrophils to the reaction site. There follows destruction of neutrophils in the form of nuclear fragmentation and activation of the clotting system that results in the conversion of fibrinogen to fibrin. Direct immunofluorescent studies of early lesions of leukocytoclastic vasculitis reveal deposits of IgG, IgM, and complement in and around the blood vessel walls. Thus, the critical factors in the development of leukocytoclastic vasculitis appear to be (1) the nature of the antigen, (2) the type of antibody produced, and (3) the size of the immune complexes formed. Electron microscopic studies have shown that in affected capillaries and venules, the immune complexes appear first and are followed by neutrophils and lastly by fibrin (Fig. 8-7). This sequence explains why fibrin cannot always be visualized in early lesions of leukocytoclastic vasculitis. In some instances no cause can be identified for leukocytoclastic vasculitis.

Special problems arise in histologic interpretation of early lesions of leukocytoclastic vasculitis because, at that stage, the only microscopic abnormality is the presence of neutrophils in and around the walls of capillaries and venules. Often there is then no observable nuclear dust or fibrin. Such findings are insufficient to make a sure diagnosis of leukocytoclastic vasculitis. A biopsy of the same lesion only hours later, however, may show neutrophils, nuclear dust, and fibrin within the walls of blood vessels, features that establish the diagnosis of leukocytoclastic vasculitis indubitably. The reason that the mere presence of inflammatory cells within the walls of *small blood vessels* is not sufficient in itself to diagnose vasculitis is that these cells may be simply passing through, on their way from the lumina of vessels to the surrounding tissues (diapedesis). On the other hand, the presence of inflammatory cells within the walls of *large blood vessels* is an undeniable sign of vasculitis.

Small Vessel Involvement, Capillary-Venule (Fig. 8-8)

Leukocytoclastic vasculitis that involves small blood vessels, particularly postcapillary venules, is the most common type of cutaneous and systemic vasculitis. The essential histologic findings in leukocytoclastic vasculitis are neutrophils, nuclear dust, and fibrin within and around capillaries and venules in the dermis. In addition, there is often a mixed inflammatory-cell infiltrate of eosinophils, lymphocytes, histiocytes, and mast cells surrounding the venules of the superficial and/or deep dermal plexuses and sometimes even those of the subcutis. The amount of nuclear dust and fibrin in a particular specimen varies tremendously and is probably dependent upon several factors, among them the site of the lesion, its duration, and its inciting agent(s).

Microscopic observation of leukocytoclastic vasculitis involving cutaneous small blood vessels gives no clue as to whether the pathologic process is wholly confined to the skin or also involves other organs. Additionally, histologic identification of leukocyto-

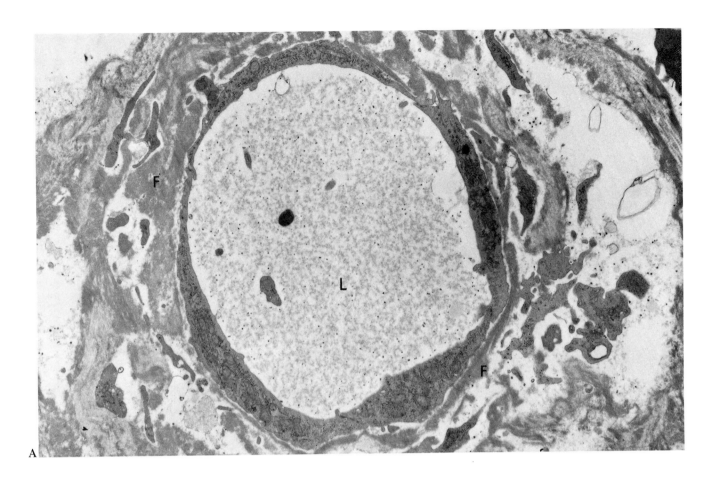

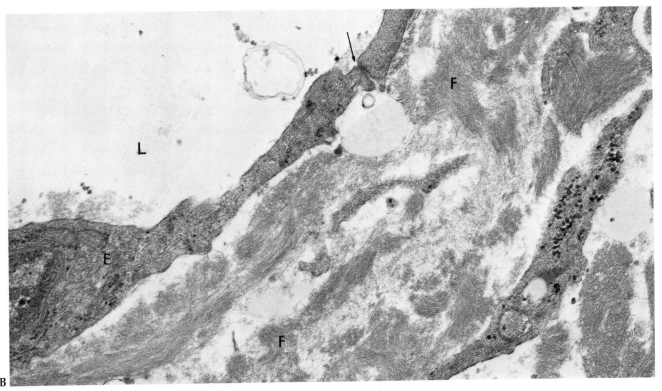

FIG. 8-7. Fibrin deposition in leukocytoclastic vasculitis. A, Deposits of fibrin (F) within and around a dermal capillary. L = lumen. (× 10,000.) B, Fibrin can be seen surrounding endothelial cells (E) in this higher magnification. (× 51,875.) Note altered tight junctions (arrow) between adjacent endothelial cells. L = lumen. (Courtesy Elaine Waldo, M.D.)

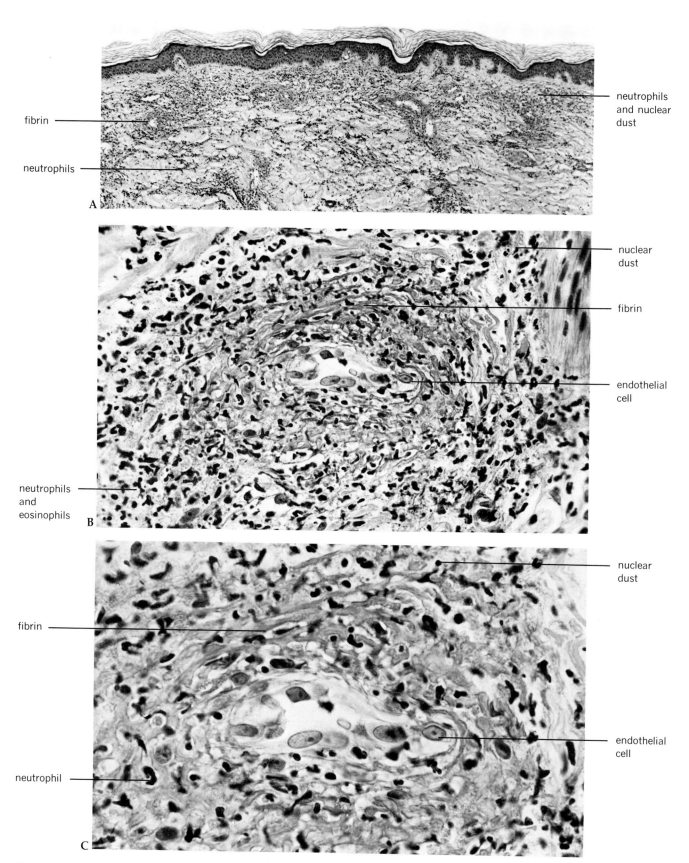

FIG. 8-8. Leukocytoclastic vasculitis. Superficial and deep infiltrate of mostly neutrophils and nuclear dust is present both around and in walls of venules where fibrin is also deposited. Endothelial lining of venule is rimmed by abundant fibrin within which are numerous neutrophils and their remnants, i.e., nuclear dust. (A, × 74; B, × 666; C, × 1080.)

clastic vasculitis suggests nothing about the specific cause of the disorder, any more than histologic diagnosis of erythema multiforme or erythema nodosum implies a specific etiologic agent. Identical appearances do not necessarily imply identical causes or mechanisms. By histologic criteria alone, the dermatopathologist cannot distinguish among the many diseases that are characterized by leukocytoclastic vasculitis. The underlying disease may be determined only by thorough examination and follow-up of each patient by the clinician. Even then, specific diseases or responsible agents are often not identified.

The clinical lesions of leukocytoclastic vasculitis, whatever their cause, are also similar in appearance. The most commonly cited clinical expression of leukocytoclastic vasculitis is "palpable purpura," that is, purpuric papules. The earliest lesions of leukocytoclastic vasculitis, however, may have no obvious purpuric component and appear only as urticarial papules. At times the vasculitic process progresses rapidly to nodules, vesicles, bullae, pustules, and ulcers. The blisters and pustules form within the epidermis (Fig. 8-9); subepidermal vesicles develop rarely. The roofs of the blisters are often gray because the epidermis is necrotic. Because of the numerous neutrophils and the abundant nuclear dust that gather at the tips of the dermal papillae, the vesiculobullous lesions of leukocytoclastic vasculitis must sometimes be differentiated histologically from dermatitis herpetiformis and bullous systemic lupus erythematosus. Although skin lesions of leukocytoclastic vasculitis may occur anywhere on the integument, formation of them on the lower extremities is commonest.

Henoch-Schönlein syndrome is a systemic leukocytoclastic vasculitis that may involve the gastrointestinal tract, joints, and kidneys in addition to the skin. The syndrome primarily affects children and young adults and frequently follows viral infections, especially of the upper respiratory tract.

The common cutaneous lesions of *systemic lupus erythematosus* are discoid plaques and evanescent malar erythema. Uncommonly, the lesions are those of leukocytoclastic vasculitis. Ulcers on the legs, periungual telangiectases, panniculitis (lupus erythematosus profundus), and digital gangrene are other rare cutaneous manifestations of systemic lupus erythematosus. Mucous membranes may also be affected by discoid lesions. There may be nonscarring, patchy, or diffuse hair loss or scarring alopecia in the discoid plaques. Arthritis, pericarditis, pleuritis, and nephritis are frequent systemic expressions of lupus erythematosus; other organs may be involved less frequently.

Rheumatoid nodules are more often seen in *rheumatoid arthritis* than are lesions of leukocytoclastic vasculitis. In rheumatoid nod-

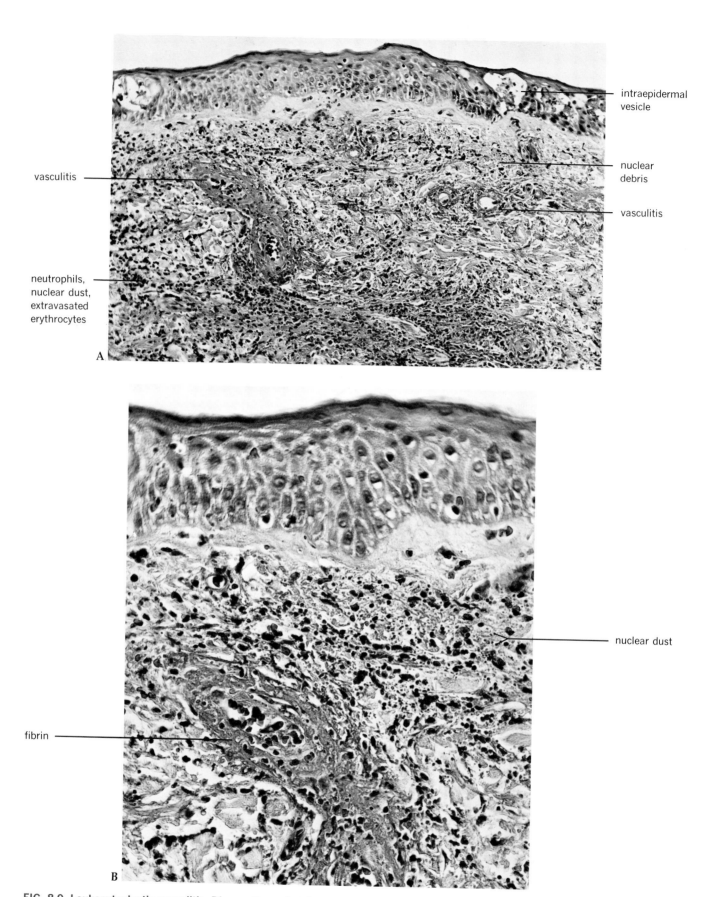

intraepidermal
vesicle

nuclear
debris

vasculitis

vasculitis

neutrophils,
nuclear dust,
extravasated
erythrocytes

nuclear dust

fibrin

FIG. 8-9. Leukocytoclastic vasculitis. Diagnostic marks pictured are fibrin, neutrophils, and nuclear dust within walls of venules. Note intraepidermal location of vesicles. (A, × 209; B, × 440; C, × 633.)

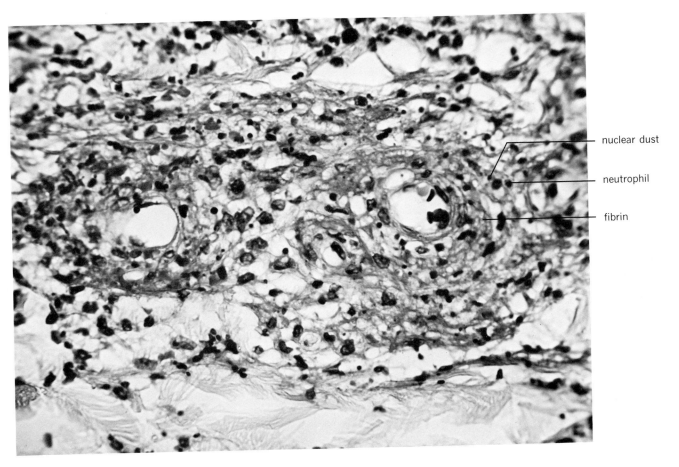

nuclear dust

neutrophil

fibrin

FIG. 8-9. C.

ules, palisaded histiocytes surround a mass of fibrin. The fibrin may be the remains of a previous severe leukocytoclastic vasculitis at that site. Digital infarcts, bullae, ulcers, and acral gangrene are other cutaneous, probably vasculitic, manifestations of rheumatoid arthritis. Pyoderma gangrenosum also develops in patients with rheumatoid arthritis. Rheumatoid leukocytoclastic vasculitis occurs primarily in patients with high titers of rheumatoid factor.

Erythema elevatum diutinum is a clinical expression of protracted leukocytoclastic vasculitis. Histologically, in early lesions of erythema elevatum diutinum there is a dense, predominantly neutrophilic infiltrate with nuclear dust within and around blood vessel walls of the superficial and deep plexuses. In time, eosinophils, lymphocytes, and histiocytes become more numerous. Eventually, in long-standing lesions, fibroblasts and fibrosis are prominent. Fibrin is usually abundant within venular walls and in former times it was dubbed "toxic hyalin." Another vestige of the terminology of earlier times is "extracellular cholesterolosis," which is now regarded as identical with erythema elevatum diutinum. In exceptional cases, there is no histologic evidence of vasculitis.

The symmetrically distributed purpuric papules and plaques of erythema elevatum diutinum favor the dorsa of the hands and the extensor surfaces overlying joints, but the lesions can occur on the skin of the trunk, buttocks, and other sites. The plaques tend to persist for months and even years. Polyarthritis and involvement of the internal organs often accompany the cutaneous lesions.

Although *polyarteritis nodosa, allergic granulomatosis,* and *Wegener's granulomatosis* are vasculitides that predominantly affect larger blood vessels, the typical changes of leukocytoclastic vasculitis of the small blood vessels may occur in each of these diseases. There is more comprehensive discussion of polyarteritis nodosa, allergic granulomatosis, and Wegener's granulomatosis later in this chapter.

Leukocytoclastic vasculitis may be a manifestation of *cryoglobulinemia* and *hyperglobulinemic purpura of Waldenström.* In addition to signs of vasculitis, there may be deposits of homogeneous eosinophilic material in the lumina of the involved small blood vessels. Cryoglobulins are present not only in some cases of systemic lupus erythematosus and rheumatoid arthritis, but also in some cases of multiple myeloma and malignant lymphomas. In other instances of cryoglobulinemia, no cause can be found. Only in mixed cryoglobulinemia does leukocytoclastic vasculitis develop.

Many *drugs*—most notably penicillin, sulfonamides, and phenylbutazone—have been implicated as causes of leukocytoclastic vasculitis. Numerous other drugs have been reported as probable causes of leukocytoclastic vasculitis.

Acute febrile neutrophilic dermatosis (Sweet's syndrome), which is treated more extensively in Chapters 7 and 9, shows all the histologic features of leukocytoclastic vasculitis except fibrin within the walls of capillaries and venules. For this reason, it is probably best considered morphologically to be a neutrophilic nodular dermatitis rather than a vasculitis.

Leprosy in reaction usually refers to Lucio's phenomenon and erythema nodosum leprosum. *Lucio's phenomenon (erythema necroticans, lazarine leprosy)* occurs in diffuse lepromatous leprosy in which the entire skin is infiltrated with foamy histiocytes filled with lepra bacilli. In this condition there are depressed cell-mediated immunity and slight resistance to the bacillus of leprosy. Consequently the skin teems with organisms. Lucio's phenomenon refers to the leukocytoclastic vasculitis that may supervene in such patients. It is characterized clinically by erythematous macules, papules, and plaques that may progress to vesicles, bullae, pustules, necrosis, and ulceration. Often the lesions heal with atrophic scars. Systemic signs and symptoms include chills and fever, epistaxis, gastrointestinal disturbances, and nerve pain.

Histologic findings of the Lucio phenomenon in the skin include leukocytoclastic vasculitis superimposed on the features of diffuse lepromatous leprosy, i.e., a dense diffuse infiltrate of foam cells throughout the dermis, sometimes extending into the subcutaneous fat. In severe ulcerative lesions of Lucio's phenomenon, the number of acid-fast bacilli, as revealed by Fite stain, is diminished, and those organisms that can be identified are fragmented and granular, an indication of nonviability. The organisms are plentiful in the surrounding skin, as is usual in lepromatous leprosy.

Erythema nodosum leprosum occurs in patients with lepromatous leprosy who have plaques and nodules, whereas the Lucio's phenomenon occurs in patients with diffuse lepromatous leprosy. It is characterized clinically by lesions that resemble erythema nodosum, but in generalized distribution. However, the nodose lesions of erythema nodosum leprosum, unlike those of erythema nodosum, occasionally become necrotic and ulcerated. Erythema nodosum leprosum is often accompanied by systemic signs and symptoms, such as fever, nerve swelling and pain, bone pain, orchitis, iritis, and polyarthritis. Erythema nodosum is primarily a septal panniculitis, whereas erythema nodosum leprosum is predominantly a vasculitis of the dermis and subcutis.

Histologic sections from lesions of erythema nodosum leprosum reveal a predominantly neutrophilic infiltrate that is dispersed among foamy histiocytes throughout the dermis and sometimes the subcutaneous fat. Then, eosinophils, lymphocytes, and plasma cells join the neutrophils. In most cases, there is vasculitis with leukocytoclasis. The number of viable acid-fast bacilli is reduced in lesions of erythema nodosum leprosum.

In rare cases livedo reticularis occurs in conjunction with papular and nodular lesions of leukocytoclastic vasculitis. Whether this represents early changes in *livedo vasculitis* that will eventuate in *atrophie blanche* has not yet been clearly established.

Granuloma faciale is a distinctive condition characterized by leukocytoclastic vasculitis during its early stages only. Initially, there is an infiltrate of neutrophils and nuclear dust within and around blood vessels throughout the dermis, especially the upper half (Fig. 8-10). Even as the infiltrate increases in density, it spares the papillary and periadnexal dermis, leaving a zone of uninvolved collagen between the epithelium and the inflammatory cells. During this neutrophilic stage, fibrin is often present within the walls of venules. Later, eosinophils appear and become the dominant inflammatory cells. Large numbers of lymphocytes, plasma cells, histiocytes, and some mast cells eventually join the eosinophils, and the number of neutrophils decreases. Ultimately, fibro-

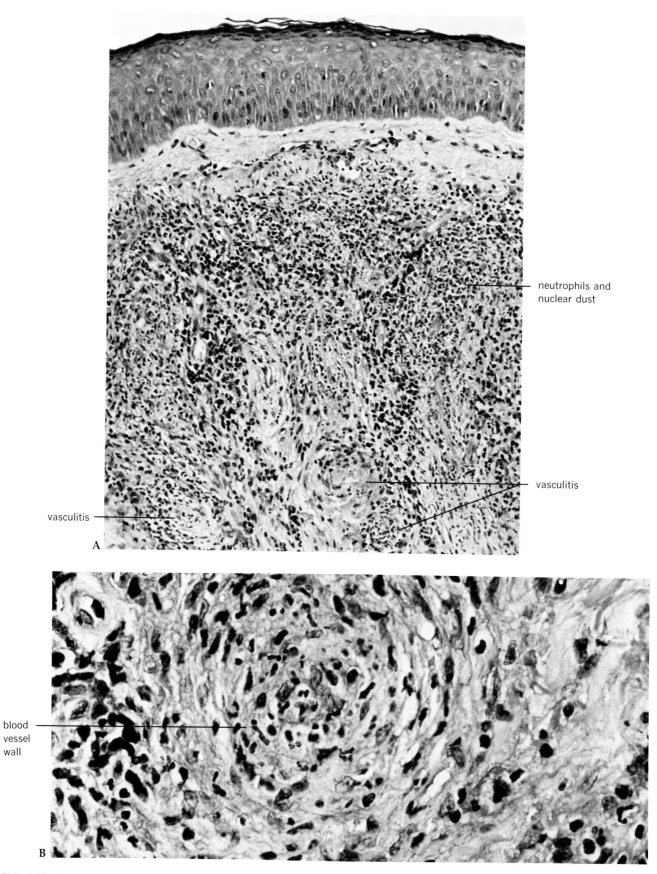

neutrophils and
nuclear dust

vasculitis

vasculitis

blood
vessel
wall

FIG. 8-10. Granuloma faciale, early lesion. Typical changes of leukocytoclastic vasculitis are present. Note that process leads to virtual occlusion of many of involved small blood vessels. (A, × 220; B, × 706.)

blasts appear and fibrosis supervenes. The term *granuloma faciale* is a misnomer because histiocytes are not the major component of the infiltrate during most of the course of each lesion, and lesions may occur on skin areas other than that of the face.

Clinically, granuloma faciale appears as one or several papules, plaques, or nodules that have patulous follicular ostia. The lesions are usually situated on the face. The consistency and color of the lesions vary with the stage of the process. Early lesions are soft and almost unchanged in skin color. Later lesions are first firm and reddish brown and finally become hard and purplish. The proportion of inflammatory-cell infiltrate to fibrosis is responsible for these clinical alterations, the more fibrosis, the more the induration. The clinical characteristics of accentuated follicular openings is probably related to sparing of the peri-infundibular connective tissue by the dense inflammatory-cell infiltrate.

In this connection, I must digress a moment to clarify the problem of vasculitis with respect to pityriasis lichenoides et varioliformis acuta (Mucha-Habermann disease). Pityriasis lichenoides et varioliformis acuta is *not* usually associated with vasculitis. Rarely will a biopsy of typical clinical lesions of pityriasis lichenoides et varioliformis acuta reveal characteristic histologic features of that disease and of leukocytoclastic vasculitis. Pityriasis lichenoides et varioliformis acuta usually consists of a superficial and deep perivascular lymphohistiocytic infiltrate that obscures the dermoepidermal junction, along which there are vacuolar alteration and numerous necrotic keratinocytes. Focal intercellular and intracellular edema may eventuate in an intraepidermal vesicle. In *exceptional* cases of pityriasis lichenoides et varioliformis acuta, in addition to these histologic findings, there are neutrophils, nuclear dust, and fibrin within and around blood vessel walls. In other *rare* cases of pityriasis lichenoides et varioliformis acuta (and lymphomatoid papulosis) a lymphocytic vasculitis with fibrin may be seen.

Typical changes of leukocytoclastic vasculitis can involve the blood vessels of the superficial plexus in some cases of *herpes simplex, herpes zoster,* and *varicella.* These vasculitic changes are found beneath the characteristic epidermal changes of herpesvirus infections (Fig. 8-11). In these instances of vasculitis there are usually severe epidermal necrosis and eventual ulceration. It may be that ulcerative and scarring lesions of herpesvirus infection result, in part, from the vasculitis. Herpesvirus infections are discussed at greater length in Chapter 10.

In some early lesions of *granuloma annulare* and *necrobiosis lipoidica* there are histologic signs of necrotizing vasculitis. Specifically, in the center of the palisade of histiocytes, nuclear debris

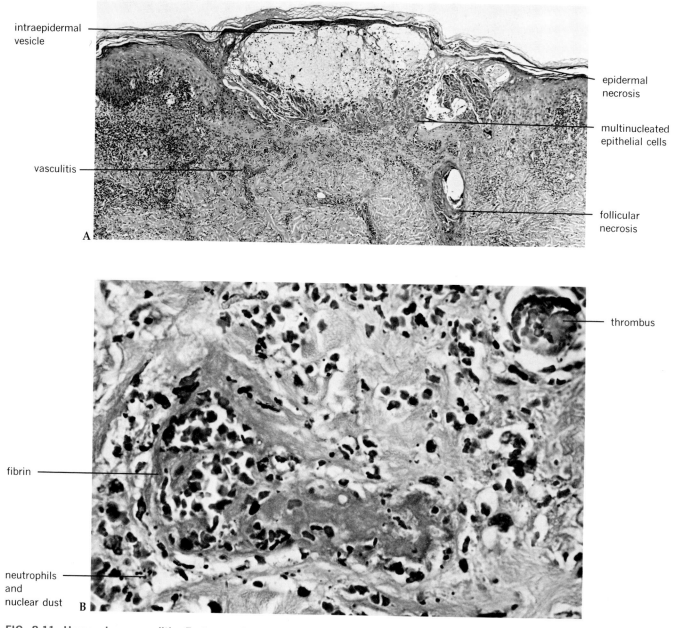

intraepidermal vesicle

epidermal necrosis

multinucleated epithelial cells

vasculitis

follicular necrosis

A

thrombus

fibrin

neutrophils and nuclear dust

B

FIG. 8-11. Herpesvirus vasculitis. Features of leukocytoclastic vasculitis may on occasion be seen in blood vessels of the superficial plexus beneath typical intraepidermal changes of herpesvirus infections. (× 61.) B, Fibrin, neutrophils, and nuclear dust are seen in wall of one venule and a thrombus within another. (× 799.)

may surround the outline of a small necrotic blood vessel (Figs. 8-12, 8-13). Perhaps the pathway of palisaded granuloma formation begins with vasculitic destruction of a small blood vessel or infarction, proceeds to ischemic alteration of the surrounding connective tissue, and eventuates in a histiocytic response to this altered connective tissue. Rheumatoid nodule, in which a central core of fibrin is encircled by histiocytes, may be the consummate example of this hypothesis. Lastly, fibrin and inflammatory cells may be seen in the walls of blood vessels subjacent to ulceration (Fig. 8-14).

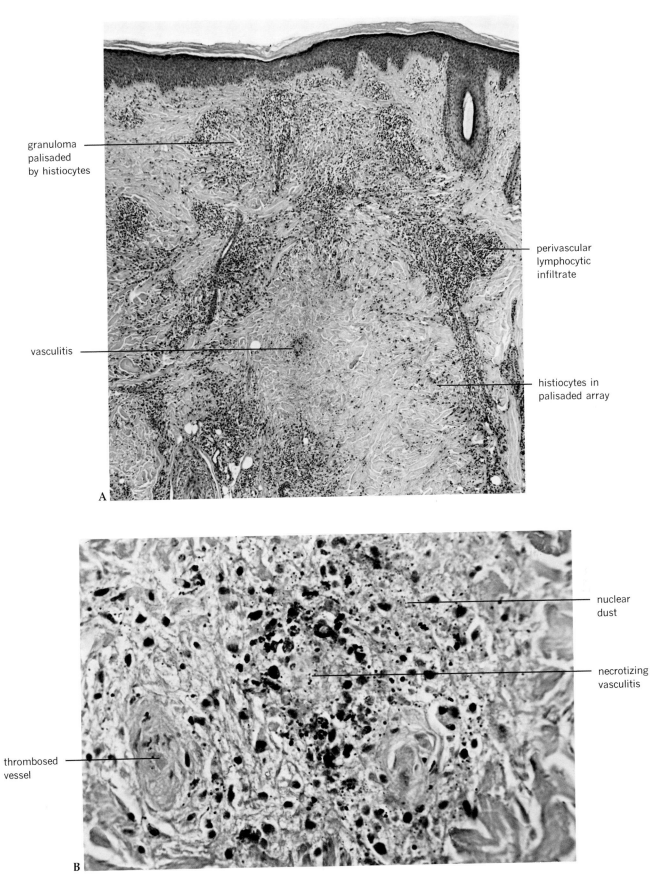

granuloma
palisaded
by histiocytes

perivascular
lymphocytic
infiltrate

vasculitis

histiocytes in
palisaded array

A

nuclear
dust

necrotizing
vasculitis

thrombosed
vessel

B

FIG. 8-12. Vasculitis in granuloma annulare. Near center of large granuloma bounded by histiocytes in palisaded array a small necrotic blood vessel is largely obscured by neutrophils and nuclear dust. (A, × 58; B, × 653.)

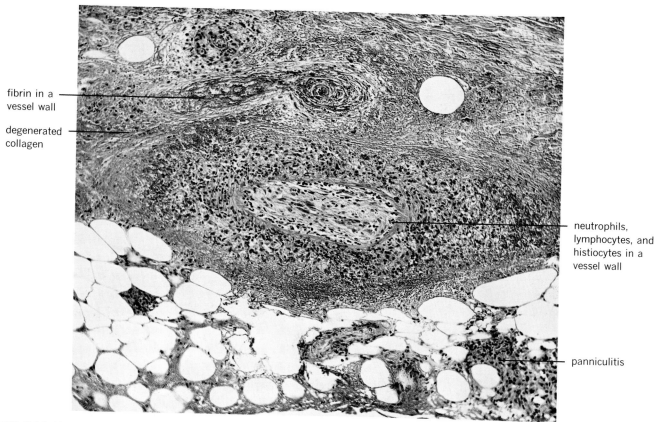

fibrin in a
vessel wall

degenerated
collagen

neutrophils,
lymphocytes, and
histiocytes in a
vessel wall

panniculitis

FIG. 8-13. Necrobiosis lipoidica. Fibrin and neutrophils in walls of small vessels as pictured are characteristic of leukocytoclastic vasculitis, and numerous histiocytes, some multinucleated, in walls of larger vessels (one is shown in center of field) are features of granulomatous vasculitis. Both may occur in necrobiosis lipoidica and concurrently in different blood vessels within the same specimen. These changes are usually most pronounced in the lower portion of the dermis as shown here. (× 164.)

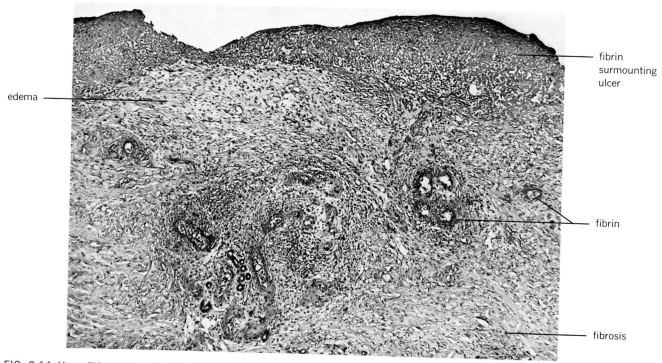

edema

fibrin
surmounting
ulcer

fibrin

fibrosis

FIG. 8-14. Vasculitis secondary to ulceration. Fibrin commonly covers an ulcer and rims the subjacent small blood vessels. The changes illustrated resulted from severe stasis. (A, × 86; B, × 431.)

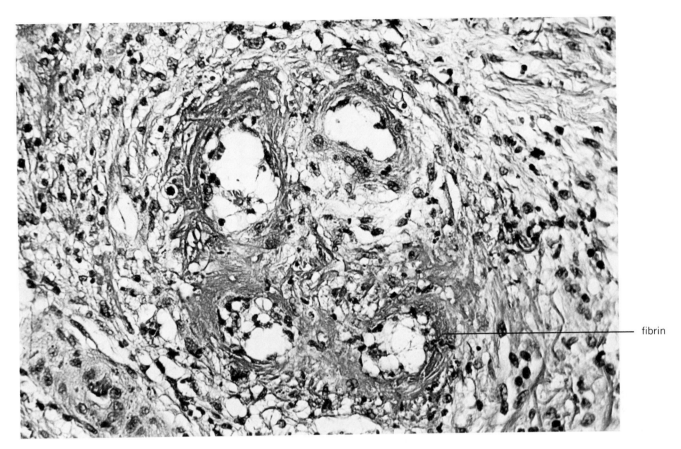

fibrin

FIG. 8-14. B.

Large Vessel Involvement, Arterial

Polyarteritis nodosa (periarteritis or panarteritis nodosa) is a disease in which leukocytoclastic vasculitis involves arteries, rather than venules, and large, rather than small, vessels (Fig. 8-15). In this condition the immune complexes are deposited in medium-sized arteries, and the resultant pathologic changes give polyarteritis nodosa its distinctive constellation of clinical symptoms and signs. Despite the predominant involvement of medium-sized arteries, especially at their bifurcations, adjacent veins, small arteries and, occasionally, even arterioles may be affected. Rarely, cutaneous lesions of polyarteritis nodosa may show leukocytoclastic changes in still smaller blood vessels.

All the histologic features of leukocytoclastic vasculitis are seen in polyarteritis nodosa: fibrin, neutrophils, fragments of neutrophil nuclei, and sometimes eosinophils. Arterial necrosis may lead to the formation of aneurysms that may subsequently rupture. The aneurysmal dilatations can be seen with the naked eye and palpated as nodules, 5 to 10 mm in size, hence the designation *nodosa*. Subcutaneous arterial aneurysms, too, may present themselves as nodules in the skin. In time, arteries may become

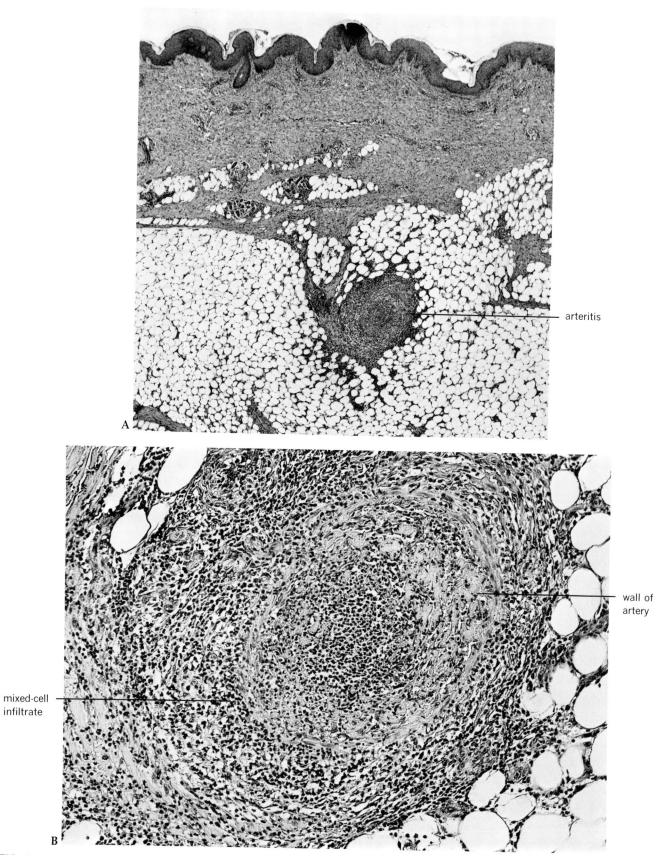

arteritis

wall of
artery

mixed-cell
infiltrate

FIG. 8-15. Polyarteritis nodosa. Unlike nodular vasculitis in which inflammatory-cell infiltrate involves not only the wall of an artery in subcutaneous fat but much of the surrounding fat, inflammatory cells in subcutaneous polyarteritis nodosa are mostly limited to wall of artery alone. (A, × 27; B, × 174.)

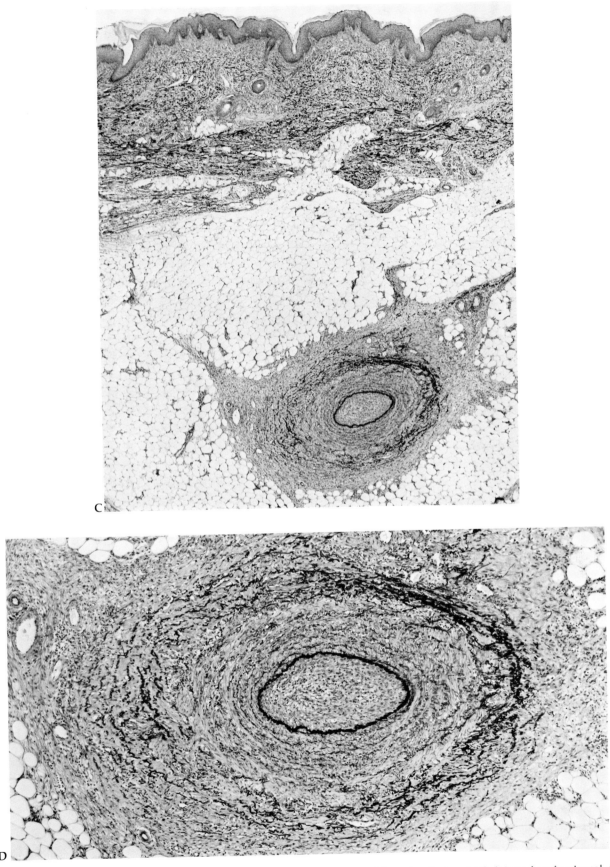

C

D

FIG. 8-15 (continued). Elastic tissue stain shows that large blood vessel in subcutis has both internal and external elastic membranes, confirming that it is an artery. (C, × 28; D, × 80.)

occluded by thrombi which result in infarction and eventual scarring. The clinical concomitants of subcutaneous arterial infarction may be purpura, bullae, ulceration, and even digital gangrene.

Although lymphocytes, histiocytes, and plasma cells may join the polymorphonuclear-cell infiltrate, histiocytes are not usually predominant in polyarteritis nodosa, nor are they congregated extravascularly. Long-standing lesions, however, may inevitably show granulomatous arteritis. The absence of extravascular granulomatous inflammation is one important feature in the differentiation of polyarteritis nodosa from allergic granulomatosis.

The arterial lesions in polyarteritis nodosa are widespread in distribution. In most patients the kidneys are affected by arteritis and glomerulonephritis, and hence renal insufficiency is the usual cause of death. Coronary arteritis may precipitate occlusion and myocardial infarction. Mesenteric arteritis can cause intestinal perforation and hemorrhage. Other gastrointestinal complications of polyarteritis nodosa result from involvement of the appendix, pancreas, gall bladder, and liver. Both the peripheral and central nervous systems may be affected by the vasculitis and resultant ischemia. The lungs, however, are not involved in polyarteritis nodosa.

Drugs (particularly some antibiotics), hepatitis-associated antigen (Australia antigen), and streptococci have been implicated as causes of polyarteritis nodosa. Australia antigen, complement, and IgM have all been demonstrated in the vasculitic lesions of polyarteritis nodosa associated with chronic Australia antigenemia. Resolution of the hepatitits is generally accompanied by disappearance of the vasculitis.

Polyarteritis nodosa may occur at any age, more commonly in adults. Men are affected four times as frequently as are women. The incidence of polyarteritis nodosa reached a peak during the time when sulfonamides were the main systemic antibacterial agent and has declined steadily since the sulfonamides were replaced by more effective antimicrobials.

Subcutaneous polyarteritis nodosa refers to a disease that involves only small arteries in the panniculus with typical changes of leukocytoclastic vasculitis (Fig. 8-16). The involved subcutaneous blood vessels show all of the histologic changes associated with classic polyarteritis nodosa, i.e., necrosis of the artery wall, either circumferentially or segmentally, fibrin, neutrophils, and nuclear dust. With time the other inflammatory cells may also be present. The necrotizing changes usually result in obliteration of the vessel and its replacement by fibrosis. There is no involvement of the internal organs.

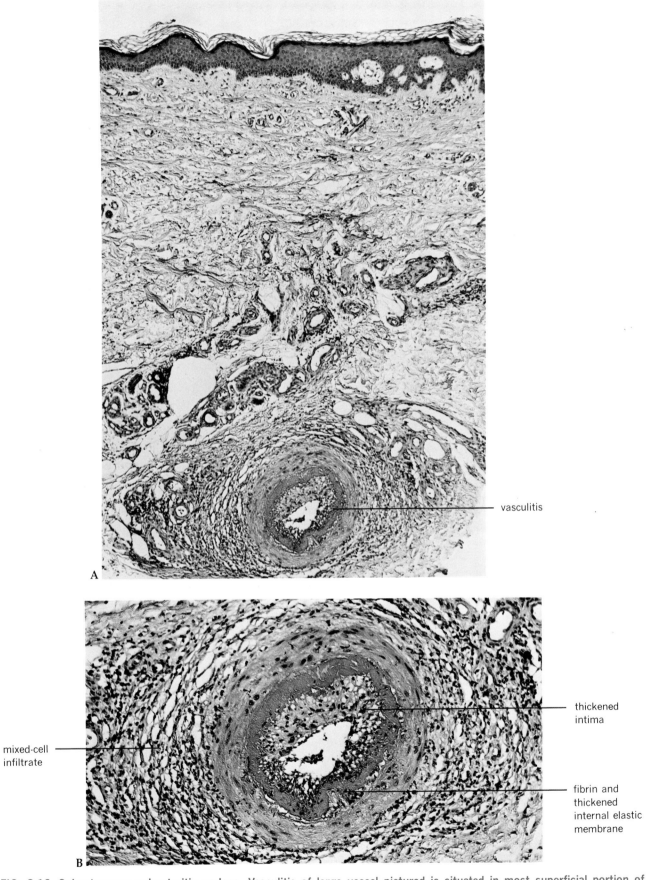

vasculitis

thickened intima

mixed-cell infiltrate

fibrin and thickened internal elastic membrane

FIG. 8-16. Subcutaneous polyarteritis nodosa. Vasculitis of large vessel pictured is situated in most superficial portion of subcutaneous fat. (A, × 89; B, × 208.)

Subcutaneous polyarteritis nodosa can be differentiated from nodular vasculitis primarily by the extensive involvement of the fat lobules with necrosis and an inflammatory-cell infiltrate in nodular vasculitis compared to the scant perivascular panniculitis secondary to the vasculitis in subcutaneous polyarteritis nodosa.

Clinically, the patient with subcutaneous polyarteritis nodosa will have painful subcutaneous nodules, usually associated with livedo reticularis, especially on the lower extremities. The nodules may become hemorrhagic and necrotic and eventually ulcerate. These lesions tend to leave and then recur. Patients with subcutaneous lesions of polyarteritis nodosa and no evidence of the disease in internal organs have an excellent prognosis, in contrast to patients with systemic polyarteritis nodosa who have concomitant involvement of the subcutaneous arteries. Subcutaneous polyarteritis nodosa is comparable to other limited forms of the disease such as polyarteritis nodosa confined to the appendix or gallbladder.

Nonleukocytoclastic Vasculitis

Although leukocytoclastic vasculitis is generally marked by the presence of neutrophilic nuclear debris, there is practically no nuclear "dust" in nonleukocytoclastic vasculitis. However, in early lesions of leukocytoclastic vasculitis, no fragments of neutrophil nuclei may be seen, and in late lesions of nonleukocytoclastic vasculitis a few nuclear fragments may be detected. Therefore, histologic differentiation between early lesions of leukocytoclastic (allergic) vasculitis and those of nonleukocytoclastic (septic) vasculitis may be difficult, if not impossible.

Small Vessel Involvement, Capillary-Venule

Septicemias, such as *gonococcemia* and *meningococcemia*, produce histologic changes in the skin that are indistinguishable from one another. The uncommon acute meningococcemia and the even more rare acute gonococcemia are associated with disseminated intravascular coagulation and are discussed later in this chapter. Early lesions of patients with chronic gonococcal or meningococcal infections show a predominantly neutrophilic infiltrate in and around blood-vessel walls throughout the dermis (Fig. 8-17). Thrombi usually occlude capillaries and venules in at least the upper dermis, and fibrin may be found within blood vessel walls

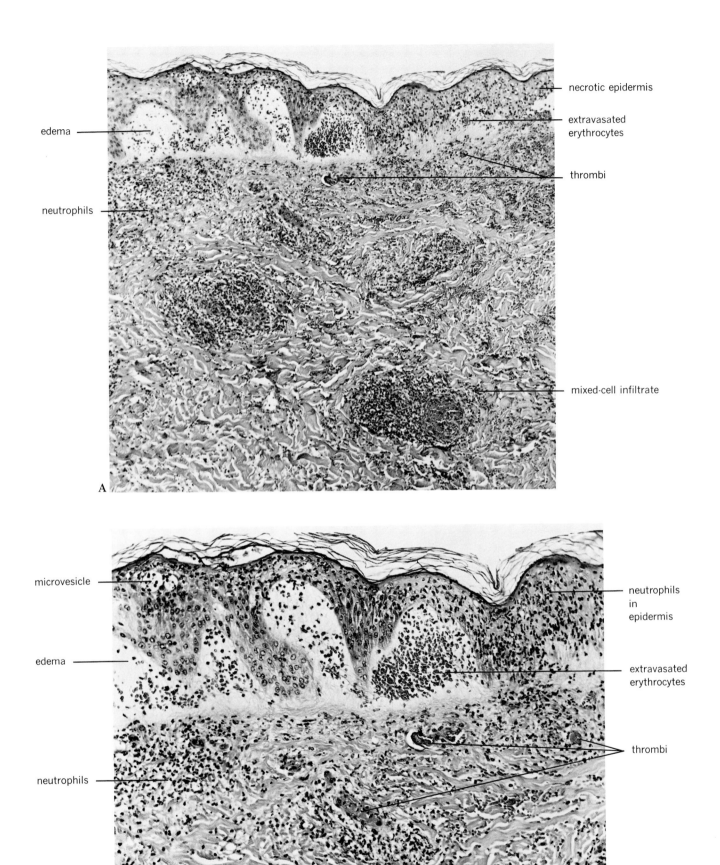

necrotic epidermis

extravasated
erythrocytes

edema

thrombi

neutrophils

mixed-cell infiltrate

A

microvesicle

neutrophils
in
epidermis

edema

extravasated
erythrocytes

neutrophils

thrombi

B

FIG. 8-17. Gonococcal vasculitis, chronic type. Thrombi in lumens of all small blood vessels pictured lead to edema of papillary dermis, extravasation of red blood cells, and necrotic epidermis containing neutrophils. (A, × 83; B, × 753.)

VASCULITIS 357

(Fig. 8-18). Arterioles in the mid and lower reticular dermis, and sometimes even in the subcutis, may be affected by the vasculitic process. The edematous papillary dermis contains numerous extravasated erythrocytes, as well as neutrophils. An intraepidermal vesiculopustule forms secondary to intracellular and intercellular edema coupled with collections of neutrophils, and a subepidermal vesicle may develop secondary to extensive edema in the papillary dermis. Necrosis of the epidermis and often of the adnexal epithelium usually accompanies these changes. Neutrophils are often present within the necrotic epidermis.

In some instances it may be impossible to distinguish the earliest lesions of a septic vasculitis, such as chronic gonococcemia, from those of a leukocytoclastic vasculitis. As a rule, however, thrombi are present more regularly in septic vasculitis, whereas nuclear dust and fibrin occur more frequently in leukocytoclastic vasculitis (Fig. 8-19). In exceptional cases, however, thrombi appear in leukocytoclastic vasculitis, and leukocytoclasis and fibrin in septic vasculitis. Only capillaries and venules are involved in leukocytoclastic vasculitis, whereas arterioles may also be affected in septic vasculitis. Eosinophils tend to be more plentiful in allergic (i.e., leukocytoclastic), rather than in septic, vasculitis. Epidermal changes, however, are more common in septic than in leukocytoclastic vasculitis. When neutrophils abound in the papillary dermis of chronic gonococcemia or meningococce-

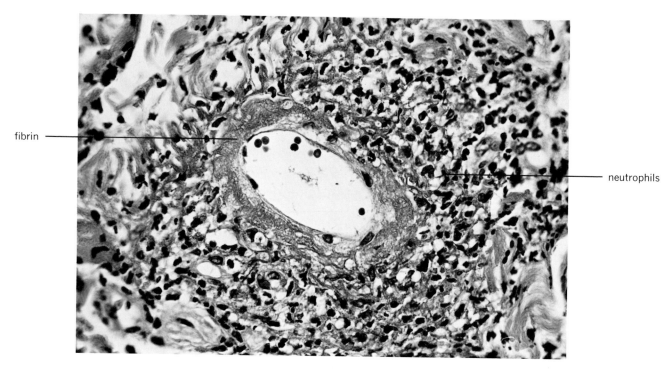

fibrin

neutrophils

FIG. 8-18. Gonococcal vasculitis, chronic type. In some lesions of septic vasculitis histologic changes may be similar to those of leukocytoclastic vasculitis as in this specimen with fibrin and neutrophils in the blood-vessel wall. ($\times$ 624.)

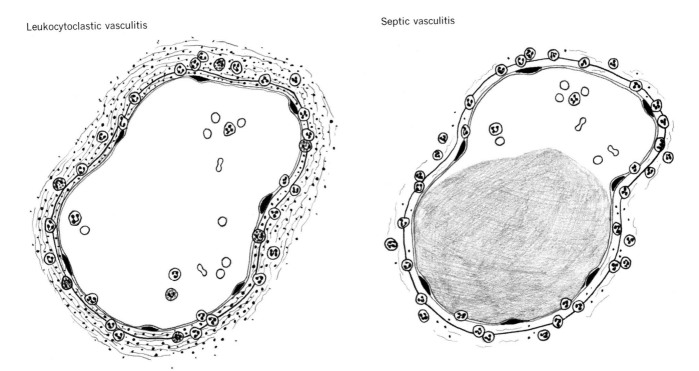

Leukocytoclastic vasculitis

Septic vasculitis

FIG. 8-19. Diagrammatic representation contrasting leukocytoclastic vasculitis and septic vasculitis.

mia, the condition must be differentiated histologically from dermatitis herpetiformis and from bullous systemic lupus erythematosus. Differentiation is possible by the finding of vasculitis in the septic lesion.

Older lesions of chronic gonococcemia and chronic meningococcemia show predominantly lymphohistiocytic infiltration with fewer neutrophilis than are found in the earlier lesions.

Clinically, untreated acute gonococcal and meningococcal septicemias are explosive, fulminant, and often fatal. Chronic gonococcemia and meningococcemia are prolonged, episodic, and nonfatal. The chronic form of these septicemias is much more common. Gram-negative diplococci are usually seen on smears and recovered easily from skin lesions of the acute septicemias, but they are practically never demonstrated by either Gram's stain of smears or of tissue sections or grown in culture from skin lesions of chronic gonococcemia and chronic meningococcemia.

Clinically, chronic gonococcemia and chronic meningococcemia are characterized by a triad of fever, migratory arthralgia that frequently settles as an arthritis of the knee, wrist, or ankle, and sparse, tender skin lesions that favor the distal parts of the extremities. The skin lesions are of three types. They may be purpuric, usually petechiae and/or small ecchymoses on the palmar and plantar surfaces, vesiculopustules that arise on broad erythematous bases, and, rarely, hemorrhagic bullae. A clinical feature of chronic gonococcal septicemia that differentiates it from chronic meningococcemia is tenosynovitis.

Acute gonococcemia and acute meningococcemia are associated with widespread purpuric skin lesions and hemorrhages in internal organs, the result of necrotizing vasculitis and disseminated intravascular coagulation. There is a paucity of inflammatory cells. Meningitis, carditis, and nephritis are among the complications that formerly inevitably led to death.

Janeway lesions and *Osler's nodes*—tiny, vividly pink, edematous macules and papules on the acral parts of patients with acute and subacute endocarditis—have histologic features indistinguishable from those of chronic gonococcal and meningococcal septicemia. Fibrin microthrombi plug the small blood vessels of the superficial plexus and are associated with a neutrophilic vasculitis, abscesses in the dermal papillae, and necrosis of the epidermis. Staphylococcus aureus has been cultured from both Janeway lesions and Osler's nodes (as have Proteus and Candida, but rarely), indicating that these skin lesions are caused in part by septic emboli originating from endocardial valves.

The histologic features of *pseudomonas vasculitis* are similar to those of acute gonococcal and acute meningococcal vasculitis with scant inflammatory cells, severe necrosis of blood vessels, and numerous thrombi. Myriad gram-negative bacilli are present within the walls of capillaries and venules, and throughout the dermis. The histologic findings in pseudomonas septicemia are usually accompanied by those of a consumptive coagulopathy. Bullae, ulcers, and eschars develop more readily in pseudomonas septicemia than in acute gonococcemia and meningococcemia.

The clinical changes of pseudomonas septicemia are known as ecthyma gangrenosum because of their tendency to progress to ulcers. These lesions begin as patches of erythema that usually become purpuric and bullous and often ulcerate. Gram-negative bacilli are readily identified in smears and tissue sections and are easily grown in culture from skin lesions. Systemic signs of pseudomonas septicemia are fever, jaundice, splenomegaly, meningitis, endocarditis, and pulmonary abscesses.

Staphylococcal septicemia with skin lesions is rare. It is recognized clinically by purpuric pustules. In addition to vasculitis, histologic sections show numerous extravasated erythrocytes within the papillary dermis and neutrophilic abscesses within the epidermis (Fig. 8-20). Gram-positive cocci are profuse in smears and tissue sections from skin lesions and are readily grown in culture.

The *spirochetal vasculitis* of secondary syphilis, incorrectly termed *malignant syphilis* or *lues maligna*, consists of a mixed inflammatory-cell infiltrate of lymphocytes, plasma cells, histiocytes,

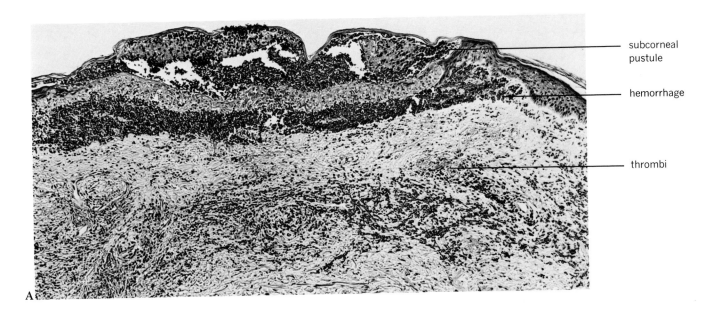

subcorneal pustule

hemorrhage

thrombi

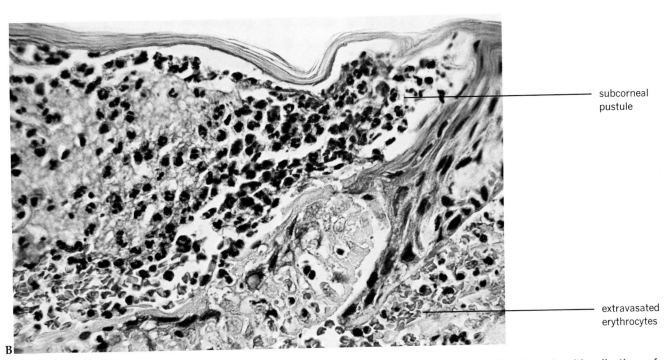

subcorneal pustule

extravasated erythrocytes

FIG. 8-20. Staphylococcal septicemia. Clinical sign of pustules and purpura together correlates histologically with collections of neutrophils within epidermis and numerous extravasated erythrocytes within dermis. The latter phenomenon follows thrombosis of small dermal blood vessels. (A, × 97; B, × 678.)

and neutrophils within and around blood vessels at all levels of the dermis. Fibrin may be present in some capillaries and venules, although many blood vessels simply have thickened walls with an increased number of plump endothelial cells. Thrombi occlude some lumina of blood vessels in the superficial plexus. Epidermal necrosis eventuates in ulceration, and collagen degeneration culminates in fibrosis. Clinically, the lesions of syphilitic vasculitis are vesiculopustular, crusted, ulcerative, and scarred. Extremely high serologic titers for syphilis are the rule in this rare vasculitic form of secondary syphilis. The vasculitis of secondary syphilis may be analogous to that of lepromatous leprosy (Lucio's phenomenon).

Large Vessel Involvement, Venous

In actuality, *migratory thrombophlebitis* (multiple segmental thrombophlebitis), which involves the superficial veins of the legs and arms, does not migrate, but multicentrically affects segments of the venous system. Biopsy specimens of involved veins show an inflammatory-cell infiltrate within the walls of the veins (Fig. 8-21). Often thrombi occlude the lumina. The clinical correlates of these histologic findings are redness, tenderness, and swelling over a well-circumscribed segment of a superficial vein. When a solid cord is formed, the thrombus can be palpated.

Migratory thrombophlebitis may signal an associated visceral malignancy, most commonly a mucin-producing adenocarcinoma of the body or tail of the pancreas and less commonly a carcinoma of the head of the pancreas, the lung, stomach, or gallbladder. Malignant lymphomas, including Hodgkin's disease, have also been associated with migratory thrombophlebitis.

Migratory thrombophlebitis tends to occur in superficial veins of middle-aged and older men. Segments of one or more veins may be involved concurrently. There is a tendency for thrombi to re-form in previously involved venous segments. Death often occurs from pulmonary emboli.

The cause of migratory thrombophlebitis is not known, although it has been shown that the carcinoma does not directly invade the walls of the involved veins. Finally, it should be noted that thromboangiitis obliterans (Buerger's disease) can be associated with a multiple segmental thrombophlebitis that is clinically and histologically indistinguishable from that associated with underlying malignant neoplasms. Buerger's disease may be nothing more than severe arteriosclerosis in young men who are prodigious cigarette smokers.

Varicose thrombophlebitis is fundamentally a phlebothrombosis with subsequent mild thrombophlebitis. Prolonged stasis leads to thrombosis within the tortuous leg veins. Eventually there is organization of the thrombus. The inflammatory-cell infiltrate within the vein wall is usually sparse. Varicose thrombophlebitis can involve the superficial, deep, and communicating veins.

Mondor's disease is a thrombophlebitis of a superficial vein in the subcutaneous fat of the breast or anterior chest wall. It appears as a subcutaneous tender cord with overlying linear depression, especially in women. The cause of the condition is unknown.

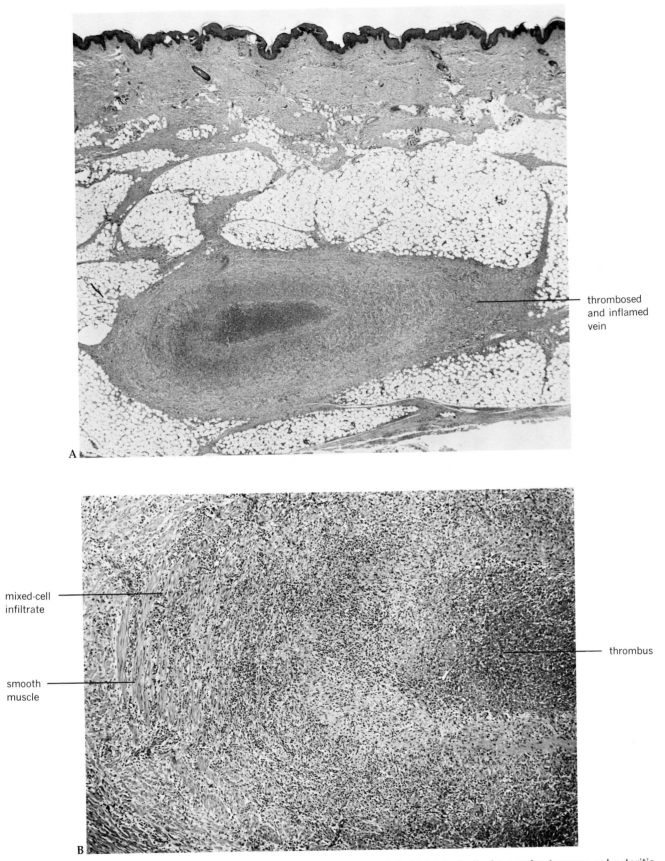

FIG. 8-21. Migratory thrombophlebitis. This condition must be differentiated histologically from subcutaneous polyarteritis nodosa. Large size and oval shape of blood vessel pictured indicate that it is a vein. The absence of an internal elastic membrane, demonstrable by stain for elastic tissue, confirms the fact. (A, × 14; B, × 77.)

Nodular vasculitis is an arteritis in the subcutis and is associated with severe panniculitis, unlike subcutaneous polyarteritis nodosa in which the inflammatory-cell infiltrate is confined mostly to the walls of the arteries. (Fig. 8-22). With time the arteritis may become granulomatous (Fig. 8-23). A dense mixed inflammatory-cell infiltrate also involves the dermis. Because nodular vasculitis is accompanied by extensive inflammatory changes in the subcutaneous fat, the disease is considered more fully in Chapter 14.

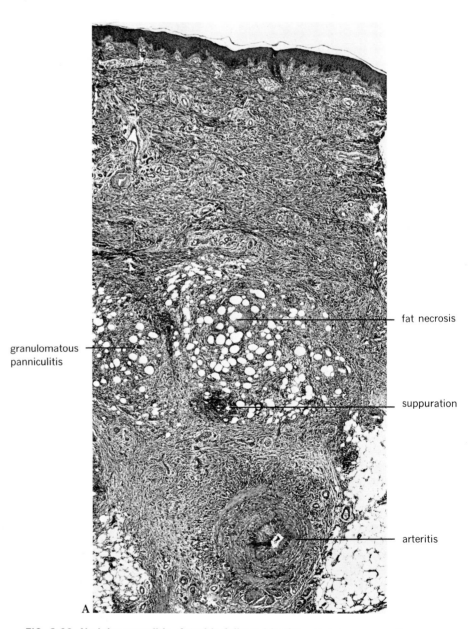

granulomatous panniculitis

fat necrosis

suppuration

arteritis

FIG. 8-22. Nodular vasculitis. Arteritis followed by fat necrosis, suppuration, granulomatous inflammation, and fibrosis are characteristic histologic features. (A, × 28; B, × 78; C, × 144.)

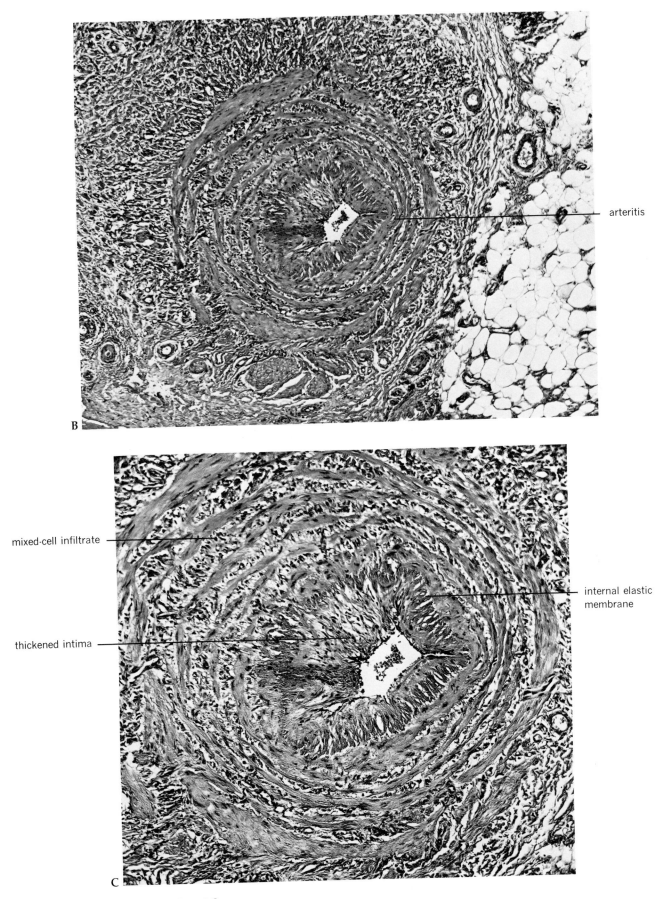

arteritis

mixed-cell infiltrate

internal elastic membrane

thickened intima

FIG. 8-22. Nodular vasculitis. B and C.

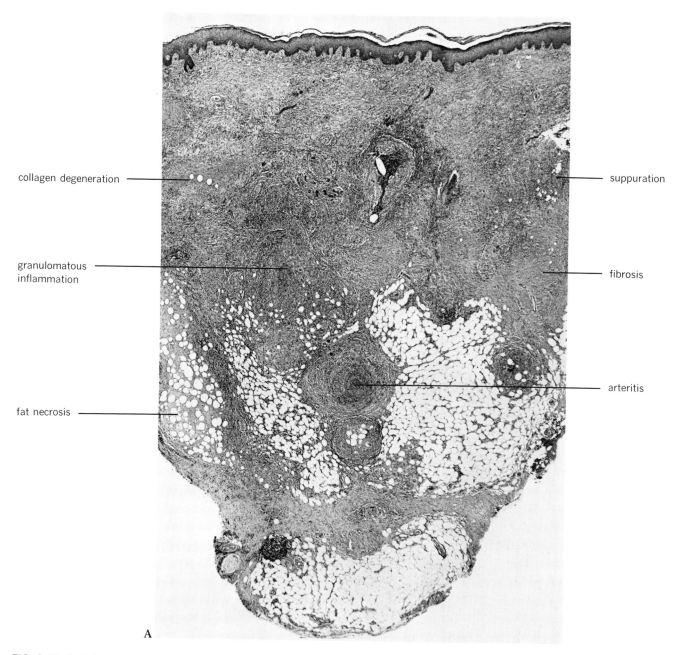

collagen degeneration

suppuration

granulomatous inflammation

fibrosis

fat necrosis

arteritis

A

FIG. 8-23. Nodular vasculitis. The original predominantly neutrophilic arteritis may evolve into granulomatous arteritis in older lesions of nodular vasculitis. (A, × 24; B, × 49; C, × 158.)

Among the earliest histologic changes in cutaneous lesions of *scleroderma* is a neutrophilic vasculitis that involves small to medium-sized arteries in the subcutaneous fat (Fig. 8-24). These critical changes are not often seen in histologic sections because the biopsy specimen is not usually taken early enough in the course of the disease and is not usually deep enough. When these conditions do obtain, however, a dense infiltrate of neutrophils can be seen within the thickened vessel wall of almost every small artery in the specimen. No vasculitis is present in the dermal blood vessels.

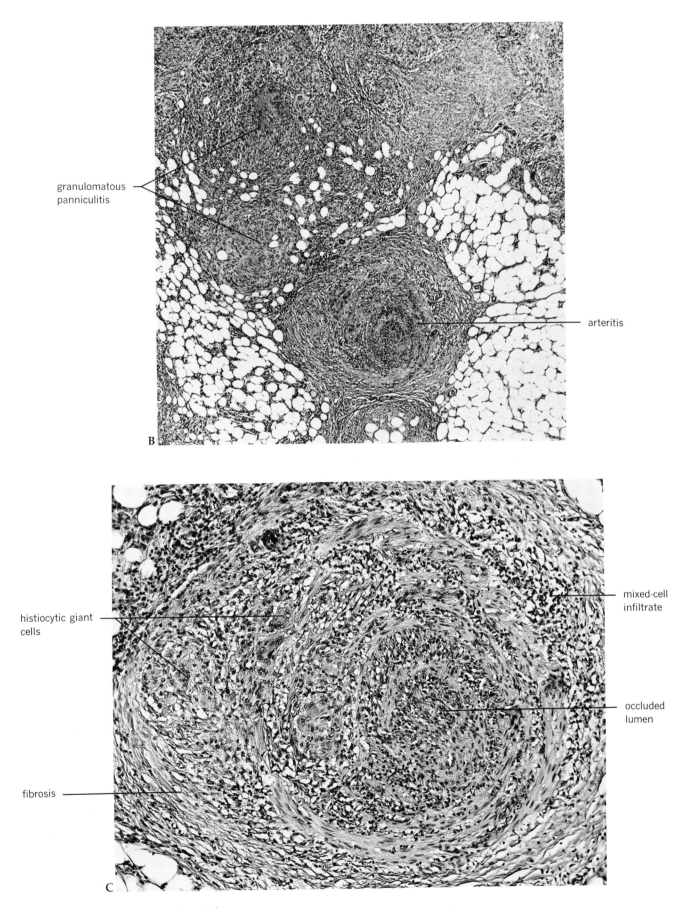

granulomatous
panniculitis

arteritis

histiocytic giant
cells

mixed-cell
infiltrate

occluded
lumen

fibrosis

FIG. 8-23. Nodular vasculitis. B and C.

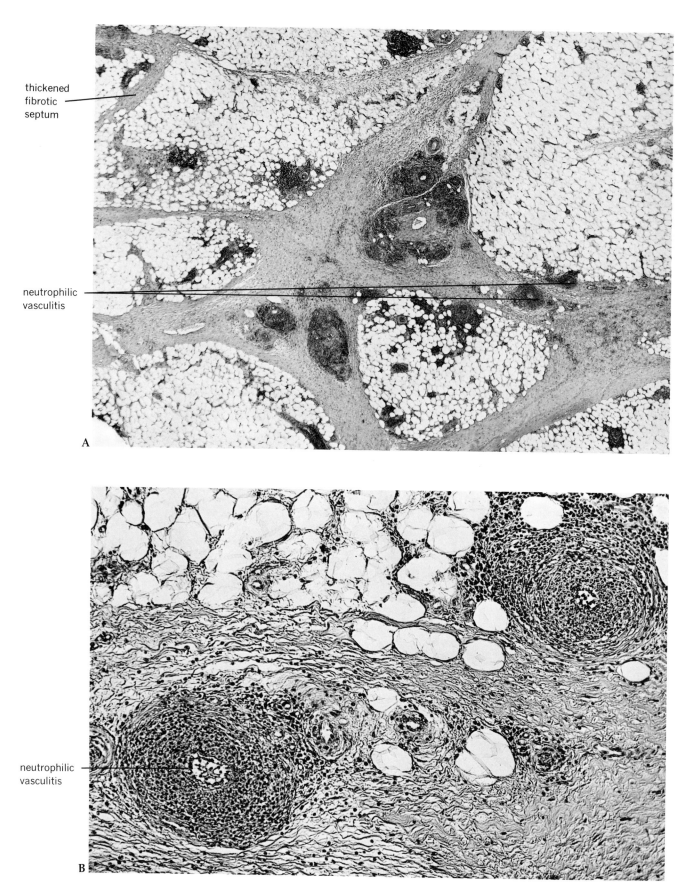

thickened
fibrotic
septum

neutrophilic
vasculitis

neutrophilic
vasculitis

A

B

FIG. 8-24. Vasculitis of scleroderma. In earliest stages, neutrophilic vasculitis occurs in medium-sized blood vessels that are housed within thickened fibrous septa of subcutaneous fat. (A, × 25; B, × 174; C, × 630.)

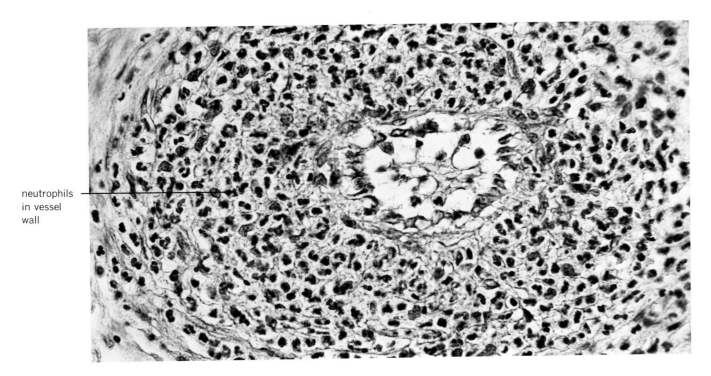

neutrophils
in vessel
wall

FIG. 8-24. C.

Lymphocytic Vasculitis

Lymphocytic vasculitis, unlike neutrophilic vasculitis, is exceptionally rare, and it is mentioned here briefly for completeness.

Small Vessel Involvement, Capillary-Venule

In a small percentage of biopsy specimens from lesions of *pityriasis lichenoides et varioliformis acuta* and *lymphomatoid papulosis*, fibrin is present within venular walls at different levels of the dermis. Lymphocytes may also be found within these blood-vessel walls, as well as surrounding them. Thus, a true lymphocytic vasculitis can *rarely* accompany both pityriasis lichenoides et varioliformis acuta and lymphomatoid papulosis. It must be reemphasized, however, that vasculitic changes are exceptional.

Clinically, lesions of pityriasis lichenoides et varioliformis acuta and some lesions of lymphomatoid papulosis have morphologic features in common—namely, hemorrhagic macules, papules, and vesicles—as well as necrotic lesions, ulcers, and scars. Pityriasis lichenoides et varioliformis acuta and lymphomatoid papulosis are more fully discussed in Chapter 7.

Occasionally, a lymphocytic vasculitis occurs in arthropod reactions caused by insect bites and scabies (Fig. 8-25). Numerous eosinophils are usually present in the inflammatory-cell infiltrate. Thrombi often occlude the lumina of the superficial capillaries and venules (Fig. 8-26).

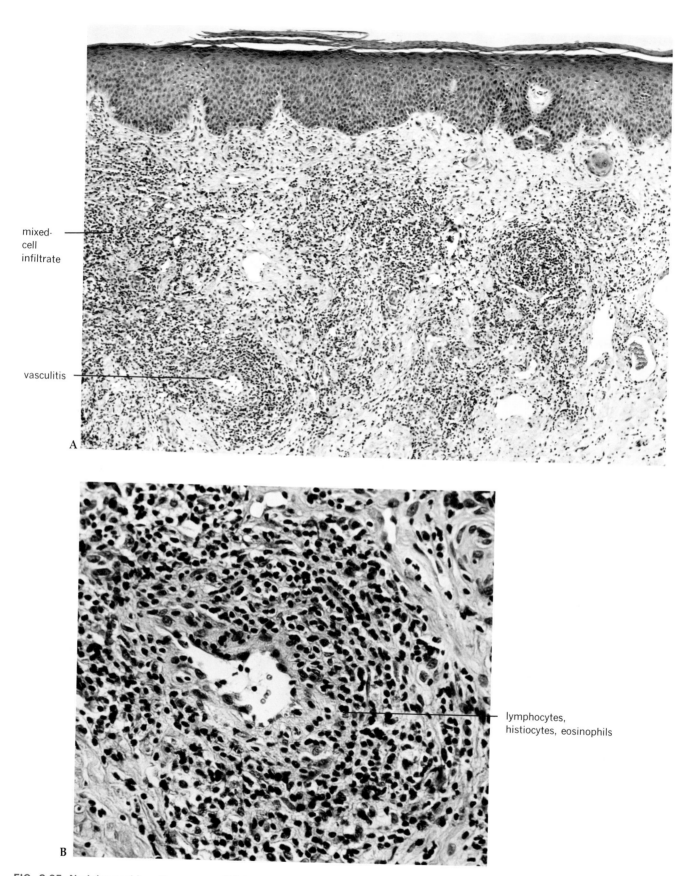

mixed-
cell
infiltrate

vasculitis

A

lymphocytes,
histiocytes, eosinophils

B

FIG. 8-25. Nodular scabies. Dense superficial and deep perivascular and interstitial infiltrate of lymphocytes, histiocytes, and eosinophils is characteristic of nodular lesions of scabies. Inflammatory cells, as shown, are often present in walls of medium-sized blood vessels in deep portion of dermis and sometimes in subcutaneous fat. (A, × 104; B, × 180.)

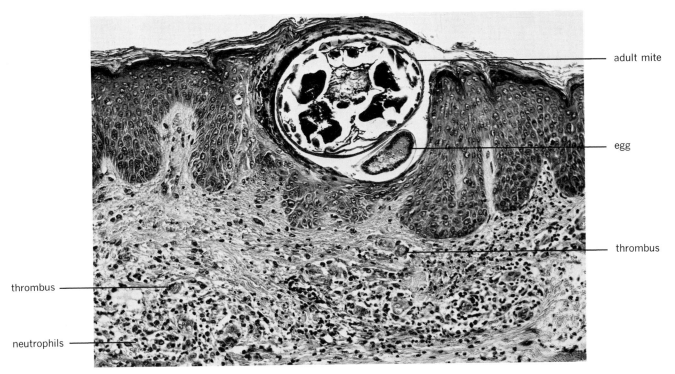

FIG. 8-26. Scabietic vasculitis. The lumen of each capillary and venule shown is plugged by a thrombus, and neutrophils are seen within and around blood vessel walls. (× 214.)

Histiocytic Vasculitis (Granulomatous Vasculitis)

No vasculitis begins with histiocytes in the walls of blood vessels. Granulomatous vasculitis represents a relatively advanced stage of the disease process. When more is learned about the early phases of necrobiosis lipoidica, allergic granulomatosis, Wegener's granulomatosis, lethal midline granuloma, and giant-cell arteritis, they can be reclassified accordingly.

Small Vessel Involvement, Capillary-Venule

At one stage in the evolution of *necrobiosis lipoidica*, histiocytes, some of them multinucleated, are present within the walls of capillaries and venules throughout the dermis. Epithelioid tubercles may obscure the tiny blood vessels in the papillary dermis and the larger vessels in the deep reticular dermis. Necrobiosis lipoidica is discussed in greater depth in Chapter 9.

Large Vessel Involvement, Arterial

Allergic granulomatosis (Churg-Strauss syndrome) has many features in common with polyarteritis nodosa. The gross anatomic findings in both diseases are indistinguishable, i.e., nodular swellings along the course of medium-sized arteries. In both diseases, the heart, kidneys, gastrointestinal tract, liver, spleen, gallbladder, and pancreas can be affected. Both diseases can be associated with cardiac failure, renal damage, hypertension, abdominal pain, and peripheral neuropathy. Purpura and subcutaneous nodules are among the common cutaneous manifestations of polyarteritis nodosa and allergic granulomatosis.

Additionally, the microscopic changes in the involved arteries of allergic granulomatosis are similar to those of polyarteritis nodosa, not only in distribution, but also in character. Both diseases display segmental fibrin deposits in arterial walls. The destruction of blood vessels may proceed to aneurysmal dilatation and rupture or to thrombosis, with resulting infarction and scarring.

Histologically, polyarteritis nodosa is a leukocytoclastic vasculitis that involves medium-sized arteries. In allergic granulomatosis, neutrophils and fibrin are generally found in the arteries. There is also a dense infiltrate of eosinophils and eosinophil nuclear dust, as well as a granulomatous infiltrate of epithelioid cells and multinucleated histiocytic cells. In addition to the granulomatous arteritis of allergic granulomatosis, there are often extravascular granulomatous foci in the connective-tissue stroma of many organs, including the skin. These extravascular collections of histiocytes are arranged in a palisade around a central focus of fibrin, collagen degeneration, necrotic neutrophils and eosinophils, histiocytes, and fibroblasts. These palisaded granulomas with central deposits of fibrin have also been described in the subcutaneous nodules of allergic granulomatosis.

Allergic granulomatosis is differentiated clinically from polyarteritis nodosa by the triad of asthma, fever, and high eosinophilia. Also, unlike polyarteritis nodosa, allergic granulomatosis is often marked by recurrent episodes of pneumonia that have the typical clinical, pathologic, and roentgenologic findings of Löffler's pulmonary infiltration. Women are affected with allergic granulomatosis more commonly than are men. Allergic granulomatosis differs from polyarteritis nodosa chiefly by its (1) pulmonary involvement, (2) granulomatous vasculitis, and (3) extravascular palisaded granulomas.

It is possible that allergic granulomatosis actually represents a variant of polyarteritis nodosa in which the patients also have asthma and eosinophilia. Furthermore, in long-standing leukocytoclastic vasculitis, a granulomatous inflammatory infiltrate may supervene. The absence of typical histologic changes of leukocytoclastic vasculitis in allergic granulomatosis could result from a sampling error, a biopsy of the lesions having been done at a later histiocytic, rather than an earlier neutrophilic, stage. Lastly, the fibrin within the seemingly extravascular palisaded granulomas may be the residue of a blood vessel destroyed beyond recognition by the vasculitic process. Such a theory links allergic granulomatosis and polyarteritis nodosa as aspects in a spectrum of leukocytoclastic vasculitis involving medium-sized arteries. Support for this thesis comes from careful clinical follow-up of patients with this constellation of disease signs. Blending of clinical manifestations tends to erase the significance of a separation of allergic granulomatosis from polyarteritis nodosa. Allergic granulomatosis is now an extremely rare disease.

The underlying pathologic process in *Wegener's granulomatosis* is severe leukocytoclastic arteritis, often with thrombosis, that results in massive tissue necrosis and ulceration. In time, granulomatous inflammation with histiocytes, lymphocytes, and plasma cells dominates the histologic scene. In some instances there is granulomatous vasculitis. The underlying vascular changes in Wegener's granulomatosis may be difficult to detect because of extensive necrosis.

The pathologic changes of Wegener's granulomatosis have a predilection for the upper and lower respiratory tracts and for the kidneys. A destructive sinusitis often is the presenting lesion of Wegener's granulomatosis, but the disease can also involve regions in the upper respiratory tract such as the nasal and oral cavities, larynx, and trachea. The lungs are affected in several ways, from necrosis of the pulmonary parenchyma to hemorrhagic infarcts secondary to thrombosis of pulmonary arteries. Renal disease in Wegener's granulomatosis is usually a focal or diffuse glomerulonephritis, and the resultant alterations lead to renal failure and rapidly fatal uremia. Other signs of Wegener's granulomatosis are fever, otitis, arthritis, and neurologic disturbances.

Skin lesions occur in about 50% of patients with Wegener's granulomatosis. These lesions are papulonecrotic, vesicular, ulcerative, and nodular. They tend to be symmetrical and to be situated on the elbows, knees, and buttocks especially. The histologic signs of leukocytoclastic vasculitis may also be noted in all blood vessels in the skin.

In several ways the generalized form of Wegener's granulomatosis resembles polyarteritis nodosa. In both conditions the renal changes are those of necrotizing glomerulitis. Histologically, Wegener's granulomatosis and polyarteritis nodosa are often indistinguishable, but Wegener's is more commonly granulomatous. The widespread arteritis of Wegener's granulomatosis exhibits the same histologic changes as does classic polyarteritis nodosa, i.e., leukocytoclastic vasculitis, thrombosis, and fibrosis.

The coronary arteritis of Wegener's granulomatosis is similar to that of polyarteritis nodosa. Wegener himself thought that the disease he described was a variant of polyarteritis nodosa.

Wegener's granulomatosis differs, however, from polyarteritis nodosa in at least two respects. Polyarteritis nodosa, as a rule, has no lung involvement, whereas Wegener's granulomatosis does. Hypertension is common in polyarteritis nodosa, but not in Wegener's granulomatosis.

Wegener's granulomatosis, in some ways, bears a striking similarity to allergic granulomatosis. Both diseases are characterized pathologically by leukocytoclastic vasculitis (neutrophil nuclear dust in Wegener's granulomatosis, eosinophil nuclear dust in allergic granulomatosis) with an associated granulomatous infiltrate. Unlike allergic granulomatosis, however, Wegener's granulomatosis is not associated with asthma, eosinophilia, or hypertension. The presenting signs and symptoms of Wegener's granulomatosis are often those of sinusitis or destructive inflammatory lesions of the nasopharynx or lungs, whereas the usual presenting complaint of the patient with allergic granulomatosis is asthma.

A limited type of Wegener's granulomatosis involves the lower, but not the upper, respiratory tract, and can be associated with skin, but not kidney, lesions. The lesion referred to as *lethal midline granuloma* represents either a form of Wegener's granulomatosis of the upper respiratory tract or a manifestation of malignant lymphoma. Death from this localized form of Wegener's granulomatosis usually results from extensive local tissue destruction, hemorrhage, or cachexia. Patients with lethal midline granuloma who survive sometimes later develop the widespread arteritis and renal disease typical of generalized Wegener's granulomatosis. Patients with lethal midline granuloma may have necrosis and ulceration in the nasal and perioral skin.

Giant-cell arteritis has been known by many different names, such as temporal arteritis, cranial arteritis, giant-cell polyarteritis, and polymyalgia rheumatica. Giant-cell arteritis is probably the preferable designation, although giant cells cannot always be demonstrated on biopsy. The disease may be widespread and involves large and medium-sized arteries of middle-aged and elderly persons.

The earliest histologic changes of giant-cell arteritis, a neutrophilic infiltrate within the vessel walls, are seen rarely because most biopsy specimens are taken from relatively advanced arterial lesions. Such advanced lesions display severely narrowed or obliterated vascular lumina, intimal proliferation, fragmentation of the internal elastic membrane, a lymphohistiocytic infiltrate with varying numbers of histiocytic giant cells within the thickened media, and scattered lymphocytes within the adventitia. No fibrin is deposited within the vessel wall.

Although many arteries, such as the renal and coronary, may be affected by giant-cell arteritis, the process most often involves the major arteries of the aortic arch and the cranial arteries, especially the temporal arteries. A characteristic physical sign of giant-cell arteritis involving the temporal artery is a hard pulseless cord along which nodules and tender areas are easily palpated. The most dramatic symptoms of temporal arteritis are headache, scalp pain, and visual disturbances, including blindness. Skin changes are uncommon in giant-cell arteritis, but erythema, edema, blisters, ulceration, and even gangrene occur as the cutaneous consequences of ischemia secondary to progressive arterial destruction.

Miscellaneous Vasculitides

Malignant atrophic papulosis, livedo vasculitis, lymphomatoid granulomatosis and hyperparathyroidism with cutaneous vascular calcification and gangrene are included in the miscellaneous category. At the present time either not enough is known about their earliest histologic changes or they do not fit neatly into the other categories in this classification of vasculitis.

Small Vessel Involvement

Malignant atrophic papulosis (Degos' disease) is a systemic vascular disease in which small and medium-sized arteries undergo progressive intimal fibrosis, causing focal infarction, especially of the skin and the gastrointestinal tract. The first manifestations of malignant atrophic papulosis usually involve the arterioles in the middle and lower portions of the dermis. Within the walls of these small arteries is an infiltrate of neutrophils, lymphocytes, and histiocytes. These cells are also present around the vessels and among the collagen bundles. Clinical concomitants of these histologic changes are pink papules distributed primarily on the trunk and extremities. Thrombosis and subendothelial sclerosis combine to occlude the lumina of these vessels, leading to infarction. The epidermis and often the adnexal epithelium become necrotic, and the collagen above the occluded arterioles undergoes degeneration. Clinically, the papular skin lesions show central necrosis, ulceration, and umbilication, but slightly elevated pink borders.

The end stage of this infarctive process is seen microscopically as wedge-shaped dermal sclerosis with severe epidermal thinning, complete loss of the rete pattern, and slight orthokeratosis and parakeratosis. Adnexal epithelium is absent in the triangular zone of sclerosis. Abundant amounts of acid mucopolysaccharide may be present in the areas of sclerosis. The clinical expression of these late histologic changes is an umbilicated lesion with a central smooth, atrophic, porcelain-white scar, sometimes covered by a fine whitish scale and surrounded by a slightly elevated pink telangiectatic rim.

Similar pathologic changes of obliterating arteriolitis and subsequent sclerosis occur in small and medium-sized arteries throughout the gastrointestinal tract. The serosal surface may also be studded with porcelain-white scars. Malignant atrophic papulosis is usually a fatal disease of young men. Death is secondary to intestinal perforation and peritonitis or to cerebral infarction. Evidences of gastrointestinal involvement, such as pain, weight loss, diarrhea, and intestinal obstruction generally follow the onset of cutaneous lesions. Other organs such as the heart, brain, eyes, and kidneys may be affected. The course of malignant atrophic papulosis may be fulminant, lasting only a few weeks, or indolent, persisting for several years.

The lesions of *livedo vasculitis-atrophie blanche* occur almost exclusively in women on the lower extremities near the ankle. In this region, the superficial dermal blood vessels are normally altered by the stasis caused by upright posture. They are seemingly increased in number (perhaps simply tortuous) and have thick walls with plump endothelial cells.

Among the earliest histologic findings in livedo vasculitis is a vasculitis (probably leukocytoclastic) involving capillaries and venules throughout the dermis, especially in the upper half (Fig. 8-27). Within the walls of these vessels there is fibrin and within the lumina there are fibrin thrombi. A sparse infiltrate of neutrophils and nuclear dust is present within the deposits of fibrin. A more dense infiltrate of lymphocytes and histiocytes surrounds the vessels. The edematous papillary dermis contains many extravasated erythrocytes. Intracellular and intercellular edema may eventuate in intraepidermal vesiculation. Frequently, the epidermis is necrotic.

Thrombi eventually occlude some of the compromised superficial capillaries and venules (Fig. 8-28), resulting in infarction and ulceration. In time, the inflammatory-cell infiltrate diminishes, but siderophages persist as evidence of prior hemorrhage. At its end stage, livedo vasculitis is known as atrophie blanche, having come to dermal sclerosis, telangiectases, and a thin epidermis devoid of

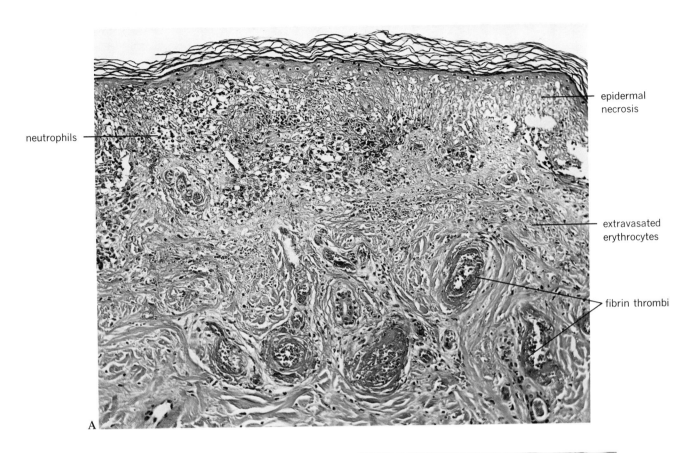

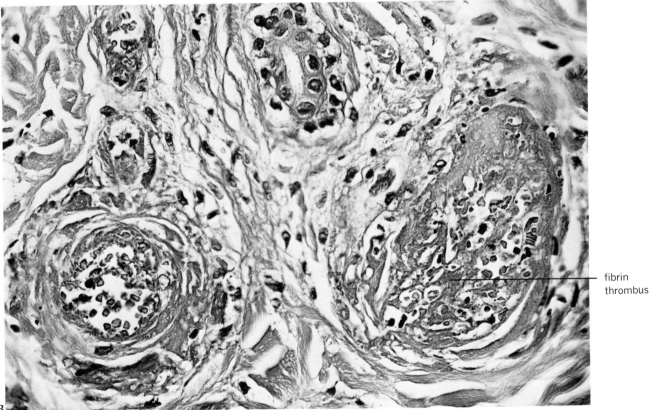

FIG. 8-27. Livedo vasculitis, early lesion. Numerous thrombi in superficial blood vessels result in extravasation of erythrocytes and necrosis of epidermis. A scant inflammatory-cell infiltrate of mostly neutrophils is present in this early lesion. Concurrent with lesions of this type, livedo reticularis may be seen on the legs. (A, × 170; B, × 580.)

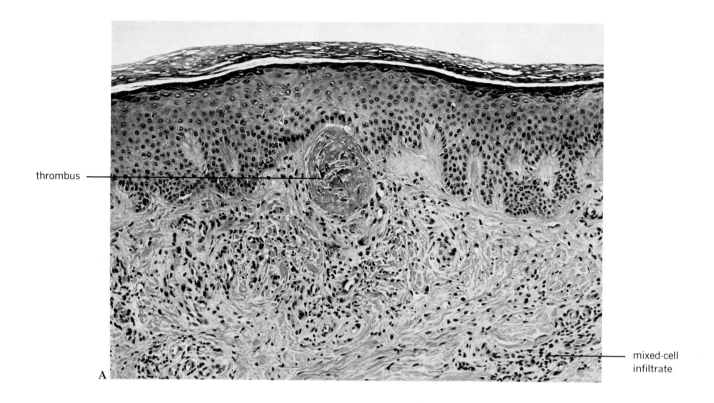

thrombus

mixed-cell
infiltrate

A

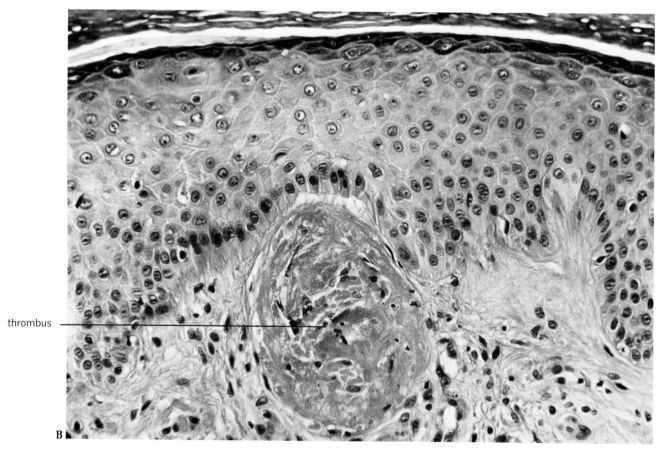

thrombus

B

FIG. 8-28. Livedo vasculitis, later lesion. Vasculitic changes of early lesions proceed inevitably to thromboses which contribute to the fibrosis responsible for characteristic clinical white scars of atrophie blanche. (A, × 173; B, × 372.)

rete-ridges and of melanin. Similar thrombotic and eventually sclerotic changes occur in skin injured by radiotherapy (Fig. 8-29).

The clinical counterparts of these histologic changes in livedo vasculitis are inflammatory purpuric papules that may evolve into hemorrhagic vesicles. Commonly, the lesions ulcerate, the ulcers being notoriously painful. Eventually, the ulcers are replaced by smooth, ivory-white, depressed, atrophic scars (atrophie blanche).

The pathologic changes of livedo vasculitis-atrophie blanche, both grossly and microscopically, are closely related to, if not identical with, those of livedo reticularis with summer ulcerations. A pathologic picture resembling atrophie blanche has on occasion been found in systemic lupus erythematosus.

Lymphomatoid granulomatosis is a disease of middle-aged men primarily affecting the lungs, but may also involve the kidneys, central nervous system, and (in approximately 50% of all patients) the skin. Two different processes are seen in histologic sections from skin lesions of lymphomatoid granulomatosis. One is a dense, diffuse, cellular infiltrate of lymphocytes, histiocytes, plasma cells, eosinophils, and numerous atypical mononuclear cells. Some of the mononuclear cells may be in mitosis, and some of the mitotic figures may be atypical. This dense infiltrate fills the dermis and may extend into the subcutaneous fat. The second process is a vasculitis of dermal arterioles in which the blood-vessel walls are infiltrated with the same cells as is the dermis.

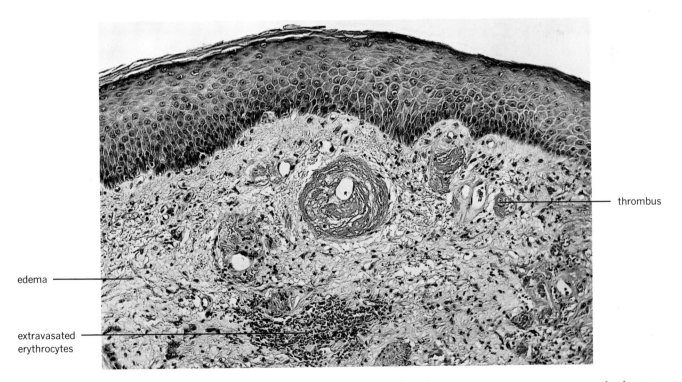

FIG. 8-29. Radiation injury, acute. Thrombi and associated extravasation of erythrocytes and edema are among early changes. Severe cases terminate in ulceration, consequent loss of substance, and sclerosis (radiation atrophy). (× 171.)

Clinically, the skin lesions of lymphomatoid granulomatosis are reddish-purple papules, plaques, nodules, and ulcerated nodules, occurring primarily on the legs. About 15% of patients with lymphomatoid granulomatosis die of an atypical malignant lymphoma. The exact nosologic niche appropriate for lymphomatoid granulomatosis (e.g., vasculitis or malignant lymphoma or both) is at present unsettled.

Hyperparathyroidism with cutaneous vascular calcification and gangrene is a rare event that usually occurs in association with a parathyroid adenoma. The cutaneous gangrene probably results from infarction secondary to calcium deposits in blood vessels throughout the dermis and the subcutaneous fat. A mixed inflammatory-cell infiltrate containing many neutrophils is present within blood vessel walls and throughout the dermis. There are also collagen degeneration and necrosis of adnexal epithelia and epidermis with resultant ulceration. Concomitant with the destructive skin lesions there are metastatic (ectopic) calcification in other organs, elevated levels of serum calcium, osteitis fibrosa, psychosis, and gastroduodenal ulcers. When cutaneous gangrene supervenes, the disease is usually fatal.

Thromboses without Vasculitis

Although thrombi commonly occur in association with vasculitis, they can also develop in the absence of vasculitis as I have defined it. Thus, strictly speaking, disseminated intravascular coagulation, Waldenström's macroglobulinemia, paroxysmal nocturnal hemoglobinuria, coumarin-induced necrosis, atheroemboli, and phlebothromboses are not vasculitides, but they are more suitably placed here than in any other chapter.

Small Vessel Involvement

Disseminated intravascular coagulation does not refer to a specific disease, but to an acquired hemorrhagic syndrome secondary to pathophysiologic events precipitated by a variety of causes (Fig. 8-30). In disseminated intravascular coagulation there is a deficiency of fibrinogen, platelets, and certain clotting factors. Fibrinolysins are increased. These abnormalities derive from an activation of the coagulation process that results in the consumption of fibrin, platelets, and certain clotting factors. Purpura fulminans, thrombotic thrombocytopenic purpura, and the hemolytic-uremic syndrome are consumption coagulopathies.

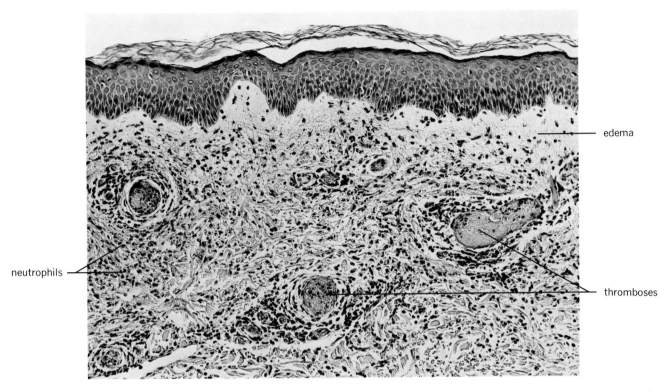

FIG. 8-30. Consumptive coagulopathy. A, Thrombi occlude almost every capillary and venule in upper part of dermis in this early lesion of patient with purpura fulminans. Shortly, there will be epidermal necrosis and subepidermal vesiculation. Note the scant, predominantly neutrophilic infiltrate. ($\times$ 184.)

The histologic features of disseminated intravascular coagulation in skin are the presence of thrombi within capillaries and venules throughout the dermis, extravasation of erythrocytes around these vessels, and subepidermal vesiculation and epidermal necrosis. Adnexal epithelia may also become necrotic. The sparseness of inflammatory cells, most of them neutrophils, is characteristic of disseminated intravascular coagulation. Histologic differential diagnosis of disseminated intravascular coagulation includes *Waldenström's macroglobulinemia, paroxysmal nocturnal hemoglobinuria, and coumarin-induced necrosis.* Thrombi in small blood vessels with little inflammatory-cell infiltrate are common to these conditions.

The corresponding clinical features of cutaneous disseminated intravascular coagulation are erythema followed rapidly by purpura and gray-roofed necrotic hemorrhagic bullae. Ulceration and eschar formation are late manifestations of this infarctive process. The lesions of purpura fulminans may be localized, but more often are widespread. The same pathologic changes of disseminated intravascular coagulation that are found in skin also occur in internal organs, most frequently in the kidneys, lungs, testes, and adrenals, and in the central nervous system.

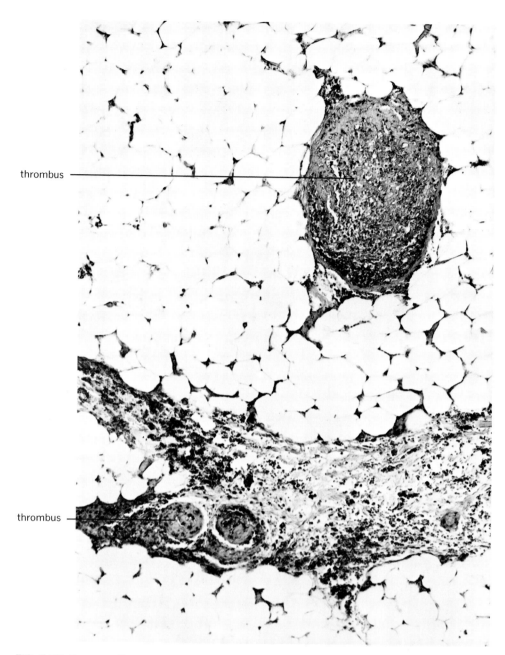

thrombus

thrombus

FIG. 8-30. Consumptive coagulopathy. B, Thromboses may form in blood vessels in subcutaneous fat as shown here. (× 104.)

The most common causes of disseminated intravascular coagulation are acute bacterial septicemias, especially by Escherichia coli, meningococci (Waterhouse-Friderichsen syndrome), and pseudomonas; viral infections, especially varicella; rickettsial infections, especially Rocky Mountain spotted fever; malaria; amniotic fluid emboli; some carcinomas; and metabolic acidosis.

Atheroemboli, emboli composed of atheromatous deposits containing cholesterol clefts, may be found in the cutaneous blood vessels of patients with severe ulcerating atherosclerosis of the aorta.

Phlebothrombosis refers to a thrombus-containing vein in which a slight inflammatory-cell infiltrate is present only perivascularly and not within the blood vessel wall. Phlebothromboses occur in varicose veins and in hemorrhoids. Hemorrhoids are tortuous, dilated, submucosal anal veins that often undergo thrombosis and subsequent organization.

Nodular and Diffuse Dermatitis

Nodular Dermatitis

Neutrophils predominate
  Acute febrile neutrophilic dermatosis
  Abscesses
Histiocytes predominate (granulomatous, tuberculoid)
  Primary cutaneous tuberculosis
  Lupus vulgaris
  Scrofuloderma
  Miliary tuberculosis
  Leishmaniasis, chronic cutaneous type
  Leprosy, tuberculoid and dimorphous types
  Syphilis, late secondary and tertiary stages
  Rosacea and perioral dermatitis, granulomatous types
Histiocytes predominate (granulomatous, sarcoidal)
  Sarcoidosis
  Silica, beryllium, and zirconium granulomas
  Lichen nitidus
  Lichen striatus
Histiocytes predominate (granulomatous, palisaded)
  Granuloma annulare
  Necrobiosis lipoidica
  Granulomatosis disciformis of face
  Rheumatoid nodule, pseudorheumatoid nodule, and rheumatic nodule
  Gout
  Juxta-articular nodes of syphilis
Histiocytes predominate (granulomatous, foreign-body reaction)
  Ruptured follicular cysts
  Metals
  Vegetable materials
  Abnormal endogenous deposits
Mixed-cell infiltrate containing atypical mononuclear cells
  Pseudolymphomas

Diffuse Dermatitis

Neutrophils predominate
  Granuloma faciale
  Erythema elevatum diutinum
  Rheumatoid neutrophilic dermatitis
  Pyoderma gangrenosum
Neutrophils and histiocytes predominate (suppurative granulomatous dermatitis)
  Deep fungal infections
  Atypical mycobacterial infections
  Halogenodermas
  Follicular-occlusion tetrad
Histiocytes with foamy or granular cytoplasm predominate
  Xanthomas
  Xanthoma disseminatum
  Xanthogranulomas, juvenile and adult
  Reticulohistiocytic granuloma
  Histiocytoma
  Mineral oil granulomas
  Lepromatous leprosy
  Leishmaniasis, acute cutaneous and disseminated anergic cutaneous types
Histiocytic giant cells predominate
  Granulomatous slack skin
  Xanthogranulomas
  Reticulohistiocytic granuloma
Plasma cells predominate
  Syphilitic chancre
  Chancroid
  Granuloma inguinale
  Lymphogranuloma venereum
  Rhinoscleroma
  Leishmaniasis
  Plasmacytoma
  Secondary syphilis
Mast cells predominate
  Urticaria pigmentosa, nodular type
Mixed-cell infiltrate containing atypical mononuclear cells
  Histiocytosis X
  Pseudolymphomas

Nodular *and* Diffuse Dermatitis

9

THE TERMS *nodular dermatitis* and *diffuse dermatitis* in the subsequent context are used to describe histologic, rather than clinical, patterns. Nodular dermatitis denotes discrete perivascular inflammatory-cell infiltrates within the dermis that are so large that they form nodules (Fig. 9-1). Nodular dermatitis usually exhibits multiple nodules of inflammatory cells, but occasionally the specimen may show only a large solitary nodule (Fig. 9-2). Diffuse dermatitis refers to a cellular infiltrate so dense that discrete cellular aggregates can no longer be recognized, and consequently the dermal collagen is almost completely obscured by the massiveness of the inflammatory-cell infiltrate (Fig. 9-3). Diffuse dermatitis may consist of an inflammatory-cell infiltrate that is uniformly dense throughout the entire thickness of the dermis or dense in the entire upper dermis and sparse or absent in the lower (Fig. 9-4).

Nodular and diffuse dermatitis can be subclassified according to the inflammatory-cell composition, i.e., predominantly neutrophils, lymphocytes, plasma cells, histiocytes, mast cells, or mixed cells. The preponderant cell in many nodular and diffuse derma-

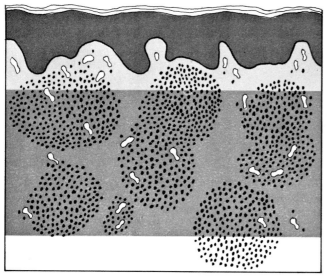

FIG. 9-1. Nodular dermatitis.

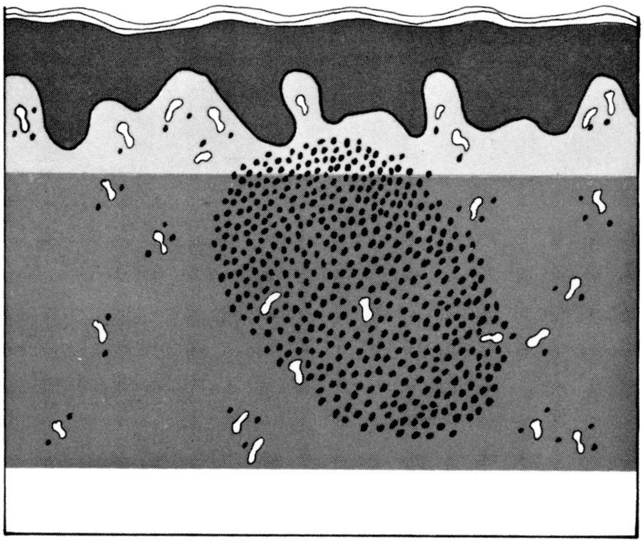

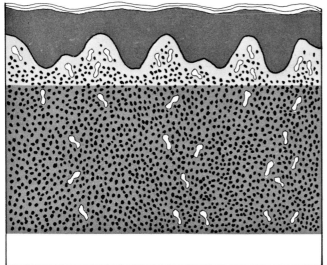

FIG. 9-2. Large solitary nodule.

FIG. 9-3. Diffuse dermatitis.

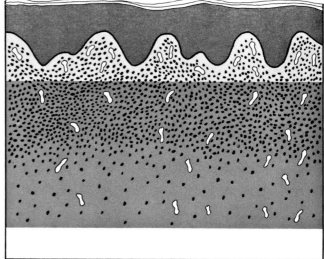

FIG. 9-4. Diffuse dermatitis in upper half of dermis.

titides is the histiocyte, and such infiltrates are termed *granulomatous*. Granulomatous infiltrates may be nodular or diffuse, but not all nodular and diffuse dermatitides are granulomatous.

Epithelioid cells are histiocytes with elongated or oval vesicular nuclei surrounded by abundant, finely granular, eosinophilic cytoplasm with poorly defined cell borders. These cells are termed *epithelioid* because, like epithelial cells, they appear to touch one another. Foam cells are histiocytes whose lipid content imparts a vacuolated appearance to their cytoplasm.

Multinucleated histiocytes (histiocytic giant cells) may or may not be present in granulomatous dermatitides. The nuclei in a Langhans' giant cell tend to form a circle or a semicircle at the periphery of the cell, whereas the nuclei in a foreign-body giant cell tend to scatter throughout the cytoplasm. A Touton giant cell is characterized by a central homogeneous, amphophilic core of cytoplasm surrounded by a wreath of nuclei, which, in turn, is surrounded by abundant foamy cytoplasm. These three types of giant cells are histiocytic variants, and each can occur in a variety of granulomatous reactions. Each of the three types can be seen in foreign-body reactions, and foreign-body giant cells can be seen in reactions that are devoid of discernible foreign objects, such as idiopathic sarcoidosis.

Certain general principles apply to the examination of all granulomatous reactions in skin. A specimen with a granulomatous infiltrate should be (1) studied with polarized light in an attempt to discover birefringent foreign material (e.g., silica is birefringent, zirconium is not), (2) stained with PAS or silver methenamine in search of fungi, and (3) stained with special techniques (e.g., Ziehl-Neelsen, Fite, auramine) to expose the organisms of tuberculosis, atypical mycobacterial diseases, and leprosy. If syphilis is suspected, a Warthin-Starry silver stain for spirochetes should be performed; and if leishmaniasis, a Giemsa stain should be done for nonflagellate protozoons (Leishman-Donovan bodies). If an infectious cause is thought possible, cultures should be obtained. If foreign bodies are under consideration, chemical analyses of biopsy specimens should be undertaken. In rare instances, should an ultramicroscopic particle be responsible, electron microscopy may provide an answer to the riddle of causation. Sometimes acid-fast bacilli can be discerned by electron microscopy in lesions of tuberculoid leprosy in which no organisms have been discovered with special stains and light microscopy.

Nodular Dermatitis

The nodular histologic pattern in which neutrophils predominate will be seen in biopsies from acute febrile neutrophilic dermatosis and abscesses. Histiocytes are the predominant cell in biopsies from a number of granulomatous dermatitides that may be divided into tuberculoid, sarcoidal, palisaded, and foreign body types. Biopsies from pseudolymphomas will have a mixed-cell infiltrate containing atypical mononuclear cells.

The decision about whether a pattern is either a dense, superficial and deep perivascular dermatitis or a nodular dermatitis is a subjective one. Most superficial and deep perivascular dermatitides are not associated with dense cellular infiltrates.

Neutrophils Predominate

Acute Febrile Neutrophilic Dermatosis (Sweet's Syndrome) (Fig. 9-5)

—Nodular infiltrate composed primarily of neutrophils, but also of some lymphocytes, histiocytes, and eosinophils, throughout the dermis
—Variable amount of nuclear dust
—Papillary dermis edematous
—Focal collagen degeneration
—Varying numbers of extravasated erythrocytes, especially in the papillary dermis

Biopsies from early lesions of acute febrile neutrophilic dermatosis show an infiltrate of neutrophils and nuclear dust around the blood vessels throughout the dermis, but especially the upper half. In time, the density of the infiltrate may increase with neutrophils both in perivascular nodules and among collagen bundles. The collagen in some foci undergoes degeneration and appears basophilic. There is usually edema of the papillary dermis in early lesions, as well as varying numbers of extravasated erythrocytes and prominently dilated capillaries and venules. Later, a few eosinophils may be seen within the infiltrate, and eventually lymphocytes and histiocytes may be preponderant. The epidermis is not usually involved, and rarely will microscopic intraepidermal abscesses form.

Histologically, acute febrile neutrophilic dermatosis resembles erythema elevatum diutinum and early granuloma faciale, but lacks specific signs of vasculitis. At first glance, acute febrile neutrophilic dermatosis resembles a leukocytoclastic vasculitis, but fibrin is not present within the blood-vessel walls, purpura is not a significant component of the lesions, and vesicles do not usually occur.

Clinically, as the title suggests, acute febrile neutrophilic dermatosis is a febrile disease of sudden onset with a course of weeks or months. A neutrophilic leukocytosis of approximately 12,000 to 20,000 cells/mm^3 is usually present. Some patients also have concurrent arthritis and conjunctivitis. Most patients are middle-aged women. The skin lesions are red, painful, and tender, sharply delimited urticarial plaques with slightly raised borders asymmetrically distributed on the face, neck, and extremities, particularly around the elbows and knees. Individual lesions persist for many days and heal without scarring. The limb lesions must be distinguished clinically from those of erythema elevatum diutinum, and the facial lesions from those of granuloma faciale.

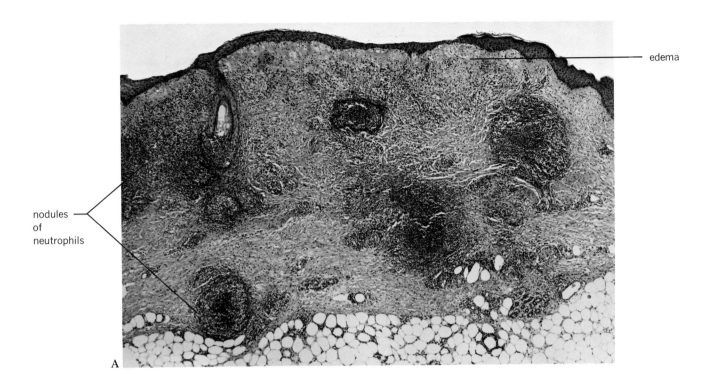

nodules
of
neutrophils

edema

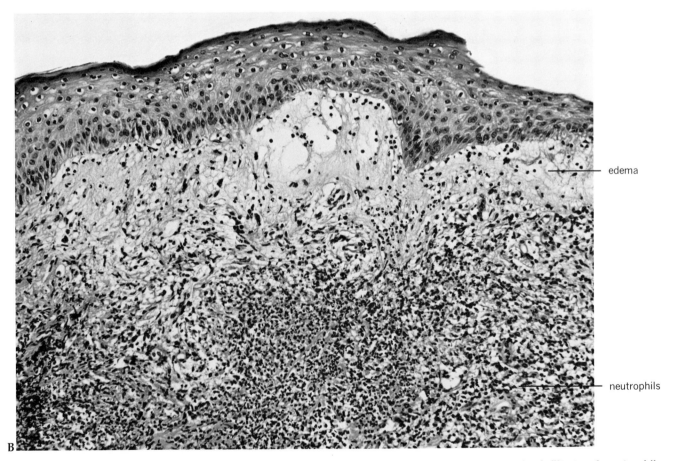

edema

neutrophils

FIG. 9-5. Acute febrile neutrophilic dermatosis (Sweet's syndrome). **A,** Dense nodular perivascular infiltrate of neutrophils throughout dermis is characteristic feature. (× 49.) **B,** Edema of papillary dermis in addition to infiltrate of neutrophils is another typical feature. (× 176.) Extensive edema in upper part of lesion is also seen in some lesions of polymorphous light eruptions, reactions to insect bites, erysipelas, and early lesions of lichen sclerosus et atrophicus.

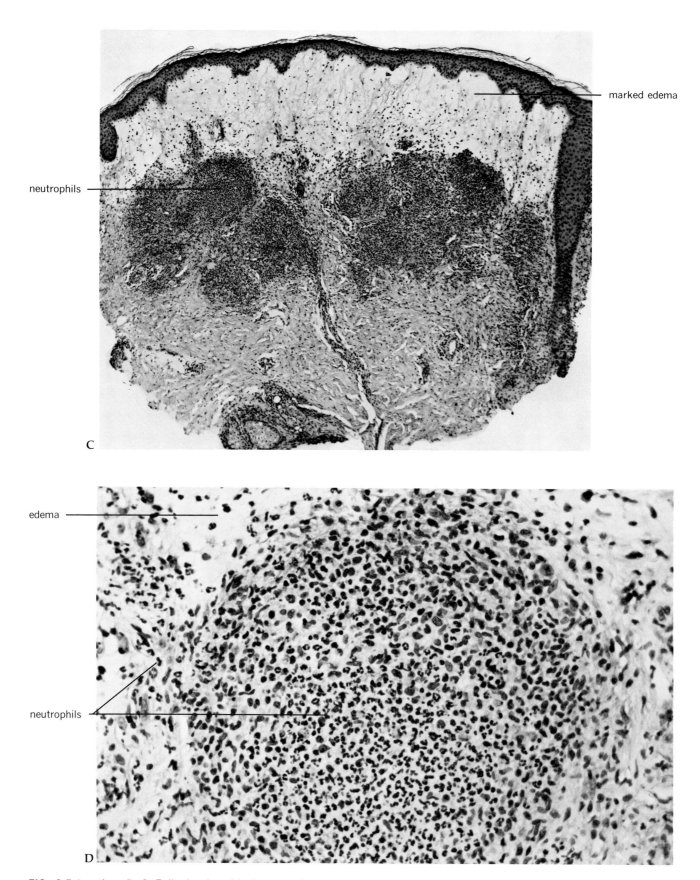

marked edema

neutrophils

edema

neutrophils

C

D

FIG. 9-5 (continued). C, Fully developed lesions may have such massive edema of papillary dermis that a subepidermal blister forms as shown here. (× 56.) D, In this higher magnification aggregations of inflammatory cells within dermis are seen to consist mostly of neutrophils. (× 353.)

Large dermal abscesses can result from a variety of infectious agents including bacteria (e.g., streptococci and staphylococci, erysipelothrix, mycobacteria, nocardia, actinomyces), fungi (e.g., sporotrichosis [Fig. 9-6], maduromycosis, dermatophytosis [Fig. 9-7]), algae (e.g., protothecosis), and protozoa (e.g., amoeba) and from foreign bodies such as cornified cells of ruptured follicular cysts (e.g., cystic acne). A search for organisms should always be made in dermal abscesses. Appropriate special stains include the Gram's stain for bacteria, PAS with prior digestion by malt diastase or amylase for sporotrichosis, PAS or silver methenamine for fungi in dermatophytic folliculitis (Majocchi's granuloma) and for yeasts in candidal abscesses, and phosphotungstic acid hematoxylin for amoeba. Acid-fast stains generally reveal tubercle bacilli in lesions of bacillus-laden tuberculoderms such as scrofuloderma. The organisms of actinomycosis and nocardiosis are easily seen in hematoxylin-eosin-stained sections as granular colonies from which mycelial filaments radiate, but Gram's stain is necessary to visualize the gram-positive bacilli Erysipelothrix rhusiopathiae, the causative organism in erysipeloid. Granules of mycetoma can also be detected in sections stained by hematoxylin and eosin. Large clumps of pseudomonas can simulate a grain of mycetoma (Fig. 9-8). In abscesses that occur in the "follicular occlusion tetrad" of acne conglobata, hidradenitis suppurativa, dissecting cellulitis of the scalp, and pilonidal sinus, the follicular epithelium is usually visible within or around the abscesses (Fig. 9-9A). In early inflammatory responses to ruptured follicular cysts, cornified cells (squames) can usually be seen within the abscesses or within multinucleated histiocytes (Fig. 9-9B, C). Another common cause of abscesses in skin is foreign bodies such as splinters (Fig. 9-10).

Eventually, the neutrophilic collections are joined at their periphery by mononuclear cells (lymphocytes, plasma cells, histiocytes), and by multinucleated histiocytes, and the suppurative dermatitis becomes a suppurative granulomatous one. The lesions generally resolve with fibrosis.

Clinically, abscesses are fluctuant nodules that often are associated with draining sinuses.

It cannot be emphasized too strongly that whenever one sees collections of neutrophils in the skin, whether in abscesses within the dermis or in pustules within the epidermis or hair follicle, one should search diligently for infectious organisms. This dictum applies equally to suppuration within the subcutaneous fat where special stains can uncover such dissimilar organisms as atypical mycobacteria and Sporotrichum.

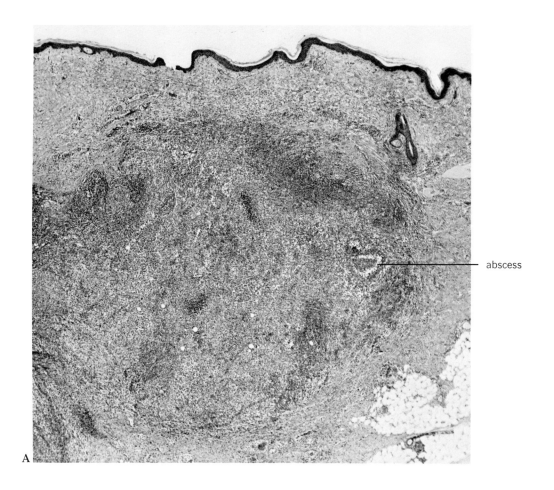

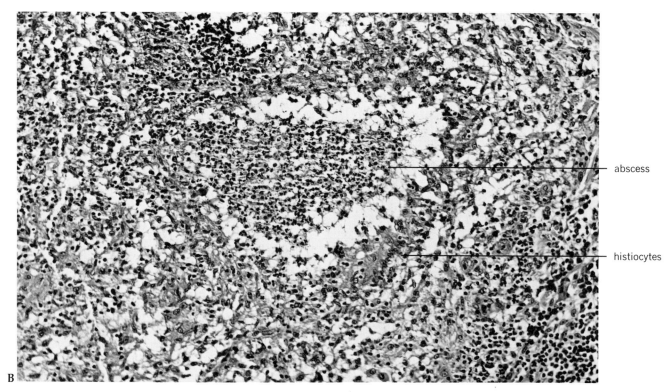

FIG. 9-6. Sporotrichosis. A, In early fluctuant lesions there is suppuration throughout dermis. Later, histiocytes and finally fibroblasts predominate in these lesions. (× 23.) B, Abscess surrounded by histiocytes. (× 205.)

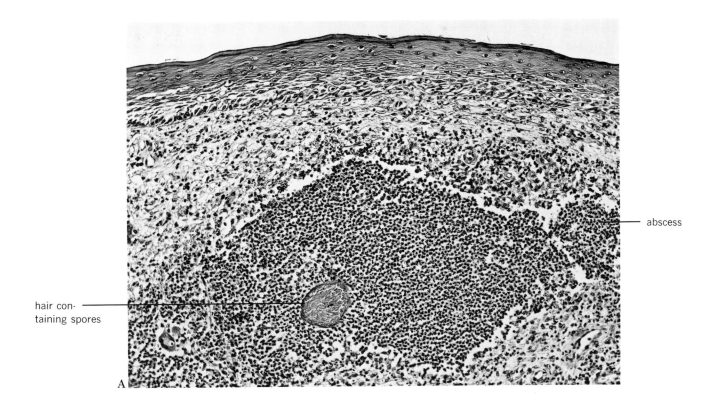

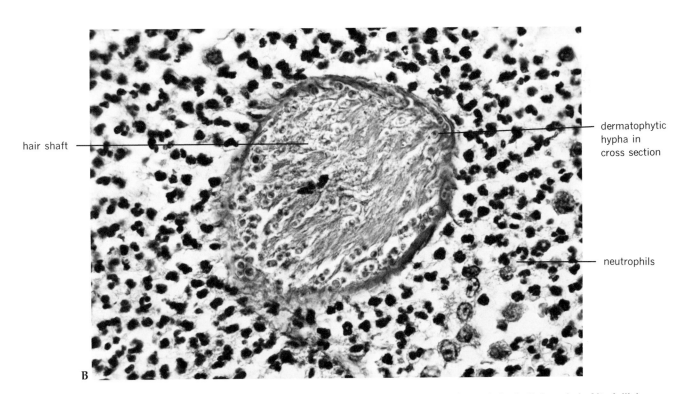

FIG. 9-7. Dermatophytic dermal abscess. Large collection of neutrophils resulted from reaction to hair shaft denuded of its follicle and invaded by many fungal elements, all of which act like foreign body. (A, × 182; B, × 826.)

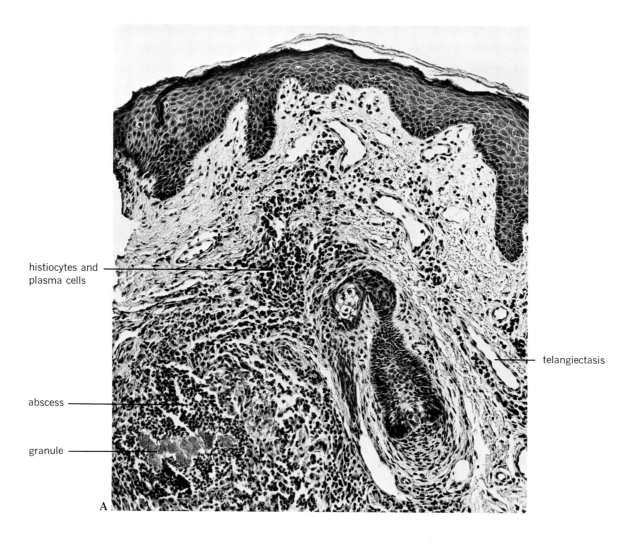

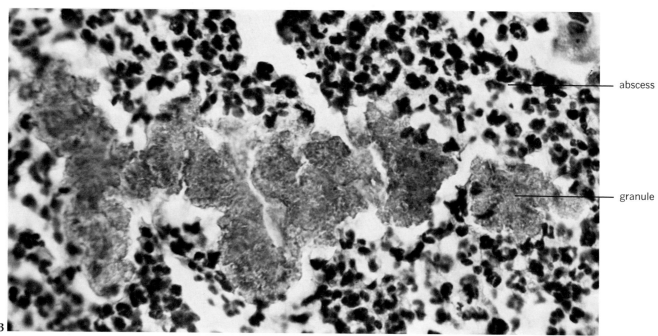

FIG. 9-8. Pseudomonas pseudomycetoma. Within the center of an abscess a colony of pseudomonas can be seen. Granule is a colony of bacteria. (A, × 166; B, × 893.)

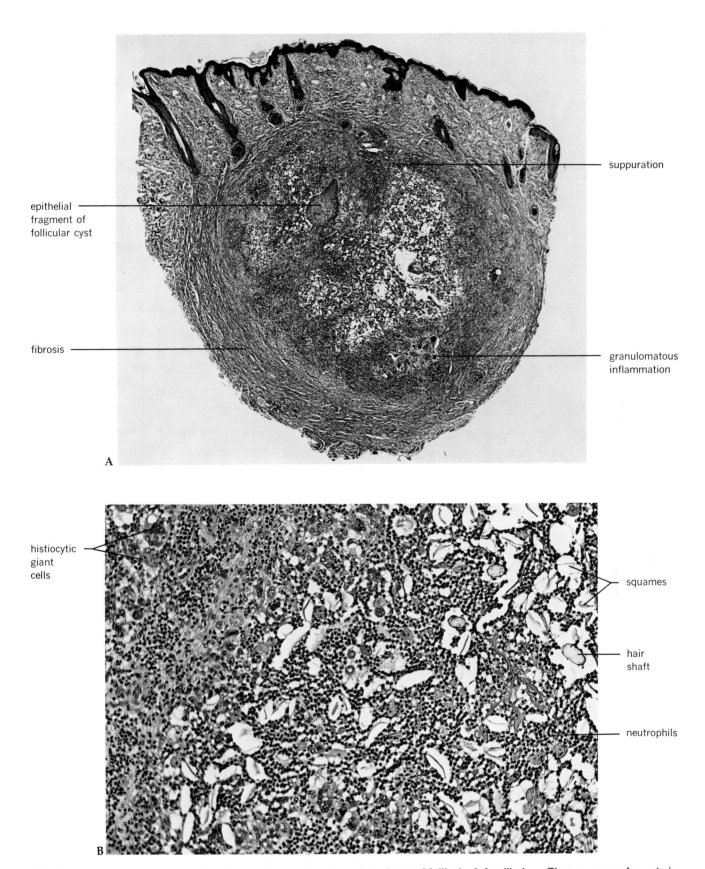

FIG. 9-9. Suppurative granulomatous dermatitis secondary to ruptured cyst of follicular infundibulum. The sequence of events in this lesion was rupture of an infundibular cyst (only a fragment of the lining can still be identified), spewing of cyst contents into the dermis (especially squames which are individually cornified cells), suppuration, granulomatous inflammation, and fibrosis. This is a foreign body reaction to the squames and hair shafts. (A, × 21; B, × 184.)

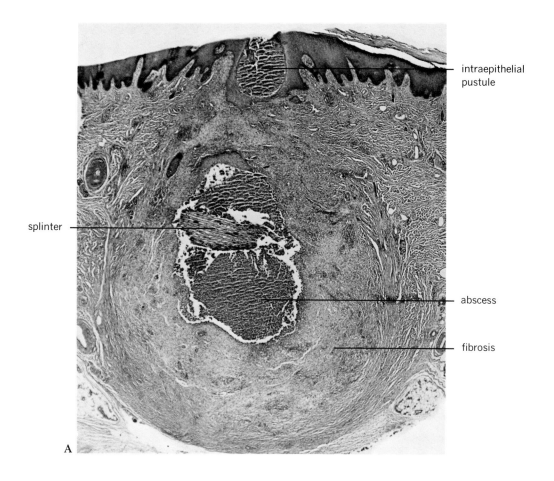

intraepithelial
pustule

splinter

abscess

fibrosis

A

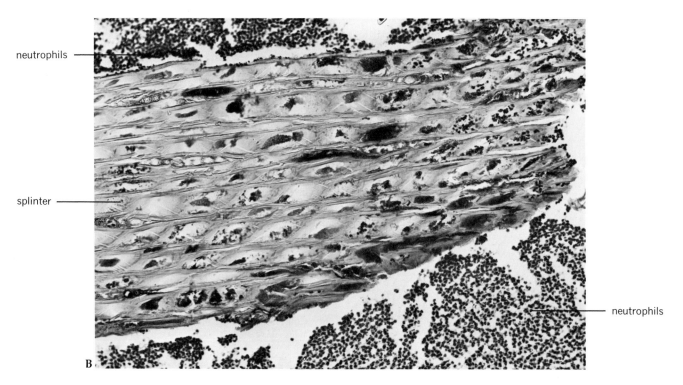

neutrophils

splinter

neutrophils

B

FIG. 9-10. Splinter in an abscess. Sliver of wood within dermis has evoked intense response by neutrophils, forming an abscess which is in turn surrounded by fibrotic pseudocapsule. (A, × 20; B, × 210.) See also Plate 5.

Histiocytes Predominate (Granulomatous, Tuberculoid) (Fig. 9-11)

Tuberculoid refers to a histologic appearance of a well-circumscribed collection of epithelioid histiocytes surrounded by a dense cuff of lymphocytes (Fig. 9-12). Varying amounts of necrosis, from none to much, can be seen in the center of the collection of cells that predominantly are histiocytes. Langhans' giant cells may be present in the epithelioid clusters. Tuberculoid granulomatous dermatitis is seen not only in tuberculoid leprosy but also in conditions such as lupus vulgaris and chronic cutaneous leishmaniasis.

Primary Cutaneous Tuberculosis (Tuberculous Chancre)

—Epithelioid tubercles, some with central caseation necrosis, surrounded by lymphocytes and varying numbers of fibroblasts
—Extensive epidermal hyperplasia
—Ulceration occasionally

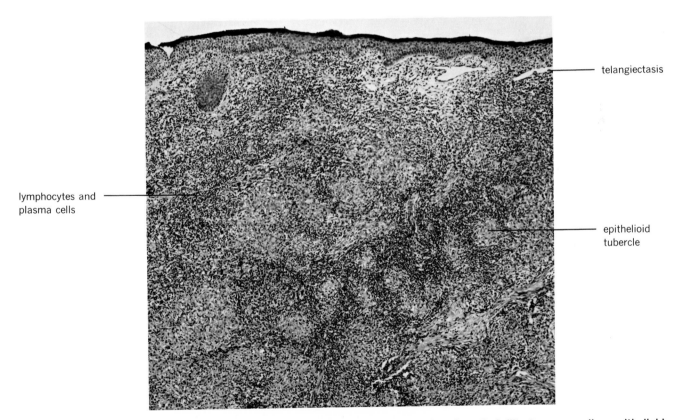

FIG. 9-11. Granulomatous dermatitis, tuberculoid type. Dense predominantly lymphocytic infiltrate surrounding epithelioid tubercles may be seen in lupus vulgaris, tuberculoid leprosy, and chronic or relapsing form of cutaneous leishmaniasis. Causative organisms are rarely found in tuberculoid granulomas stained for them. (× 62.)

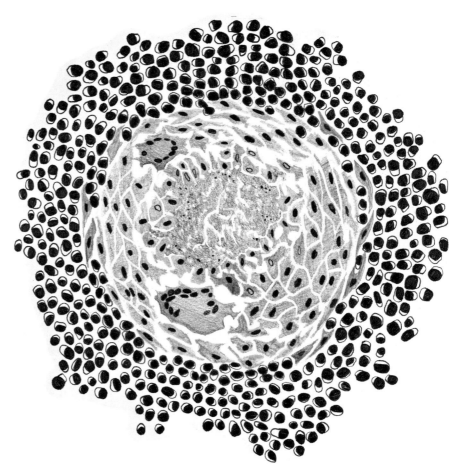

FIG. 9-12. Tuberculoid granuloma.

The histologic changes are characteristic of fully developed lesions of primary cutaneous tuberculosis. In early stages, neutrophils predominate.

The acid-fast bacilli of tuberculosis (*Mycobacterium tuberculosis,* tubercle bacilli) are slender, curved rods measuring approximately 4 microns in length and less than 1 micron in diameter. These organisms are present within the tubercles of primary tuberculosis, in the centers of which are epithelioid cells surrounded by multinucleated epithelioid cells (Langhans' giant cells), which in turn, are surrounded by lymphocytes and finally by fibroblasts. Acid-fast bacilli can usually be demonstrated by the Ziehl-Neelsen stain within early skin lesions of primary tuberculosis.

The necrosis in tuberculosis is referred to as caseation necrosis, a gross pathologic term for the cheesy material that is characteristic of tuberculosis. Histologically, caseation appears as pink, granular material in the center of the tubercles. All cellular outlines are lost in caseation necrosis.

Primary tuberculosis is always exogenous, occurring primarily in children who have not been previously exposed to the tubercle bacillus. The lesion is commonly referred to as a "tuberculous chancre" because it often is an ulcerated nodule that follows inoculation of the skin with tubercle bacilli in a previously uninfected person. The tuberculous chancre is accompanied by prominent regional lymphadenopathy.

Lupus Vulgaris (Fig. 9-13)

—Epithelioid tubercles surrounded by lymphocytes in the upper half of the dermis, impinging upon the epidermis
—Thin epidermis
—Prominent fibrosis and telangiectases in long-standing lesions

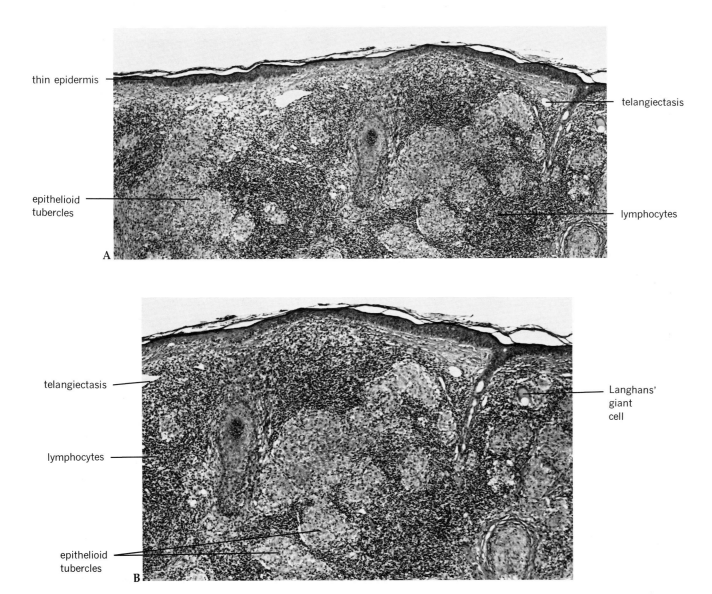

FIG. 9-13. Lupus vulgaris. A, Well-circumscribed epithelioid tubercles are surrounded by dense infiltrate of lymphocytes. (× 65.) B, Granulomas are indistinguishable from those of chronic leishmaniasis and tuberculoid leprosy. (× 81.)

Lupus vulgaris is characterized clinically by tiny papules with "apple-jelly" appearances surrounding atrophic scars. Clinical variants include plaques, nodules, and vegetative and ulcerative forms. Biopsy of the papules reveals tuberculoid granulomas, usually devoid of caseation necrosis. The "apple-jelly" appearance of the papules is due to epithelioid tubercles situated immediately beneath a thinned epidermis. Acid-fast bacilli cannot be demonstrated in most cases of lupus vulgaris.

Scrofuloderma

—Tuberculoid granulomas, with abundant caseation necrosis, at periphery of lesion
—Central abscess occasionally

Tubercles with caseation and suppuration appear clinically as fluctuant, dusky-purple nodules that ulcerate and discharge pus. The draining sinuses finally heal with scars. Scrofuloderma results from direct extension of tubercle bacilli into the skin from underlying tuberculous foci in lymph nodes, bones, or joints.

Tubercle bacilli can usually be demonstrated after diligent study of sections stained for acid-fast organisms.

Miliary Tuberculosis

Some tendency to tubercle formation and caseation occurs within the dermis of nonulcerated skin in miliary tuberculosis. Acid-fast bacilli can be found within necrotic foci.

Leishmaniasis, Chronic Cutaneous Type (Recidivans)

Chronic cutaneous leishmaniasis has all of the features of a tuberculoid granuloma and frequently has numerous plasma cells. The typical clinical lesions of chronic cutaneous leishmaniasis resemble those of lupus vulgaris, having an atrophic center with orange-tan papules at the periphery that resemble "apple-jelly" on diascopy. Nonflagellate organisms of Leishmania are not usually found in long-standing lesions, even after careful scrutiny of Giemsa-stained sections.

Leprosy, Tuberculoid and Dimorphous Types

Tuberculoid leprosy is characterized histologically by epithelioid tubercles surrounded by lymphocytes and, occasionally, plasma cells (Fig. 9-14A, B). Multinucleated histiocytes may also be pres-

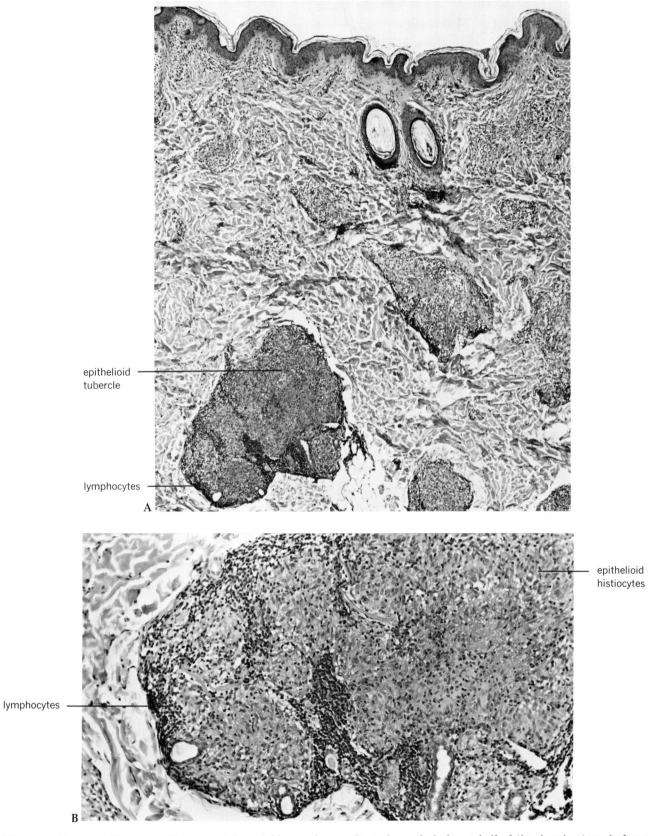

epithelioid
tubercle

lymphocytes

A

epithelioid
histiocytes

lymphocytes

B

FIG. 9-14. Tuberculoid leprosy. Elongated tuberculoid granulomas situated mostly in lower half of the dermis strongly favor diagnosis of tuberculoid leprosy. Serial sections will almost always reveal histiocytes within small dermal nerves. Although acid-fast organisms cannot usually be demonstrated in tuberculoid leprosy by special stains, they can be detected by examination with the electron microscope. (A, × 58; B, × 182.)

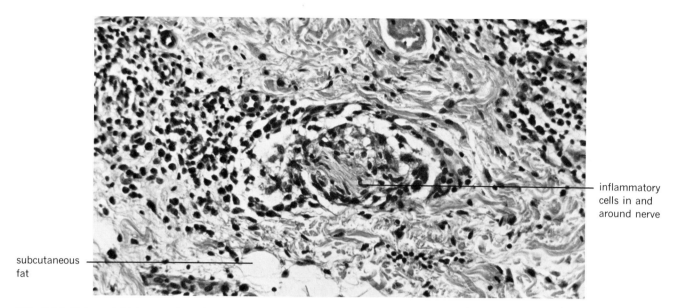

subcutaneous fat

inflammatory cells in and around nerve

FIG. 9-14. Tuberculoid leprosy (continued). C, Note mononuclear cells around and within small nerves, especially in the deep reticular dermis. Eventually the nerves are destroyed and sensation is lost. ($\times$ 374.)

ent. The critical histologic clue to the diagnosis of tuberculoid leprosy is the tendency of the histiocytic infiltrate to involve small cutaneous nerves. The infiltrate is usually present not only around the nerves but within them (Fig. 9-14C). In evaluating granulomatous dermatitides, it is imperative to study cutaneous nerves for this important sign of leprosy. Lepra bacilli are practically never demonstrable in tuberculoid leprosy, but, when found, there are but a few at the periphery of active lesions.

The infiltrate of cells in tuberculoid leprosy, unlike that of cutaneous sarcoidosis, tends to involve nerves and the hair erector muscles, consists of many more lymphocytes and plasma cells around the epithelioid tubercles, and is unassociated with fibrin in the center of some tubercles. The epithelioid tubercles of tuberculoid leprosy are often elliptically elongated (Fig. 9-15), whereas those of sarcoidosis are rounded.

Tuberculoid leprosy characteristically consists clinically of a few, large, asymmetrically arranged, sharply circumscribed, hypopigmented, anesthetic patches or plaques. Progressive involvement of peripheral nerves by histiocytic infiltrates can lead to fibrosis which is often manifested clinically as palpable cords.

Dimorphous leprosy has histologic features of both tuberculoid and lepromatous leprosy, i.e., foam cells admixed with tuberculoid granulomas (Fig. 9-16). The lepra bacilli are found within the foamy histiocytes, and small cutaneous nerves are often involved by the process. Clinically, dimorphous leprosy, which is also termed "borderline" leprosy, shares gross features of tuberculoid and lepromatous types.

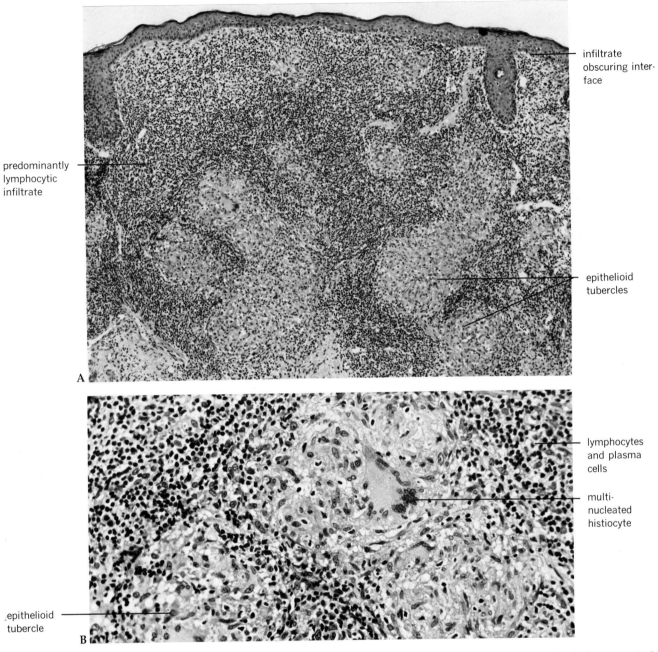

predominantly
lymphocytic
infiltrate

infiltrate
obscuring inter-
face

epithelioid
tubercles

lymphocytes
and plasma
cells

multi-
nucleated
histiocyte

epithelioid
tubercle

A

B

FIG. 9-15. Tuberculoid leprosy. A, Note tendency to confluence of elongated tubercles and their multiplicity in lower part of dermis. The process tends to destroy adnexal structures, especially nerves. (× 92.) B, Elongated tubercles are surrounded by predominantly lymphocytic infiltrate in which plasma cells are commonly found. Even with special stains, such as Fite's, acid-fast bacilli are rarely found. They may be demonstrated, however, with the electron microscope. (× 350.)

Syphilis, Late Secondary and Tertiary Stages (Fig. 9-17)

The tuberculoid structure of late secondary and tertiary syphilis can often be distinguished from the granulomas of tuberculosis by the presence of numerous plasma cells around the tubercles of epithelioid cells and the tendency of blood vessels in syphilis to have thick walls with an increased number of large endothelial

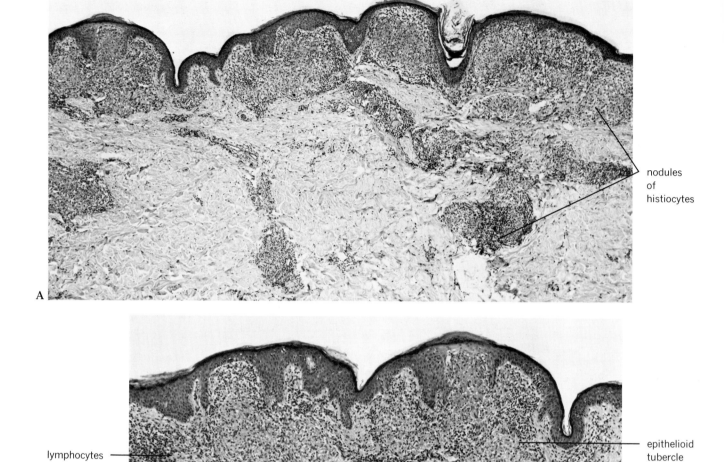

A

lymphocytes

epithelioid
tubercle

foamy and
epithelioid
histiocytes

nodules
of
histiocytes

B

FIG. 9-16. Borderline (dimorphous) leprosy. Note combination of foamy histiocytes of lepromatous leprosy and epithelioid histiocytes of tuberculoid leprosy. Numerous acid-fast bacilli can be demonstrated within foam cells by a special stain like Fite's. (A, × 47; B, × 85.)

cells. The gummatous necrosis in tertiary syphilis differs from caseation necrosis by the faint persistence of shadowy cell outlines. No leukocytes are present in these avascular necrotic centers. At the margins are epithelioid cells, lymphocytes, plasma cells, and plump fibroblasts. Obliterative endarteritis narrows the blood vessel walls at the periphery. Spirochetes are exceedingly difficult to demonstrate. Clinically, the granulomatous lesions of late secondary syphilis consist of widespread papules and nodules. Gummatous lesions of tertiary syphilis consist of few crusted atrophic plaques.

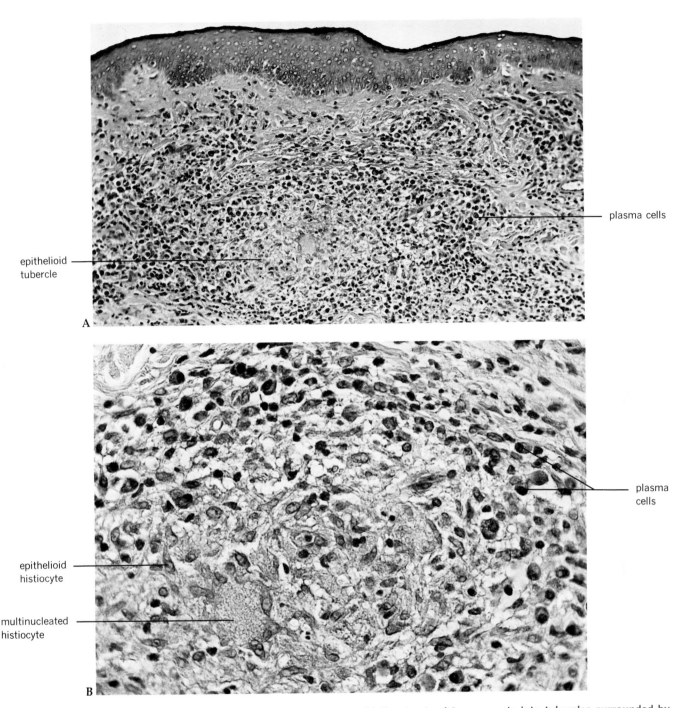

labels on image:
plasma cells
epithelioid tubercle
A
epithelioid histiocyte
multinucleated histiocyte
plasma cells
B

FIG. 9-17. Secondary syphilis, granulomatous. During late stage, histiocytes tend to aggregate into tubercles surrounded by many plasma cells as illustrated. The abundance of plasma cells helps to differentiate late lesions from other granulomatous skin diseases characterized by collections of epithelioid cells such as sarcoidosis and tuberculoid leprosy. (A, × 198; B, × 600.)

In addition to the gumma, another type of cutaneous lesion in tertiary syphilis is the juxta-articular node. These tiny papules on the fingers, near joints, are characterized histologically by fibrosis, histiocytes, and plasma cells, as well as by vascular changes. Under the scanning objective, these lesions sometimes resemble histiocytomas and dermatofibromas (see Chapter 13). Spirochetes are detected rarely, if at all, in juxta-articular nodes.

Rosacea and Perioral Dermatitis, Granulomatous Types (Fig. 9-18)

—Well-circumscribed epithelioid tubercles, usually contiguous to hair follicles, surrounded by lymphocytes
—Necrosis occurring within the tubercles
—Some tubercles impinging upon the thinned epidermis
—Slight spongiosis occasionally within the infundibular epithelium

Yellow-brown to reddish follicular papules of various sizes, as well as pustules, develop on the forehead, nose, cheeks, and chin

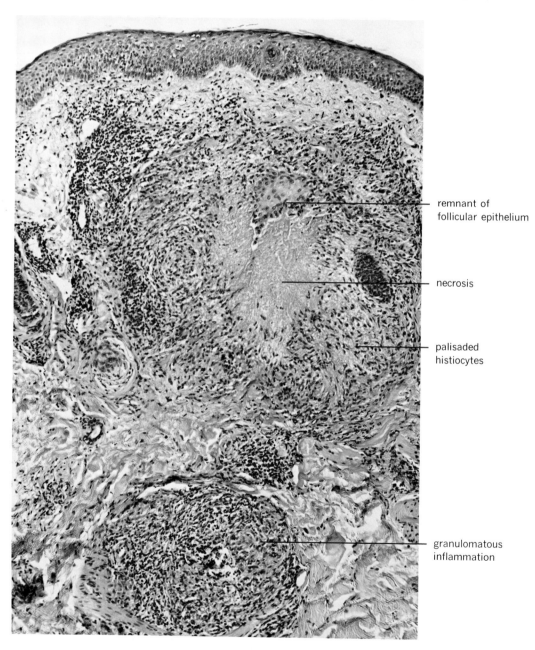

remnant of follicular epithelium

necrosis

palisaded histiocytes

granulomatous inflammation

FIG. 9-18. Perioral dermatitis. Rupture of follicular infundibulum pictured results in necrosis, suppuration, and granulomatous inflammation. (A, × 113; B, × 198.)

of patients with granulomatous rosacea. When similar lesions are present mainly around the mouth, especially of young adult women, the condition is called perioral dermatitis. Like rosacea, perioral dermatitis is fundamentally an inflammatory process involving hair follicles. Initially, both conditions are suppurative folliculitides that progress to granulomatous folliculitis and dermatitis. Often the face is covered by telangiectases, and the nose may be rhinophymatous. The granulomatous papules of rosacea may resolve with hyperpigmented atrophic scars.

It is probable that the so-called rosacealike tuberculid, lupus miliaris disseminatus faciei, and acnitis are related to rosacea, rather than to tuberculosis.

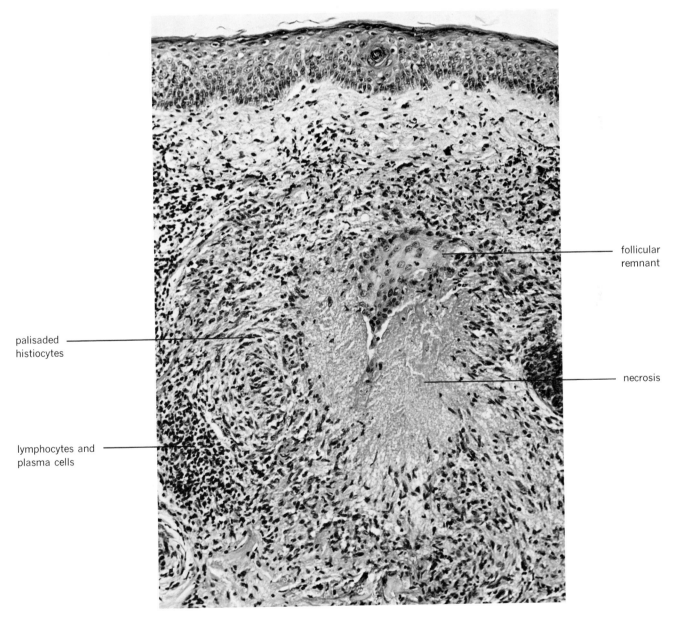

FIG. 9-18. Perioral dermatitis (continued). B.

Histiocytes Predominate (Granulomatous, Sarcoidal)(Fig. 9-19)

Sarcoidal refers to a well-circumscribed collection of epithelioid cells with a sparse or absent lymphocytic infiltrate ("naked tubercle"), in contrast with tuberculoid granulomas, in which the epithelioid tubercles are surrounded by a conspicuous lymphocytic infiltrate. However, it is an oversimplification to think that sarcoidosis in skin consists only of naked tubercles. The fact is that in exceptional cases cutaneous sarcoidosis may be characterized by tuberculoid granulomas in which dense lymphocytic infiltrates surround epithelioid tubercles. A helpful clue to the differentiation of true sarcoidosis from other sarcoidal granulomatous dermatitides is the occasional finding of fibrin in the center of some tubercles of sarcoidosis.

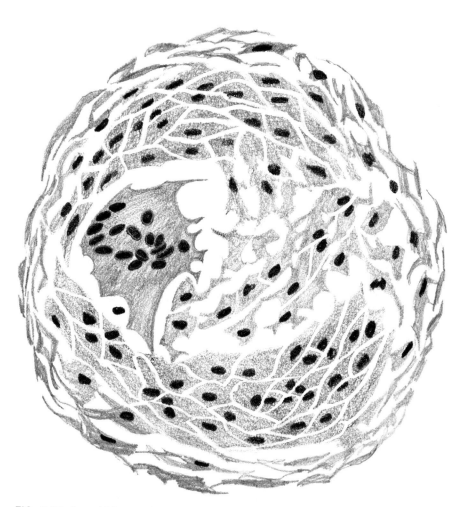

FIG. 9-19. Sarcoidal granuloma.

—Noncaseating tubercles throughout the dermis and sometimes subcutaneous fat

—Large, plump epithelioid cells in well-circumscribed clusters

—Usually scant or absent lymphocytes at the periphery of the epithelioid tubercles, but tuberculoid granulomas with numerous lymphocytes may occur

—Occasional multinucleated histiocytes in the epithelioid tubercles

—Inclusions often within the epithelioid and/or multinucleated histiocytes: (1) asteroid bodies, i.e., eosinophilic star-shaped bodies (Fig. 9-21), (2) Schaumann bodies, i.e., basophilic laminated concentric whorls

—Fibrin often in the center of epithelioid tubercles

—Epithelioid tubercles usually spare the epidermis, making ulceration rare

The diagnosis of idiopathic sarcoidosis is one of exclusion. Its causative agent has not yet been discovered. Therefore, the skin biopsy must be examined for known causes of granulomas that

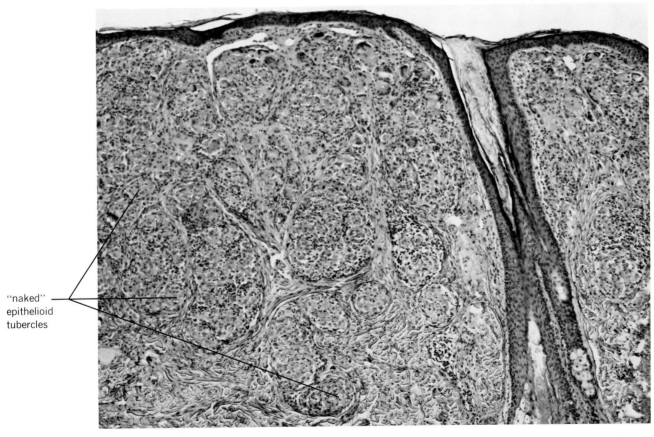

"naked" epithelioid tubercles

FIG. 9-20. Sarcoidosis. A, Typical features illustrated are numerous "naked" tubercles within dermis and sometimes in subcutaneous fat. A tubercle is "naked" if it is not surrounded by a significant number of lymphocytes and plasma cells. (× 74.)

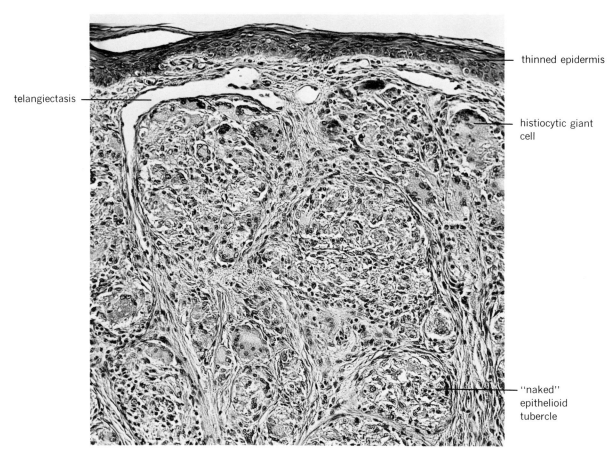

FIG. 9-20. Sarcoidosis. B, Changes similar to those of idiopathic sarcoidosis can be seen in cutaneous lesions caused by silica, beryllium, and zirconium. Silica and beryllium may be detected by examining the specimen with polarized light. (× 169.)

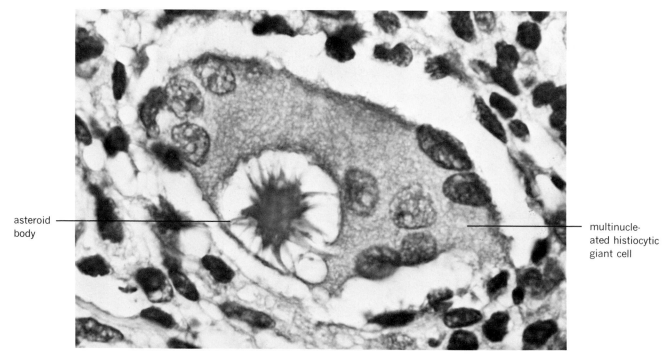

FIG. 9-21. Asteroid body in multinucleated histiocytic giant cell from lesion of sarcoidosis. Asteroid bodies are not specific for any one granulomatous disease but may occur in such diverse processes as sporotrichosis and Miescher's granulomatosis. (× 1785.) See also Plate 4.

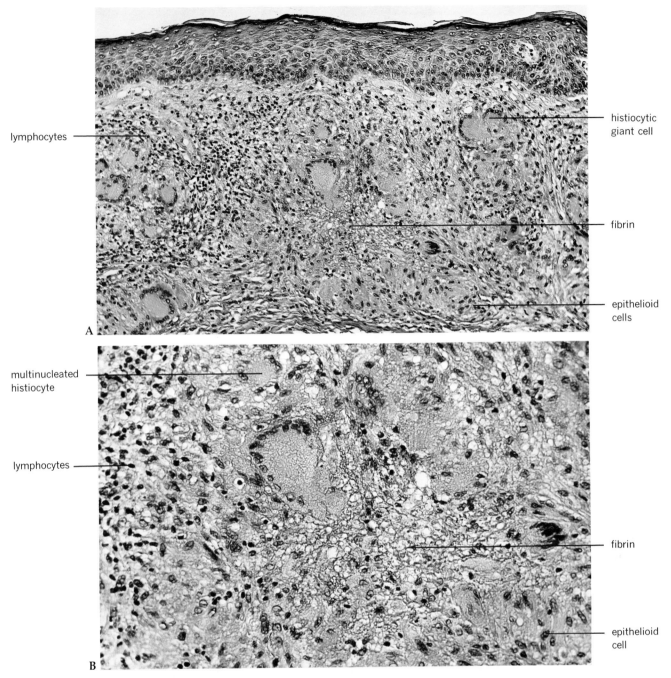

lymphocytes

histiocytic giant cell

fibrin

epithelioid cells

A

multinucleated histiocyte

lymphocytes

fibrin

epithelioid cell

B

FIG. 9-22. Sarcoidosis. Fibrin in center of some epithelioid tubercles is common feature pictured. Number of multinucleated histiocytic giant cells varies greatly. A diagnosis cannot be made solely on basis of histologic changes. (A, × 170; B, × 317.)

mimic those of sarcoidosis. First, the specimen should be examined with polarized light for materials that induce sarcoidal granulomas; if silica (usually from glass or sand) or beryllium (from cuts incurred from broken fluorescent light bulbs) is present, it will be revealed as brilliant, doubly refractile crystals. Zirconium, entering the skin from application of deodorants and poison ivy remedies, does not polarize, and the causative material can only be uncovered by chemical, incineration, or spectrophotometric techniques. If no foreign matter can be demonstrated with polarizing lenses, a variety of staining methods should be employed, namely, PAS or methenamine silver for superficial and deep fungi, Ziehl-Neelsen stain for the acid-fast rods of tuberculosis cutis, Fite stain for leprosy, Giemsa stain for the protozoon of leishmaniasis, and Warthin-Starry silver stain for the spirochetes of syphilis. If all of these studies prove to be negative, the granulomatous dermatitis characterized by naked epithelioid tubercles, often with central fibrin, is diagnosed as sarcoidosis (Fig. 9-22). However, if this convention of designating diseases of unknown cause having epithelioid tubercles as sarcoidosis were carried to its logical conclusion, then lichen nitidus would become sarcoidosis. For this reason, several criteria, in addition to the histologic ones, are required for the diagnosis of sarcoidosis. Histologic sections of a positive Kveim-test site show epithelioid tubercles within the dermis, similar to findings in sarcoidosis.

Clinically, the most common skin lesions of idiopathic sarcoidosis are multiple, firm, grouped papules and nodules that usually have no signs of epidermal alteration. Other forms of cutaneous sarcoidosis are scaly patches, plaques, widespread erythema, subcutaneous nodules, scarring alopecia, and, rarely, ulcerated nodules. The hue of the papules and nodules ranges from skin-colored to purple, often being orange-tan or pink. The papules tend to spread peripherally and heal in the center. The resultant annular sarcoidosis is especially common in black people. All of these various clinical forms of cutaneous sarcoidosis show the typical histologic pattern of sarcoidal granulomas upon biopsy. Follicular papules result when granulomas are around hair follicles.

Lichen Nitidus (Fig. 9-23)

—Circumscribed collections of histiocytes in widened dermal papillae
—Histiocytic multinucleated cells, some containing melanin, within the histiocytic aggregates
—Adjacent epidermal rete ridges sometimes forming a pincer to partially enclose the collections of histiocytes, giving a "ball-and-claw" appearance
—Vacuolar alteration of the dermoepidermal interface overlying each collection of histiocytes, sometimes resulting in dermoepidermal separation
—Focal parakeratosis above the dermal histiocytic aggregates
—Superficial perivascular lymphohistiocytic infiltrate with melanophages

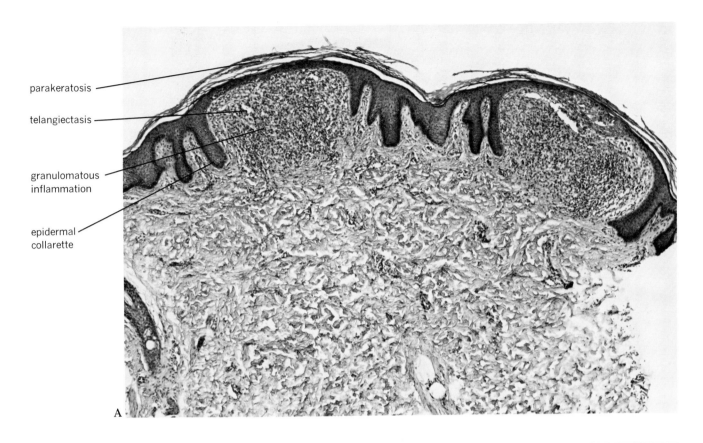

parakeratosis

telangiectasis

granulomatous
inflammation

epidermal
collarette

A

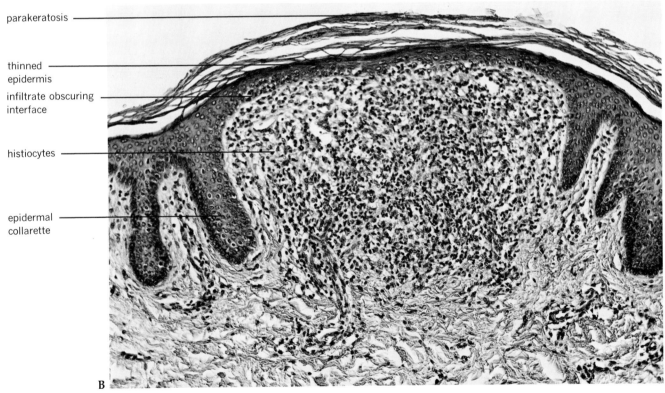

parakeratosis

thinned
epidermis

infiltrate obscuring
interface

histiocytes

epidermal
collarette

B

FIG. 9-23. Lichen nitidus. A, Each well-circumscribed collection of histiocytes and lymphocytes in the papillary dermis gives rise to a tiny clinical papule. Dermal papillae are widened by lymphohistiocytic infiltrates which in turn are partially enclosed by peripheral rete ridges, giving the impression of "balls and claws." This is a relatively early lesion because histiocytes are but slightly preponderant. (× 70.) B, Parakeratosis, thinned epidermis, discrete arrangement of inflammatory cells, and predominantly histiocytic, rather than lymphocytic, quality of infiltrate differentiate lichen nitidus from lichen planus. (× 169.)

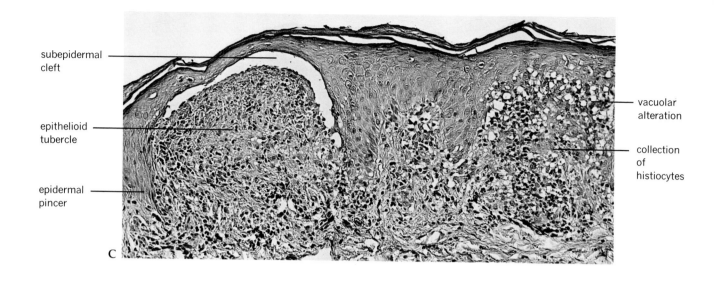

subepidermal cleft

epithelioid tubercle

epidermal pincer

vacuolar alteration

collection of histiocytes

C

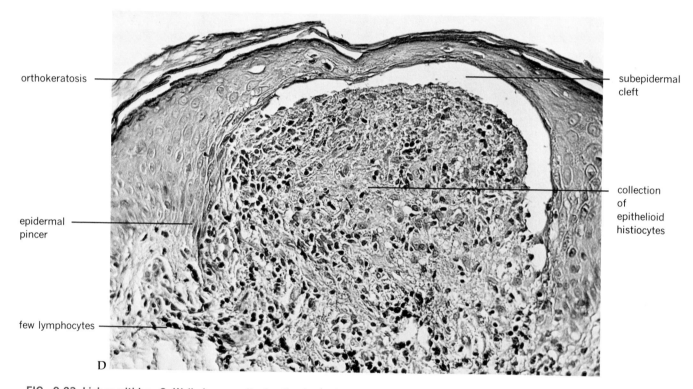

orthokeratosis

subepidermal cleft

epidermal pincer

collection of epithelioid histiocytes

few lymphocytes

D

FIG. 9-23. Lichen nitidus. C, Well-circumscribed collections of epithelioid cells (i.e., "naked" tubercles, sarcoidal granulomas) in widened dermal papillae partially enclosed by epidermal rete ridges are virtually diagnostic of lichen nitidus. This is a relatively advanced lesion because the inflammatory-cell infiltrate consists almost wholly of histiocytes. (× 216.) D, Clefts that result from severe vacuolar alteration at the dermoepidermal junction are often seen. (× 376.)

Each tiny, shiny, flat-topped papule, ranging from skin-colored to pink, of lichen nitidus represents a conglomerate of histiocytes that has widened and elevated a single dermal papilla. The histologic pattern of lichen nitidus is distinctive. Because the infiltrate is focal and granulomatous, lichen nitidus is easily differentiated histologically from lichen planus in which the predominantly lymphocytic infiltrate forms a band across the papillary dermis.

—Focal collections of histiocytes and occasional multinucleated histiocytes within dermal papillae

—Prominent vacuolar alteration of the dermoepidermal interface, often forming subepidermal clefts above the histiocytic collections

—Clumps of homogeneous eosinophilic material, presumably dyskeratotic cells, within the histiocytic aggregates of the papillary dermis

—Dyskeratotic cells, sometimes within the epidermis, especially at the dermoepidermal interface

—Slight focal spongiosis

—Slight focal parakeratosis

—Lymphohistiocytic infiltrate around the blood vessels of the superficial plexus

Lichen striatus is a linearly arranged, papular eruption of children that appears suddenly and disappears spontaneously in weeks or months. Some of the papules are flat-topped; others are scaly. Histologically, lichen striatus bears some resemblance to lichen nitidus, with the addition of spongiosis and dyskeratotic cells. Lichen striatus is also discussed in Chapter 6.

Histiocytes Predominate (Granulomatous, Palisaded) (Fig. 9-24)

Palisaded refers to the alignment of histiocytes like staves around a central focus of mucin (granuloma annulare), fibrin (rheumatoid nodule), degenerated collagen (necrobiosis lipoidica), urates (gout), lipids (eruptive xanthoma), or other foreign materials such as calcium. In their classic histologic presentations, some palisaded granulomatous diseases, e.g., rheumatoid nodule, show at least one altered focus that is rimmed by histiocytes. In other instances, however, no palisade of histiocytes can be seen, especially in granuloma annulare, necrobiosis lipoidica, and granulomatosis disciformis. Rather, the histiocytes are focally scattered among collagen bundles and are not distributed in palisaded array. It is important to be aware that not all "palisaded" granulomas are truly palisaded in every instance. Another variation that may occur in a single biopsy specimen, such as that of granuloma annulare, is the presence of histiocytes both in palisaded array and interposed between collagen bundles.

Most textbooks claim that it is often impossible to differentiate histologically among granuloma annulare, necrobiosis lipoidica, and rheumatoid nodule. In my opinion, these diseases are as distinguishable histologically as they are clinically. One serious

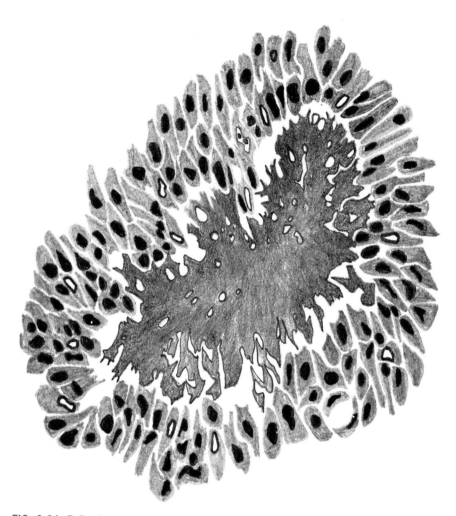

FIG. 9-24. Palisaded granuloma.

limiting factor in the histologic differentiation of these three diseases in the past has been the erroneous application of the nebulous term *necrobiosis* to the changes. Although there is some degeneration of collagen (and elastic tissue) in all of these diseases, it is usually negligible compared to deposits of mucin in granular annulare and of fibrin in rheumatoid nodule.

Granuloma Annulare (Fig. 9-25)

—Histiocytes arranged in rings and also distributed among collagen bundles in discrete foci throughout the dermis
—Areas of normal dermis among palisaded granulomas
—Granular and fibrillary, slightly basophilic material (mucin) around collagen bundles in various degrees of degeneration in the foci of histiocytic aggregation (Plate 1)
—Superficial and deep perivascular lymphohistiocytic infiltrate
—Overlying epidermis usually normal

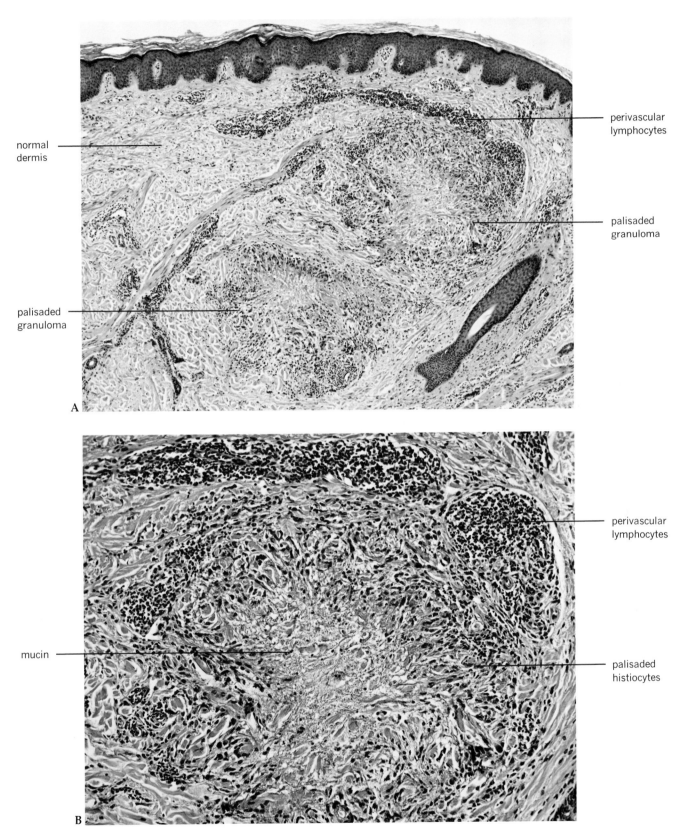

normal
dermis

palisaded
granuloma

perivascular
lymphocytes

palisaded
granuloma

A

mucin

perivascular
lymphocytes

palisaded
histiocytes

B

FIG. 9-25. Granuloma annulare. A, Two well-circumscribed palisaded granulomas in upper half of dermis are typical. In contrast to necrobiosis lipoidica, note intervening and adjacent areas of normal dermis, abundant mucin in center of palisaded areas, and normal epidermis. ($\times$ 61.) B, In higher magnification note deposition of plentiful mucin within zone of palisaded histiocytes. Most of material pictured here is mucin which displaced collagen, little of which has undergone degeneration. In contrast, there is practically no mucin but considerable degeneration of collagen in early lesions of necrobiosis lipoidica ($\times$ 156.)

Although there are variations in the histologic presentation of granuloma annulare, the common denominators in all instances are histiocytes—dispersed (Fig. 9-26), palisaded (Fig. 9-27), and aggregated in well-circumscribed areas—scattered among collagen bundles that are separated from one another by mucin. The amount of mucin varies greatly from scarce to abundant. Mucin is recognized in preparations stained with hematoxylin and eosin as a slightly basophilic, granular, and fibrillary material. Its presence can be confirmed by staining with toluidine blue or colloidal iron. A common misconception about granuloma annulare is that there is always destruction of collagen bundles. Although some degeneration of collagen does occur, collagen is usually not significantly destroyed, but rather displaced by mucin (Fig. 9-25). The fact that the collagen is largely unaltered in most cases of granuloma annulare is witnessed by healed lesions that resolve without clinical or histological scarring, although elastic fibers are lost from the centers of the palisades. However, in exceptional cases there may be considerable collagen degeneration and deposits of fibrin and mucin in granuloma annulare (Fig. 9-28).

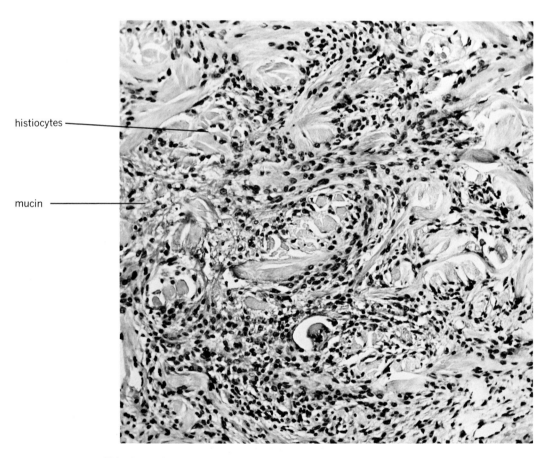

FIG. 9-26. Granuloma annulare. Not all lesions have histiocytes in palisaded array. Many such as that shown here, consist of discrete collections of histiocytes interposed between collagen bundles. Note presence of mucin, a consistent finding. ($\times$ 187.)

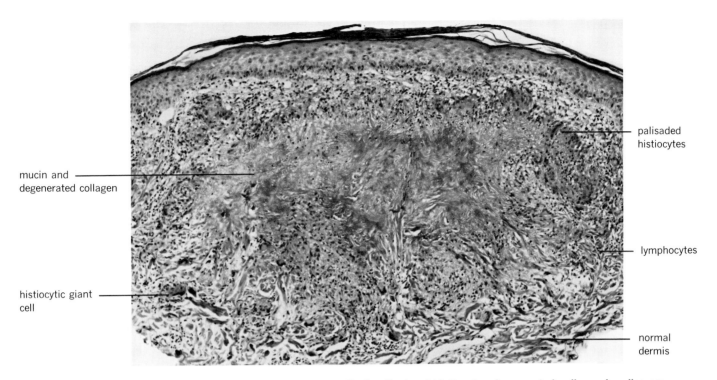

FIG. 9-27. Granuloma annulare. In center of sharply circumscribed palisade of histiocytes degenerated collagen bundles are pushed apart by abundant mucin. Numerous multinucleated histiocytic giant cells are present in this section. Therefore finding many giant cells is not a differential feature in favor of necrobiosis lipoidica. (× 90.)

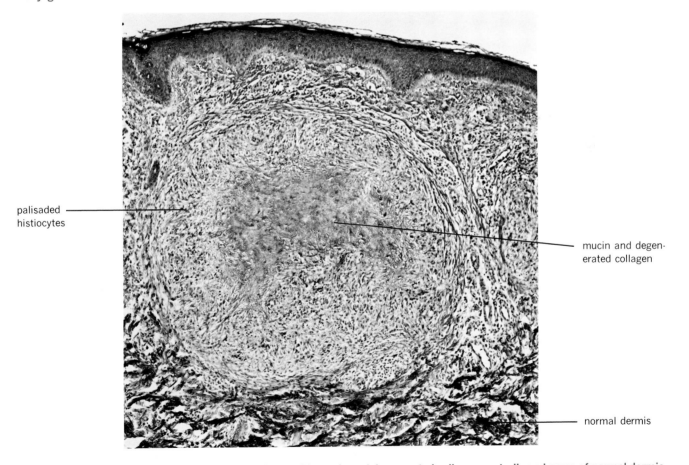

FIG. 9-28. Granuloma annulare. Palisaded granuloma with mucin and degenerated collagen centrally and areas of normal dermis peripherally are diagnostic features. In this photomicrograph the extent of degeneration of collagen is exceptional. (× 74.)

The palisaded granulomas in granuloma annulare are situated focally in otherwise normal dermis, whereas the pathologic changes of necrobiosis lipoidica tend to involve the entire dermis diffusely. The focal granulomas of granuloma annulare are usually situated in the upper half of the dermis, whereas in necrobiosis lipoidica the diffuse process favors the lower half and the subcutis. Increased mucin within the dermis is a consistent finding in granuloma annulare, but not in necrobiosis lipoidica. Mast cells which as a general phenomenon always accompany increase of connective-tissue mucin also do so in granuloma annulare. Although necrotizing vasculitis occurs in early lesions of both diseases (Fig. 9-29), granulomatous vasculitis is not seen in granuloma annulare, whereas blood-vessel walls are often obscured by a predominantly histiocytic infiltrate in necrobiosis lipoidica. Plasma cells, a common feature of necrobiosis lipoidica, are uncommon in granuloma annulare. Early in the development of both granuloma annulare and necrobiosis lipoidica one may see necrotizing vasculitis of small blood vessels surrounded by degeneration of collagen and, peripherally, necrotic histiocytes in palisaded pattern. The fact that necrotizing vasculitis is found so uncommonly in histologic sections of granuloma annulare may be explained by the stage of the lesion at the time of the biopsy (vascu-

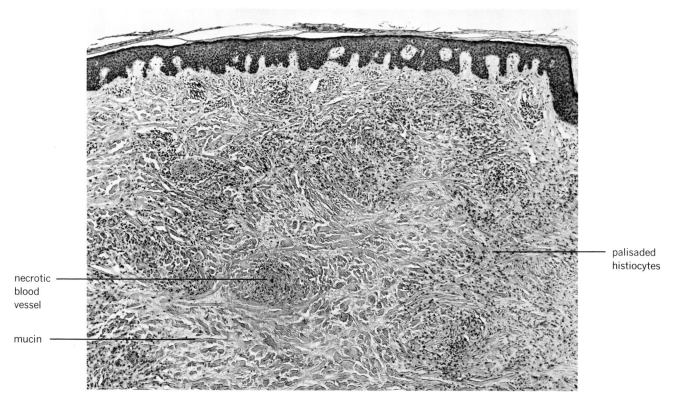

necrotic blood vessel

mucin

palisaded histiocytes

FIG. 9-29. Vasculitis is granuloma annulare. A, In center of palisade of histiocytes necrotizing vasculitis may often be seen. (× 72.)

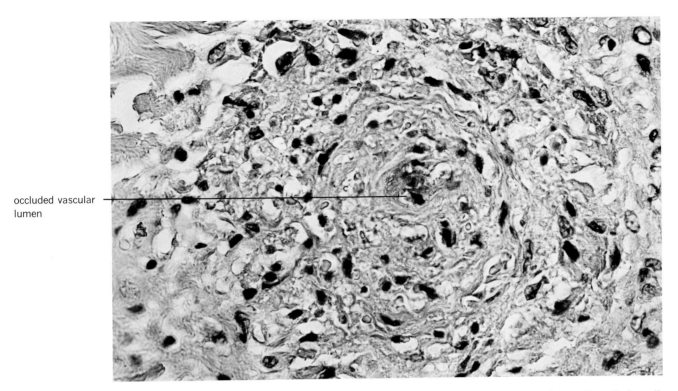

occluded vascular
lumen

FIG. 9-29. Vasculitis in granuloma annulare. B, Higher magnification of inflammatory cells within and around necrotic wall of small blood vessel. (×629.)

litis being an early event) and the randomness of the sectioning (the vasculitis being but dot-sized in the center of a large palisade and therefore likely to be missed).

Sometimes it may be difficult to differentiate histologically between granuloma annulare and eruptive xanthoma. The critical difference is deposits of extracellular lipids in the center of a palisade of histiocytes in the latter condition in contrast to deposits of mucin in the former.

Rarely, the histologic alterations of granuloma annulare may develop so superficially within the dermis that the overlying epidermis is also involved either by thinning or by focal ulceration giving the impression of "perforation" of the skin surface by the granulomatous process (Fig. 9-30). Another unusual histologic variant of granuloma annulare resembles sarcoidosis by formation of "naked" epithelioid tubercles (Fig. 9-31). Sometimes, the nuclei of histiocytes in granuloma annulare are atypical, suggesting to an inexperienced observer a histologic diagnosis of mycosis fungoides or metastatic carcinoma. Still more uncommon are numerous eosinophils in the infiltrate of granuloma annulare, which may give it the appearance of an arthropod reaction. At first glance with scanning magnification, some lesions of granuloma annulare may appear to be perivascular lymphocytic infiltrates, but closer inspection will reveal some histiocytes scattered interstitially.

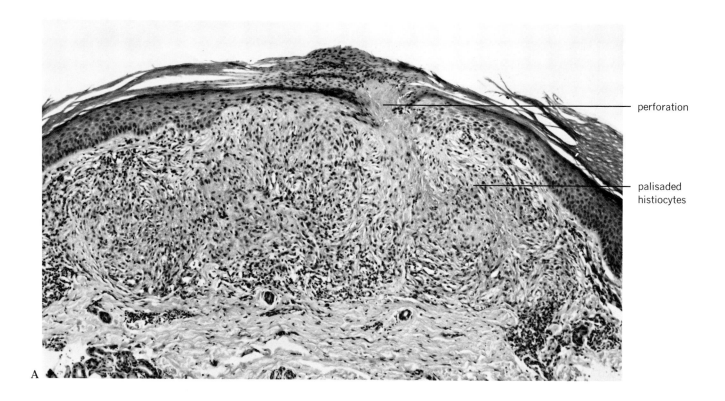

perforation

palisaded
histiocytes

A

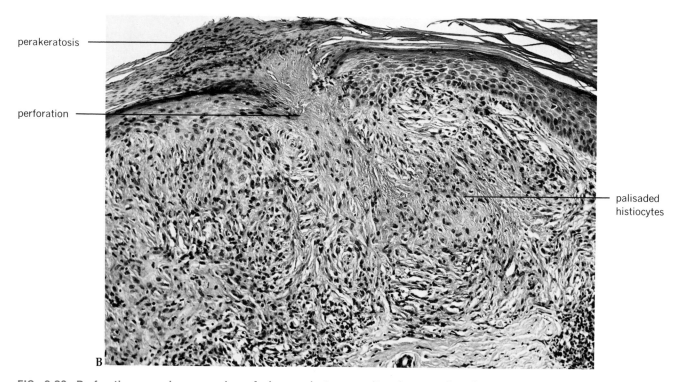

perakeratosis

perforation

palisaded
histiocytes

B

FIG. 9-30. Perforating granuloma annulare. A, In rare instances, altered connective tissue extends from dermis through epidermis, a phenomenon aptly termed "perforation." (× 102.) B, Higher power view to show altered collagen (and mucin) extending from the dermis through the epidermis, which is capped by parakeratosis. Palisade of histiocytes surrounding altered connective tissue establishes this perforating phenomenon as that of granuloma annulare. (× 181.)

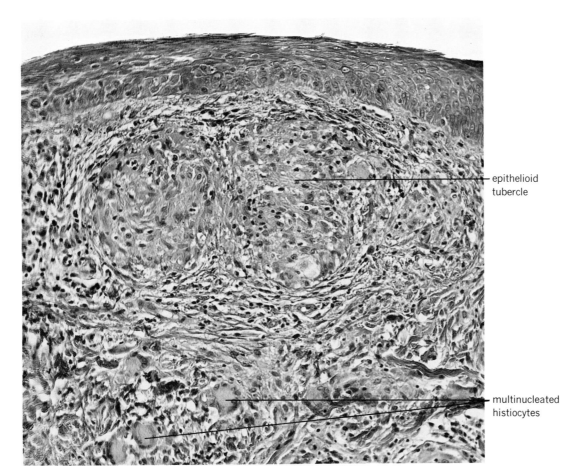

epithelioid
tubercle

multinucleated
histiocytes

FIG. 9-31. Granuloma annulare with sarcoidal features. Rarely will there be "naked tubercles" suggestive of idiopathic sarcoidosis or one of the conditions whose histopathology is granulomatous in the sarcoidal manner. A stain for acid mucopolysaccharide will reveal increased mucin between collagen bundles, confirming diagnosis of granuloma annulare. (× 203.)

There are several clinical presentations of granuloma annulare, namely, one or several rings composed of contiguous confluent skin-colored papules; plaques with tiny papules at the periphery and hyperpigmentation in the center; innumerable discrete, tiny papules, some with central dells, in generalized distribution; and subcutaneous nodules. All of these manifestations of granuloma annulare have histologic features in common.

Granuloma multiforme, a disease that affects women mostly, occurs in Central Africa and is probably a plaque type of granuloma annulare. The term *actinic granuloma* has been given to a granulomatous dermatitis in which histiocytes have engulfed elastotic material in the dermis. It is more likely that in most instances, actinic granuloma is merely granuloma annulare occurring in skin that has been damaged by sunlight. The presence of elastotic fibers within histiocytic giant cells is an adventitious, nonspecific finding, and it is unlikely that actinic granuloma is a disease sui generis.

Acute Necrobiosis Lipoidica (Fig. 9-32)

—Superficial and deep perivascular and interstitial infiltrate of neutrophils
—Neutrophils in the fat septa and at the peripheries of fat lobules
—Necrotizing vasculitis of blood vessels in the mid and lower dermis; thrombi in some of the necrotic vessels
—Degeneration of collagen around the necrotic blood vessels
—Necrosis of adnexal epithelium and inflammatory cells in the vicinity of the necrotic blood vessels

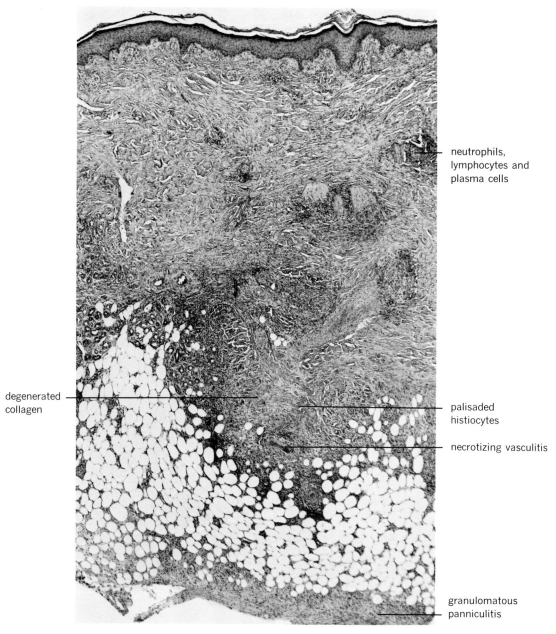

neutrophils, lymphocytes and plasma cells

degenerated collagen

palisaded histiocytes

necrotizing vasculitis

granulomatous panniculitis

FIG. 9-32. Necrobiosis lipoidica, acute. A, Among relatively early changes is necrotizing vasculitis that involves small blood vessels in mid and lower dermis. Degeneration of collagen occurs in zone around necrotic vessels. (× 33.)

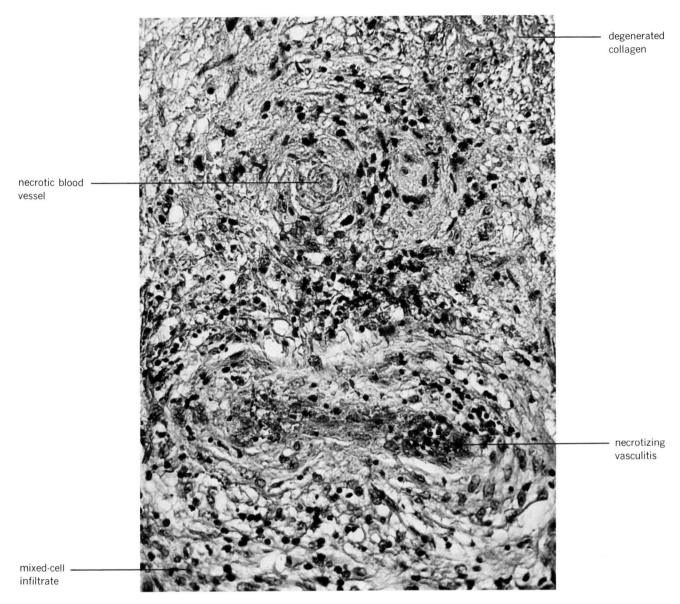

degenerated collagen

necrotic blood vessel

necrotizing vasculitis

mixed-cell infiltrate

FIG. 9-32. Necrobiosis lipoidica, acute. B, Higher magnification shows thrombi within lumina of necrotic blood vessels. Note collagen degeneration of reticular dermis. (× 360.)

Subacute Necrobiosis Lipoidica (Fig. 9-33)

—Superficial and deep perivascular infiltrate, mainly of plasma cells and lymphocytes
—Histiocytes, some epithelioid and some multinucleated, in and around blood vessels throughout the dermis (granulomatous vasculitis) and in the thickened septa of the subcutis (granulomatous panniculitis)
—Histiocytes radially arranged around foci of collagen degeneration at all levels of the dermis, especially the lower reticular dermis
—Thinning of the epidermis with flattening of the pattern formed by rete ridges and dermal papillae

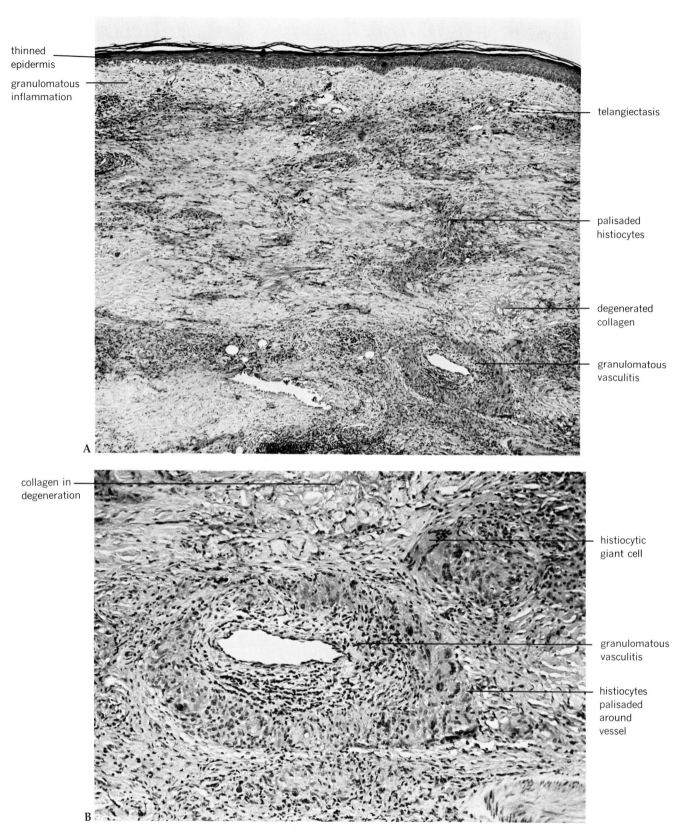

thinned epidermis

granulomatous inflammation

telangiectasis

palisaded histiocytes

degenerated collagen

granulomatous vasculitis

A

collagen in degeneration

histiocytic giant cell

granulomatous vasculitis

histiocytes palisaded around vessel

B

FIG. 9-33. Necrobiosis lipoidica, subacute. A, Entire dermis from superficial vascular plexus to within subcutaneous fat is affected. Unlike granuloma annulare, in which there are regions of unaffected normal dermis interspersed among zones of granulomatous inflammation, there is no area of normal reticular dermis. (× 58.) B, Early necrotizing vasculitis results in degeneration of collagen and necrosis of epithelial structures. With time, as shown in this higher magnification, there is granulomatous vasculitis and finally sclerosis of entire dermis. (× 182.)

—Dermal sclerosis, especially of the mid and lower reticular dermis
—Thickened sclerotic septa in the subcutaneous fat
—Obliteration of dermal blood vessels of various sizes by granulomatous infiltrate and sclerosis
—Sparse superficial and deep perivascular infiltrate of lymphocytes, histiocytes, and plasma cells
—Telangiectases in the upper dermis
—Thin epidermis with little or no pattern of interdigitation of rete ridges and dermal papillae

Because the lesions of necrobiosis lipoidica evolve for years before resolving with scar, the many different histologic features simply reflect the slowly changing pathologic process. In the earliest reddish plaques of necrobiosis lipoidica, there is a neutrophilic necrotizing vasculitis which is followed by degeneration of collagen and necrosis of adnexal epithelial structures in the region of the compromised vessel. Biopsies of lesions at the stage of necrotizing vasculitis are rare, and thus histologic material from such early lesions is not commonly seen by pathologists. Biopsies of older evolving (granulomatous) and resolving (sclerotic) lesions are more common, and these lesions are seen to consist of patches with smooth, shiny, yellowish, telangiectatic, depressed centers

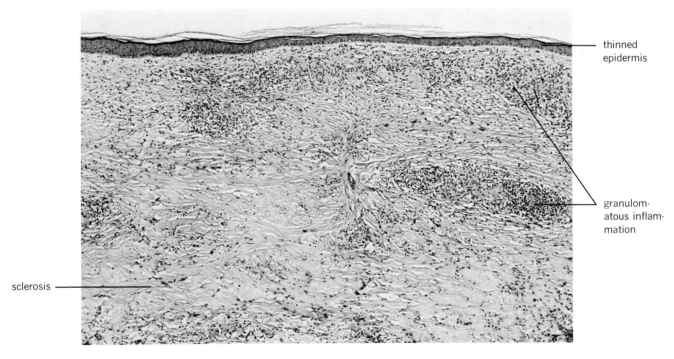

thinned epidermis

granulomatous inflammation

sclerosis

FIG. 9-34. Necrobiosis lipoidica, chronic lesion. Sclerosis of reticular dermis is prominent in this relatively longstanding lesion. That the process is still active may be inferred by persistence of granulomatous infiltrate. In "burned-out" lesions, there is no inflammatory-cell component, only sclerosis. (× 80.)

(atrophic scars) and violaceous, slightly elevated peripheries. Histologically, the burned-out central portion shows a sclerotic dermis beneath a thin epidermis. The sclerosis is most striking in the lower part of the reticular dermis which appears thickened because much of the subcutis has also been replaced by sclerotic collagen. Biopsy of the active violaceous periphery reveals a mixture, in varying proportions, of necrotizing vasculitis, collagen degeneration (Fig. 9-35), necrosis of hair follicles and sweat apparatuses, a dense perivascular infiltrate of plasma cells, palisaded granulomatous dermatitis (Fig. 9-36), panniculitis, and sclerosis. The blood vessels in the lowest part of the dermis, at the junction with the subcutis, are prominently involved by the initially neutrophilic and subsequently granulomatous vasculitis (Fig. 9-33). The superficial dermal blood vessels also are often obliterated by granulomatous inflammation and sclerosis (Fig. 9-37). The yellow color of necrobiosis lipoidica is imparted by deposits of lipid in the upper part of the dermis. The fatty material is easily demonstrated with the oil red O or Sudan black stains.

In most instances, the histologic diagnosis of necrobiosis lipoidica can be made with reasonable certainty in sections stained by hematoxylin and eosin. In rare instances it is difficult to distinguish necrobiosis lipoidica from granuloma annulare. A critical histologic feature that helps to differentiate necrobiosis lipoidica from granuloma annulare is the diffuseness of the pathologic process throughout the entirely abnormal dermis in necrobiosis lipoidica (Fig. 9-38). In granuloma annulare there are multiple palisaded granulomatous foci interspersed among normal dermis. The major change in granuloma annulare is in the upper part of the dermis, but in necrobiosis lipoidica the lower part of the dermis is most markedly involved. The subcutaneous fat is usually involved in necrobiosis lipoidica, and usually not in granuloma annulare (Fig. 9-43). There are little mucin deposition and extensive degeneration of collagen in necrobiosis lipoidica, but much mucin deposition and usually relatively little collagen degeneration in granuloma annulare.

In instances in which necrobiosis lipoidica and granuloma annulare cannot be differentiated from one another with the hematoxylin and eosin stain, a stain for mucin (e.g., colloidal iron, alcian blue) may be decisive. If abundant mucin is present, the diagnosis is granuloma annulare. Mucin is not increased in necrobiosis lipoidica. There is an annular form of necrobiosis lipoidica that may be difficult to distinguish clinically from granuloma annulare, but it too has the typical histologic features of necrobiosis lipoidica which involve the entire reticular dermis, in contrast to granuloma annulare.

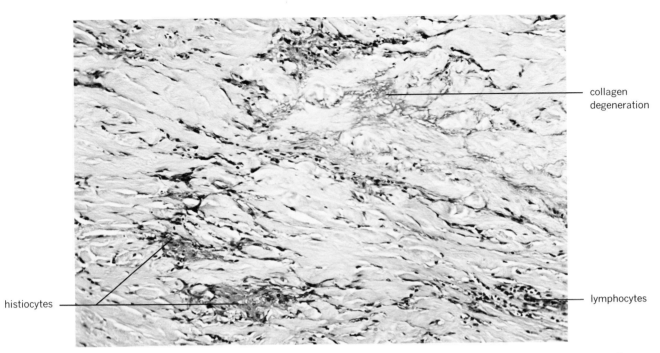

FIG. 9-35. Necrobiosis lipoidica. Small clusters of histiocytes form arc around irregularly shaped puddles of degenerated collagen. Both are consistent findings in relatively early lesions. (× 187.)

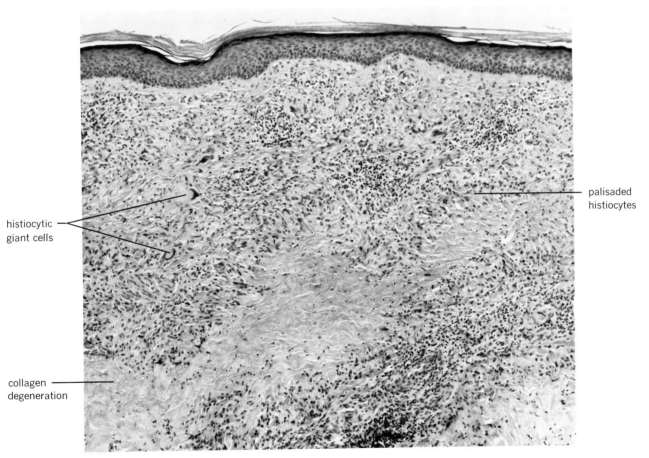

FIG. 9-36. Necrobiosis lipoidica. Unlike in granuloma annulare, there is always significant degeneration of collagen and no deposition of mucin, and entire dermis is affected by process with no intervening zones of normal dermis. (× 95.)

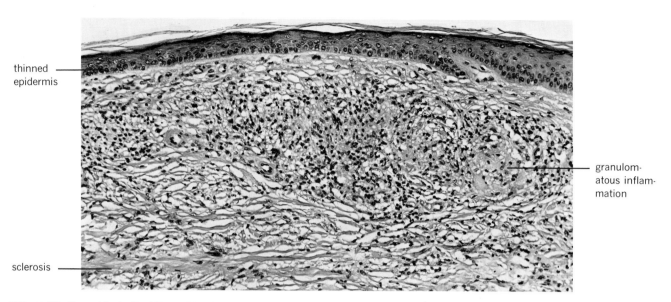

thinned epidermis

granulom- atous inflam- mation

sclerosis

FIG. 9-37. Necrobiosis lipoidica with obliteration of small blood vessels of superficial plexus and dermal sclerosis. (× 185.)

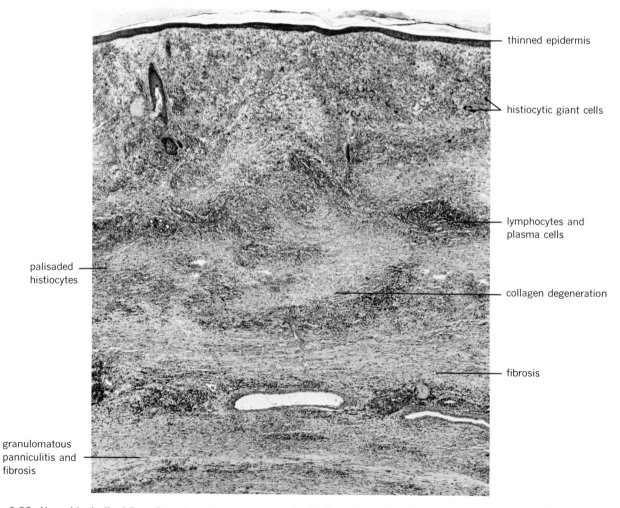

thinned epidermis

histiocytic giant cells

lymphocytes and plasma cells

palisaded histiocytes

collagen degeneration

fibrosis

granulomatous panniculitis and fibrosis

FIG. 9-38. Necrobiosis lipoidica. Granulomatous process extends from beneath epidermis well into subcutaneous fat. Note diverse histologic features: superficial and deep perivascular infiltrates of lymphocytes and plasma cells, histiocytes in palisaded array around zones of collagen degeneration, numerous multinucleated histiocytes in upper part of dermis, and fibrosis predominantly in lower half of dermis and what was formerly the subcutis. (× 28.)

Granuloma annulare heals spontaneously in months without sequelae, whereas necrobiosis lipoidica eventuates in scarring. These dramatically different clinical courses are paralleled by specific histologic differences, i.e., sclerosis in necrobiosis lipoidica and resumed "normal" dermis in granuloma annulare.

Granulomatosis Disciformis of the Face (Miescher's Granuloma) (Fig. 9-39)

Granulomatosis disciformis of the face has many histologic features of granuloma annulare, i.e., histiocytes in palisaded array and among collagen bundles especially in the upper half of the dermis. However, unlike the situation in granuloma annulare, asteroid bodies are usually present within some histiocytes (Fig. 9-40), and there is no significant mucin deposition. Unlike necrobiosis lipoidica, there is little or no collagen degeneration or sclerosis in Miescher's granuloma of the face.

Clinically, granulomatosis disciformis appears as reddish plaques, many of them annular with hypopigmented and hyperpigmented centers. The lesions develop on the face and scalp, especially on the brows of women, and they resolve spontaneously in months or years, without scarring. At present it is probably best to regard Miescher's granuloma as a distinctive palisaded granulomatous dermatitis.

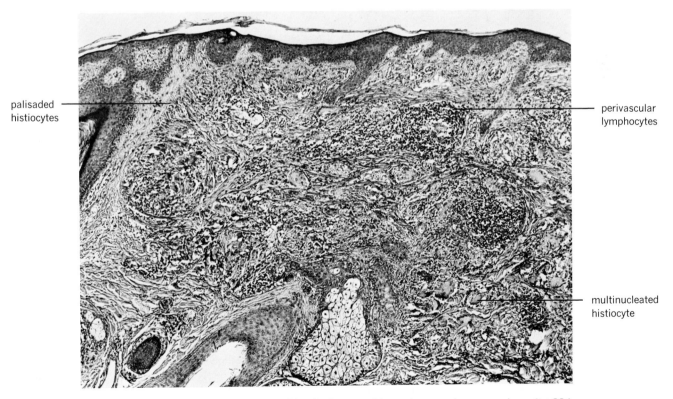

palisaded histiocytes

perivascular lymphocytes

multinucleated histiocyte

FIG. 9-39. Granulomatosis disciformis of face. Note histologic resemblance to granuloma annulare. (× 88.)

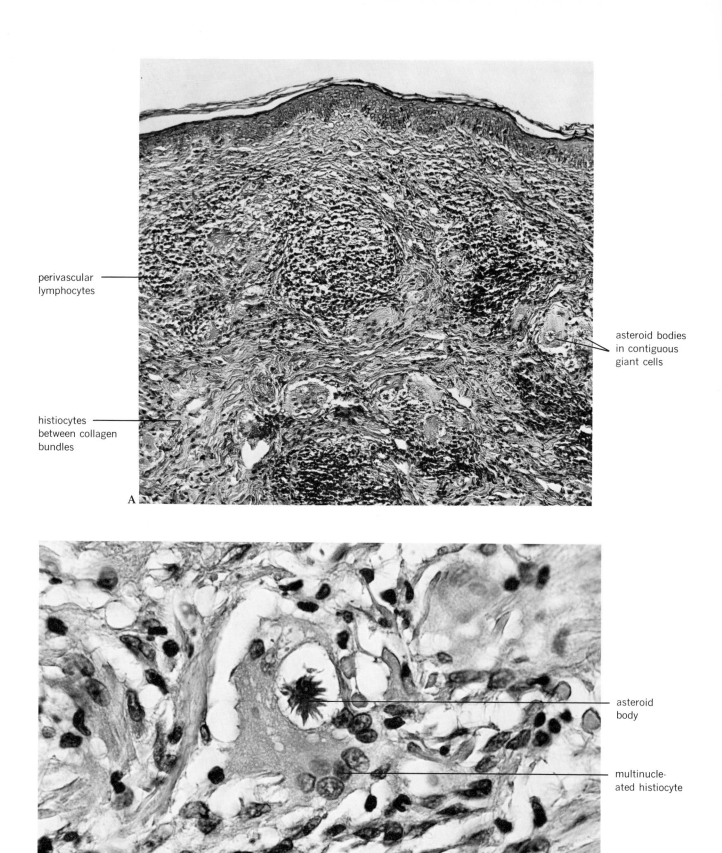

perivascular lymphocytes

asteroid bodies in contiguous giant cells

histiocytes between collagen bundles

A

asteroid body

multinucleated histiocyte

B

FIG. 9-40. Granulomatosis disciformis of face. A, Asteroid bodies within histiocytes and absence of abundant mucin differentiate this palisaded lesion from granuloma annulare. ($\times$ 166.) B, Higher magnification of asteroid body within multinucleated histiocytic giant cell. Asteroid bodies are not specific for this condition but may also occur in such disparate diseases as sarcoidosis and sporotrichosis. ($\times$ 817.)

Color Plates

Plate 1. *Special Stains*

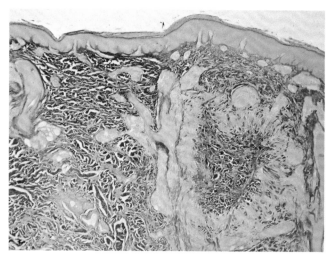

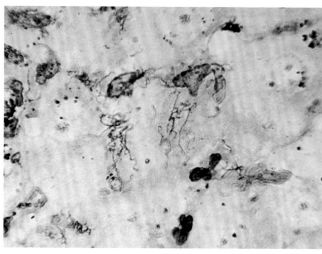

1. Colloidal iron stain for acid mucopolysaccharides (granuloma annulare; × 27)

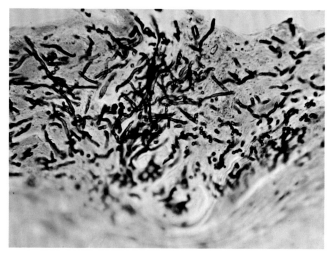

2. Silver methenamine stain for fungi (Candida albicans; × 353)

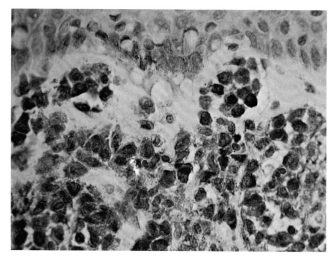

3. Giemsa stain for mast cells (urticaria pigmentosa; × 450)

4. Warthin-Starry stain for spirochetes (secondary syphilis; × 1000)

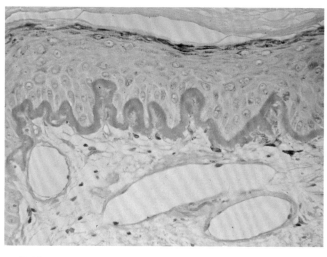

5. PAS stain for thickened basement membrane (chronic discoid lupus erythematosus; × 220)

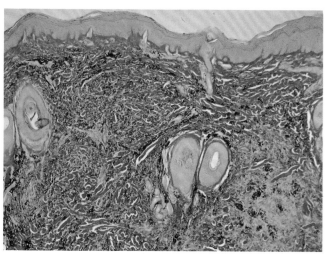

6. Perls' stain for hemosiderin (histiocytoma-dermatofibroma; × 27)

Plate 2. *Organisms Within the Epidermis*

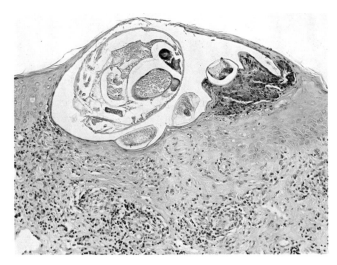

1. Mite, Sarcoptes scabiei, and ova in cornified layer in lesion of scabies (× 110)

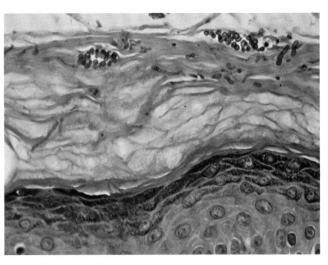

4. Hyphae and spores of Malassezia furfur in cornified layer of epidermis in lesion of tinea versicolor (× 460)

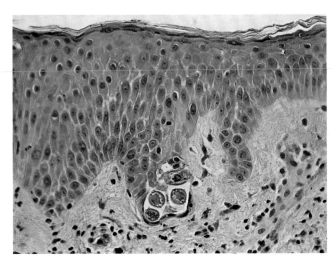

2. Larva of species of Ancylostoma above basal layer of epidermis in lesion of creeping eruption (× 220)

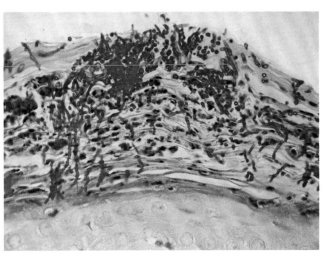

5. Hyphae and spores of Candida albicans in cornified layer of epidermis in lesion of candidiasis (PAS stain) (× 353)

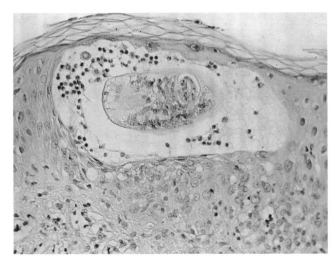

3. Cercaria in spinous zone of epidermis in lesion of swimmer's itch (× 220)

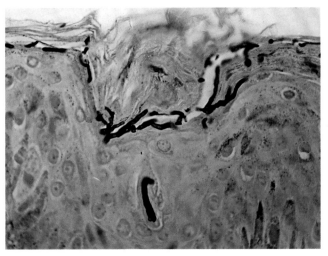

6. Hyphae of Trichophyton rubrum in cornified layer of epidermis in lesion of dermatophytosis (silver methenamine stain) (× 353)

Plate 3. Organisms Within the Dermis

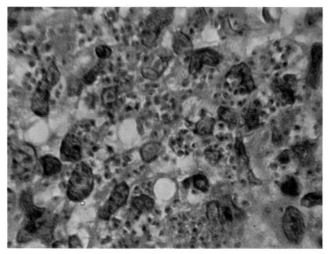

1. Organisms of Leishmania tropica in histiocytes of cutaneous leishmaniasis (H & E; × 1000)

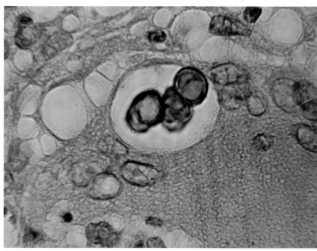

4. "Copper pennies" of chromomycosis in multinucleated histiocyte (H & E; × 1000)

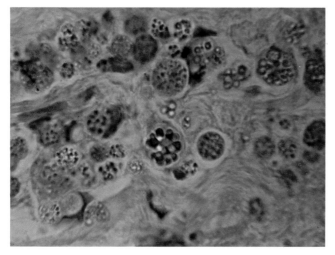

2. Refractile bodies of prototheca lying free in dermis of protothecosis (H & E; × 1000)

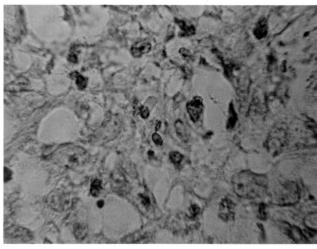

5. Budding of Sporotrichum schenckii in lesion of sporotrichosis (PAS with prior digestion by diastase; × 1000)

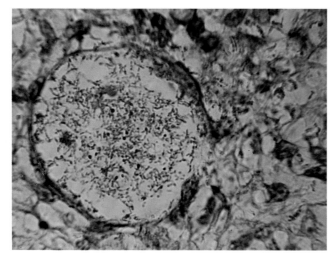

3. Lepra bacilli in huge histiocyte (globus) of lepromatous leprosy (Fite stain; × 1000)

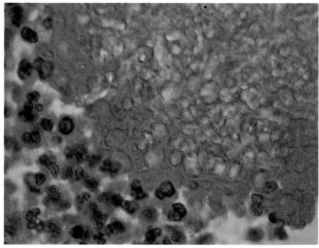

6. Fungal elements of Allescheria boydii in mycetoma (PAS; × 1000)

Plate 4. *Giant Cells in the Skin*

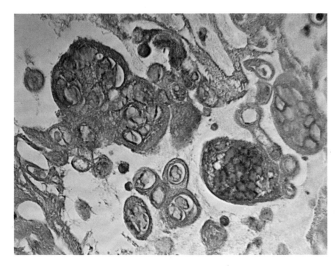

1. Multinucleated epithelial giant cells in herpesvirus infection (× 418)

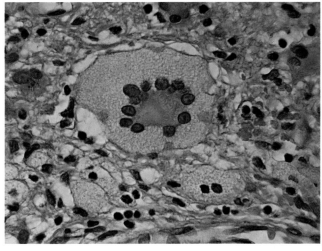

4. Touton giant cell, a histiocyte with wreath of nuclei in foamy cytoplasm, in xanthogranuloma (× 418)

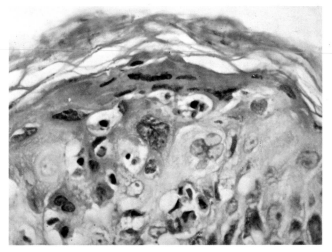

2. Multinucleated epithelial giant cells in measles (× 418)

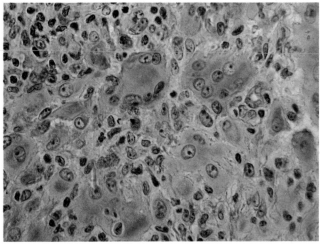

5. Histiocytic giant cells with "ground glass" cytoplasm in reticulohistiocytic granuloma (× 418)

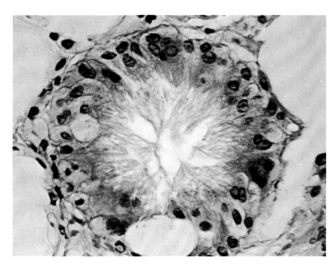

3. Multinucleated histiocytic giant cell containing starburst of crystals in subcutaneous fat necrosis of newborn (× 418)

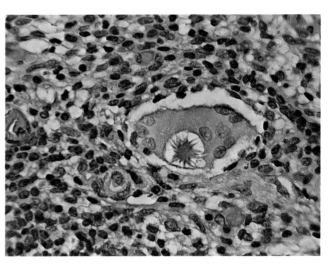

6. Asteroid body in foreign body giant cell (× 418)

Plate 5. *Materials Visualizable by Polarized Light*

CONVENTIONAL ILLUMINATION   PARTIAL POLARIZATION   FULL POLARIZATION

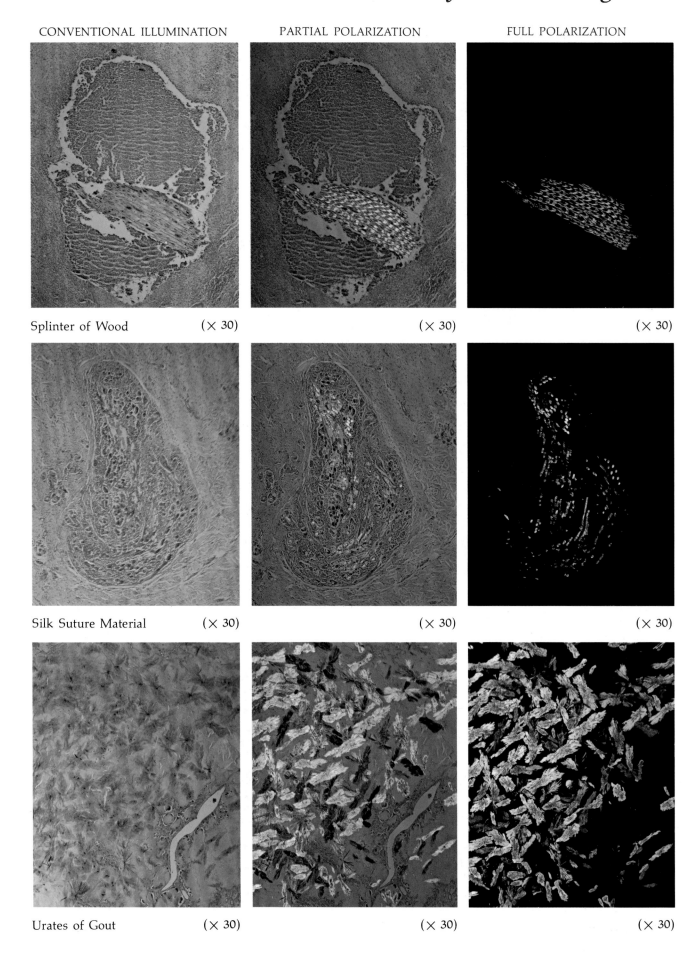

Splinter of Wood   (× 30)   (× 30)   (× 30)

Silk Suture Material   (× 30)   (× 30)   (× 30)

Urates of Gout   (× 30)   (× 30)   (× 30)

Plate 6. *Three Distinctive Subepidermal Blistering Diseases*

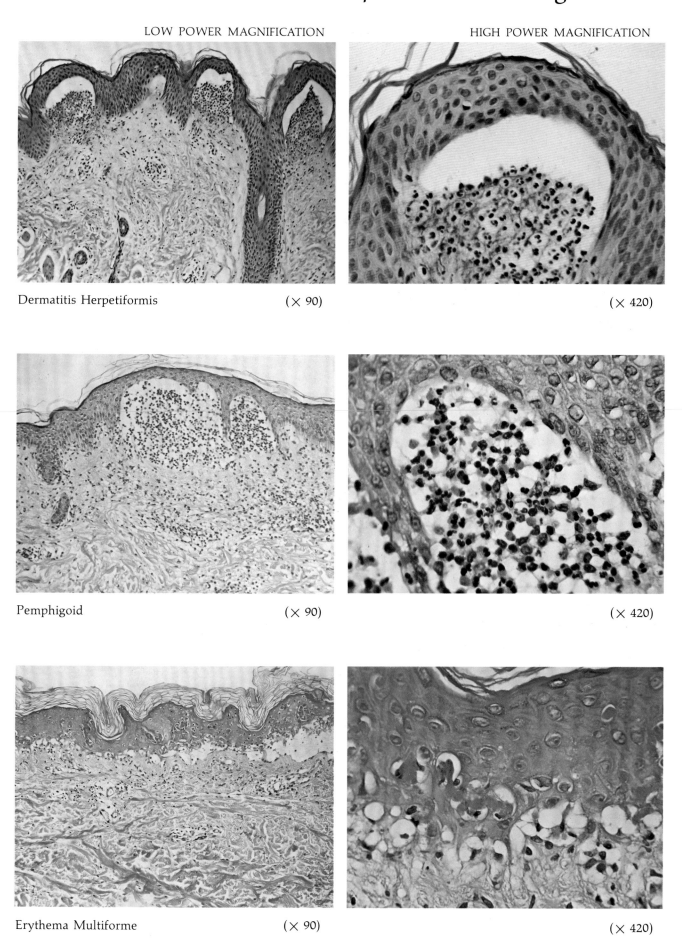

Dermatitis Herpetiformis   (× 90)   (× 420)

Pemphigoid   (× 90)   (× 420)

Erythema Multiforme   (× 90)   (× 420)

Rheumatoid Nodule (Fig. 9-41), Pseudorheumatoid Nodule, and Rheumatic Nodule

—Dense deposit(s) of fibrin within the subcutaneous fat and/or within the dermis
—Palisades of histiocytes around the fibrin

Rheumatoid, pseudorheumatoid, and rheumatic nodules are quite distinct from the other types of palisaded granulomas. Fibrin is deposited in them, whereas deposition of mucin characterizes granuloma annulare and degeneration of collagen marks necrobiosis lipoidica. These nodules in most instances form subcutaneously, whereas the lesions of granuloma annulare and necrobiosis lipoidica develop mainly in the dermis.

Pseudorheumatoid (nonrheumatoid) nodule is another lesion to be distinguished from rheumatoid nodule. It is identical histologically, but the pseudorheumatoid nodule is located mostly in the dermis, rather than in the subcutis. The pseudorheumatoid nodule is usually solitary, unassociated with rheumatoid arthritis, and in sites other than over joints. So-called pseudorheumatoid nodules situated in the subcutis usually prove to be changes of subcutaneous granuloma annulare. Special stains reveal abundant mucin in subcutaneous granuloma annulare, but not in rheumatoid or pseudorheumatoid nodules.

The subcutaneous nodules that form in some patients with rheumatic fever are histologically indistinguishable from those of rheumatoid arthritis and from the pseudorheumatoid nodule. Rheumatic nodules tend to resolve spontaneously, whereas their histologic simulators tend to persist.

Clinically, rheumatoid nodules are firm, dome-shaped, skin-colored lesions usually seated near or over larger joints. They occur in approximately 10% of children with rheumatoid arthritis and in about 20% of adults with the disease.

Gout (Fig. 9-42)

Urate deposits in a feathery basophilic matrix and surrounded by multinucleated histiocytic giant cells are the characteristic histologic features of gout. Sodium urate deposits can be seen best in specimens fixed in alcohol rather than in formalin. Urate is magnificently multicolored and refractile with polarlized light. In formalin-fixed gouty tissues, the urate can be demonstrated with the De Galantha stain. Gouty lesions in skin, tophi, appear as firm papules or nodules, especially on the ears and near small joints

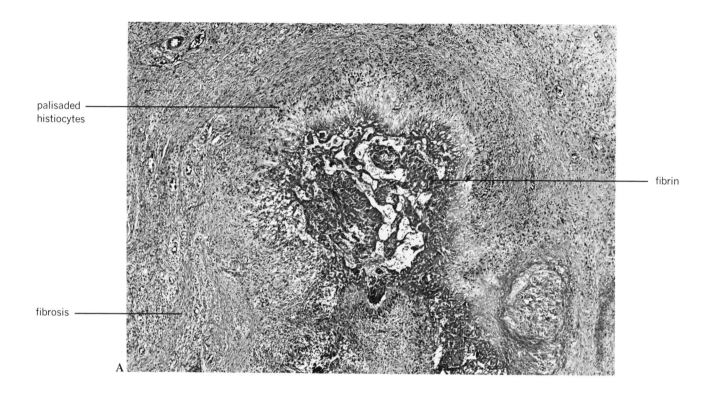

palisaded
histiocytes

fibrin

fibrosis

A

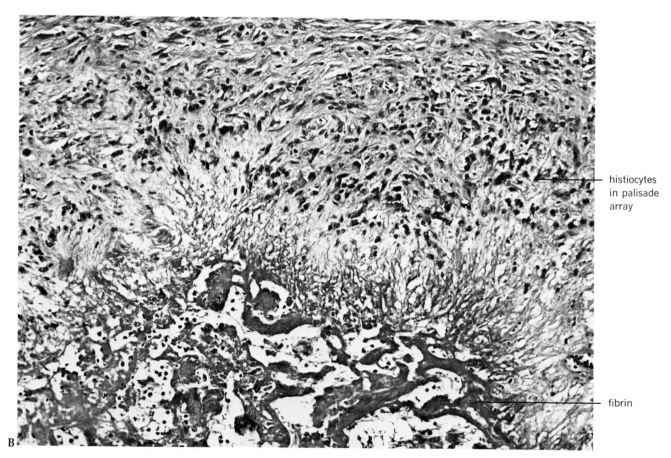

histiocytes
in palisade
array

fibrin

B

FIG. 9-41. Rheumatoid nodule. In contrast to granuloma annulare wherein histiocytes surround deposits of mucin in a palisade and to necrobiosis lipoidica wherein histiocytes surround degenerated collagen in a palisade, the histiocytes of rheumatoid nodule encircle lakes of fibrin. (A, × 60; B, × 203.)

such as that of the big toe. Gout is included as a palisaded granuloma because of the tendency of histiocytes to be arranged in radial fashion around the urate deposits. Gout can also be considered a foreign-body granuloma (Plate 5).

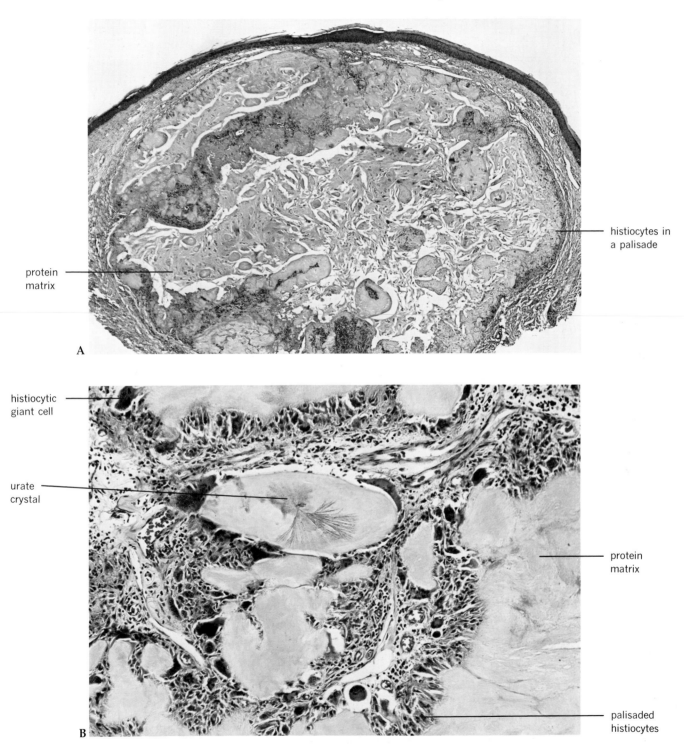

FIG. 9-42. Gout. A, Histiocytes in palisaded array surround urate crystals embedded in protein matrix. Only a few urate crystals are usually preserved in a specimen that has been fixed in formalin, as the one shown here. A better fixative for preservation of urates is absolute alcohol. (× 32.) B, In sections stained with hematoxylin and eosin, bright yellow crystals of sodium urate can be seen within basophilic protein matrix. Histiocytes, some multinucleated, surround each irregularly shaped aggregate. (× 187.)

Juxta-articular Nodes of Syphilis

In late lesions of secondary or early tertiary syphilis that occur near joints, histiocytes are often arranged in palisades within the dermis as well as scattered between collagen bundles. Important clues to diagnosis of juxta-articular nodes are the plasma cells around the blood vessels of the superficial and deep plexuses and the fibrosis of the reticular dermis. In some lesions the combination of histiocytes and fibrosis resembles the architecture of a histiocytoma—dermatofibroma.

Histiocytes Predominate (Granulomatous, Foreign-body Reaction) (Fig. 9-43)

The most common foreign-body reactions in skin are those resulting from *ruptured follicular cysts* (Fig. 9-44). Histologically, these reactions are usually diagnosed with facility because the epithelial-lined cyst or portions of it are readily recognized. Even in long-standing foreign-body granulomas secondary to ruptured follicular cysts, cornified cells (squames) can usually be detected within individual multinucleated histiocytes. If abundant lipid is present within the cyst, foamy histiocytes will be found where

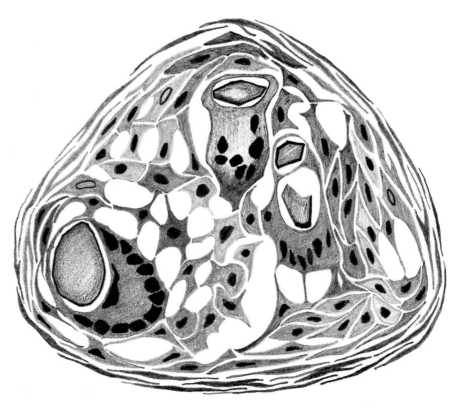

FIG. 9-43. Foreign body granuloma.

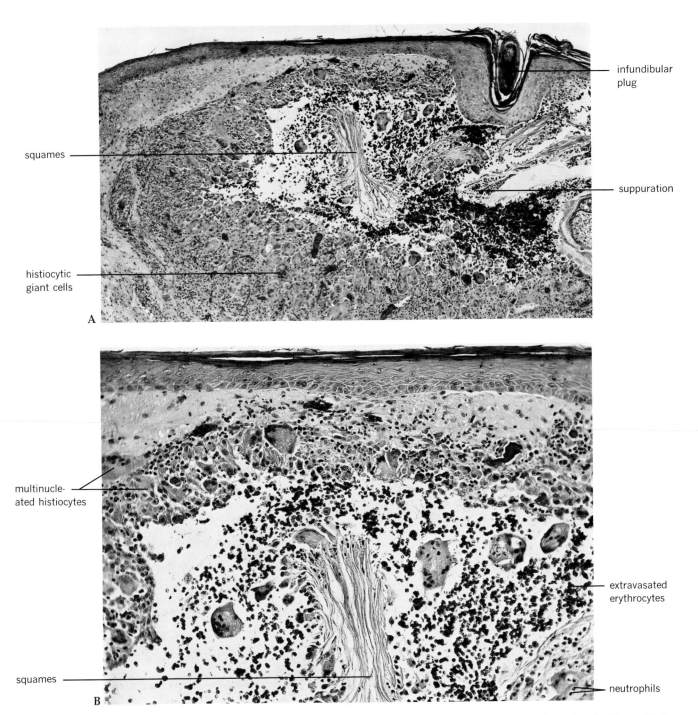

labels on image:
- infundibular plug
- squames
- suppuration
- histiocytic giant cells
- A
- multinucle-ated histiocytes
- extravasated erythrocytes
- squames
- neutrophils
- B

FIG. 9-44. Granulomatous dermatitis following rupture of infundibular cyst. Note spewing of squames into dermis. (A, × 63; B, × 176.)

rupture has occurred. The earliest inflammatory response to rup-tured cysts is suppuration followed by granuloma formation and lastly by fibrosis.

The commonest follicular cyst in skin is lined by epithelium indistinguishable from that of the epidermis and of the hair-fol-licle infundibulum (i.e., epidermoid or infundibular cyst). Milia are tiny infundibular cysts. "Cystic" acne results from rupture of

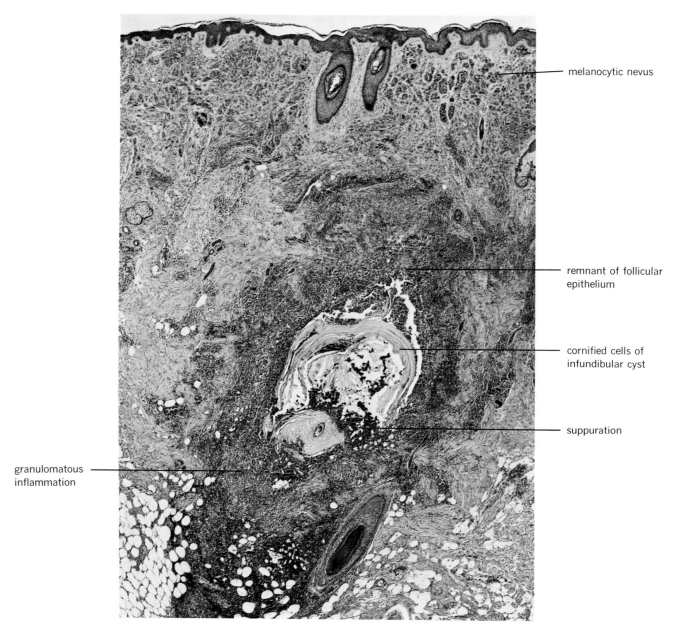

melanocytic nevus

remnant of follicular epithelium

cornified cells of infundibular cyst

suppuration

granulomatous inflammation

FIG. 9-45. Suppurative granulomatous dermatitis secondary to ruptured infundibular cyst beneath intradermal melanocytic nevus. Sequence of rupture, subsequent suppuration, granulomatous inflammation, and fibrosis is not uncommon. Sudden change in pigmented lesion may prompt both patient and physician to suspect malignant melanoma clinically. ($\times$ 29.)

infundibular cysts. A rather common phenomenon is rupture of an infundibular cyst that underlies a melanocytic nevus (Fig. 9-45). A less common follicular cyst occurs predominantly on the scalp, and its epithelial lining is identical to that of the hair follicle isthmus or of a catagen hair (i.e., isthmus-catagen cyst). This cyst has also been termed "trichilemmal cyst" and incorrectly "sebaceous cyst." The only true sebaceous cyst in skin is steatocystoma multiplex whose lining resembles the sebaceous duct.

Beryllium, zirconium and *silica* have been discussed previously in this chapter under sarcoidal granulomas. Mercury used to impart a red color to tattoos also can cause sarcoidal granulomas, as can carbon (Fig. 9-46). In histologic sections, however, most tattoo materials appear black and not all of them elicit an inflammatory response.

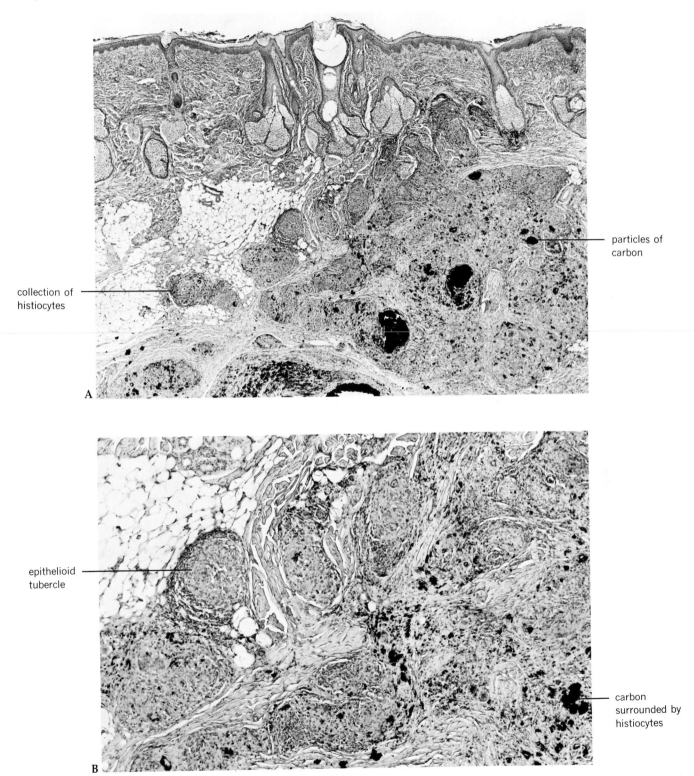

FIG. 9-46. Foreign-body granuloma. Particles of carbon in dermis and subcutaneous fat, seen here as jet black masses of various sizes, are foreign bodies that induce histiocytes to engulf them. (A, × 27; B, × 83.)

Splinters and *sutures* are common foreign bodies in skin. Slivers of wood are recognized histologically by the "stepladder" pattern of cellulose (Fig. 9-10). Sutures are seen as homogeneous pale yellow materials that are refractile with polarizing light (Plate 5). When the bristle of a *cactus* is withdrawn from the skin, its rearward angulated barbs are torn loose, and these induce a granulomatous dermatitis (Fig. 9-47).

Starch is also uncovered by polarizing light and appears as particles in the shape of Maltese crosses. Starch granulomas in skin usually result from starch that is introduced into a wound by surgical gloves.

Abnormal Endogenous Deposits (Urates, Calcium)

Histiocytes may form a palisade around abnormal endogenous deposits such as urates or calcium.

Urates have already been discussed in this chapter under gout (Fig. 9-42).

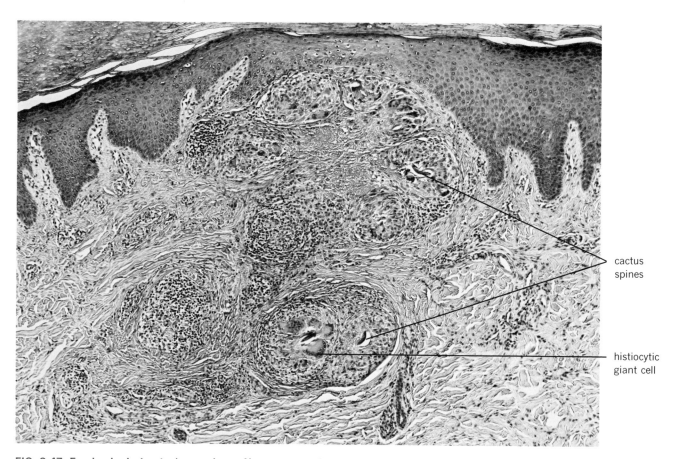

cactus
spines

histiocytic
giant cell

FIG. 9-47. Foreign-body (cactus) granuloma. Note cactus spines surrounded by histiocytes, some of which are multinucleated. Histiocytes in granulomatous focus beneath epidermis are aligned in palisaded array, resembling at first glance the changes in granuloma annulare. (A, × 85; B, × 646.)

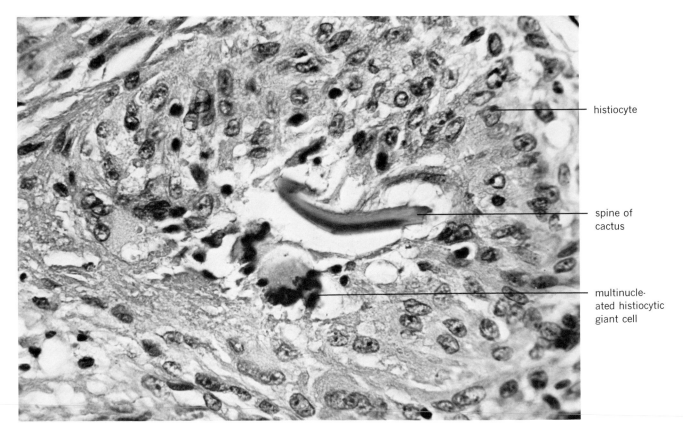

histiocyte

spine of
cactus

multinucle-
ated histiocytic
giant cell

FIG. 9-47. Foreign body (cactus) granuloma. B.

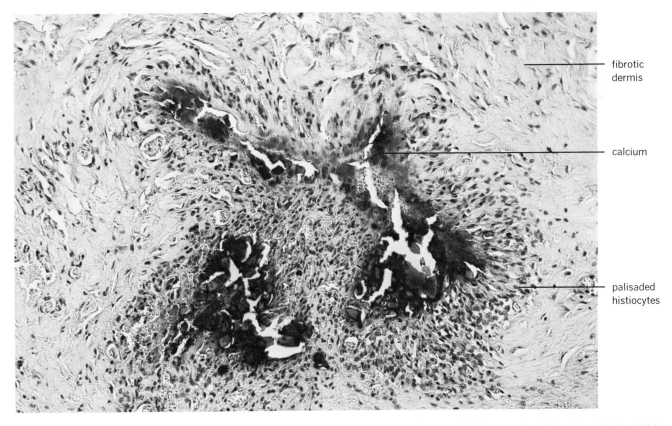

fibrotic
dermis

calcium

palisaded
histiocytes

FIG. 9-48. Calcinosis cutis with palisaded granulomatous dermatitis. Histiocytes form palisade around calcium deposit. ($\times$ 200.)

Calcium may be deposited secondary to tissue injury (dystrophic calcification) in inflammatory processes such as acne vulgaris, tuberculosis, systemic lupus erythematosus, dermatomyositis, and systemic sclerosis and secondary to systemic hypercalcemia as a manifestation of abnormal calcium and/or phosphorus metabolism (metastatic calcification) such as in hyperparathyroidism, hypervitaminosis D, and sarcoidosis. Calcium can elicit a granulomatous reaction when huge calcific deposits occur near joints (pseudotumoral calcinosis, calcific "gout") (Fig. 9-48). In many instances, however, calcium does not evoke an inflammatory response.

Mixed-cell Infiltrate Containing Atypical Mononuclear Cells

In nodular dermatitis with a mixed-cell infiltrate eosinophils and plasma cells are usually seen in addition to lymphocytes and histiocytes. The atypical mononuclear cells are generally lymphoblasts or prolymphocytes, but occasionally they may be immature forms in the histiocytic series.

Pseudolymphomas (Fig. 9-49)

—Dense nodular and/or diffuse mixed inflammatory-cell infiltrate, especially of small lymphocytes, as well as histiocytes, atypical mononuclear cells, and often eosinophils and plasma cells
—Involvement of upper dermis equal to or greater than that of the lower dermis and subcutis
—Prominent vasculature with an increased number of blood vessels having plump endothelial cells
—Polychrome bodies (tingible bodies, nuclear dust) common
—Germinal centers occasionally
—Ectopic lipocytes (adipose metaplasia) sometimes within the infiltrate of the upper dermis
—Epidermal hyperplasia occasionally

Perhaps the most difficult diagnostic problem in cutaneous histopathology concerns the distinction between inflammatory pseudolymphomas and malignant lymphomas (excluding mycosis fungoides and Hodgkin's disease). Pseudolymphoma simply indicates a benign inflammatory simulation of malignant lymphoma and implies nothing about the cause. Pseudolymphomas are dense dermatitides that can be either nodular or diffuse and may extend into the subcutaneous fat.

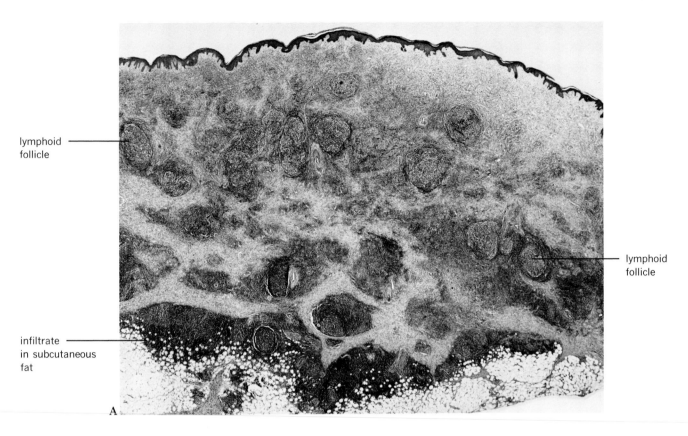

lymphoid
follicle

lymphoid
follicle

infiltrate
in subcutaneous
fat

A

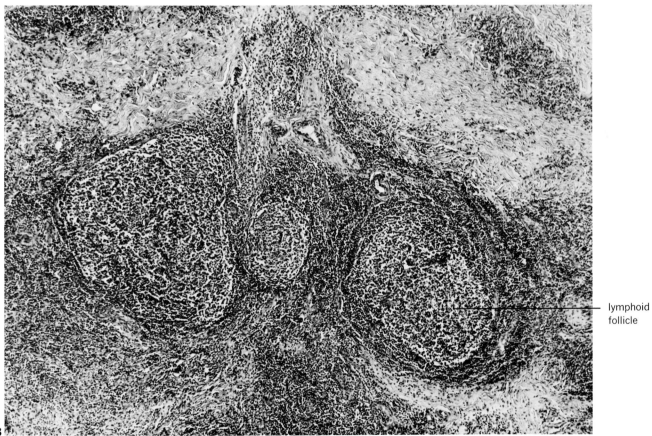

lymphoid
follicle

B

FIG. 9-49. Pseudolymphoma. A, Lymphoid follicles (germinal centers) in nodular infiltrate that is equally dense in upper and lower portions of specimen are diagnostic features. (× 14.) B, Higher magnification of three lymphoid follicles. (× 77.)

In contrast with these histologic features of cutaneous pseudolymphoma, cutaneous malignant lymphoma (Fig. 9-50) has a monomorphous cellular infiltrate, often of blasts rather than small lymphocytes; involvement of the lower part of the dermis is approximately equal to or greater than that of the upper part of the dermis; the vasculature is not prominent; the germinal centers are absent (except for the rare giant follicular malignant lymphoma); polychrome bodies are rare, and epidermal hyperplasia is unusual. Necrosis of blood vessels and adnexal structures, however, is common in malignant lymphoma.

Cytologic features, such as nuclear atypia, increased numbers of mitotic figures, and atypical mitotic figures, are not decisive in differentiating cutaneous pseudolymphoma from cutaneous malignant lymphoma. However, numerous atypical mitotic figures per high power field do favor the diagnosis of malignant lymphoma. The criteria based largely upon architectural pattern outlined above are helpful in most, but not all, cases (Fig. 9-51). The ultimate criterion is biologic behavior, i.e., the clinical course of the disease. Pseudolymphomas behave in a benign fashion, which is in contrast with malignant lymphomas.

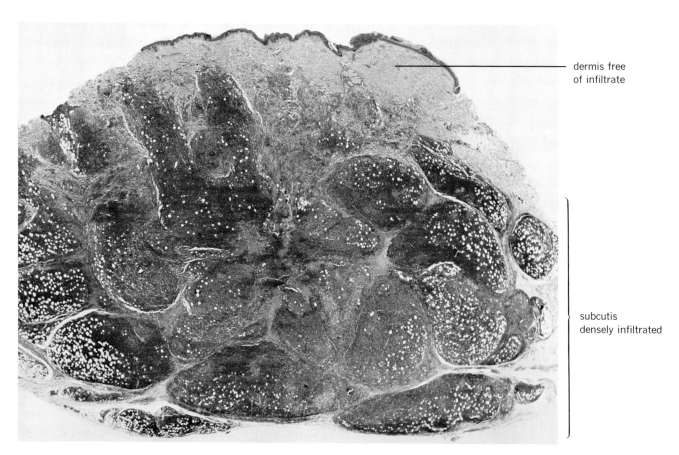

dermis free
of infiltrate

subcutis
densely infiltrated

FIG. 9-50. Cutaneous malignant lymphoma. Salient features are monomorphous mononuclear cell infiltrates denser in lower portion of specimen than in upper part. (× 9.)

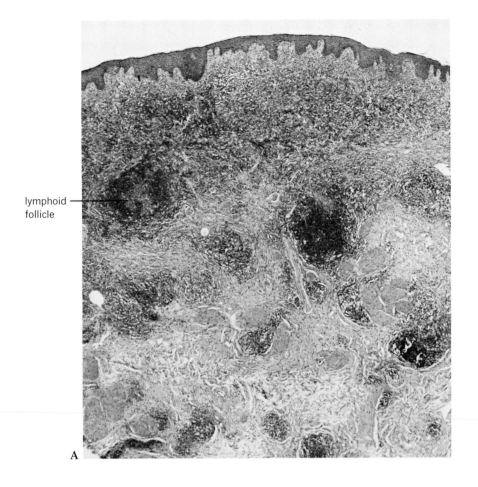

lymphoid
follicle

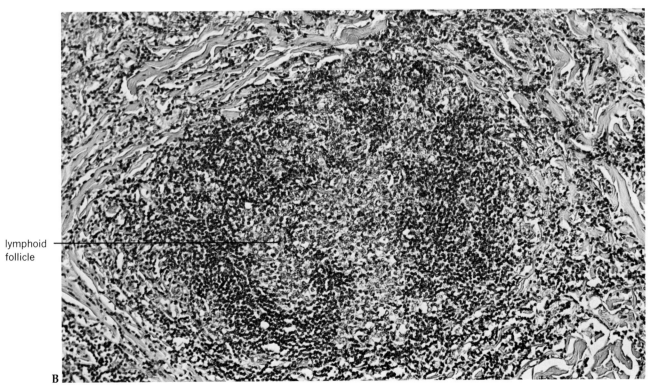

lymphoid
follicle

FIG. 9-51. Pseudolymphoma. This is not a malignant lymphoma because infiltrate is clearly more dense in upper than lower part of dermis and lymphoid follicles (germinal centers) are present. (A, × 27; B, × 174.)

Pseudolymphoma of the skin (lymphocytoma cutis, lymphadenosis benigna cutis or Spiegler-Fendt sarcoid, cutaneous lymphoplasia, cutaneous lymphoid hyperplasia, lymphadenoid granuloma) has been reported to develop following trauma, insect bites (Fig. 9-52), vaccinations, hyposensitization injections, and drug administration (such as of hydantoin and hydantoin-like drugs), although in most patients the cause remains obscure. Nodular lesions of scabies, which are nodular both clinically and histologi-

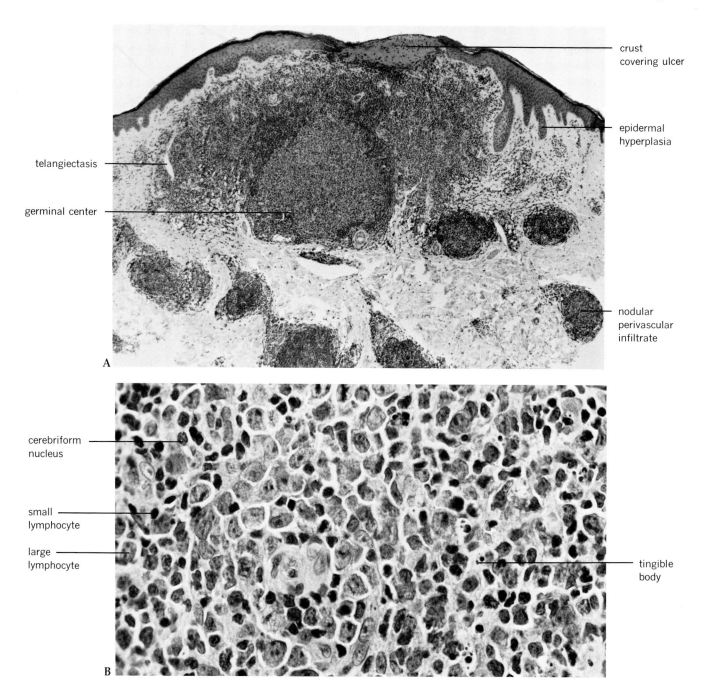

FIG. 9-52. Pseudolymphoma induced by tick bite. Ulcer indicates point of entry, and dense nodular inflammatory infiltrates containing lymphoid follicles harboring atypical mononuclear cells represent response to products of insect. Note dense infiltrate in upper part of dermis and many germinal centers, features of pseudolymphomas. (A, × 82; B, × 766.)

cally, often have the histologic appearance of pseudolymphoma (Fig. 9-53). Cutaneous pseudolymphoma, unlike cutaneous malignant lymphoma, is usually wholly confined to the skin. Although malignant lymphoma, except for mycosis fungoides, can in rare instances originate in the skin, the majority of cutaneous lymphomatous lesions are secondary to known or occult systemic involvement.

Just as cutaneous pseudolymphoma may histologically mimic cutaneous malignant lymphoma, so, too, these processes may be dificult to distinguish from one another clinically. Both may be either solitary or multiple nodules, reddish-purple or plum-colored. Nodules of malignant lymphoma tend to ulcerate, whereas those of pseudolymphoma do not.

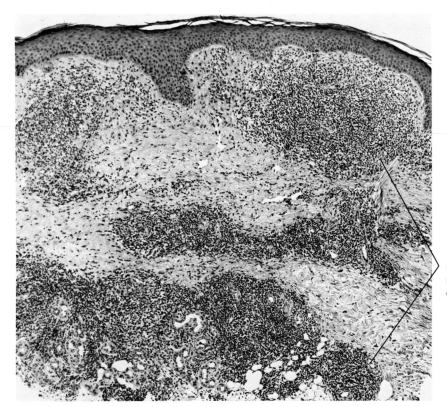

nodules of
mixed inflammatory
cells

FIG. 9-53. Nodular scabies. Dense dermal infiltrate consists of lymphocytes, histiocytes, plasma cells, and usually numerous eosinophils. ($\times$ 66.)

Diffuse Dermatitis

As in dermatitides with the nodular histologic pattern, those with the diffuse histologic pattern may be subdivided according to the type of inflammatory cells that are prominent in the infiltrate: neutrophils, histiocytes, plasma cells, mast cells, and a mixture of them.

Neutrophils Predominate

Granuloma Faciale (Fig. 9-54)

Granuloma faciale is a dense diffuse dermatitis with a distinctive histologic pattern because its infiltrate spares the papillary-periadnexal dermis. Only during the early phase of this long-standing pathologic process is the infiltrate primarily composed of neutrophils, usually in concert with leukocytoclastic vasculitis (see Chapter 8). Later, eosinophils are the predominant cells, and they are followed by lymphocytes, plasma cells, and finally by fibroblasts. The process begins as a leukocytoclastic vasculitis and ends with fibrosis but is usually not granulomatous.

Clinically the solitary or multiple papules, nodules, or plaques of granuloma faciale are of different colors, ranging from pink-orange to yellow-brown, depending upon the stage of the disease, and are characterized by widened, patulous follicular openings.

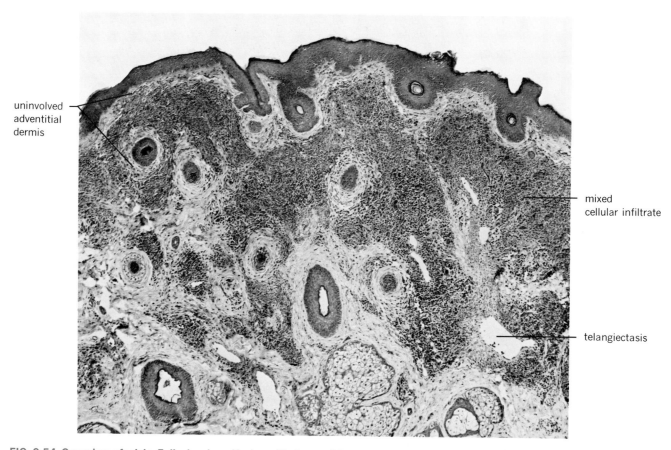

uninvolved adventitial dermis

mixed cellular infiltrate

telangiectasis

FIG. 9-54. Granuloma faciale. Fully developed lesion with dense, diffuse, mixed inflammatory-cell infiltrate of lymphocytes, plasma cells, histiocytes, and numerous eosinophils. Characteristically the infiltrate spares the papillary and periadnexal dermis (adventitial dermis). (A, × 75; B, × 352.)

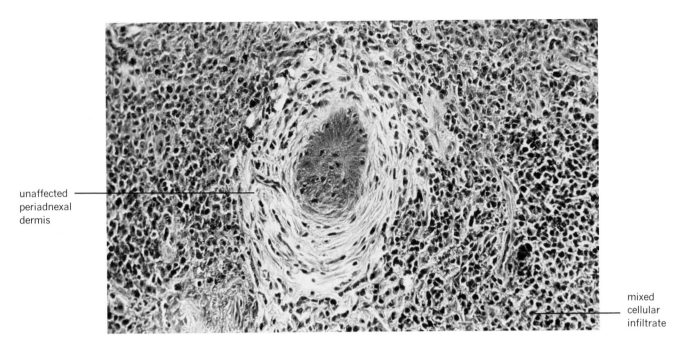

unaffected periadnexal dermis

mixed cellular infiltrate

FIG. 9-54. Granuloma faciale (continued). B.

Erythema Elevatum Diutinum

Erythema elevatum diutinum, a nodular and plaque expression of chronic leukocytoclastic vasculitis, may appear histologically as a dense predominantly neutrophilic dermatitis in which eosinophils, lymphocytes, plasma cells, and histiocytes can be found (see Chapter 8). In rare instances only a diffuse neutrophilic dermatitis without vasculitis is seen.

Clinically, erythema elevatum diutinum consists of symmetrical red-purple plaques and nodules overlying joints, especially the phalangeal joints, on the dorsa of the hands, the elbows, and knees. The lesions tend to persist for months and even years.

Rheumatoid Neutrophilic Dermatitis (Fig. 9-55)

Rheumatoid neutrophilic dermatitis is a rare disease that occurs only in patients with severe "malignant" rheumatoid arthritis and consists histologically of a dense, diffuse, predominantly neutrophilic infiltrate that involves the entire dermis. The neutrophils are so numerous in the dermal papillae that they form abscesses resembling those of dermatitis herpetiformis. Lymphocytes, plasma cells, histiocytes, multinucleated histiocytes, and eosinophils are scattered throughout the dense diffuse dermal neutrophilic infiltrate. Capillaries and venules are widely dilated, but there is no vasculitis.

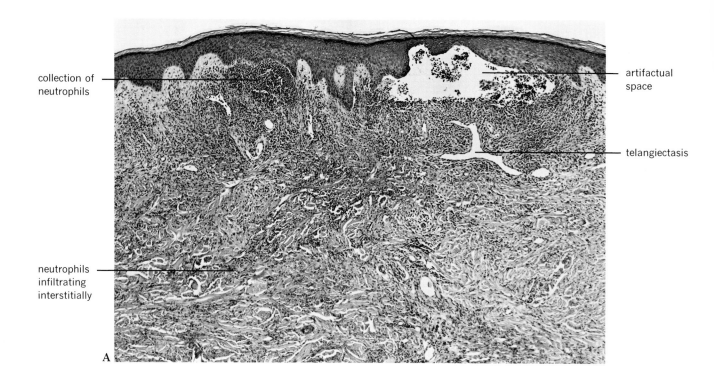

collection of neutrophils —

artifactual space

telangiectasis

neutrophils infiltrating interstitially —

A

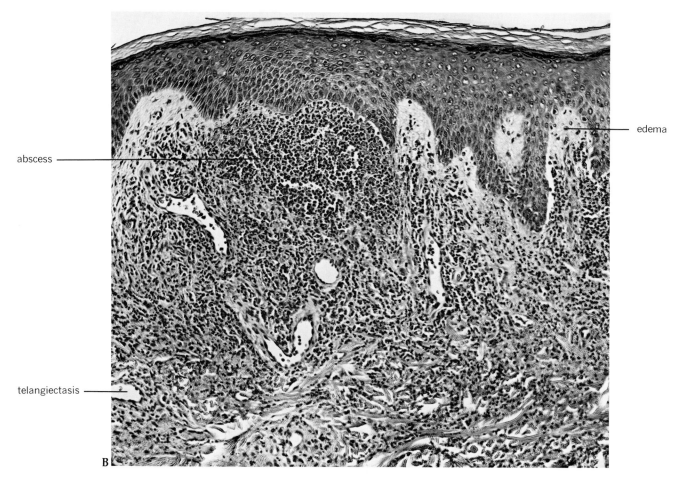

edema

abscess —

telangiectasis —

B

FIG. 9-55. Rheumatoid neutrophilic dermatitis. Note dense diffuse infiltrate of neutrophils. Space beneath epidermis is site where neutrophils were lost in processing. The condition resembles erythema elevatum diutinum except for lack of vasculitic features such as fibrin within walls of capillaries and venules. (A, × 70; B, × 190.)

Clinically, rheumatoid neutrophilic dermatitis closely resembles erythema elevatum diutinum and consists of symmetrical red-purple plaques and nodules overlying the joints, especially those of the dorsa of the hands, as well as the joints of the elbows and knees. Rheumatoid neutrophilic dermatitis differs from erythema elevatum diutinum histologically by the lack of vasculitis.

Pyoderma Gangrenosum (Fig. 9-56)

Fully developed lesions of pyoderma gangrenosum show ulceration; beneath the ulcer is a dense, diffuse, predominantly neutrophilic infiltrate extending throughout the dermis and sometimes into the subcutaneous fat. The papillary dermis is edematous and contains many neutrophils and extravasated erythrocytes. Subepidermal vesiculation results from massive papillary dermal edema; intraepidermal vesiculation results from intracellular edema; and pustules from collections of neutrophils within epidermis.

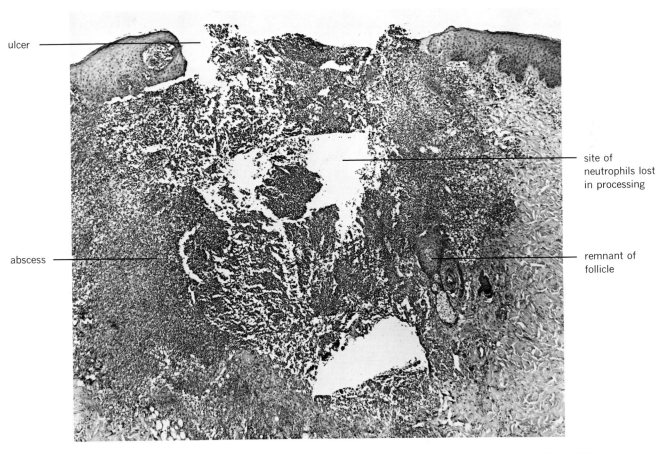

FIG. 9-56. Pyoderma gangrenosum. A, Early ulcerated lesion apparently the result of rupture of hair follicle with consequent suppuration which then drained to skin surface. Spaces in dermis are artifacts of preparation. (× 39.)

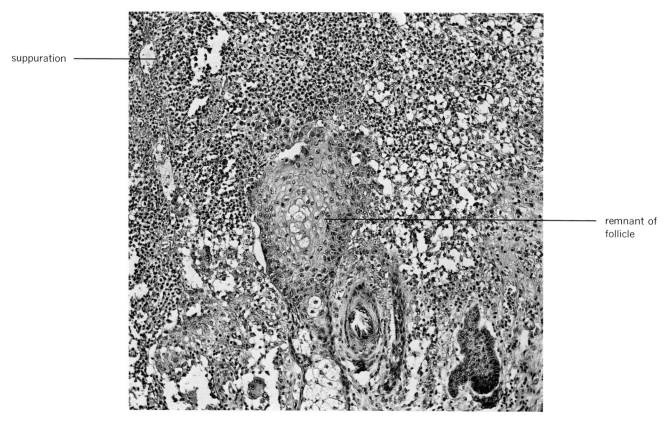

suppuration

remnant of follicle

FIG. 9-56. Pyoderma gangrenosum. B, Higher magnification of follicular remnant and surrounding abscess. (× 134.)

Because biopsies of this destructive process are usual only during its ulcerative phase, the critical early histologic changes are not commonly appreciated. Biopsy of early lesions of pyoderma gangrenosum may reveal necrotizing vasculitis that involves small blood vessels in the dermis and in the subcutis. The histologic expression of this necrotizing vasculitis is fibrin deposition and neutrophils in blood-vessel walls. In other early lesions, there is suppuration both within and around a ruptured follicular unit (Fig. 9-57). These findings suggest that pyoderma gangrenosum may begin as either a vasculitis or a folliculitis.

Clinically, pyoderma gangrenosum begins as a vesiculopustular process extending peripherally, leaving a slightly depressed central crust. These nummular crusted lesions ulcerate, and the ulcer develops distinctive undermined edges, a dusky bluish-violet border, and a red areola. The ulcers slowly advance centrifugally, some attaining a diameter as large as 10 or more centimeters. They heal with atrophic scars.

Crops of vesiculopustules that simulate the clinical lesions of dermatitis herpetiformis may be associated with pyoderma gangrenosum. The tense vesiculopustules do not necessarily proceed to necrosis and ulceration, but may resolve spontaneously, leaving no sequellae.

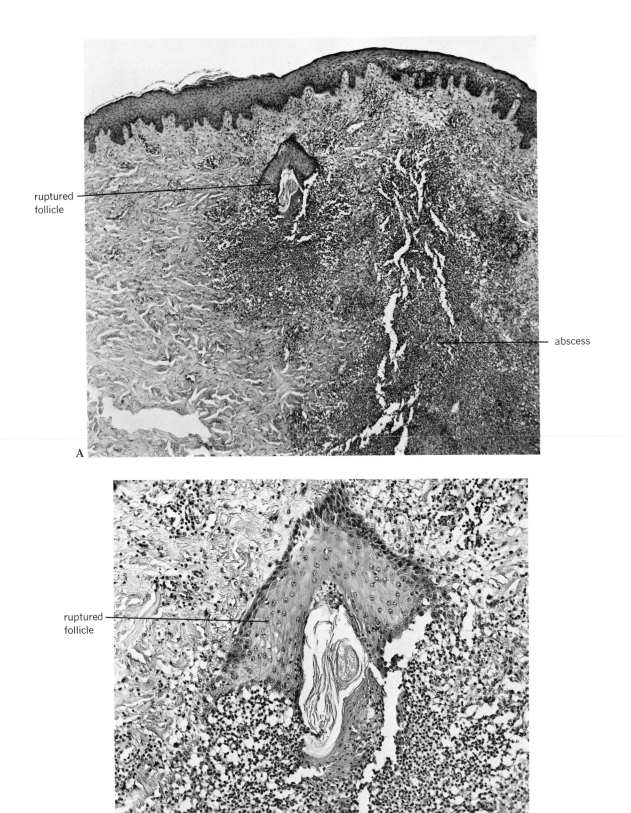

FIG. 9-57. Pyoderma gangrenosum. Early, nonulcerated lesions often show dense infiltrate of neutrophils adjacent to ruptured hair follicle. (A, × 38; B, × 134.)

Many patients with pyoderma gangrenosum have ulcerative colitis, and some rheumatoid arthritis. The condition has also appeared in association with regional enteritis, chronic active hepatitis, and paraproteinemias.

Neutrophils and Histiocytes Predominate (Suppurative Granulomatous Dermatitis) (Fig. 9-58)

Suppurative granulomatous dermatitis describes an inflammatory process that has both granulomatous (i.e., composed predominantly of histiocytes) and suppurative (i.e., composed of neutrophils that form abscesses) features. The suppurative granulomatous dermatitides include (1) deep fungal infections, candida granuloma, and kerion; (2) atypical mycobacterial infections and tuberculosis verrucosa cutis; (3) actinomycosis, nocardiosis, and mycetoma; (4) protothecosis; (5) halogenodermas; and (6) the follicular-occlusion tetrad.

With Epidermal Hyperplasia (Fig. 9-59)

The suppurative granulomatous dermatitides can be subdivided according to the presence or absence of significant epidermal hyperplasia. The commonest histologic presentation of the suppurative type with epidermal hyperplasia is typified by the deep fungal and atypical mycobacterial infections. In fact, in the absence of identifiable organisms, it may be impossible to differentiate histologically between some deep fungal infections, such as sporotrichosis, and some atypical mycobacterial infections, such as swimming-pool granuloma.

—Severe papillated epidermal and often trichilemmal hyperplasia
—Infundibula widely dilated by scale-crust
—Abscesses within the hyperplastic epidermis and the infundibular epithelium
—Dense diffuse mixed inflammatory-cell infiltrate involving at least the superficial dermis and composed of neutrophils, histiocytes, multinucleated histiocytes, plasma cells, lymphocytes, and often eosinophils
—Abscesses in the superficial dermis
—Epithelioid tubercles occasionally
—Widely dilated thick-walled blood vessels with plump endothelial cells
—Varying degrees of edema and fibrosis in the upper part of the dermis, depending on the stage of the disease

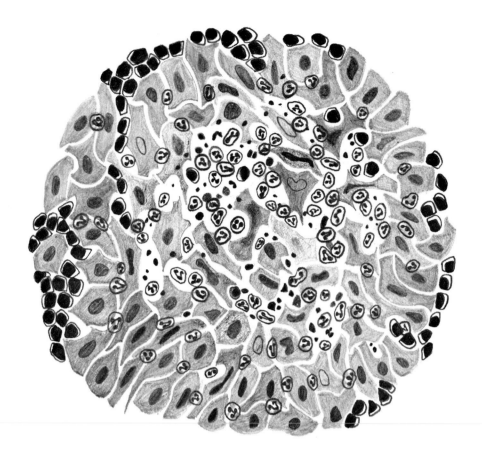

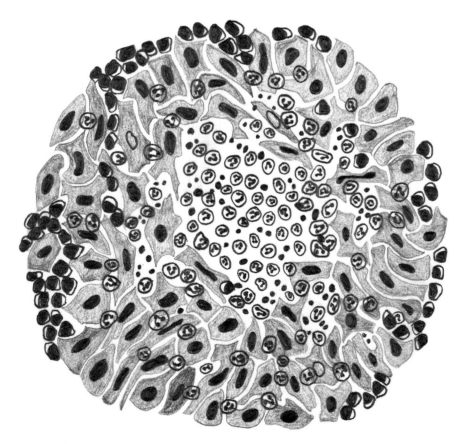

FIG. 9-58. Suppurative granulomas.

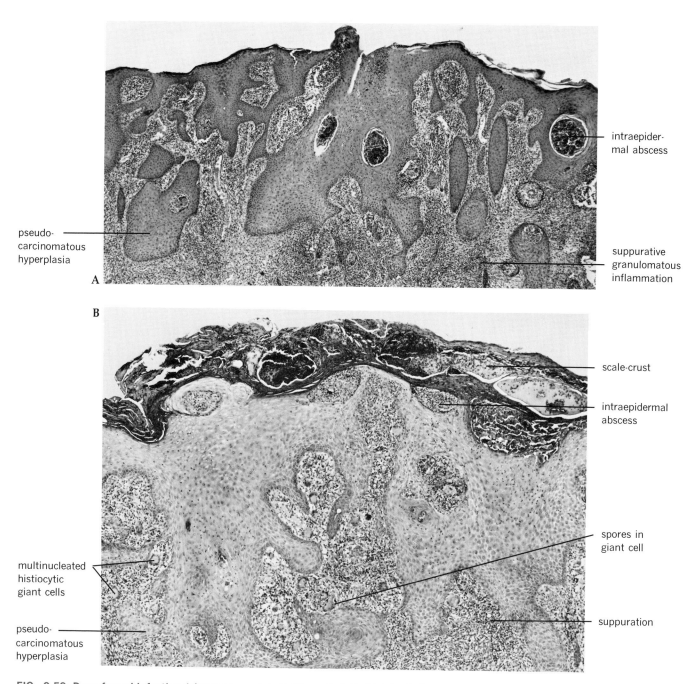

FIG. 9-59. Deep fungal infection (chromomycosis). A, Characteristic histologic feature is combination of pseudocarcinomatous hyperplasia overlying suppurative granulomatous dermatitis. (× 50.) B, Spores, in this case of chromomycosis, are most readily found in histiocytic giant cells and in abscesses. (× 66.) See also Plate 3.

Histologically, these fungal and bacterial diseases are characterized initially by a neutrophilic response, followed by a predominantly histiocytic infiltrate that also contains neutrophils, eosinophils, lymphocytes, and plasma cells and, eventually, by fibrosis. The clinical counterparts to these histologic changes of fungal and atypical mycobacterial granulomas are verrucous, sometimes pustular, nodules covered by vegetative scales and crusts that in time resolve with scar.

Deep Fungal and Atypical Mycobacterial Infections. The unequivocal diagnosis of deep fungal and atypical mycobacterial infections requires the demonstration of a causative organism (Fig. 9-60). When fungi are present, they can usually be detected in hematoxylin-and-eosin-stained sections. This is especially true of the thick-walled budding spores of *North American blastomycosis*, the single and multiple budding spores of *paracoccidioidomycosis* that resemble a mariner's wheel, the dark brown oval spores of *chromomycosis* that have been compared to copper pennies (Fig. 9-61), the groups and chains of round spores connected to one another by short tubes of *keloidal blastomycosis* (Lobo's disease), and the large thick-walled spores of *coccidioidomycosis* that contain endospores (Fig. 9-62). The huge sporangia of *rhinosporidiosis*, containing hundreds of round spores, are also distinctive, as are the lymphocyte-like spores of *cryptococcosis*, surrounded by their huge clear capsules. The hyphae and spores of *candidal granuloma* can be recognized by budding yeast cells and pseudomycelia (Fig. 9-63). The organisms of each of these diseases often can be found lying free within abscesses or within the cytoplasm of histiocytes, especially multinucleated ones. These various spores and hyphae are sometimes better demonstrated with PAS or silver methenamine stains. In the case of sporotrichosis the spores are best seen when diastase has first been applied to the tissue section, followed by staining with PAS (Fig. 9-64).

Ziehl-Neelsen stain is necessary to demonstrate the acid-fast rods of *atypical mycobacterial infections. Swimming pool granuloma* is caused by the direct inoculation of the skin by Mycobacterium marinum. In size the atypical mycobacteria are longer and broader than the tubercle bacilli. However, even with a special stain, it may be impossible to visualize the organisms in tissue sections. They are best detected in foci of necrosis and suppuration.

Tuberculosis Verrucosa Cutis. Tuberculoid granulomas with prominent papillated epidermal hyperplasia and hyperkeratosis are seen in tuberculosis verrucosa cutis. Varying amounts of suppuration and fibrosis can be seen, depending on the stage of the disease. Tubercle bacilli cannot usually be detected even with acid-fast stains. Clinically, the verrucous plaques are also called "anatomic tubercle" or "prosector's wart" because in days past they resulted from direct inoculation of tubercle bacilli into a previously sensitized person who had handled diseased tissue.

Actinomycosis, Nocardiosis, Mycetoma, and Botryomycosis. The microorganisms of actinomycosis appear histologically as granular colonies composed of filaments from which club-shaped processes radiate. In sections stained by hematoxylin and eosin the central portion of the granules appears bluish, and the peripheral

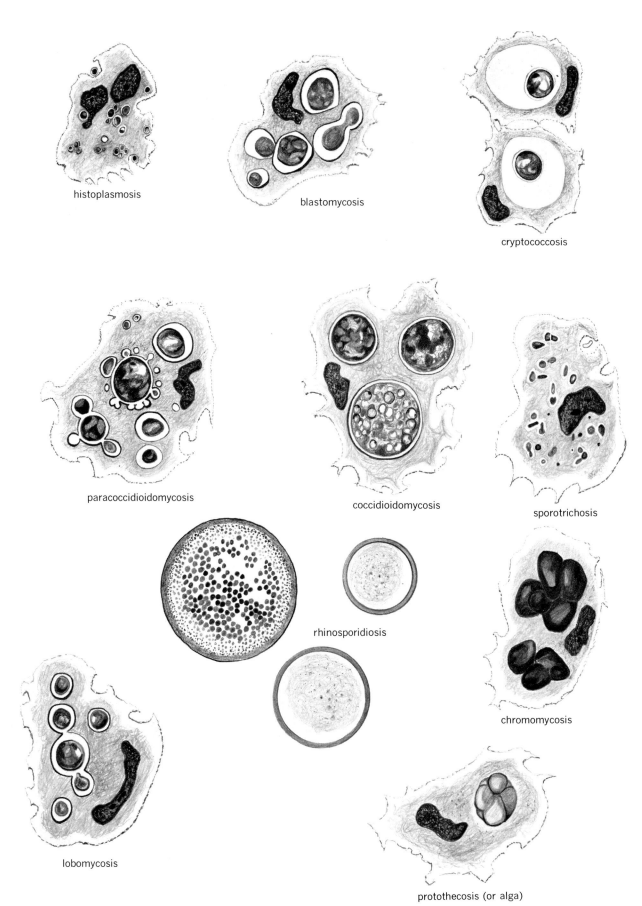

histoplasmosis

blastomycosis

cryptococcosis

paracoccidioidomycosis

coccidioidomycosis

sporotrichosis

rhinosporidiosis

chromomycosis

lobomycosis

protot500thecosis (or alga)

FIG. 9-60. Fungal organisms. Protot501thecosis is an alga.

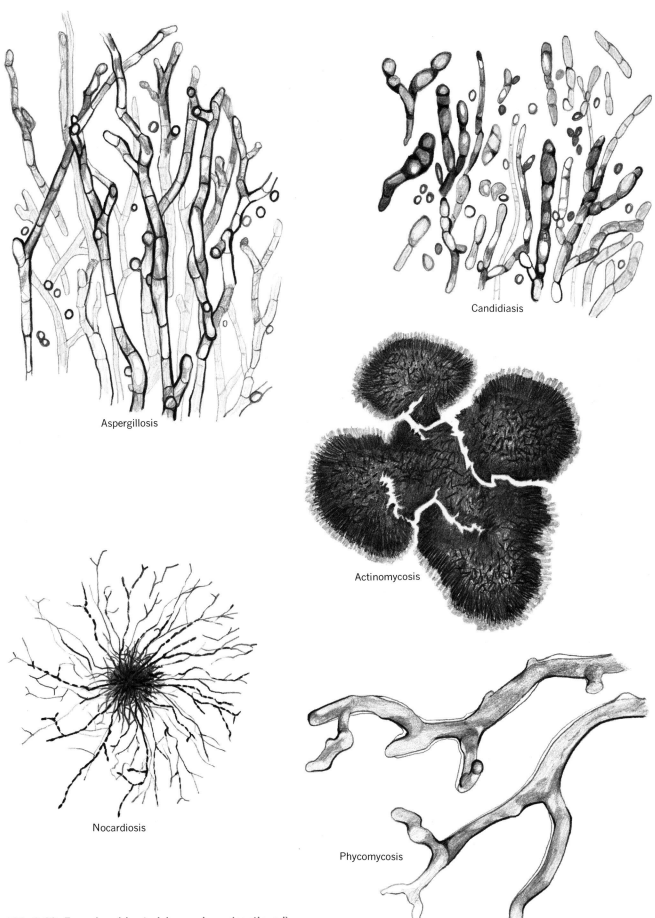

Aspergillosis

Candidiasis

Actinomycosis

Nocardiosis

Phycomycosis

FIG. 9-60. Fungal and bacterial organisms (continued).

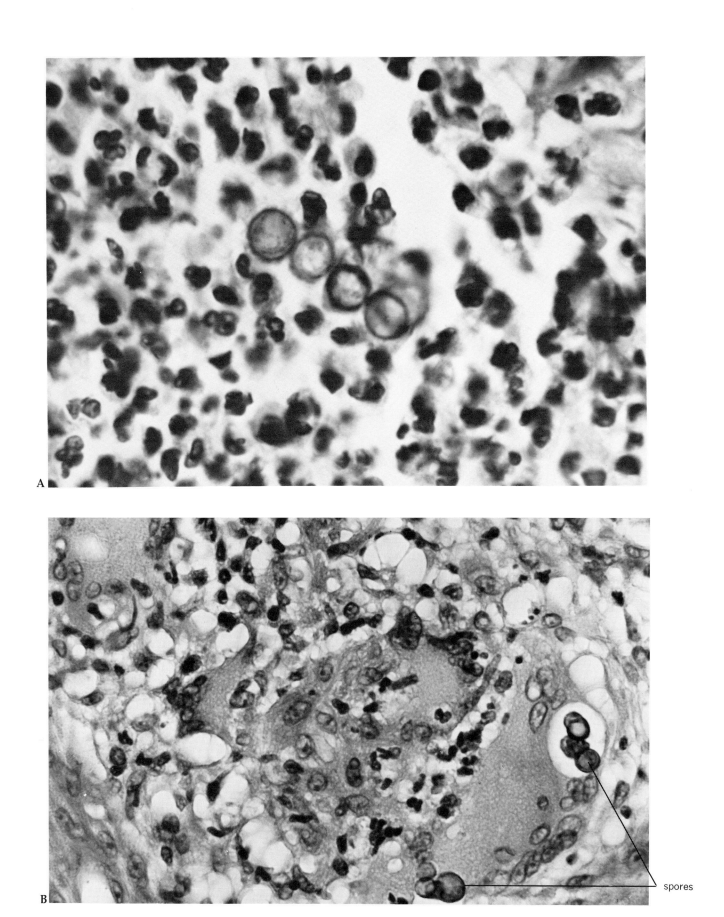

FIG. 9-61. Chromomycosis. A, Four large, round, brown spores are seen within dermal abscess. (× 1,700.) B, Note spores in histiocytic giant cells.

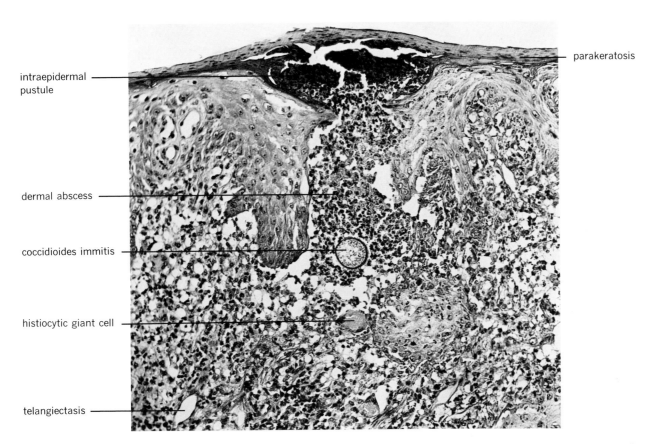

intraepidermal pustule

parakeratosis

dermal abscess

coccidioides immitis

histiocytic giant cell

telangiectasis

FIG. 9-62. Coccidioidomycosis. Within abscess surrounded by pseudocarcinomatous hyperplasia and granulomatous inflammation sits endospore containing spherules of Coccidioides immitis. (× 180.)

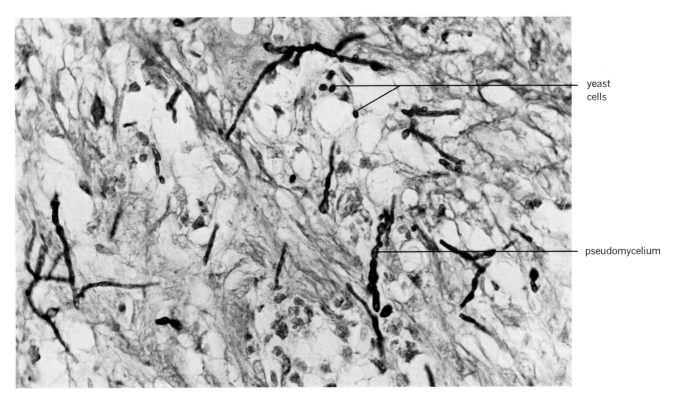

yeast cells

pseudomycelium

FIG. 9-63. Candida granuloma. Typical morphologic features in section stained by PAS are budding yeast cells and pseudomycelia, which are budding yeast cells that remain attached and give appearance of filament. (× 635.)

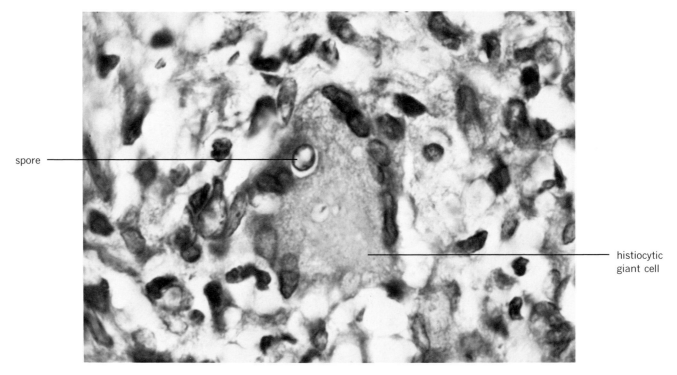

spore

histiocytic giant cell

FIG. 9-64. Sporotrichosis. Round spore engulfed by multinucleated histiocytic giant cell has been demonstrated by first applying diastase to section to remove other obscuring materials that are PAS positive and then staining it with PAS. (× 1950.)

clubs are reddish. The filaments are gram-positive, but not acid-fast. The granules are lodged in dermal abscesses that are surrounded by successive zones of granulomatous inflammation and fibrosis. Sinus tracts tend to extend from the abscesses to the skin surface. By contrast, the filamentous organisms of *nocardiosis* are partly acid-fast and have less tendency to form granules. Abscesses with sinus tracts, granulomas, and fibrosis also occur in nocardiosis. *Mycetomas* can also be caused by a variety of fungi that have in common the production of granules and of suppurative granulomatous inflammation (Plate 3). The most common cause of mycetoma in the United States is Allescheria boydii. *Botryomycosis* is a bacterial mycetoma. Within the abscesses of this chronic suppurative granulomatous dermatitis and panniculitis are granules composed of innumerable staphylococci. A pseudomycetoma may result from infections of skin caused by Pseudomonas aeruginosa (Fig. 9-8).

Protothecosis is caused by algae that are capable of growing, not only in the dermis, but also in subcutaneous tissue and lymph nodes. Prototheca are identified in histologic sections as nonbudding spores with characteristic septations (Fig. 9-65). Clinical manifestations of protothecosis vary from verrucous hyperkeratoses to ulcerations. The organisms may enter lymphatics and induce granulomatous lymphadenitis.

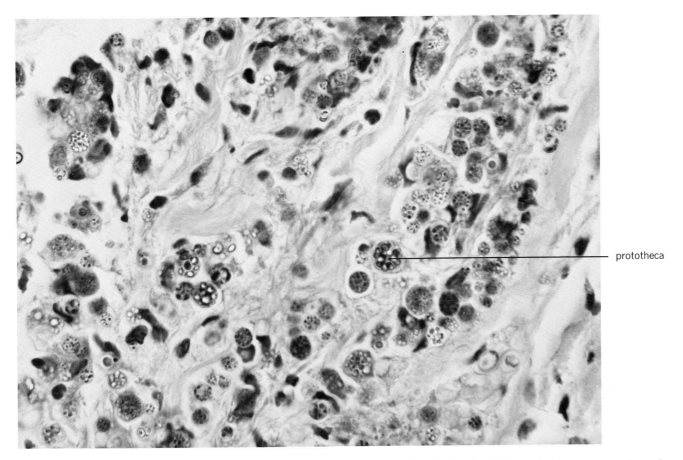

prototheca

FIG. 9-65. Protothecosis. Opalescent algae pictured here may be found inside and outside of histiocytes. Each sporangium of protothecosis contains endospores within which there are at most eight daughter cells. See also Plate 3.

Halogenodermas. The halogenodermas are differentiated from the deep fungal infections of skin by the absence of organisms and by the primarily follicular nature of the process. The follicular infundibula in halogenodermas are widely dilated and filled with cornified cells and numerous neutrophils. Abscesses form within infundibular epithelium and in the upper part of the dermis. Rupture of the dilated infundibula precipitates a neutrophilic reaction within the superficial dermis. When elastic fibers are intimately associated with the tiny abscesses at the base of the ruptured infundibula, which can occur in other folliculitides, there is a striking resemblance histologically to elastosis perforans serpiginosa. These early changes are followed by a mononuclear-cell reaction and ultimately by fibrosis.

Some early lesions in florid eruptions caused by iodides and bromides have little or no epidermal hyperplasia, but rather a dense dermal nodular or diffuse mixed inflammatory-cell infiltrate that consists mostly of neutrophils (Fig. 9-66). Within these suppurative lesions there are often numerous eosinophils and atypical mononuclear cells. These atypical mononuclear cells, with large

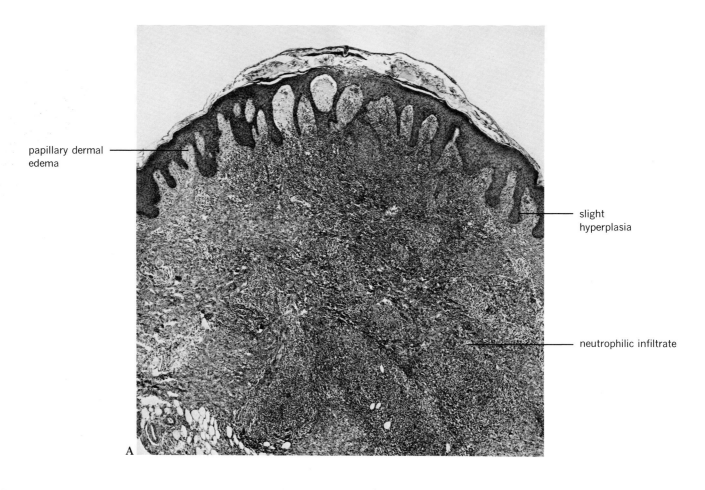

papillary dermal
edema

slight
hyperplasia

neutrophilic infiltrate

A

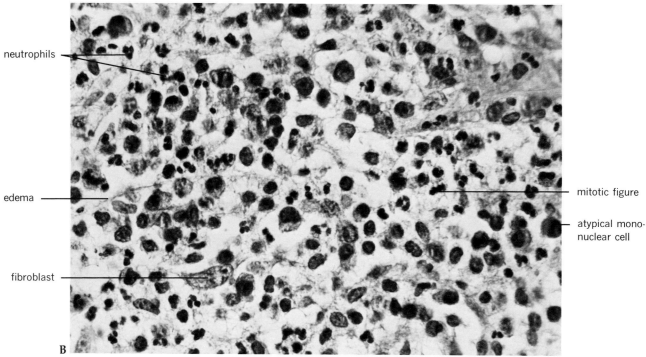

neutrophils

edema

fibroblast

B

mitotic figure

atypical mono-
nuclear cell

FIG. 9-66. Halogenoderma. A, In early lesion caused by ingestion of iodides, dermal infiltrate is dense, diffuse, and composed mostly of neutrophils and epidermis is only slightly hyperplastic. (× 29.) B, Still higher magnification shows mixed inflammatory-cell infiltrate composed mostly of neutrophils but also containing many atypical mononuclear cells, some of which are in mitosis, in an edematous dermis. (× 836.)

nuclei and prominent nucleoli, are sometimes in mitosis. The neutrophils may enter the epidermis where they form spongiform pustules. The papillary dermis of these lesions is usually edematous, and subepidermal vesiculation may develop. Clinically, the halogenodermas, like the deep fungal infections, are usually crusted, verrucous nodules and plaques whose surfaces may be peppered with follicular pustules. The early florid lesions consist of indurated papulopustules and nodulopustules.

Follicular-occlusion Tetrad. The follicular-occlusion tetrad includes acne conglobata, dissecting cellulitis of the scalp, hidradenitis suppurativa, and pilonidal sinus. Each of these processes has in common rupture of a follicular unit or cyst with resultant abscess formation. In some instances sinuses form in an attempt to contain the exuberant suppuration. These conditions proceed through granuloma formation to scarring. Hidradenitis is a misnomer because the eccrine and apocrine glands are affected only secondarily as a consequence of follicular rupture and abscess development. The only clue to the follicular relationship of these diseases may be the finding of either individual cornified cells (squames) within histiocytes or multinucleated histiocytes in the dermis. Sometimes hyperplastic or fragmented epithelium, the remains of the original follicular unit, may be visible, and often the infiltrate of mixed inflammatory cells is so dense that the inciting hair follicle cause can only be presumed, not detected.

Without Epidermal Hyperplasia

Included in the suppurative granulomatous dermatitides without epidermal hyperplasia are ruptured follicular cysts and other foreign body reactions. These were described earlier in the chapter.

Histocytes with Foamy or Granular Cytoplasm Predominate (Fig. 9-67)

Xanthomas

—Foamy histiocytes (foam cells) in nodular or diffuse dermal accumulations
—Sprinkling of lymphocytes perivascularly
—Epidermis usually thin

Xanthomas can be thought of as inflammations, hyperplasias, neoplasias, or deposits. Because they can mimic other granulomatous dermatitides, e.g., lepromatous leprosy, they are discussed

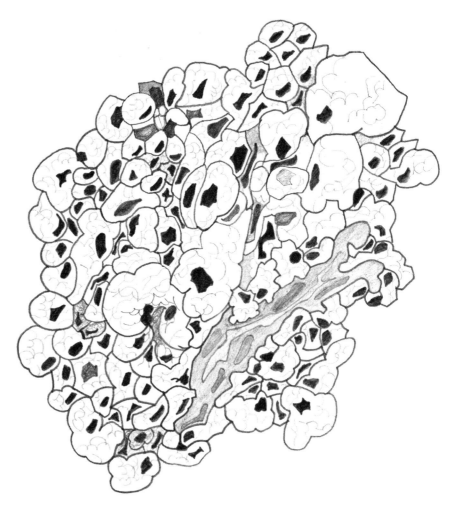

FIG. 9-67. Xanthogranuloma.

here. Fundamental to all xanthomas are foamy histiocytes whose lipid content imparts a yellowish hue to the skin lesions. Initially, these histiocytes are perivascular, and their progressive accumulation leads to nodular and diffuse configurations. The many morphologic variants of xanthoma can usually be distinguished grossly and microscopically. Clinical forms of xanthomas are termed tuberous, tuberoeruptive, eruptive, striate, palmar, plane, nodular, and tendon. The differing sizes of these xanthomas are a function of the number and distribution of foamy histiocytes within the dermis. In addition to the foamy histiocytes in eruptive xanthomas, there is an inflammatory-cell mixture of predominantly neutrophils and lymphocytes (Fig. 9-68). In xanthelasmas a sparse infiltrate of lymphocytes is often scattered among the many large foamy histiocytes (Fig. 9-69). Lipochrome pigment is often visible within the cytoplasm of foam cells in xanthelasmas, yellow plaques that occur invariably on the eyelids.

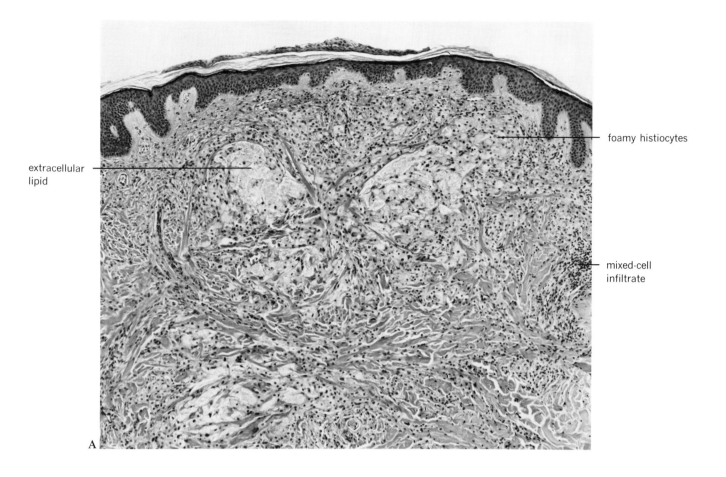

extracellular
lipid

foamy histiocytes

mixed-cell
infiltrate

A

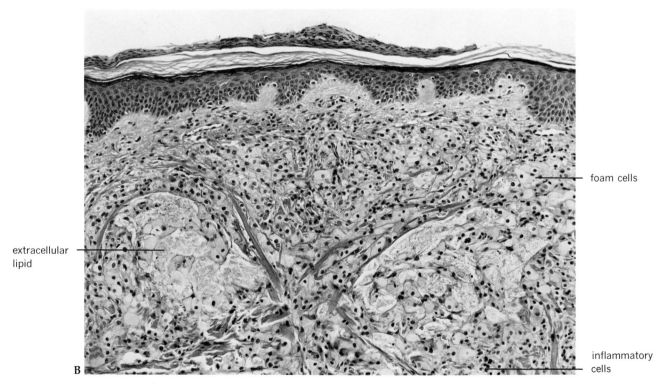

extracellular
lipid

foam cells

inflammatory
cells

B

FIG. 9-68. Eruptive xanthoma. Histologic characteristics are lipid both within histiocytes and extracellularly and sprinkling of lymphocytes and neutrophils. Interposition of histiocytes between collagen bundles must be differentiated from histiocytes of granuloma annulare in which cytoplasm is not foamy. (A, × 92; B, × 180.)

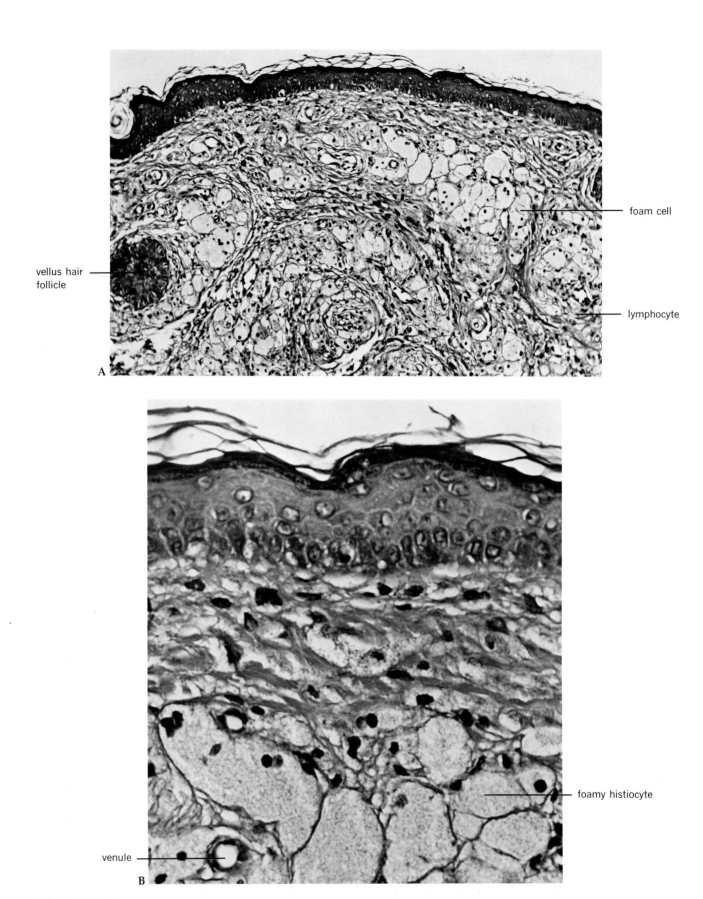

FIG. 9-69. Xanthelasma. Histiocytes of various sizes and shapes, whose cytoplasm is laden with abundant lipid, are present throughout upper part of dermis in lesion from an eyelid. Lymphocytes are sparsely scattered among foamy histiocytes. (A, × 187; B, × 600.)

All patients with xanthomas should undergo serum tests for fasting levels of triglycerides and cholesterol and for lipoprotein electrophoresis which may indicate the type of abnormality in lipid metabolism. Some lipid abnormalities and associated xanthomas may be reversible by dietary and medical therapy. Not all xanthomas, however, are associated with hyperlipoproteinemia.

In some xanthomas, such as eruptive ones, the dermal lipid presumably spills over from the blood. In the case of histiocytomas, the dermal lipid originates from serum and erythrocytes that enter the skin secondary to injury. In other foam cell infiltrates, such as in lepromatous leprosy, the lipid results from intracellular bacterial components. In still other foam cell diseases in skin, such as xanthogranulomas, reticulohistiocytic granulomas, and xanthoma disseminatum, the source of the lipid that comes to be deposited in the skin is unknown.

Xanthoma Disseminatum (Fig. 9-70)

Histologically, these lesions are xanthogranulomas that consist of foamy cells and multinucleated foam cells, some of them of the Touton type. Unlike the juvenile and adult xanthogranulomas, those of xanthoma disseminatum are not associated with eosinophils and plasma cells, do not undergo prominent fibrosis, and do not resolve spontaneously. Unlike the situation in reticulohistiocytic granulomas, the cytoplasm of histiocytes does not resemble ground glass.

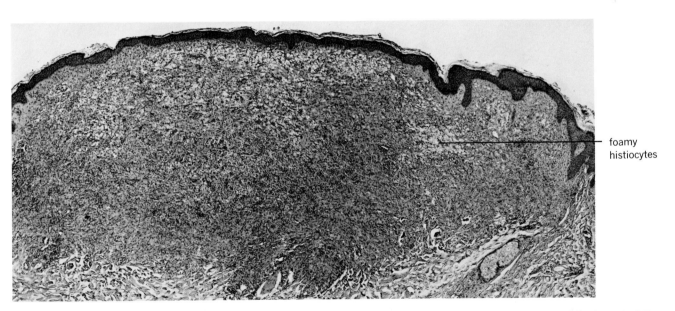

foamy
histiocytes

FIG. 9-70. Xanthoma disseminatum. Dense diffuse infiltrate of foamy histiocytes, some of them multinucleated, is characteristic. Note that the more foamy histiocytes are concentrated in upper part of dermis. (A, × 35; B, × 174.)

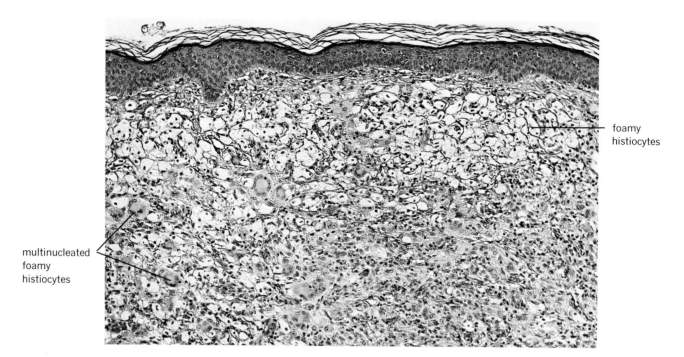

foamy
histiocytes

multinucleated
foamy
histiocytes

FIG. 9-70. Xanthoma disseminatum (continued). B.

Clinically, the yellow, yellow-pink, or yellow-brown papules and plaques of xanthoma disseminatum symmetrically involve the major creases, especially the axillary, inguinal, antecubital and popliteal fossae, as well as the eyelids and perinasal and perioral regions. Mucous membranes of the respiratory, gastrointestinal, and genitourinary tracts are often affected. Diabetes insipidus occurs in about one-half of all patients with this often fatal disease. Plasma lipids are normal. The failure to demonstrate Langerhans' granules by electron microscopy in the histiocytes of xanthoma disseminatum indicates that, despite clinical similarities, it is a process different from Hand-Schüller-Christian disease (chronic idiopathic xanthomatosis).

Xanthogranulomas, Juvenile and Adult (Fig. 9-71)

—Histiocytes, many of them foam cells, throughout the dense infiltrate
—Touton giant cells in variable numbers throughout the dense infiltrate (Plate 3)
—Eosinophils, lymphocytes, and plasma cells often scattered among the histiocytes
—Cellular infiltrate abutting against the usually thin epidermis, but often with hyperplastic rete at the periphery
—Fibrosis in older lesions

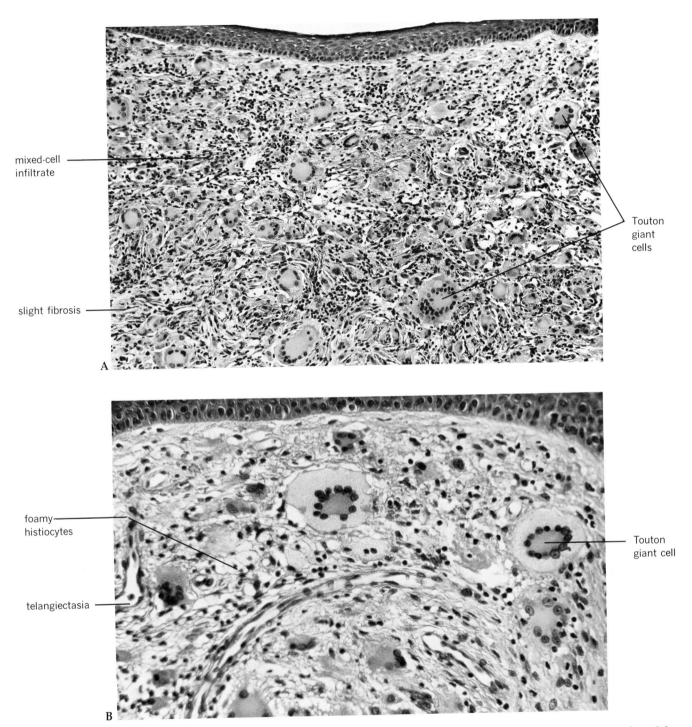

FIG. 9-71. Xanthogranuloma, early lesion. Note multinucleated giant histiocytes (Touton giant cells) whose rings of nuclei separate central homogeneous cores from foamy peripheries. In addition, there is mixed inflammatory-cell infiltrate of neutrophils, eosinophils, lymphocytes, and plasma cells. Fibroblasts with fibrosis dominate older lesions. (A, × 148; B, × 288.)

Xanthogranulomas in children and adults are fundamentally xanthomas that are unassociated with hyperlipoproteinemia. Histologically, early lesions consist preponderantly of foam cells and distinctive foamy multinucleated histiocytes (Touton giant cells are two-toned—amphophilic centrally and foamy peripherally). Older lesions resolve by fibrosis and resemble histiocytomas.

Juvenile xanthogranulomas consist of yellow-orange-tan papules, plaques, and nodules in infants and children. Clinically, they must be distinguished from childhood lesions of nodular urticaria pigmentosa. The last-mentioned urticate upon rubbing. Lesions of juvenile xanthogranuloma disappear spontaneously in months to years. Xanthogranulomas that develop in adults resemble clinically the papular lesions that arise in childhood. The adult form of xanthogranuloma differs from the juvenile by usually being a solitary lesion, tending to persist, and being confined entirely to the skin. Juvenile xanthogranulomas arise in many organs besides the skin, most notably the iris, where hemorrhage into the anterior chamber of the eye can lead to blindness. Ophthalmologists should be aware of the association of ocular and cutaneous xanthogranulomas in youngsters. Misinterpretation of juvenile xanthogranuloma for malignant melanoma or retinoblastoma has led in rare instances to orbital exenteration.

Reticulohistiocytic Granuloma (Reticulohistiocytoma) (Fig. 9-72)

—Histiocytes, some slightly foamy, throughout the dermis
—Histiocytic multinucleated cells usually numerous
—Some histiocytes with atypical nuclei
—Distinctive histiocytic cytoplasm with a granular, dark eosinophilic center and light eosinophilic periphery ("ground-glass cytoplasm")
—Neutrophils, lymphocytes, and plasma cells around the dilated superficial blood vessels and scattered among the histiocytes
—Thin epidermis separated from the dense infiltrate by a thin zone of collagen
—Fibrosis in older lesions

Reticulohistiocytic granuloma is distinguished from juvenile and adult xanthogranuloma by histiocytes with atypical nuclei and a distinctive purplish hue in the cytoplasm and by the absence of Touton giant cells. In other respects the lesions are similar histologically. The reddish-brown papules and nodules of reticulohistiocytic granuloma occur primarily as multiple lesions on the face and the hands, especially along the sides of the fingers. A mutilating arthritis of the distal interphalangeal joints usually accompanies the lesions of this multicentric form of reticulohistiocytic granuloma. The lesions of reticulohistiocytic granuloma have been found in the internal organs, such as the heart and lungs, as well as in the skin and joints. One or more lesions of reticulohistiocytic granuloma can develop in the skin alone, unassociated with systemic disease.

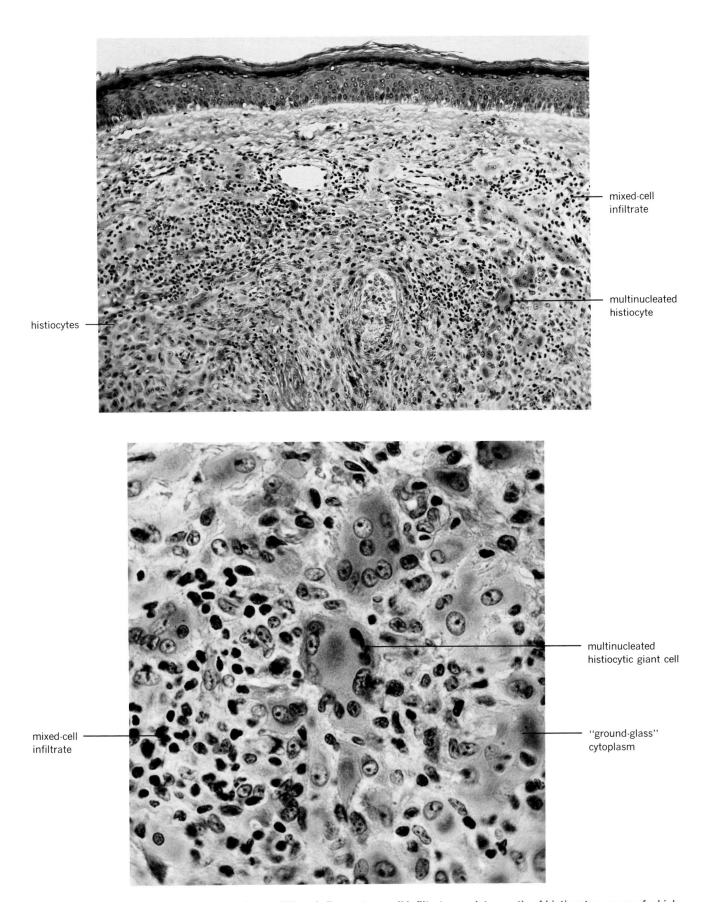

FIG. 9-72. Reticulohistiocytic granuloma. Dense diffuse inflammatory cell infiltrate consists mostly of histiocytes, many of which are multinucleated with characteristic cytoplasms resembling ground glass. (A, × 198; B, × 780.) See also Plate 4.

Histiocytoma (Fig. 9-73, 9-74)

—Histiocytes, some containing foamy cytoplasm, others containing
hemosiderin (siderophages), throughout the dermis
—Histiocytic multinucleated cells, also with foamy cytoplasm and/or
containing hemosiderin
—Fibrosis intermingled with the dense diffuse histiocytic infiltrate
—Epidermis usually hyperplastic and hyperpigmented

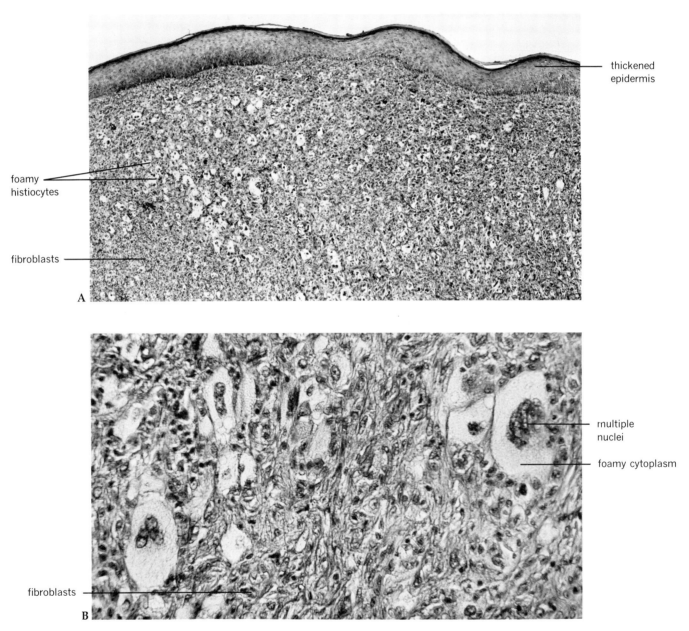

FIG. 9-73. Histiocytoma. A, Some fibroblasts are mingled with dense diffuse infiltrate of foamy histiocytes. (× 63.) B, Histiocytes
with multiple nuclei and foamy cytoplasm resulted from ingestion by macrophages of lipids, which were spilled into dermis along
with extravasation of blood secondary to traumatic event that initiated this process. (× 380.)

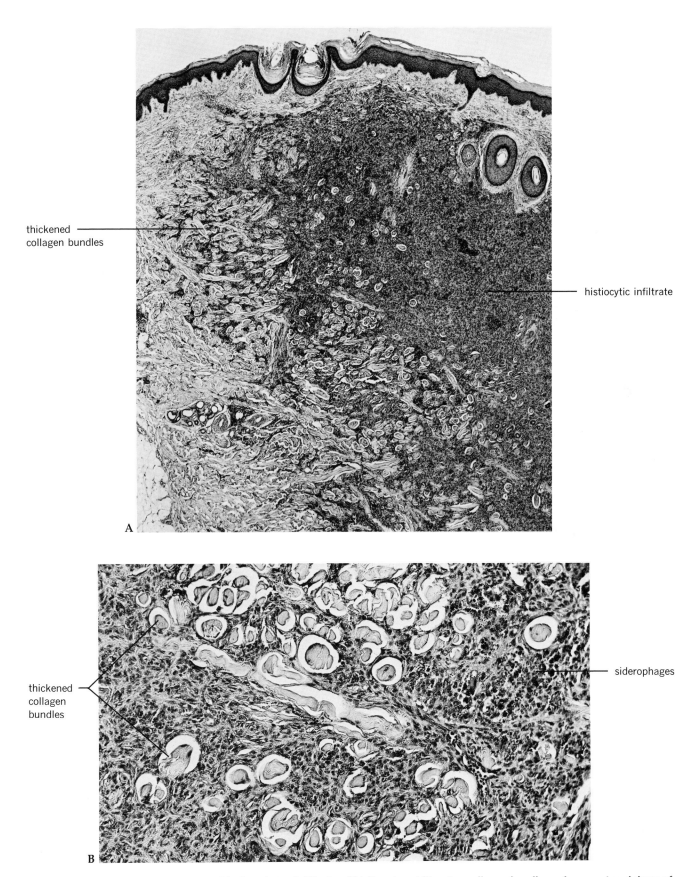

thickened collagen bundles

histiocytic infiltrate

A

thickened collagen bundles

siderophages

B

FIG. 9-74. Histiocytoma. A, In center of lesion, dense infiltrate of histiocytes obliterates collagen bundles, whereas at periphery of lesion histiocytes surround thickened collagen bundles. ($\times$ 27.) B, Siderophages (histiocytes containing hemosiderin) surround thickened collagen bundles. Hemosiderin derives from erythrocytes extravasated by trauma, usually a puncture. ($\times$ 173.)

In histiocytoma, the pattern is a dense nodular or diffuse histiocytic infiltrate. The histiocytes often contain lipid and hemosiderin. In dermatofibroma, fibroblasts and fibrosis, rather than lipid- or hemosiderin-laden histiocytes, are the dominant findings. The two lesions, histiocytoma and dermatofibroma, can usually be distinguished histologically by what most of their cells seem to be doing: storing foreign matter or manufacturing collagen. It may be that histiocytoma and dermatofibroma are merely different stages of the same pathologic process: histiocytes predominant during the phagocytic stage, fibroblasts outnumbering histiocytes during the fibrotic phase. When the plump fibroblasts of dermatofibroma resemble histiocytes or when histiocytes in histiocytoma are associated with prominent fibrosis, the two conditions, histiocytoma and dermatofibroma, overlap histologically. Irrespective of designation, these are inflammatory reactions and not neoplastic processes. Other synonyms for dermatofibroma and histiocytoma are sclerosing hemangioma, subepidermal nodular fibrosis, nodulus cutaneus, and fibroma durum.

A lesion to be differentiated histologically from histiocytoma is histoid leprosy, a manifestation of lepromatous leprosy in which fibroblasts and foam cells are intermixed. Acid-fast stains reveal vast numbers of bacteria within histiocytes of histoid leprosy.

Histiocytoma is indistinguishable clinically from dermatofibroma. Both are firm brownish nodules, usually on the legs, and both presumably result from some sort of trauma (e.g., arthropod assaults, puncture wounds, ruptured follicular cysts) in which blood containing lipids is released into the dermis.

Mineral Oil Granulomas

Paraffin once was deposited in the skin in plastic surgical procedures and is still injected by emotionally disturbed patients. The usual histologic picture consists of clear spaces in the dermis and subcutaneous fat that represent sites from which the paraffin has been removed from the specimen by processing (Fig. 9-75). Initially, the paraffin is surrounded by histiocytes and multinucleated histiocytes, as well as by varying numbers of lymphocytes. Later there are fibrosis and prominent sclerosis. This pattern of clear spaces of various sizes in a sclerotic stroma resembles that of Swiss cheese.

Silicone injected into the skin induces somewhat different histologic changes from those of paraffin. Silicone is found as granules within histiocytes scattered throughout the dermis (Fig. 9-76). There are relatively few large holes within the dermis like those

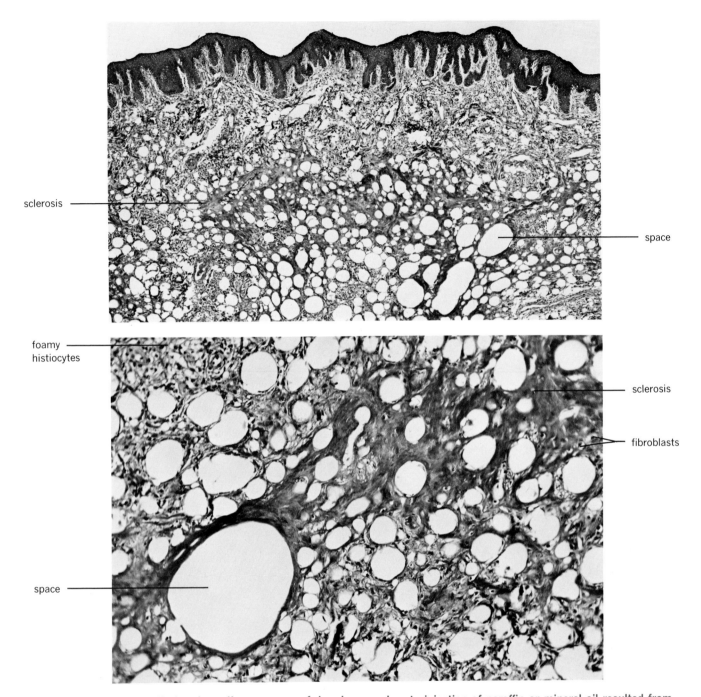

sclerosis

space

foamy
histiocytes

sclerosis

fibroblasts

space

FIG. 9-75. Paraffinoma. "Swiss-cheese" appearance of dermis secondary to injection of paraffin or mineral oil resulted from large, variously sized and shaped spaces created by droplets that were removed during tissue processing. (A, × 56; B, × 187.)

found after injections of paraffin. Furthermore, the reaction to silicone, unlike that to paraffin, is not associated with much fibrosis.

Grease-gun injuries occur particularly on the hands, and the hydrocarbons introduced thereby produce a histologic picture similar to that of paraffinoma. Various oils such as cottonseed or olive oil have been injected into the skin of genitals by disturbed persons dissatisfied with the size and shape of their organs.

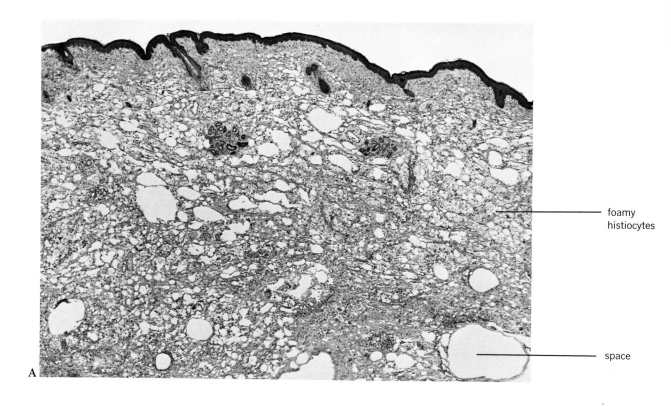

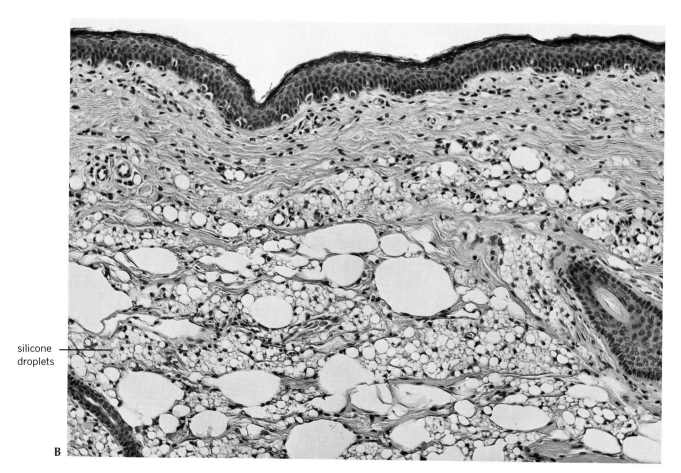

FIG. 9-76. Silicone granuloma. Note diffuse infiltrate of foamy histiocytes containing silicone throughout dermis as well as some scattered clear spaces of various sizes. (A, × 36; B, × 180.)

—Aggregates of foam cells, some forming large nodules throughout the dermis
—Gray cytoplasms in foam cells
—Inflammatory-cell infiltrate usually separated from epidermis by a narrow zone of collagen
—Few inflammatory cells in small dermal nerves

Sections of lepromatous leprosy stained by hematoxylin and eosin show foam cells, suggesting that the condition is a type of xanthoma. This impression is confirmed by exposing fresh tissue from the nodules of lepromatous leprosy to oil red O or Sudan black stains. The lipid-containing acid-fast organisms that fill the cytoplasms of histiocytes and are responsible for their foamy appearance are well demonstrated by the Fite stain. The masses of densely packed acid-fast bacilli within histiocytes are called "globi." A clue to the diagnosis of lepromatous leprosy in sections stained with hematoxylin and eosin, in contrast with other types of xanthomatous lesions, is a grayish hue to the cytoplasm of the

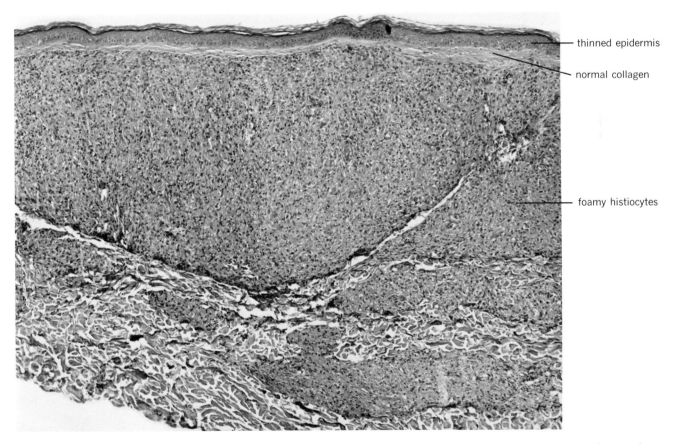

thinned epidermis

normal collagen

foamy histiocytes

FIG. 9-77. Lepromatous leprosy. A, Zone of normal collagen separates nodular and diffuse infiltrate of foamy histiocytes from thinned epidermis. (× 84.)

foam cells. This grayish color results from the way acid-fast rods in the globi take the stain. Small dermal nerves are also infiltrated with bacilli.

The clinical lesions of lepromatous leprosy are papules and nodules that vary in size depending upon the density and distribution of the foam cells within the dermis. Nodules of lepromatous leprosy, also called "lepromas," commonly form in the face and produce the so-called leonine facies.

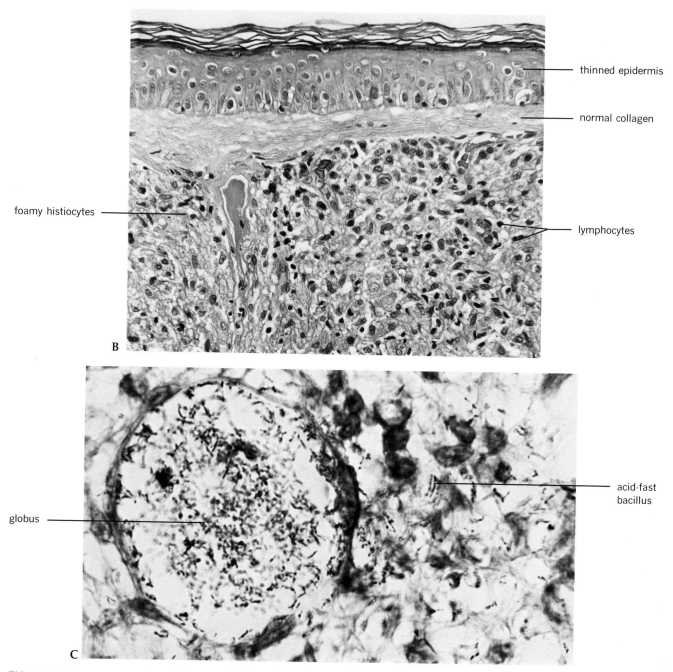

FIG. 9-77. Lepromatous leprosy. B, Higher magnification shows that some lymphocytes and plasma cells are scattered throughout infiltrate of predominantly foamy histiocytes. (× 357.) C, Fite's stain for acid-fast organisms reveals globus, single large histiocyte containing numerous acid-fast lepra bacilli. (× 1900.) See also Plate 3.

Leishmaniasis, Acute Cutaneous and Disseminated Anergic Cutaneous Types
(Fig. 9-78)

The acute lesions of cutaneous leishmaniasis are marked by dense, diffuse, dermal infiltrates of histiocytes in whose cytoplasms the organisms that cause the disease, the Leishman-Donovan bodies (Donovan bodies), are packed. In addition to these characteristically laden histiocytes, there is also a smattering of lymphocytes and plasma cells. When ulceration occurs, neutrophils are present.

Acute lesions of cutaneous leishmaniasis, exotically memorable as Aleppo or Delhi boil and oriental sore, develop shortly after a bite by a carrier sandfly (of the genus Phlebotomus) that transmits the flagellate leptomonad stage of the protozoan, Leishmania tropica. In human tissues so infested the organisms then appear as nonflagellated round or ovoid bodies within cells. The organisms are readily and well stained by hematoxylin and eosin, and also by Giemsa stain or Wright's stain. Acute nodular lesions usually ulcerate, but gradually resolve in months by scarring. In some hosts, however, in and around the scar, new lesions develop that clinically and histologically resemble the apple-jelly nodules of

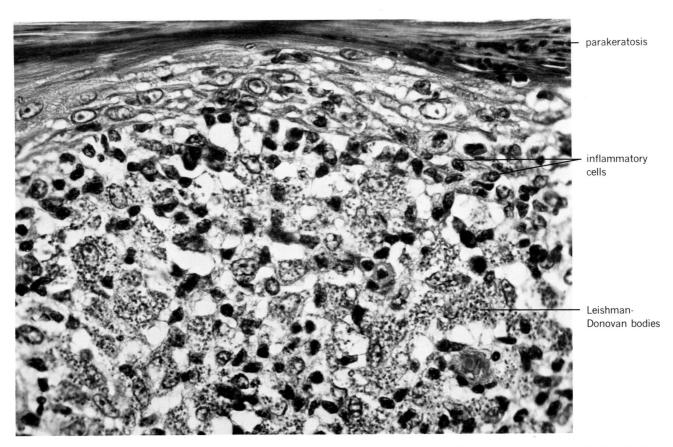

parakeratosis

inflammatory cells

Leishman-Donovan bodies

FIG. 9-78. Cutaneous leishmaniasis, early, nonulcerated lesion. Round- to oval-shaped Donovan bodies are easily visualized as dark-staining dots within histiocytes of section stained by hematoxylin and eosin. (A, × 644; B, × 653.)

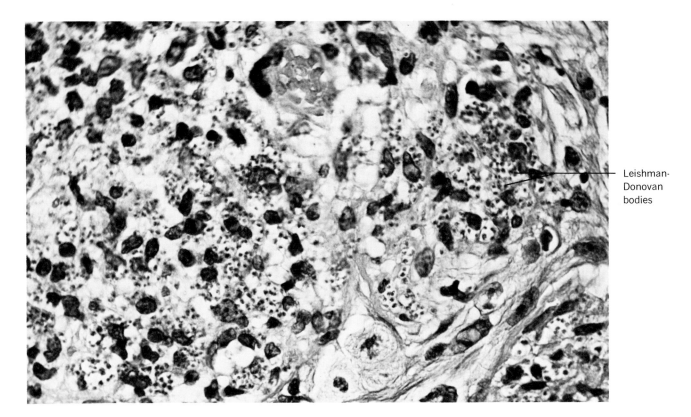

Leishman-
Donovan
bodies

FIG. 9-78. Cutaneous leishmaniasis (continued).

lupus vulgaris. Such tuberculoid granulomatous lesions are known as chronic cutaneous leishmaniasis or leishmaniasis recidivans.

Disseminated anergic cutaneous leishmaniasis clinically and histologically resembles lepromatous leprosy. The histiocytes in the dense nodular and diffuse dermal infiltrates of this form of the disease contain numerous organisms of Leishmania braziliensis, which can be readily seen in sections stained by hematoxylin and eosin, whereas the individual organisms of lepromatous leprosy can be recognized only with the aid of special stains, such as the Fite. The organisms of the species Leishmania braziliensis are indistinguishable from those of Leishmania tropica in histologic sections (Plate 3).

Intracellular organisms that must be differentiated from those of Leishmaniasis are those of histoplasmosis, rhinoscleroma, and granuloma inguinale. All but those of granuloma inguinale can be visualized in sections stained by hematoxylin and eosin.

Histiocytic Giant Cells Predominate

Three conditions characterized by numerous histiocytic giant cells are the exceedingly rare granulomatous slack skin, the uncommon reticulohistiocytic granuloma, and the relatively common xanthogranuloma.

—Histiocytes, many multinucleated, scattered throughout the entire dermis and subcutis
—Epithelioid tubercles associated with numerous lymphocytes, plasma cells, and eosinophils throughout the dermis and subcutis
—Calcified bodies of various sizes and shapes within histiocytic giant cells and in a fibrotic stroma; some matter polarizable
—Fibrotic stroma replacing the normal dermis and the subcutaneous fat
—Fibrotic collagen mostly aligned parallel to the skin surface
—Bandlike mixed inflammatory-cell infiltrate in the upper part of the dermis and a few mononuclear cells within the epidermis

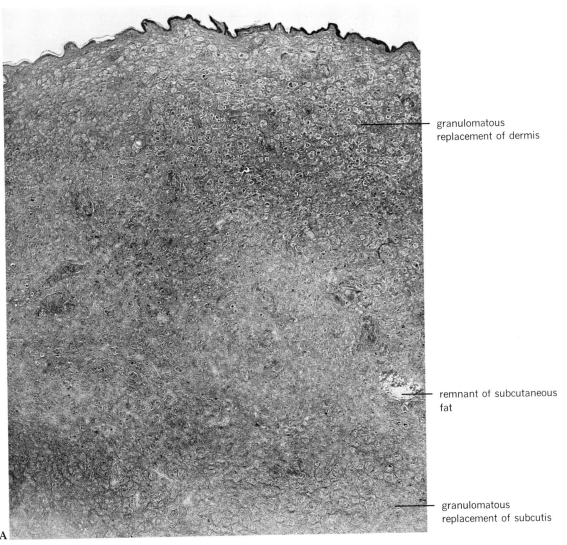

granulomatous
replacement of dermis

remnant of subcutaneous
fat

granulomatous
replacement of subcutis

A

FIG. 9-79. Granulomatous slack skin. Diagnostic histologic feature is dense diffuse inflammatory-cell infiltrate in which multinucleated histiocytic giant cells predominate. The infiltrate, in conjunction with fibrosis, completely replaces the normal dermis and subcutis. (A, × 8; B, × 292; C, × 440; D, × 595.)

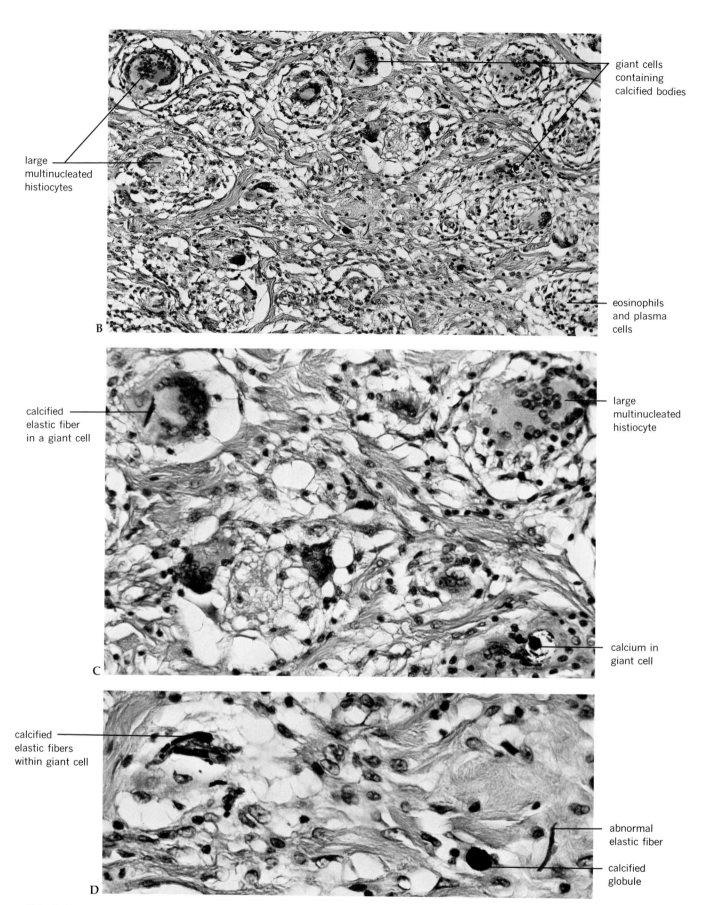

large
multinucleated
histiocytes

giant cells
containing
calcified bodies

eosinophils
and plasma
cells

B

calcified
elastic fiber
in a giant cell

large
multinucleated
histiocyte

calcium in
giant cell

C

calcified
elastic fibers
within giant cell

abnormal
elastic fiber

calcified
globule

D

FIG. 9-79. Granulomatous slack skin (continued).

This rare condition seems to have a predilection for young adult men who, over several years, progressively develop pendulous skin that droops on the arms near the axillae and on the flanks. The skin is not only slack like that of cutis laxa, but it has surface features of parapsoriasis en plaques. Whether this distinctive condition of granulomatous slack skin inevitably eventuates in malignant lymphoma has yet to be determined.

The calcified material within histiocytic giant cells and in the fibrotic stroma is both globular and elongated and appears to be calcified elastic fibers. Loss of normal elastic tissue would account in part for the extreme slackness of the affected skin.

Xanthogranulomas (page 465)

Reticulohistiocytic Granuloma (page 472)

Plasma Cells Predominate

Dense diffuse dermatitides in which plasma cells predominate tend to ulcerate (Fig. 9-80). This is especially true of the venereal diseases (e.g., syphilitic chancre, chancroid, granuloma inguinale, and lymphogranuloma venereum), as well as other infectious diseases such as rhinoscleroma and acute leishmaniasis. Before ulceration occurs, the epidermis may be hyperplastic, even pseudocarcinomatous.

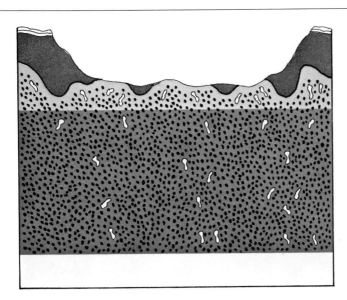

FIG. 9-80. Dense diffuse dermatitis with ulcer.

Syphilitic chancre, chancroid, granuloma inguinale, lymphogranuloma venereum, rhinoscleroma, leishmaniasis (cutaneous and mucocutaneous types), and granuloma gluteale (nodular diaper dermatitis infantum) have a number of histologic features in common (Fig. 9-81).

—Frequently ulceration and cover of fibrin on the surface of the skin
—Granulation tissue at the base of the ulceration
—Dense, diffuse dermal infiltrate of plasma cells, histiocytes, lymphocytes, and occasionally neutrophils and eosinophils
—Edema often in the superficial dermis
—Increased number of widely dilated thick-walled blood vessels with plump endothelial cells

The histologic diagnosis of chancre, chancroid, granuloma inguinale, and lymphogranuloma venereum can only be suspected, rather than made with certainty, in preparations stained by hematoxylin and eosin. Warthin-Starry silver stain should reveal the spirochete of syphilis or the bacillus of granuloma inguinale. These diseases have microscopic findings in common. The pres-

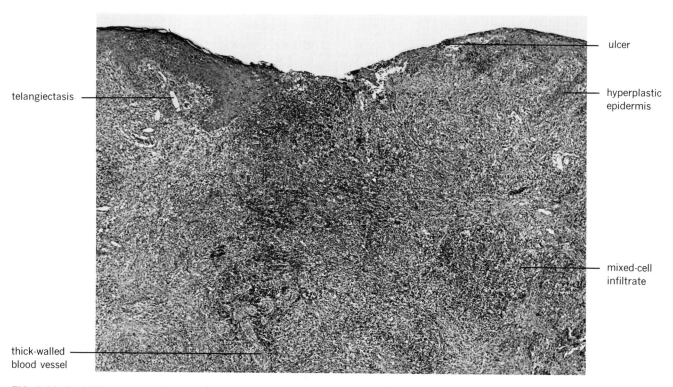

FIG. 9-81. Syphilitic chancre. Histologic changes of ulceration and dense diffuse mixed inflammatory-cell infiltrate of neutrophils, histiocytes, lymphocytes, and plasma cells are not diagnostic of chancre, but may also be seen in other venereal diseases such as chancroid, granuloma inguinale, and lymphogranuloma venereum. (× 63.)

ence of Russell bodies does not help in diagnosis because these round, refractile, homogeneous, eosinophilic-staining bodies merely represent aggregates of immunoglobulins in plasma-cell cytoplasm (Fig. 9-82). Thick-walled blood vessels with plump endothelial cells have been said to be characteristic of chancre and chancroid, but similarly altered blood vessels are also seen in each of the other diseases. Thrombi are said to be more common in the chancre of syphilis. In short, to make the diagnosis of an infectious disease with certainty, it is necessary to demonstrate the causative organism.

Morphologic identification of the spirochete of syphilis is best obtained by darkfield examination of fresh tissue and of the Donovan bodies of granuloma inguinale by smears of crushed fresh tissue.

Syphilitic Chancre. The spirochete of syphilis, Treponema pallidum, is approximately 7 microns long, and its spirals vary in number from 6 to 24. Spirochetes of this species are the causative organism of syphilitic chancre, which is an indurated, reddish papule or nodule, usually single but sometimes multiple, primarily located in the genital region. The chancre is usually eroded or ulcerated and is covered by serous fluid or crust. The Warthin-Starry silver stain is excellent for demonstration of spirochetes. The spirochete of syphilis is best discovered in the epidermis and

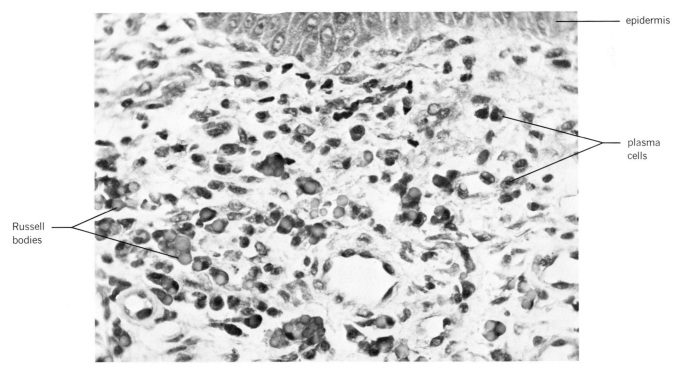

FIG. 9-82. Russell bodies. These accumulations of glycoprotein within cytoplasm of plasma cells are not specific for any one disease. ($\times$ 600.)

around blood vessels of the papillary dermis. Numerous spiro-chetes are usually present in a chancre, whereas relatively few are present in lesions of later secondary syphilis, with the exception of condylomata lata and rupial syphilis (Plate 1).

Chancroid. The causative organism of chancroid is a gram-negative coccobacillus, Hemophilus ducreyi. The bacillus of Ducrey cannot be identified with certainty in either histologic preparations or smears, but only by special cultural techniques. Thus, the histologic diagnosis of chancroid is of necessity one of exclusion, made only when the organisms of the other suspected diseases cannot be confirmed by morphologic, serologic, or cultural methods. The clinical lesions of chancroid are usually multiple, exquisitely tender genital ulcers with dirty, gray, purulent bases. The edges of the ulcer may be punched out, undermined, or ragged.

Granuloma Inguinale. Granuloma inguinale is caused by a gram-negative bacillus termed Calymmatobacterium granulomatis. These bacilli are 1 to 2 microns in diameter and are located within large histiocytes. These intracytoplasmic bacterial inclusions, termed Donovan's bodies, are best demonstrated with Giemsa stain, when they appear red, or by silver stain, when they are black. Donovan's bodies have been compared with a closed safety pin because of their oval shape with accentuation of the staining at each end. There may be more than a dozen of Donovan's bodies within each histiocyte. The diagnosis of granuloma inguinale can be made only if Donovan's bodies are found within the cells. In addition to the large histiocytes, the mixed-cell infiltrate contains numerous plasma cells, many lymphocytes and neutrophils, and rarely eosinophils; there are also tiny abscesses throughout the dense diffuse infiltrate. Clinically, granuloma inguinale is characterized by ulcers from which project beefy-red exuberant granulation tissue. The vegetations are often covered by purulent material.

Rhinoscleroma. Rhinoscleroma is caused by the bacillus Klebsiella rhinoscleromatis or the Frisch bacillus. The organisms, short gram-negative rods, approximately 1 to 2 microns long, and surrounded by a narrow capsule, are found within the cytoplasm of large histiocytes. These histiocytes, named Mikulicz cells, are not specific for rhinoscleroma. Clinically, the lesions of rhinoscleroma are stony-hard nodules located on the nose, upper lip, and palate. The nodules coalesce to become sclerotic plaques and often ulcerate.

Leishmaniasis. The three organisms that cause leishmaniasis, L. tropica (cutaneous or Oriental leishmaniasis), L. braziliensis (mucocutaneous or American leishmaniasis), and L. donovani (kala-azar) are indistinguishable from one another morphologically, although they differ immunologically. In human tissue, the protozoon is a nonflagellated form, 2 to 3 microns in cross section, with a large round nucleus and small rodlike kinetoplast. The round-to-oval bodies are best seen with Giemsa stain which colors the nucleus red, but they can also be visualized with hematoxylin-eosin stain as gray-blue dots within histiocytes. Stained by hematoxylin and eosin they are similar to the organisms of histoplasmosis, which are better visualized with Gomori's stain.

The cutaneous and mucocutaneous forms of leishmaniasis are associated with skin lesions. Both forms consist of slowly growing, firm, reddish papules that enlarge to become nodules and eventually ulcerate and scar. The mucocutaneous form tends to be more persistent and progressive, and often eventuates in widespread ulceration of the mucous membranes. A rare complication of kala-azar is a widespread granulomatous disease that involves the skin (post-kala-azar leishmaniasis) of patients who have been inadequately treated.

Granuloma Gluteale. The discrete, reddish-brown to purple nodules of granuloma gluteale infantum (nodular diaper dermatitis) occur in the diaper area of babies. The cause is not known for sure, but is thought to be a combination of the effects of urine, Candida albicans, and prolonged irritation. The nodules are not always eroded or ulcerated.

Without Ulceration

Some dense diffuse dermatitides composed mostly of plasma cells usually do not ulcerate. Examples are plasmacytoma and some lesions of secondary syphilis.

Plasmacytoma. Although plasmacytoma in most instances denotes multiple myeloma and consists of a dense, diffuse dermal infiltrate of atypical plasma cells, in rare cases a dense nodular or diffuse dermal infiltrate of normal-appearing plasma cells can be seen in patients who never develop myeloma. Examinations of bone marrow reveal a normal marrow. Primary cutaneous plasmacytoma, a benign chronic inflammatory disease, is usually manifested clinically as a solitary papule or nodule.

Secondary Syphilis. One of the many histologic presentations of secondary syphilis is a dense diffuse inflammatory-cell infiltrate composed mostly of plasma cells, with only a few histiocytes. In these instances, a lesion of secondary syphilis may be misinterpreted as a plasmacytoma or a pseudolymphoma. Plasma cells should always call to mind the possibility of syphilis.

Mast Cells Predominate

Urticaria Pigmentosa, Nodular Type (Fig. 9-83). In urticaria pigmentosa, a highly distinctive, possibly benign neoplastic, rather than inflammatory condition, there is a dense diffuse infiltrate of mast cells that involves at least the upper half of the dermis and sometimes the entire dermis. Mast cells are easily recognized by their distinctive round or oval, darkly staining nuclei and tiny amphophilic cytoplasmic granules. If a nodule of urticaria pigmentosa is rubbed within minutes before biopsy, numerous eosinophils will be scattered among the mast cells and within capillaries and venules throughout the dermis. The diagnosis of urticaria pigmentosa can usually be made with a hematoxylin and eosin stain by both pattern and cytologic features, but it is worthwhile to confirm the diagnosis with special stains such as Giemsa's or toluidine blue (Plate 5).

The nodular and bullous types of urticaria pigmentosa are primarily found in infants and children, but rarely nodules composed of mast cells may be seen in adults. The yellow-tan nodules closely resemble those of juvenile xanthogranuloma, but the latter do not urticate when rubbed. In both nodular urticaria pigmentosa and juvenile xanthogranuloma the skin lesions tend to resolve spontaneously and may have internal organ concomitants.

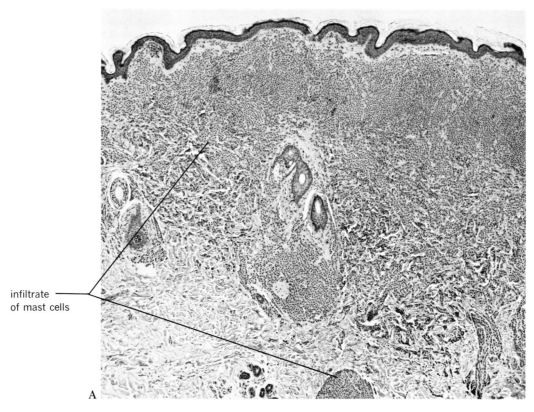

infiltrate of mast cells

FIG. 9-83. Urticaria pigmentosa, nodular lesion. Dense, diffuse, monotonous infiltrate of mast cells is diagnostic feature. (A, × 58; B, × 173; C, × 763.)

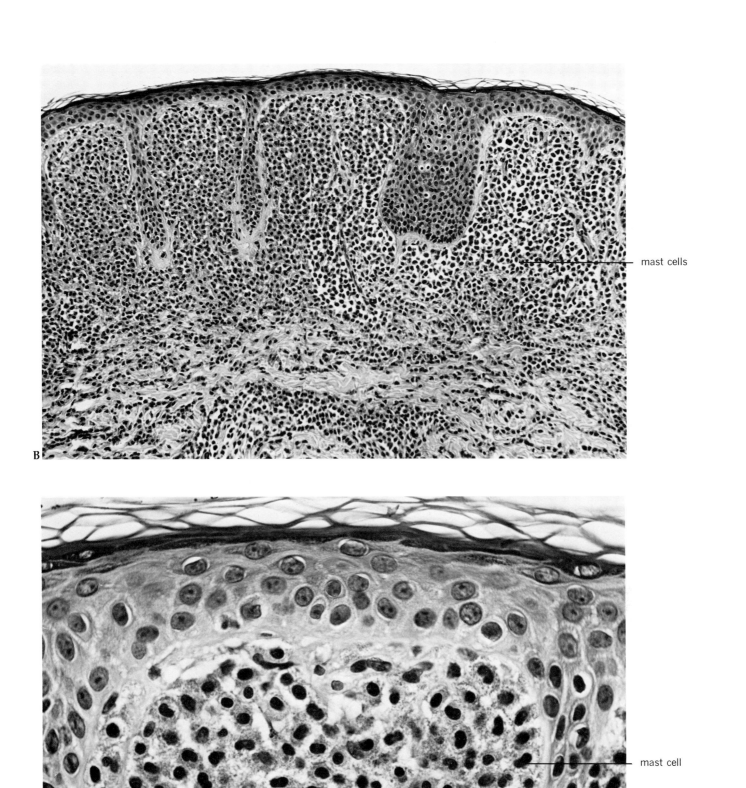

FIG. 9-83. Urticaria pigmentosa (continued).

Histiocytosis X. The spectrum of diseases that includes Letterer-Siwe disease, Hand-Schüller-Christian disease, and eosinophilic granuloma is characterized histologically by a more or less dense, diffuse dermal infiltrate (sometimes confined only to the upper part of the dermis) (Fig. 9-84), composed of eosinophils, neutrophils, plasma cells, lymphocytes, foamy histiocytes, multinucleated histiocytes, and atypical histiocytes having large, indented, kidney-shaped nuclei and abundant, deep-staining eosinophilic cytoplasms. When the atypical histiocytes of histiocytosis X are present within the epidermis, as they often are, they may resemble the collections of atypical lymphocytes within the epidermis of mycosis fungoides (i.e., Pautrier microabscesses). Fibroblasts are numerous in older lesions.

Whether histiocytosis X is truly a neoplastic process, as is generally believed, or an unusual inflammatory process is not yet settled. It is certain, however, that the lesions contain many in-

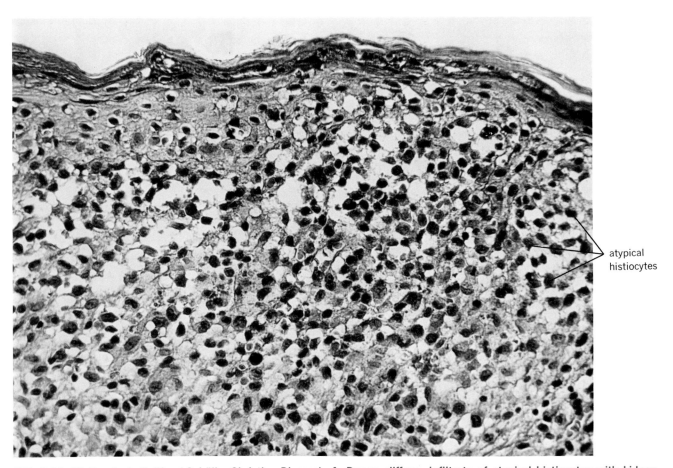

atypical histiocytes

FIG. 9-84. Histiocytosis-X (Hand-Schüller-Christian Disease). A, Dense, diffuse, infiltrate of atypical histiocytes with kidney-shaped nuclei that fills upper part of dermis, obscures dermoepidermal interface, and extends into epidermis, is virtually diagnostic of Histiocytosis-X. (× 445.)

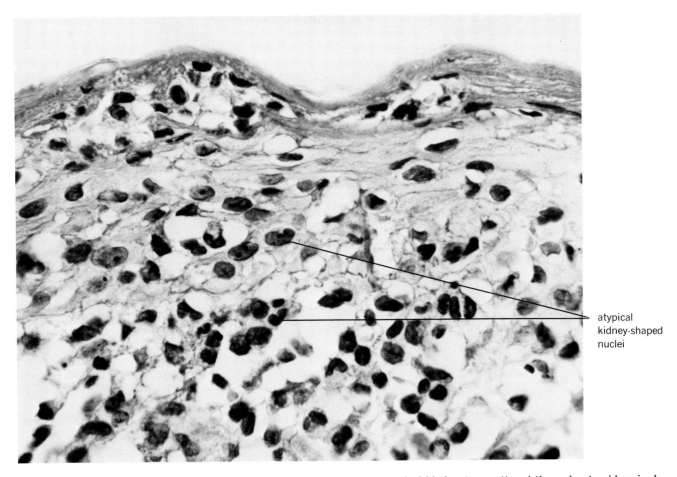

atypical
kidney-shaped
nuclei

FIG. 9-84. Histiocytosis-X. B, This higher power magnification shows atypical histiocytes scattered throughout epidermis. In contrast to convoluted, raisin-shaped nuclei in lymphocytes of mycosis fungoides, note that nuclei in histiocytes of histiocytosis-X are reniform. (× 966.)

flammatory cells and may be confused with lesions of truly inflammatory conditions, and hence the inclusion of histiocytosis X in this chapter.

The histologic common denominator of the triad of clinical conditions that now go under the title of histiocytosis X is a large, atypical histiocyte with a reniform nucleus and abundant, darkly staining eosinophilic cytoplasm. These atypical histiocytes have another characteristic, namely, Langerhans' granules visualizable by electron microscopy. In other conditions, the absence of Langerhans' granules from the cytoplasms of the foamy histiocytes—in xanthoma disseminatum, for example—indicates that they are not of the nature of histiocytosis X.

Clinically, the conditions that are variants of histiocytosis X affect children, predominantly, but adults are not exempt. The lesions are reddish-yellow, brown, or purpuric papules and plaques that may be slightly scaly and occasionally ulcerated, with the appearance of beefy granulation tissue. The cutaneous lesions of Letterer-Siwe disease tend to involve the skin of the scalp, face, neck, trunk, and buttocks; internally, organs such as the spleen, liver, lymph nodes, and bones are affected. The lesions of Hand-Schüller-Christian disease favor intertriginous sites such as the neck, axillae, and groin, but the scalp, face, and trunk may be affected. In Hand-Schüller-Christian disease, exophthalmos, diabetes insipidus, and defects in the cranial bones are usually more prominent than cutaneous lesions. Finally, the lesions of eosinophilic granuloma may be wholly confined to the bones, with no cutaneous involvement whatsoever. Of the three forms of histiocytosis X, eosinophilic granuloma has by far the best prognosis. About 50% of the patients with Letterer-Siwe disease and Hand-Schüller-Christian disease die of the conditions.

Pseudolymphomas (Fig. 9-85). See page 440. The histologic differentiation of some pseudomalignant lymphomas from authentic malignant lymphomas is perhaps the most difficult challenge in dermatopathology, with the possible exception of the differentiation of some atypical melanocytic nevi from malignant melanomas.

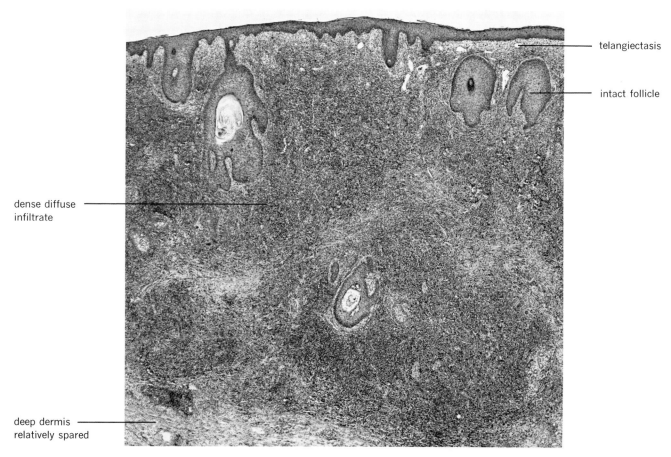

FIG. 9-85. Pseudolymphoma. A, By pattern, this is a pseudolymphoma because infiltrate is more dense in upper part of dermis than in lower part, adnexal structures are preserved, and there is prominent vascular dilation. (× 28.)

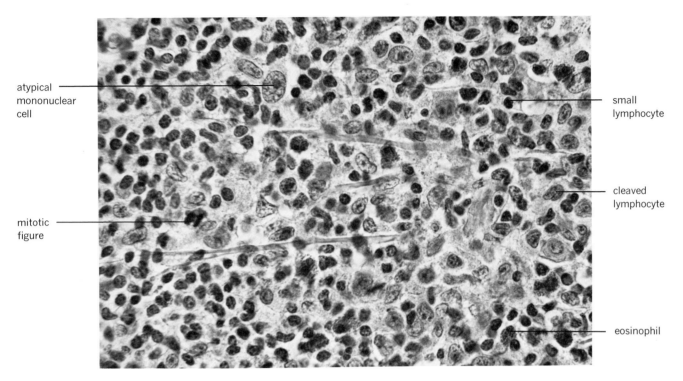

atypical mononuclear cell

mitotic figure

small lymphocyte

cleaved lymphocyte

eosinophil

FIG. 9-85. Pseudolymphoma. B, By cytologic criteria this is a pseudolymphoma because of mixture of different types of cells within infiltrate. Only two types of malignant lymphoma have infiltrates of mixed cells: mycosis fungoides and Hodgkin's disease. This is not mycosis fungoides because of absence of atypical mononuclear cells within epidermis and it is not Hodgkin's disease because of absence of Reed-Sternberg cells. (× 819.)

Intraepidermal Vesicular and Pustular Dermatitis

Spongiotic Vesicular Dermatitis

Lymphocytic spongiosis
  With superficial infiltrate
    Allergic contact dermatitis, acute
    Nummular dermatitis, acute
    Id reaction, acute
    Dyshidrotic dermatitis, acute
    Dermatophytosis, vesicular lesions
  With superficial and deep infiltrate
    Photoallergic contact dermatitis
    Hydroa vacciniforme
    Reactions to arthropods
Eosinophilic spongiosis
    Incontinentia pigmenti
    Pemphigus vulgaris
    Pemphigoid
    Herpes gestationis
    Allergic contact dermatitis
    Arthropod reactions
Spongiotic psoriasiform dermatitis, superficial
    Allergic contact dermatitis, subacute
    Nummular dermatitis, subacute

Ballooning Vesicular Dermatitis

Superficial infiltrate
    Vaccinia and variola
    Milker's nodule and orf
    Hand, foot, and mouth disease
    Herpesvirus infections
    Necrolytic migratory erythema
    Pellagra
    Acrodermatitis enteropathica
    Pachyonychia congenita
    Immersion blister
    Erythema multiforme
    Irritant contact and phototoxic types
Superficial and deep infiltrate
    Fixed drug eruption, acute
    Pityriasis lichenoides et varioliformis
      acuta

Acantholytic Vesicular Dermatitis

Suprabasal
    Pemphigus vulgaris and vegetans
    Benign familial chronic pemphigus
    Keratosis follicularis
    Transient acantholytic dermatosis
Intraspinous
    Herpesvirus infections
    Blister beetle dermatitis

Subcorneal
    Pemphigus foliaceus and erythematosus
    Staphylococcal scalded-skin syndrome
    Bullous impetigo
    Pyoderma gangrenosum

Intragranular Vesicular Dermatitis

    Friction blisters
    Weber-Cockayne disease

Intrabasal Vesicular Dermatitis

    Epidermolysis bullosa simplex

Intraepidermal Vesiculopustular Dermatitis

Superficial infiltrate
    Dermatophytosis, vesicular lesions
    Irritant contact dermatitis
    Impetiginized vesicular dermatitides
    Vesiculopustular dermatitis (volar skin)
    Vesiculopustular dermatitis of childhood
Superficial and deep infiltrate
    Reactions to fleabites
    Leukocytoclastic and septic vasculitis

Intraepidermal Pustular Dermatitis

Unilocular
    Fire-ant stings and fleabites
    Keratotic-crusted scabies
Spongiform pustular dermatitis
    Pustular psoriasis and its variants
    Syphilis (rupial, condyloma latum)
    Halogenodermas
    Pyoderma gangrenosum
    Candidiasis and dermatophytosis, acute
Subcorneal pustular dermatitis
    Subcorneal pustular dermatosis
    Miliaria crystallina
    Impetigo and bullous impetigo
    Pemphigus foliaceus and erythematosus
    Staphylococcal scalded-skin syndrome
    Candidiasis and dermatophytosis, acute
    Toxic erythema of newborn
    Pyoderma gangrenosum
    Psoriasis, guttate and pustular types
Intracorneal pustular dermatitis
    Psoriasis, eruptive lesions
    Candidiasis, subacute
    Dermatophytosis, subacute

Intraepidermal

Vesicular *and* Pustular

Dermatitis

10

THERE ARE three major morphologic expressions of the mechanisms whereby intraepidermal vesicles are formed: (1) intercellular edema (spongiosis) (Fig. 3-6A), (2) intracellular edema (ballooning) (Fig. 3-6B), and (3) acantholysis (Fig. 3-7). In some diseases more than one of these mechanisms may be operative simultaneously, e.g., acantholysis may occur within epidermal pustules (impetigo, subcorneal pustular dermatosis); acantholysis and ballooning may occur together in vesicles caused by herpesviruses (herpes simplex, herpes zoster, varicella); spongiosis and ballooning may develop simultaneously (erythema multiforme, acute fixed drug eruption); and spongiosis and acantholysis may appear concurrently (transient acantholytic dermatosis).

Spongiosis and ballooning usually involve the spinous zone of the epidermis so that blisters formed by these mechanisms tend to appear in the midepidermis. Acantholysis can involve cells at all levels of the epidermis, but the separation in acantholytic blisters tends to occur in either the very superficial epidermis (i.e., subcorneal or intragranular zones) or in the very deep epidermis (i.e., suprabasalar zone).

497

Intraepidermal pustules tend to localize within the cornified layer (intracorneal pustules), immediately beneath the cornified layer in well-circumscribed collections (subcorneal pustules), or between epidermal cell membranes in the upper half of the epidermis (spongiform pustules). The site of pustule formation within the epidermis is related, in part, to the time in the evolution of the pustular process when a biopsy is taken. Early in the development of a pustule, neutrophils will be found scattered in the lower portions of the epidermis, whereas later the neutrophils come to rest in the upper parts of the epidermis.

The classification of intraepidermal vesicular and pustular dermatitides that follows is based on (1) the dominant morphologic expression of the mechanism of vesicle or pustule formation (spongiosis, ballooning, acantholysis); (2) the site of the vesicle within the epidermis (subcorneal, intraspinous, suprabasalar, or intrabasalar); (3) position and composition of inflammatory-cell infiltrate within the dermis (superficial or superficial and deep).

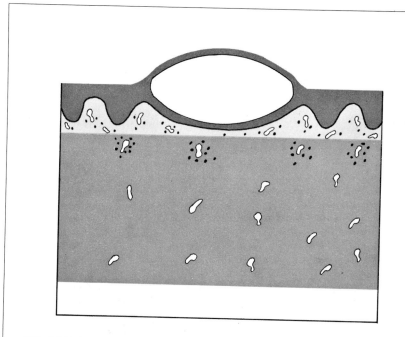

FIG. 10-1. Intraepidermal vesicular and pustular dermatitis.

Spongiotic Vesicular Dermatitis

Before beginning this section, the reader should review the pages devoted to spongiotic dermatitis in Chapter 6.   pg 218

Spongiotic vesicular lesions result when the degree of intercellular edema is sufficient to form blisters that can be detected clinically. However, not every disease in which there is histologic spongiosis is inevitably associated with clinical vesiculation. Examples of diseases distinguished microscopically by spongiosis and by no grossly visible vesicles are seborrheic dermatitis, guttate parapsoriasis, and pityriasis alba. Diseases in which spongiosis rarely, if ever, progresses to actual vesiculation are pityriasis rosea, miliaria rubra, and erythema annulare centrifigum.

Spongiotic vesicular dermatitis can be subclassified into five types: lymphocytic spongiosis, eosinophilic spongiosis, neutrophilic spongiosis, spongiosis with keratinocytic necrosis, and spongiotic psoriasiform dermatitis. These subclassifications may be further subdivided on the basis of whether the infiltrate is superficial or superficial and deep.

Lymphocytic Spongiosis

It is usually impossible to distinguish histologically among *acute allergic contact dermatitis, nummular dermatitis, id reaction,* and *dyshidrotic dermatitis* (Fig. 10-2). Each is characterized by spongiotic vesicles and a superficial, perivascular, predominantly lymphohistiocytic infiltrate. Eosinophils are sometimes present in the infiltrate of allergic contact or nummular dermatitis, id reactions, and dyshidrotic dermatitis. Some vesicular lesions caused by dermatophytes may also be difficult to differentiate histologically

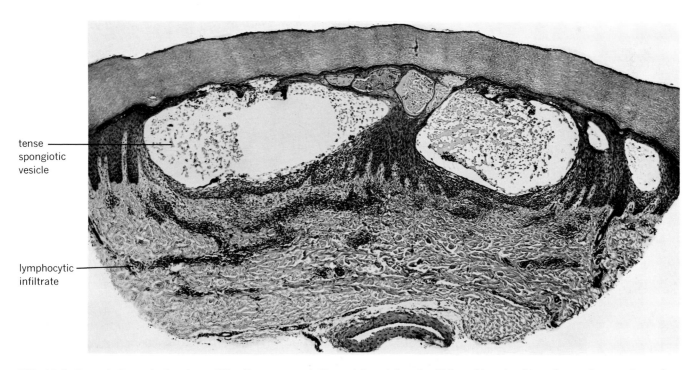

tense
spongiotic
vesicle

lymphocytic
infiltrate

FIG. 10-2. Spongiotic vesicular dermatitis. Tense spongiotic vesicles pictured within epidermis of specimens from palms of two patients are not diagnostic of a single disease, but may be found in acute lesions of allergic contact dermatitis, nummular dermatitis, dyshidrotic dermatitis, id reactions, or vesicular dermatophytic infections. A, Allergic contact dermatitis. ($\times$ 43.)

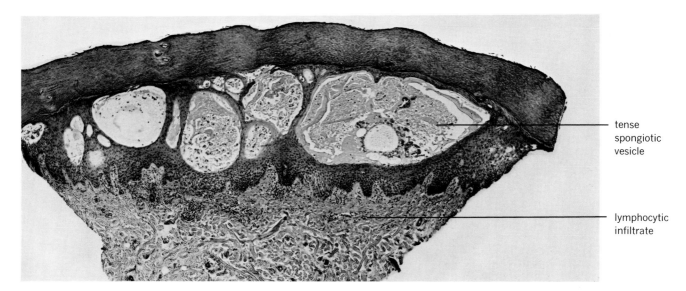

tense
spongiotic
vesicle

lymphocytic
infiltrate

FIG. 10-2. B, Dyshidrotic dermatitis. (× 43.)

from allergic contact dermatitis, nummular dermatitis, id reaction, and dyshidrotic dermatitis. The cornified layer of such lesions, especially those on palms and soles, should be scrutinized for hyphae. Usually they can be spotted in sections stained with hematoxylin and eosin more readily when transmitted light is reduced by lowering the condenser of the microscope. The organisms then appear opalescent. Special stains for fungi should be done in all suspicious cases.

A histologic feature helpful in the differentiation of *photoallergic contact dermatitis* from the other types of lymphocytic spongiotic vesicular dermatitis is the depth of the dermal infiltrate. The lymphocytes and histiocytes tend to be present around the blood vessels of both the superficial and deep plexuses in photoallergic contact dermatitis, in contrast to allergic contact dermatitis in which all of the infiltrate lies superficially. Another differentiating feature is the occasional presence of necrotic keratinocytes in the epidermis of photoallergic contact dermatitis. Histologically, *hydroa vacciniforme* is similar to photoallergic contact dermatitis (Fig. 10-3). The superficial and deep inflammatory cell infiltrate in *reactions to arthropod assaults* usually contains eosinophils, but the tense vesicle may sometimes result from lymphocytic spongiosis rather than from eosinophilic spongiosis (Fig. 10-4).

It is much easier to distinguish among these diseases clinically than histologically. Allergic contact dermatitis is characterized by papulovesiculobullous lesions that are sharply confined to areas of contact with the causative agent. Dyshidrotic dermatitis consists of tiny, tense vesicles formed almost exclusively along the sides of the fingers and on the palms. Nummular dermatitis consists of tense vesicles in coin-shaped clusters. An id reaction usually

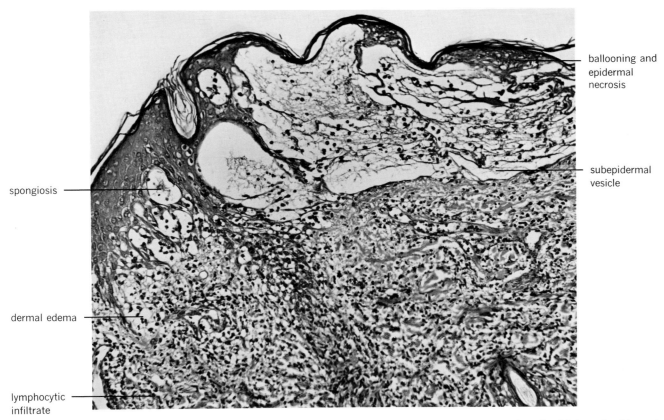

FIG. 10-3. Hydroa vacciniforme. Vesicular process began as spongiotic intraepidermal vesicle and evolved into subepidermal vesicle following rupture of vesicle through basal epidermal cells and into dermis. This specimen came from child with clinical features of erythropoietic protoporphyria, but without laboratory confirmation thereof. (× 160.)

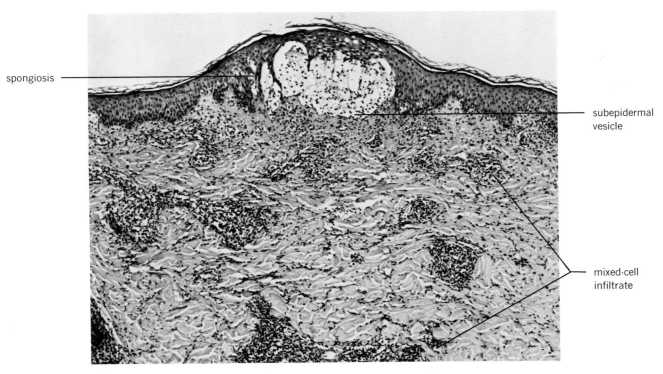

FIG. 10-4. Reaction to insect bite. Well-circumscribed tense vesicle marks actual point of insect bite which began as spongiotic intraepidermal vesicle and became subepidermal consequent to "blow-out" of vesicular contents. Note superficial and deep perivascular and interstitial inflammatory-cell infiltrate containing many eosinophils, a characteristic of reaction to arthropod assault. (× 74.)

INTRAEPIDERMAL VESICULAR AND PUSTULAR DERMATITIS 501

appears as an eruption of tense vesicles on the hands if it results from concurrent acute dermatophytic infection of the feet, or as a generalized papulovesicular eruption when it is associated with a florid, localized dermatitis, such as overtreated allergic contact dermatitis. Rarely, pityriasis rosea may become vesicular in black people and resemble a widespread id reaction. Scaly or vesicular lesions caused by dermatophytic infections tend to be annular and to extend centrifugally. Photoallergic contact dermatitis and photoallergic dermatitis resemble allergic contact dermatitis morphologically, but the light-related lesions are sharply confined to uncovered surfaces. *Hydroa vacciniforme* is a vesicular photodermatitis that can be confused clinically with congenital porphyria and even erythropoietic protoporphyria.

Eosinophilic Spongiosis

Spongiosis is inevitably accompanied by inflammatory cells. Compared to lymphocytic spongiosis, eosinophilic spongiosis is a relatively uncommon phenomenon. Spongiotic vesicles filled with eosinophils occur in the vesicular stage of *incontinentia pigmenti*, in urticarial lesions of *pemphigus vulgaris, pemphigoid,* and *herpes gestationis* and, rarely, in the intraepidermal vesicles of *allergic contact dermatitis* and *arthropod reactions.*

Only in vesicles of *incontinentia pigmenti* is eosinophilic spongiosis a consistent finding. In *pemphigus vulgaris,* the usual histologic change is a suprabasal intraepidermal blister containing acantholytic cells. Eosinophilic spongiosis may occur in the epidermis lateral to the suprabasalar blister (Fig. 10-5). In exceptional cases

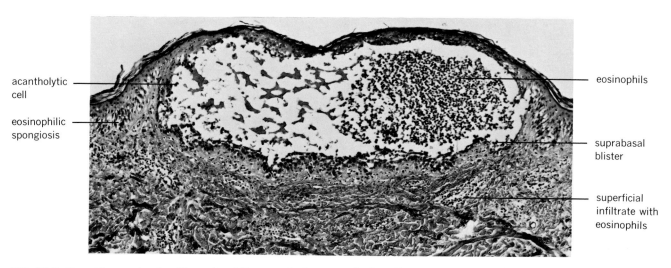

acantholytic cell

eosinophilic spongiosis

eosinophils

suprabasal blister

superficial infiltrate with eosinophils

FIG. 10-5. Pemphigus vulgaris with eosinophilic spongiosis, a rare finding. Numerous eosinophils within some lesions of pemphigus vulgaris are but one link of that condition to pemphigus vegetans. (A, × 110; B, × 173.)

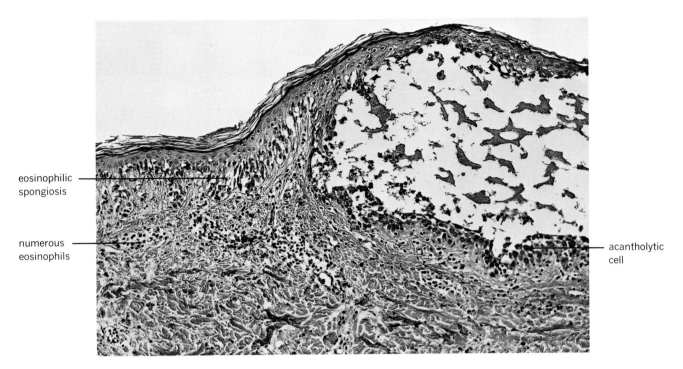

eosinophilic spongiosis

numerous eosinophils

acantholytic cell

FIG. 10-5. Pemphigus vulgaris. B.

of pemphigus vulgaris, biopsy of papular and plaque lesions may disclose eosinophilic spongiosis with none of the typical histologic features of pemphigus (suprabasal blisters and acantholytic cells). The usual histologic findings in vesicular or bullous lesions of *pemphigoid* and *herpes gestationis* are a subepidermal blister containing numerous eosinophils and a superficial perivascular infiltrate of eosinophils, lymphocytes, histiocytes, and, occasionally, neutrophils. Biopsy of the urticarial lesions of pemphigoid and of herpes gestationis reveals an edematous papillary dermis containing a mixed inflammatory-cell infiltrate with eosinophils. In such plaques, eosinophils may be scattered within the epidermis and grouped in spongiotic foci. Similar foci of eosinophilic spongiosis in pemphigoid and in herpes gestationis may appear occasionally in the epidermis lateral to the subepidermal blister.

The tense vesicle that sometimes accompanies a *reaction to an arthropod* histologically displays extensive focal spongiosis beneath which there is often intense subepidermal edema and a dense superficial and deep perivascular infiltrate of eosinophils, lymphocytes, and histiocytes. When sufficiently tense, the originally intraepidermal vesicle explodes into the dermis, resulting in subepidermal vesiculation (Fig. 10-6). Eosinophils are also interspersed among collagen bundles at all levels of the dermis. Biopsy of the edematous area that may surround the vesicle usually reveals dermal changes only. The focus of eosinophilic spongiotic vesiculation marks the actual spot of the insect bite.

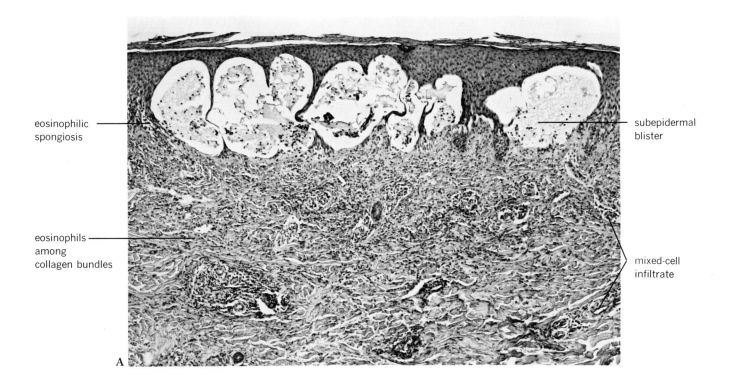

eosinophilic
spongiosis

eosinophils
among
collagen bundles

subepidermal
blister

mixed-cell
infiltrate

A

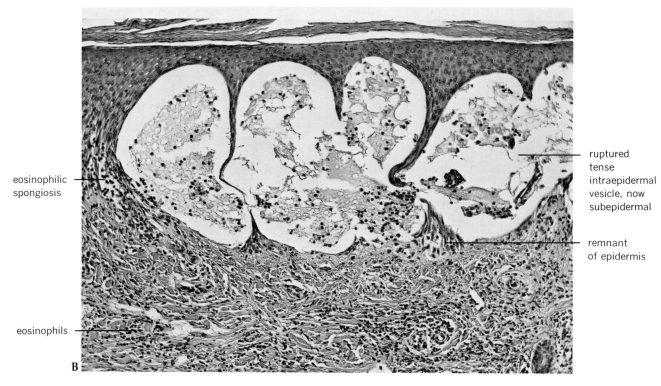

eosinophilic
spongiosis

eosinophils

ruptured
tense
intraepidermal
vesicle, now
subepidermal

remnant
of epidermis

B

FIG. 10-6. Reaction to arthropod assault, vesicular type. A, Subepidermal blister formed when pressure lifted epidermis from dermis of original spongiotic vesicular type intraepidermal blister. Numerous eosinophils are seen around blood vessels and among collagen bundles throughout the dermis. The spongiotic vesicles may contain lymphocytes and eosinophils and sometimes neutrophils. (× 87.) B, Transition from tense spongiotic intraepidermal vesicles to subepidermal positions. Strips of epidermis divide the originally multiloculated intraepidermal blister. (× 169.)

Similar spongiotic vesicles containing lymphocytes and variable numbers of eosinophils may be seen beneath burrows in the cornified layer harboring the mites of scabies (Fig. 10-7), above the channel near the base of the epidermis containing larvae of creeping eruption, and in association with cercariae in "swimmer's itch." Widespread reactions to insect bites that occur especially in children are also known as papular urticaria. Eosinophilic spongiosis must be differentiated from eosinophilic "abscesses" that are seen in toxic erythema of the newborn, pemphigus vegetans, and rarely in lesions caused by dermatophytes.

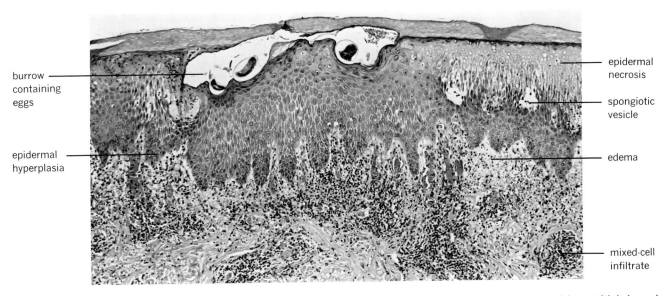

FIG. 10-7. Scabies burrow. Spongiotic vesicles are seen in vicinity of burrow, along with perivascular and interstitial dermal infiltrate containing eosinophils. (× 110.)

Neutrophilic Spongiosis

Neutrophilic spongiosis frequently eventuates in vesiculopustules. For that reason, it is treated under the section on intraepidermal vesiculopustular dermatitis later in this chapter. Very exceptional lesions of acute guttate psoriasis may show slight spongiosis in association with intraepidermal neutrophils.

Spongiosis with Keratinocytic Necrosis

The histologic clues to *irritant contact dermatitis* and *phototoxic contact dermatitis,* such as phytophotodermatitis, are spongiosis and ballooning plus keratinocytic necrosis. Intercellular edema coexists with the predominant intracellular edema. Neutrophils, as well as lymphocytes and histiocytes, are the inflammatory cells. Initially, the epidermis contains individually necrotic keratinocytes, but, in time, the entire epidermis may become necrotic.

Exceptional cases of cutaneous *erythema multiforme* are characterized by intraepidermal spongiotic vesiculation with individual necrotic keratinocytes, rather than by subepidermal vesiculation. Intracellular and intercellular edema are common, but not dominant, features in most instances of erythema multiforme in skin, but these intraepithelial changes tend to predominate in erythema multiforme of mucous membranes.

Spongiotic Psoriasiform Dermatitis

Spongiotic psoriasiform dermatitis is a specific histologic pattern that should call to mind both *subacute allergic contact dermatitis* and *subacute nummular dermatitis.* The degree of spongiosis in both of these conditions ranges from slight and wholly microscopic to extensive and clearly macroscopic. Usually, only the early lesions of nummular dermatitis have intact vesicles. Later lesions are covered by scale-crusts and have lymphocytes, histiocytes, and, not uncommonly, eosinophils in the upper dermis. Because of the often extreme pruritus of nummular dermatitis, the vesicles may be scratched away, and the epidermis may be eroded or ulcerated. Nummular dermatitis is easily diagnosed clinically because the lesions are shaped like coins of various sizes.

The distinctive exudative discoid and lichenoid chronic dermatosis described by Sulzberger and Garbe probably represents chronically rubbed nummular dermatitis, i.e., nummular dermatitis with superimposed lichen simplex chronicus.

Ballooning Vesicular Dermatitis

Ballooning vesicular dermatitis can be subclassified into two types: (1) with superficial infiltrate and (2) with superficial and deep infiltrate.

Superficial Infiltrate

Vaccinia (cowpox) consists histologically of intraepidermal vesicles formed by rupture of spinous cells due to pronounced intracellular edema (Fig. 10-8). The edematous ballooned keratinocytes in the spinous zone have abundant pale-gray cytoplasm in hematoxylin-eosin-stained sections. Small intracytoplasmic inclusions (Guarnieri bodies) are often visible. Some of the spinous cells are necrotic. Most of the epidermal nuclei are large and vesicular with

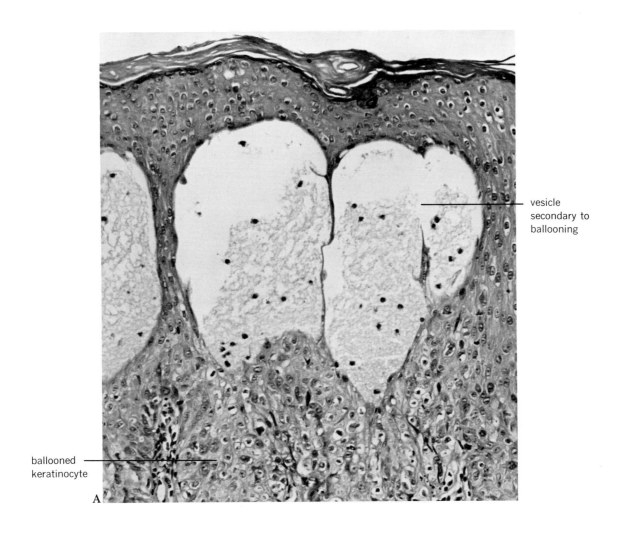

vesicle
secondary to
ballooning

ballooned
keratinocyte

A

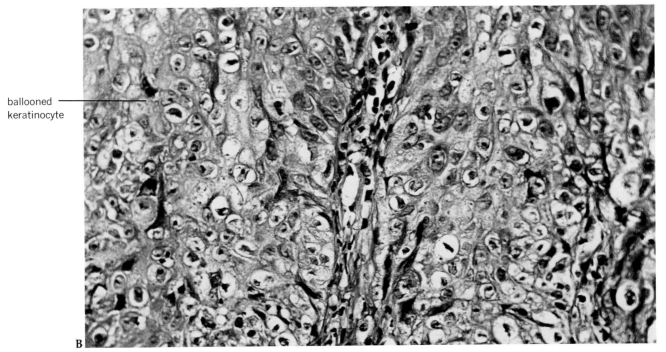

ballooned
keratinocyte

B

FIG. 10-8. Vaccinia. Intraepidermal vesicle resulted from intense ballooning of keratinocytes of the spinous zone, seen here as large cells with pale cytoplasm. (A, × 220; B, × 440.)

prominent nuclear membranes. The inflammatory-cell infiltrate of lymphocytes, histiocytes, and occasional neutrophils is usually confined to the upper part of the dermis. The histiologic features of vaccinia resemble those of *variola* (smallpox) but differ from lesions caused by herpesvirus by the absence of multinucleated epithelial giant cells.

Clinically, vaccinia consists of umbilicated vesiculopustules situated on red indurated bases. The individual clinical lesions of variola and vaccinia are also similar. Variola is differentiated clinically from varicella by the tendency of the eruption to affect the periphery of the body, whereas in varicella the lesions have a more central distribution.

Milker's nodule and orf (echthyma contagiosum) are poxvirus diseases that humans contract from cows and sheep, respectively. Both diseases are characterized by ballooning and spongiosis that eventuate in multilocular intraepidermal vesicles. There is also severe epidermal hyperplasia with varying degrees of necrosis, intraepidermal pustule formation, and a dense mixed inflammatory-cell infiltrate of lymphocytes, histiocytes, plasma cells and scattered neutrophils in the often extremely edematous upper dermis (Fig. 10-9). The lesions of milker's nodule and orf also have similar clinical features, beginning as reddish-blue papules that become nodular and then are surmounted by gray bullae. The lesions are rimmed by erythema.

Ballooning and reticulation are frequent concomitants of blistering diseases caused by viruses. The earliest pathologic changes that determine the site of blister formation in *hand, foot, and mouth disease* (a condition caused by Coxsackie viruses A-5, A-10, and A-16) develop within the epidermis where there is severe intracellular and intercellular edema (Fig. 10-10). When the ballooning and spongiosis create sufficient pressure, the intraepidermal vesicle explodes through the basal layer, forcing the epidermis to be lifted from the dermis and converting the initially intraepidermal vesicle into a subepidermal one (Fig. 10-11). Epidermal necrosis usually follows. The papillae beneath the blister are usually well preserved. An infiltrate of lymphocytes and histiocytes is present around the blood vessels of the superficial plexus.

Clinically, the skin lesions occur on the dorsal and ventral surfaces of the hands and feet, appearing as tiny, tense, gray, vesicles oblong in shape, surrounded by a distinct red rim. The gray color of the vesicle roofs is a sure sign of epidermal necrosis.

The herpesvirus vesicle results from ballooning and acantholysis. Because the diagnostic feature of *herpes simplex, herpes zoster,* and *varicella*—multinucleated epithelial giant cells—is usually associated with acantholysis, the histologic changes of herpesvirus

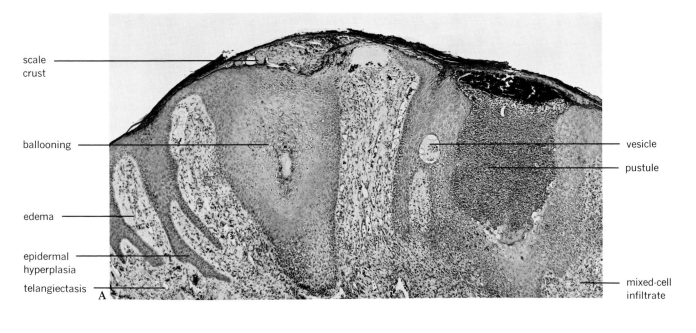

scale
crust

ballooning

edema

epidermal
hyperplasia

telangiectasis

A

vesicle

pustule

mixed-cell
infiltrate

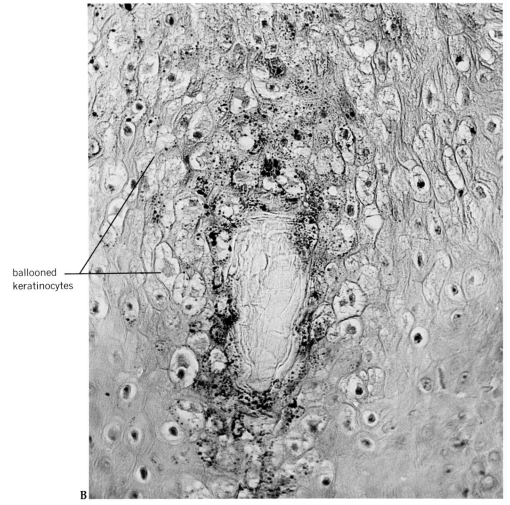

ballooned
keratinocytes

B

FIG. 10-9. Milker's nodule. A, Changes in keratinocytes pictured are characteristic of all poxvirus infections of humans that are contracted from animals. Ballooning often progresses to intraepidermal vesicles, generally multilocular. Pustules probably result from secondary bacterial infection. ($\times$ 60.) B, Severe ballooning of cytoplasm of keratinocytes should suggest a viral infection as one possible cause. ($\times$ 370.)

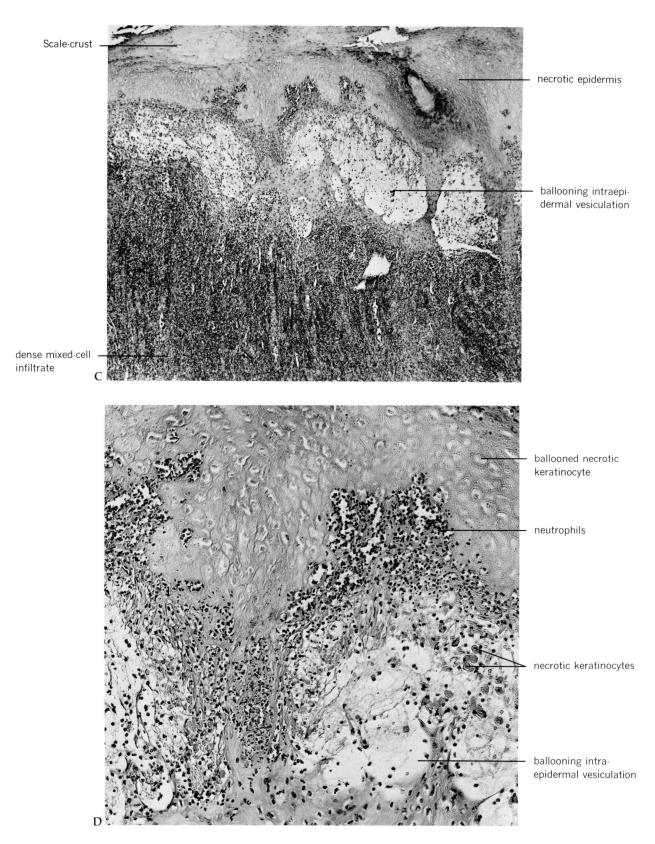

Scale-crust

necrotic epidermis

ballooning intraepidermal vesiculation

dense mixed-cell infiltrate

C

ballooned necrotic keratinocyte

neutrophils

necrotic keratinocytes

ballooning intra-epidermal vesiculation

D

FIG. 10-9. Milker's nodule. C, Fully developed blisters are characterized by multiloculated intraepidermal vesicles secondary to massive ballooning of keratinocytes. Dense, diffuse inflammatory-cell infiltrate consists mostly of lymphocytes, plasma cells, and histiocytes. (× 46.) D, In higher magnification of C, ballooned and necrotic keratinocytes are seen to better advantage. The necrosis is chemotactic for neutrophils which are numerous. (× 176.)

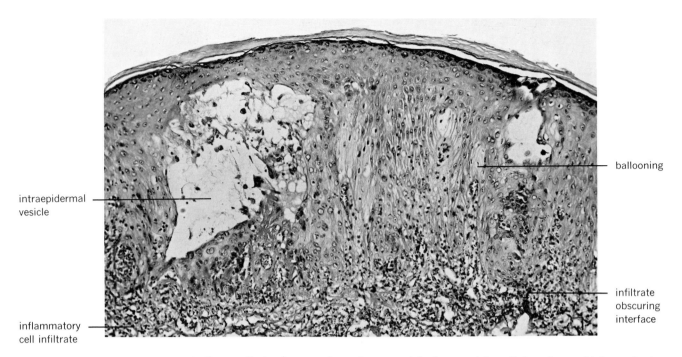

intraepidermal vesicle

inflammatory cell infiltrate

ballooning

infiltrate obscuring interface

FIG. 10-10. Hand, foot, and mouth disease. Early changes shown here consist of severe intracellular edema which eventuates in intraepidermal vesiculation. Similar changes occur in mucous membrane epithelium that is infected by the causative Coxsackie virus. (× 140.)

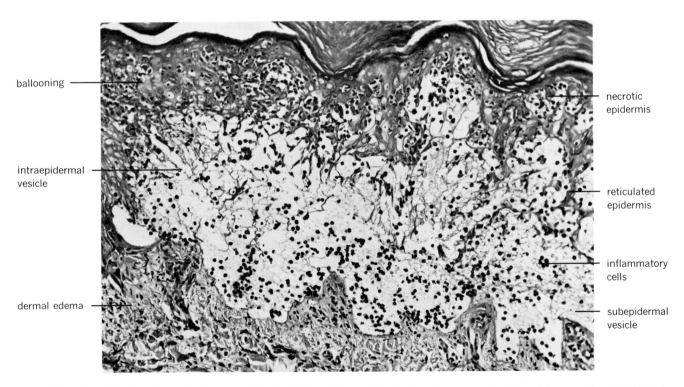

ballooning

intraepidermal vesicle

dermal edema

necrotic epidermis

reticulated epidermis

inflammatory cells

subepidermal vesicle

FIG. 10-11. Hand, foot, and mouth disease. Note that intraepidermal blister has become subepidermal because intraepidermal pressure has forced epidermis to be lifted from dermis. Also shown is severe intracellular edema accompanied by reticular alteration of epidermis. (× 209.)

infections will be discussed under acantholytic vesicular dermatitis. Before vesiculation occurs, however, ballooning, nuclear changes, and even formation of multinucleated epithelial giant cells appear and enable histologic diagnosis of herpesvirus infection (Fig. 10-12; Plate 4).

Necrolytic migratory erythema (glucagonoma bullous dermatitis) is characterized histologically by intracellular edema in the upper half of the epidermal spinuous zone that sometimes may be so extensive that a blister forms (Fig. 10-13A). The epidermis beneath the blister is usually hyperplastic, and a sparse lymphohistiocytic infiltrate is present around the widely dilated capillaries and venules of the edematous papillary dermis. When the ballooned keratinocytes become necrotic, neutrophils are attracted into the epidermis, and the intraepidermal blister is accompanied by features of a spongiform pustule (Fig. 10-13B). The histologic differential diagnosis includes pellagra, acrodermatitis enteropathica, and other diseases caused by nutritional deficiencies.

The skin lesions of necrolytic migratory erythema begin as reddish patches in which flaccid bullae arise. As the lesions spread peripherally, annular and gyrate patterns are formed. Necrolytic migratory erythema is rare and seemingly develops only in patients who have a glucagon-producing islet cell neoplasm of the pancreas. The neoplasm may be benign or a carcinoma that metastasizes. Diabetes mellitus is a common consequence of a glucagonoma.

Serum amino acids are decreased in patients with necrolytic migratory erythema. Interestingly, other deficiency diseases such as *pellagra* (nicotinamide deficiency) and *acrodermatitis enteropathica* (zinc deficiency) are characterized histologically by large pale keratinocytes in the superficial epidermis reminiscent of those in necrolytic migratory erythema. These three diseases also have clinical features in common: cheilitis, stomatitis, diarrhea, and vesiculobullous skin lesions that tend to appear around the body orifices as well as on acral parts.

The skin and mucous membrane lesions of *pachyonychia congenita*, a dominantly inherited disorder, are characterized by intracellular edema in the covering epithelium that becomes so great that the ballooned cells rupture and a blister forms. These changes occur most prominently within the spinous layer. Clinically, there are associated hyperkeratoses of the palms, soles, hair follicles, and nail beds.

When the skin is immersed in water for about 96 hours, intraepidermal *immersion blisters* develop secondary to extensive intracellular edema. A sparse inflammatory-cell infiltrate surrounds the dilated blood vessels of the edematous upper portion of the dermis.

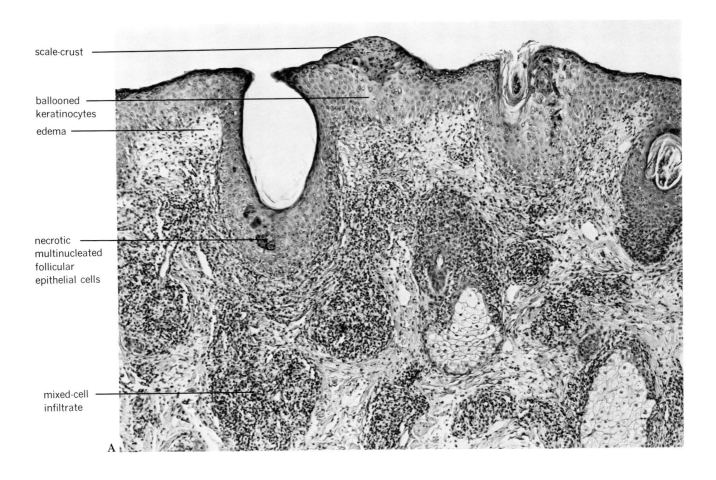

scale-crust

ballooned
keratinocytes

edema

necrotic
multinucleated
follicular
epithelial cells

mixed-cell
infiltrate

A

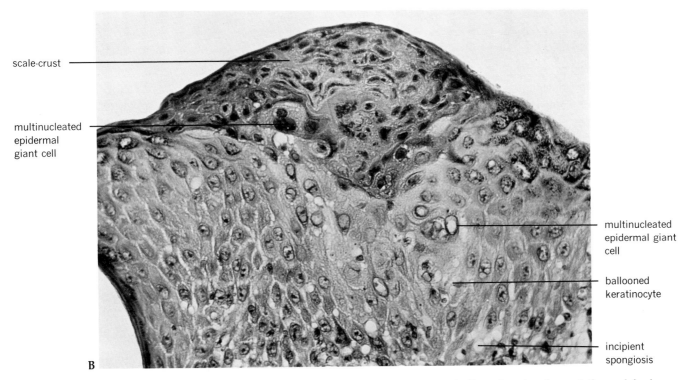

scale-crust

multinucleated
epidermal
giant cell

multinucleated
epidermal giant
cell

ballooned
keratinocyte

incipient
spongiosis

B

FIG. 10-12. Herpesvirus infection. A, Diagnostic histologic changes seen are concentration of nucleoplasm at the peripheries of ballooned keratinocytes and formation of multinucleated epithelial giant cells in both epidermal and follicular epithelium. (× 94.) B, Note accentuation of peripheral nucleoplasm, slate gray nuclei, and ballooned cytoplasm of spinous cells. Several multinucleated epidermal cells can be detected in this field. In some instances, such as this one, no blisters ever develop, the lesions appearing clinically as papules rather than vesicles. (× 440.)

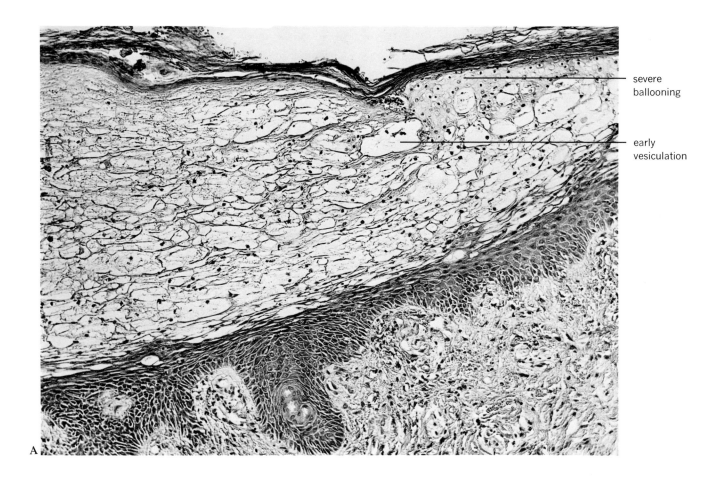

severe
ballooning

early
vesiculation

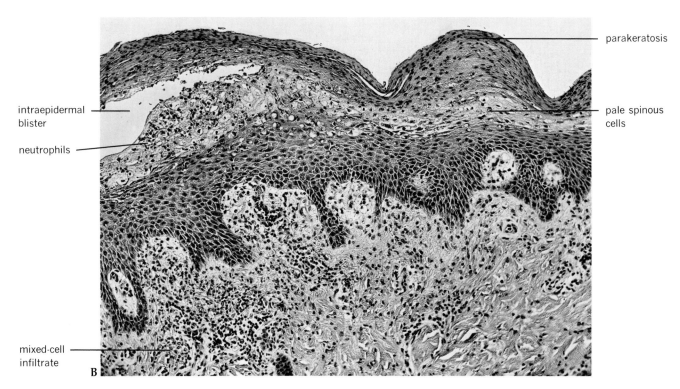

parakeratosis

intraepidermal
blister

pale spinous
cells

neutrophils

mixed-cell
infiltrate

B

FIG. 10-13. Necrolytic migratory erythema. A, Extensive ballooning pictured is characteristic of this disease. ($\times$ 174.) B, Neutrophils form spongiform pustules in this older lesion. Ballooned keratinocytes are also undergoing necrosis, and these necrotic cells are chemotactic for neutrophils. ($\times$ 166.)

Intraepidermal vesicles, a consequence principally of ballooning, sometimes develop in *erythema multiforme,* which is usually a subepidermal vesicular dermatitis (Fig. 10-14). This aspect of erythema multiforme is also covered in Chapter 6.

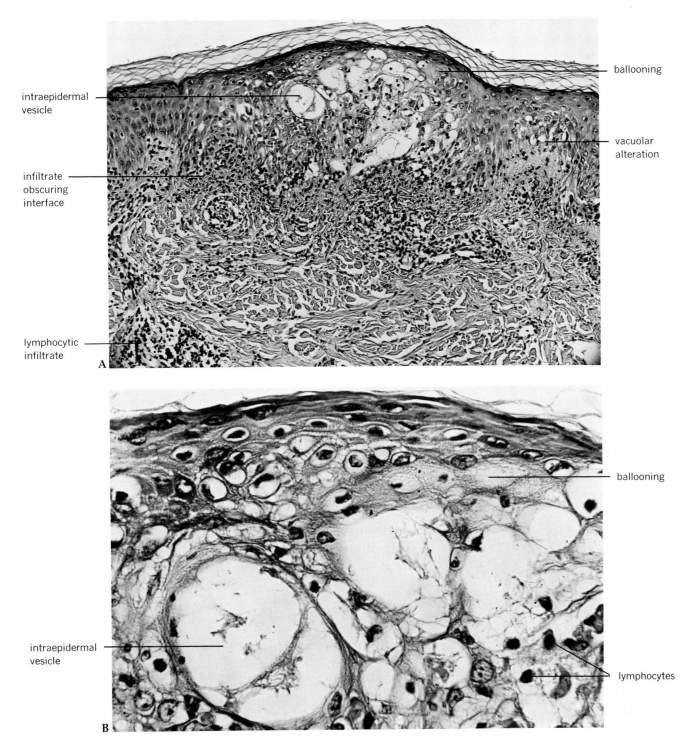

FIG. 10-14. Erythema multiforme, early lesions. Severe intracellular edema leading to intraepidermal vesiculation, vacuolar alteration giving rise to subepidermal vesiculation, necrotic keratinocytes, and superficial lymphohistiocytic infiltrate that obscures dermoepidermal interface are present. The fact that the cornified layer is normal indicates that the process shown here is, at most, a few days old. (A, × 163; B, × 763.)

Ballooning is also a prominent feature of irritant contact dermatitis, phototoxic contact dermatitis, and phototoxic dermatitis. Each of these conditions may be associated with intraepidermal vesiculation caused by severe intracellular edema, usually with concurrent necrosis of epidermal keratinocytes. Each has been considered previously in Chapter 6.

Superficial and Deep Infiltrate

The epidermis in the acute vesicular stage of a *fixed drug eruption* is characterized by both ballooned spinous cells and numerous necrotic keratinocytes (Fig. 10-15). Initially, the necrotic cells are found in the basal zone where there is also prominent vacuolar alteration. In time, there are individual necrotic keratinocytes throughout the epidermis. Later, massive intracellular edema progresses to intraepidermal vesiculation, often with a honeycomb appearance (Fig. 10-16). There is often edema of the papillary dermis, which, when extreme, can proceed to subepidermal vesiculation. Thus, intraepidermal and subepidermal vesicles can coexist in vesicular lesions of a fixed drug eruption. The mixed inflammatory-cell infiltrate is situated around the blood vessels of both the superficial and deep plexuses and interstitially between collagen bundles. Numerous neutrophils and eosinophils are present, in addition to lymphocytes, histiocytes, and mast cells. Melanophages are commonly present in the edematous papillary dermis.

The earliest epidermal changes of an acute fixed drug eruption may be indistinguishable from the epidermal changes of erythema multiforme. Both diseases demonstrate numerous necrotic keratinocytes and prominent vacuolar alteration at the dermoepidermal junction, and both may show concomitant ballooning and spongiosis within the epidermis. The most significant histologic features that distinguish fixed drug eruption from erythema multiforme reside in the dermis. In fixed drug eruption, a mixed inflammatory-cell infiltrate containing many neutrophils and eosinophils is present around blood vessels of both the superficial and deep plexuses, whereas in erythema multiforme, a lymphohistiocytic infiltrate surrounds vessels of the superficial plexus only. Additionally, in fixed drug eruption, the vesicle is usually intraepidermal, and only rarely is it also subepidermal because of massive subepidermal edema. Conversely, in erythema multiforme the blister is usually subepidermal, and only rarely is it also intraepidermal because of ballooning and spongiosis. Intraepidermal vesiculation in erythema multiforme occurs more commonly on mucous membranes than on skin.

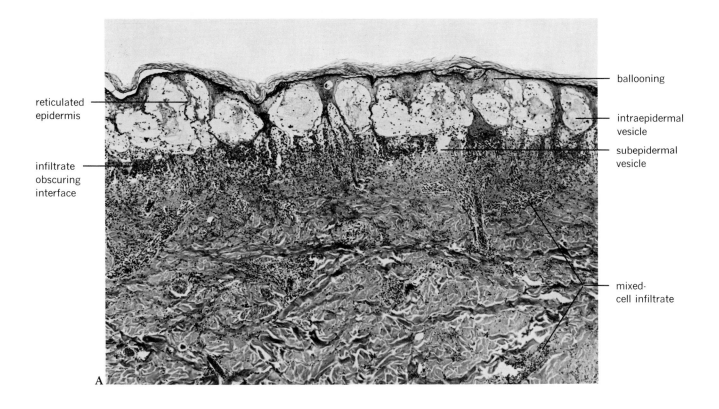

reticulated
epidermis

infiltrate
obscuring
interface

ballooning

intraepidermal
vesicle

subepidermal
vesicle

mixed-
cell infiltrate

A

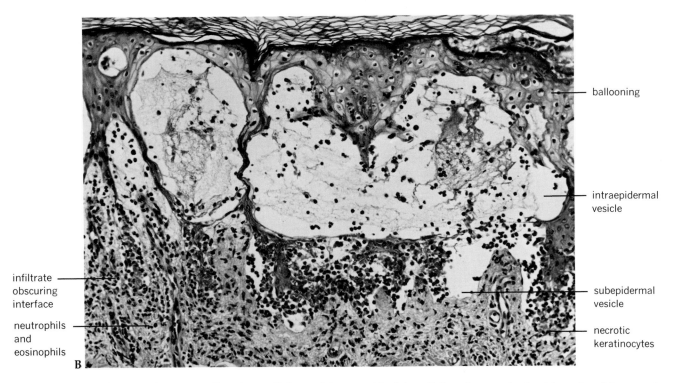

ballooning

intraepidermal
vesicle

infiltrate
obscuring
interface

neutrophils
and
eosinophils

subepidermal
vesicle

necrotic
keratinocytes

B

FIG. 10-15. Fixed drug eruption, acute. Note intracellular vesicle caused by intracellular edema and subepidermal vesicle caused by excessive tension in intraepidermal vesicle. Critical epidermal features seen are ballooning and numerous individual necrotic keratinocytes, especially in lower half of epidermis. Crucial dermal findings are superficial and deep perivascular and interstitial mixed inflammatory-cell infiltrate containing many neutrophils and eosinophils. (A, × 67; B, × 209.)

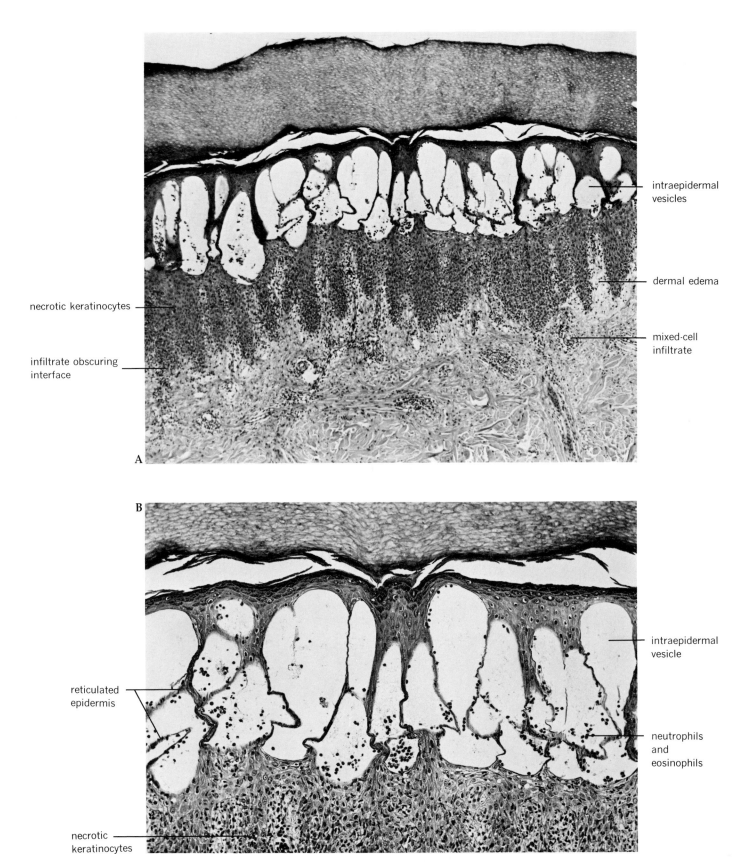

FIG. 10-16. Fixed drug eruption, acute. Honeycomb appearance caused by vesicles between reticulated strands of epidermis is typical. Viral vesicular dermatitides, such as caused by herpesvirus, may produce a similar pattern within the epidermis, but in herpetically infected epithelium there are also characteristic nuclear alterations such as steel-gray hues to the nuclei, concentration of the nucleoplasm at the peripheries, and formation of multinucleated cells. (A, × 70; B, × 184.)

Clinically, the lesions of acute fixed drug eruptions begin as dusky, reddish-purple papules that become indurated plaques surmounted by vesicles and/or bullae. The gray color of the blister roof is due to epidermal necrosis.

Intraepidermal vesiculation occurs in *pityriasis lichenoides et varioliformis acuta* (Mucha-Habermann disease) as a result of both ballooning and spongiosis (Fig. 10-17). Occasionally concomitant

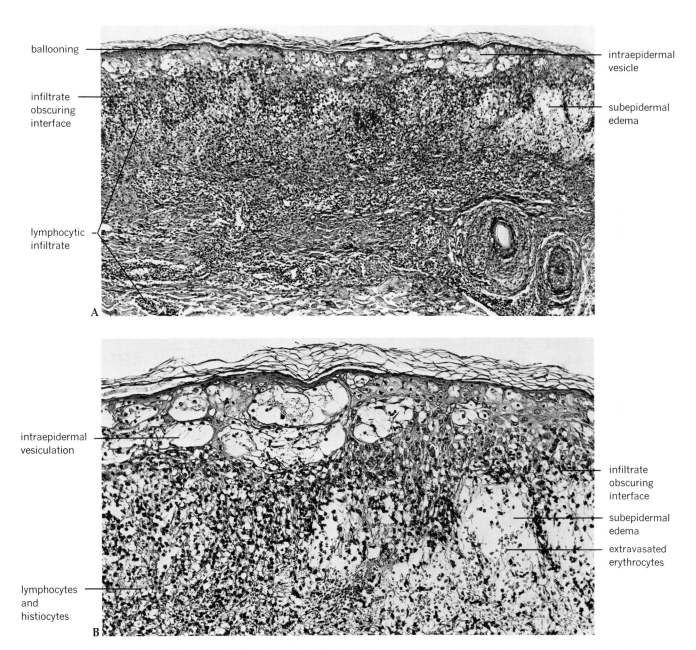

FIG. 10-17. Pityriasis lichenoides et varioliformis acuta (Mucha-Habermann disease). A, Diagnostic features pictured are superficial and deep perivascular, predominantly lymphocytic infiltrate obscuring dermoepidermal interface where there is vacuolar alteration and in the epidermis spongiosis and ballooning which evolve into intraepidermal vesiculation. (× 87.) B, In higher power view intraepidermal vesicles that result from spongiosis and ballooning can be seen. The netlike pattern of epidermis around vesicles is also described as reticular alteration. Note that inflammatory cells and extravasated erythrocytes obscure dermoepidermal junction and are present within epidermis. The fact that the cornified layer has maintained its basket-weave appearance indicates that this lesion is only a few days old. (× 180.)

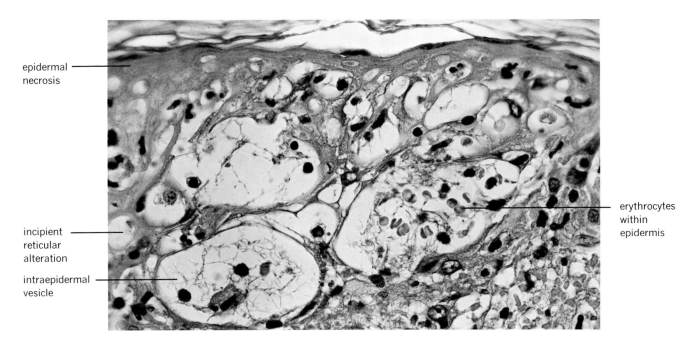

epidermal necrosis

erythrocytes within epidermis

incipient reticular alteration

intraepidermal vesicle

FIG. 10-17. Pityriasis lichenoides et varioliformis acuta. C, Still higher magnification shows intraepidermal vesicles, reticular alteration, inflammatory cells, and erythrocytes within epidermis. (× 624.)

subepidermal vesiculation develops secondary to the vacuolar alteration at the dermoepidermal junction, which is an almost constant histologic feature of this disease. The lesions are often covered by scales which consist of parakeratotic cells and neutrophils or by scale-crusts which, in addition, contain serum (Fig. 10-18).

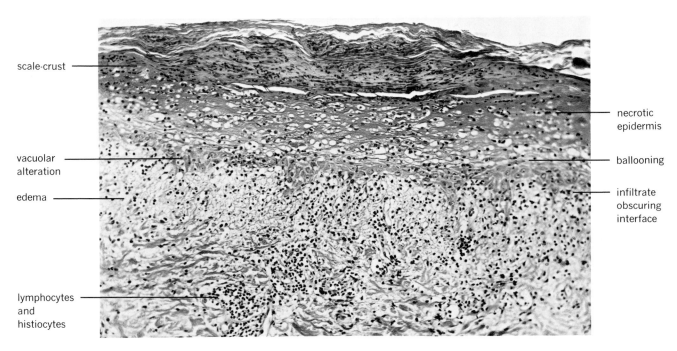

scale-crust

necrotic epidermis

vacuolar alteration

ballooning

edema

infiltrate obscuring interface

lymphocytes and histiocytes

FIG. 10-18. Pityriasis lichenoides et varioliformis acuta (Mucha-Habermann disease). Scale-crust containing neutrophils is common feature of acute lesion that is but several days old. Note other characteristic features: lymphohistiocytic infiltrate that obscures dermoepidermal interface, vacuolar alteration, ballooning of keratinocytes, and epidermal necrosis. (× 167.)

The clinical features of pityriasis lichenoides et varioliformis acuta are widespread pink-red macules and papules, some purpuric, as well as vesicles that sit atop the papules. These lesions may heal with atrophic scars that resemble those of smallpox, and thus the term *varioliformis.*

Something that somewhat resembles ballooning is the histologic change that occurs within the epidermis of *bullous congenital ichthyosiform erythroderma,* a widespread epidermal nevus that is devoid of a significant inflammatory-cell infiltrate. These histologic features, picturesquely described as epidermolytic hyperkeratosis, differ from ballooning by the presence of clear spaces of various sizes around nuclei in the spinous and granular zones; reticulated, lightly amphophilic cytoplasmic material forming indistinct, feathery cell boundaries; a thickened granular zone containing an increased number of small and large, irregularly-shaped, basophilic bodies resembling keratohyalin, and homogeneous eosinophilic bodies resembling trichohyalin; and, lastly, compact hyperkeratosis (Fig. 10-19). The clear areas within the epidermal cells do not result from edema, as in ballooning, but from overproduction of cell organelles. Blisters may develop within the epidermis secondary to coalescence and subsequent rupture of groups of large pale-staining spinous cells (Fig. 10-19B).

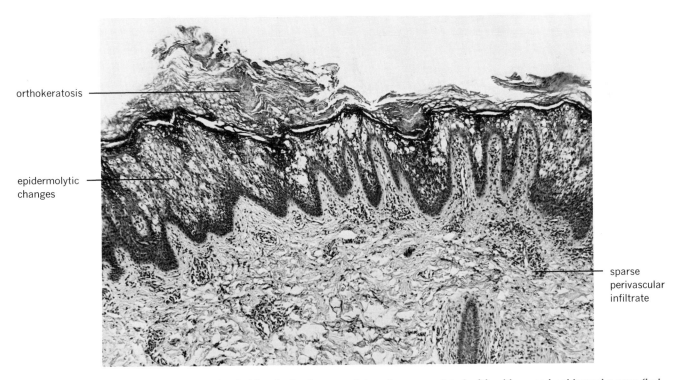

orthokeratosis

epidermolytic changes

sparse perivascular infiltrate

FIG. 10-19. Epidermolytic hyperkeratosis. A, Histologic changes pictured are associated with widespread epidermal nevus (bullous congenital ichthyosiform erythroderma), circumscribed epidermal nevi (e.g., ichthyosis hystrix), widespread follicular papules, solitary keratoses (e.g., epidermolytic acanthomas), the epithelial lining of rare follicular cysts, and incidentally in discrete epidermal foci above or to the side of various other pathologic processes. (× 94.)

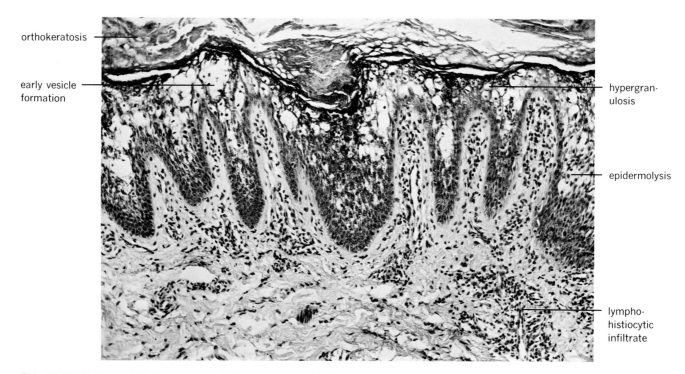

orthokeratosis

early vesicle formation

hypergran- ulosis

epidermolysis

lympho- histiocytic infiltrate

FIG. 10-19. Epidermolytic hyperkeratosis. B, Vesicles and bullae tend to occur only in epidermolytic hyperkeratosis associated with bullous congenital ichthyosiform erythroderma. (× 171.)

The precise mechanism of blister formation in bullous congenital ichthyosiform erythroderma is not known. Bacterial infection of these lesions has been reputed to be a causative factor. An alternative theory is that bullae form from exaggeration of the underlying pathologic process, without the supervention of bacteria.

The histologic changes of epidermolytic hyperkeratosis are not only found in bullous congenital ichthyosiform erythroderma, but in other epidermal nevi (e.g., ichthyosis hystrix, including some linear and systematized nevi), in widespread follicular papules, rarely in the lining of follicular cysts, solitary keratoses, and as an incidental finding, confined to a single rete ridge, in association with other seemingly unrelated pathologic processes. The variant features of epidermolytic hyperkeratosis are analogous to those of focal acantholytic dyskeratosis which is discussed later in this chapter.

Acantholytic Vesicular Dermatitis (Fig. 10-20)

Acantholytic vesicular dermatitis may be subdivided on the basis of the level in the epidermis at which the dominant separation occurs: (1) suprabasal, (2) intraspinous, and (3) subcorneal.

A useful adjunctive technique to biopsy for identification of acantholytic cells within the epidermis is the Tzanck smear. It is

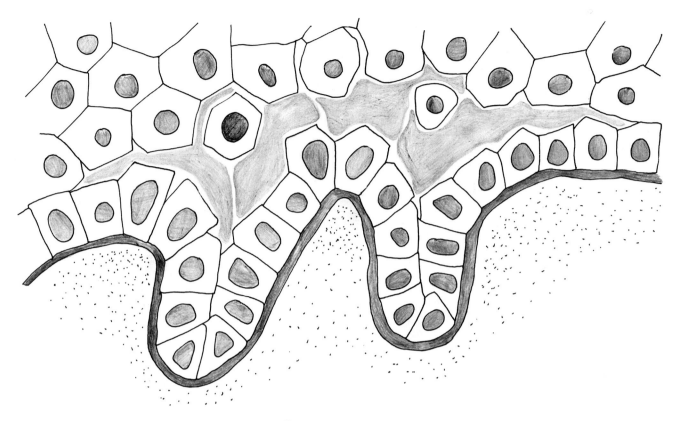

FIG. 10-20. Suprabasal vesicle with acantholytic cells.

multinucleated
epithelial
giant
cell

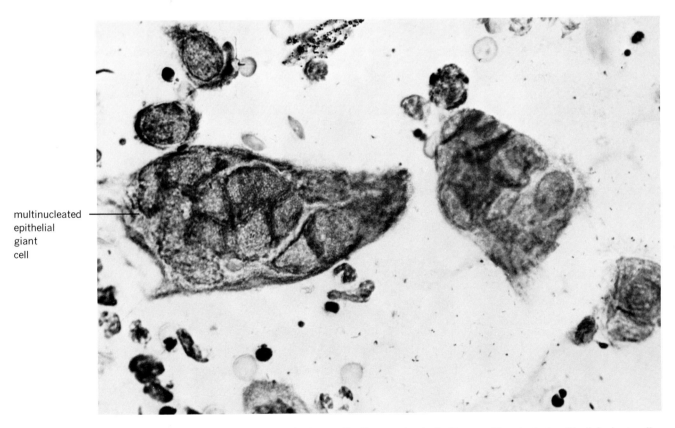

FIG. 10-21. Tzanck smear of multinucleated epithelial giant cells (herpesvirus). A, Two multinucleated epithelial giant cells, diagnostic of herpesvirus infection, are pictured. (Giemsa stain; × 1000.)

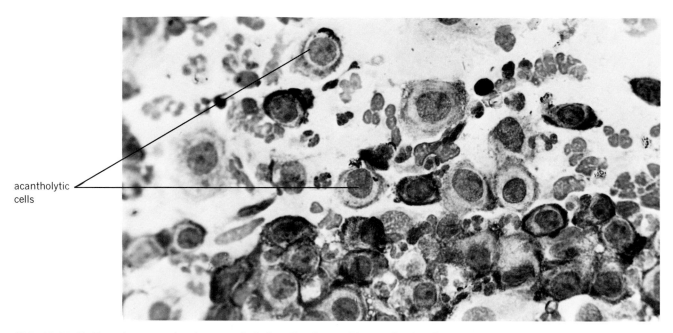

acantholytic
cells

FIG. 10-21. B, Tzanck smear showing acantholytic cells of pemphigus vulgaris. The acantholytic epidermal cells pictured are characterized by round shapes, large round nuclei, perinuclear pallor, and concentration of cytoplasm at the peripheries of the cells. (Giemsa stain; × 642.)

performed by unroofing a vesicle or bulla, reflecting the roof, and scraping with a blade the floor of the blister and the undersurface of the roof. The cells thus obtained are then smeared on a glass slide and stained by either Wright's or Giemsa's stain (Fig. 10-21). An especially effective manner of demonstrating the multinucleated epithelial cells of infections by herpesvirus is to employ the staining method of the Papanicolaou test.

The Tzanck smear is particularly helpful in the diagnosis of herpesvirus infections of skin where multinucleated epithelial giant cells, many of them acantholytic, are specific features. With this technique, in just a few minutes chickenpox may be differentiated from suspected cases of smallpox and herpetic from vaccinial Kaposi's varicelliform eruption. The Tzanck smear is also of benefit in quickly differentiating between pemphigus vulgaris and pemphigoid because numerous acantholytic cells are seen in smears of pemphigus but not in those of pemphigoid.

Any disease that shows acantholytic cells in histologic sections will also reveal them on properly done smears. However, except for herpesvirus infections, the diagnosis of other acantholytic vesiculobullous diseases of skin should always be confirmed by histologic examination and often by immunofluorescent studies.

As an aside it should be mentioned that acantholytic cells may be found in the subepidermal zone above abscesses in the papillary dermis of dermatitis herpetiformis. This is the only subepidermal vesicular dermatitis that is commonly associated with acantholytic cells.

—A continuous separation of basal cells from spinous cells (Fig. 10-22)
—Acantholytic keratinocytes within the suprabasalar space
—Generally intact epidermis above suprabasalar clefts (Fig. 10-23)
—Suprabasalar clefts extending down adnexal structures, e.g., down the follicular units, even to the bases of the trichilemmal sheaths and into eccrine sweat ducts within the dermis (Fig. 10-24)
—Sparse superficial perivascular mixed inflammatory-cell infiltrate of lymphocytes, histiocytes, and varying numbers of neutrophils, eosinophils, and plasma cells.

The intraepidermal separation in pemphigus vulgaris is not always confined to the zone immediately above the basal layer. The cleft can also occur in the middle portion of the spinous zone and within the granular zone. In fact, the same biopsy specimen of pemphigus vulgaris may show separations at different levels of the epidermis. Rarely, the earliest changes in pemphigus vulgaris may be eosinophilic spongiosis; later, acantholytic cells and numerous eosinophils are found in the suprabasal blister (Fig. 10-5).

It is sometimes difficult to distinguish histologically between pemphigus vulgaris and benign familial chronic pemphigus, inasmuch as the blisters in both acantholytic diseases form above the basal-cell layer (Figs. 10-23, 10-25). One helpful differentiating feature is that there is a tendency of the acantholytic keratinocytes in benign familial chronic pemphigus to involve most of the overlying epidermis, giving it the appearance of a "crumbling brick wall," unlike the situation in pemphigus vulgaris where the epidermis overlying the blister is mostly cohesive. Another distinction is that usually in pemphigus vulgaris, the acantholytic process involves adnexa, whereas in benign familial chronic pemphigus the adnexa are usually spared. Furthermore, the epidermis in Hailey-Hailey disease tends to become hyperplastic in contrast to pemphigus vulgaris where it does not. It must be noted, however, that these distinctions are not absolute.

Clinically, pemphigus vulgaris presents flaccid bullae that are surrounded by normal-appearing skin and mucous membranes. If downward pressure is applied to a cutaneous blister of pemphigus vulgaris, it extends peripherally; if friction is exerted on apparently normal skin, typical blisters can be induced (Nikolsky's sign). Blisters in pemphigus readily rupture and reveal a dermis that weeps because it is protected by only a single layer of basal cells.

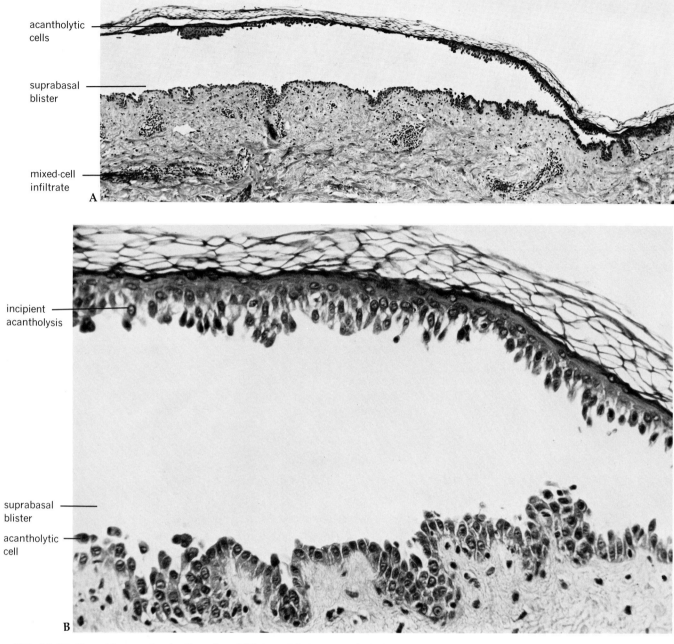

acantholytic cells

suprabasal blister

mixed-cell infiltrate

A

incipient acantholysis

suprabasal blister

acantholytic cell

B

FIG. 10-22. Pemphigus vulgaris. Suprabasal blister with few acantholytic cells above basal layer and below separated epidermis is typical. (A, × 63; B, × 340.)

The oozing serum congeals to form a crust beneath which re-epithelization proceeds. Pemphigus vulgaris varies widely from a few lesions that are relatively innocuous to an extensive disease that is fatal.

Direct and indirect immunofluorescent studies are positive in pemphigus vulgaris, with fluorescence occurring in the intercellular spaces of the epidermis. These findings indicate the presence of an antibody capable of binding an antigen in the intercellular spaces of the lesions in pemphigus vulgaris.

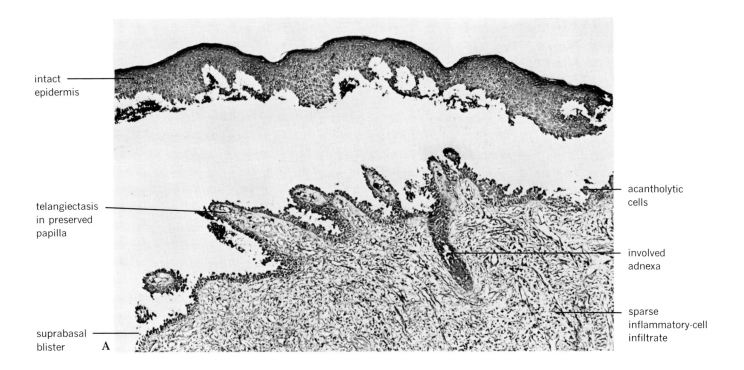

intact epidermis

telangiectasis in preserved papilla

suprabasal blister

A

acantholytic cells

involved adnexa

sparse inflammatory-cell infiltrate

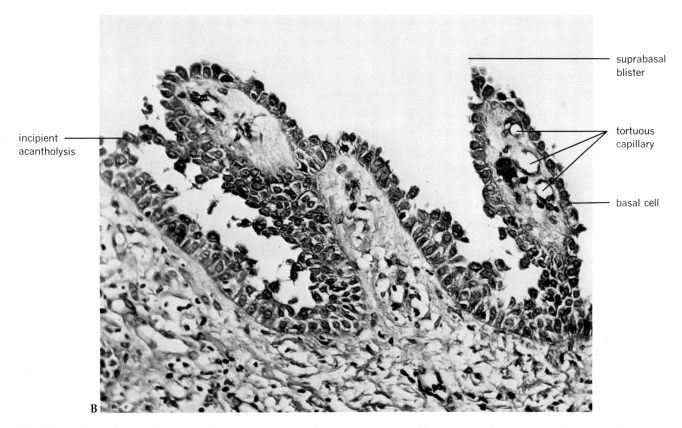

incipient acantholysis

suprabasal blister

tortuous capillary

basal cell

B

FIG. 10-23. Pemphigus vulgaris. A, Diagnostic features shown are suprabasal blister containing few acantholytic cells above which separated epidermis is mostly in normal cohesion, but beneath which the adnexal epithelium is often affected by acantholytic process. (× 85.) B, In this higher magnification there are relatively few acantholytic cells in the blister above the basal layer. (× 360.)

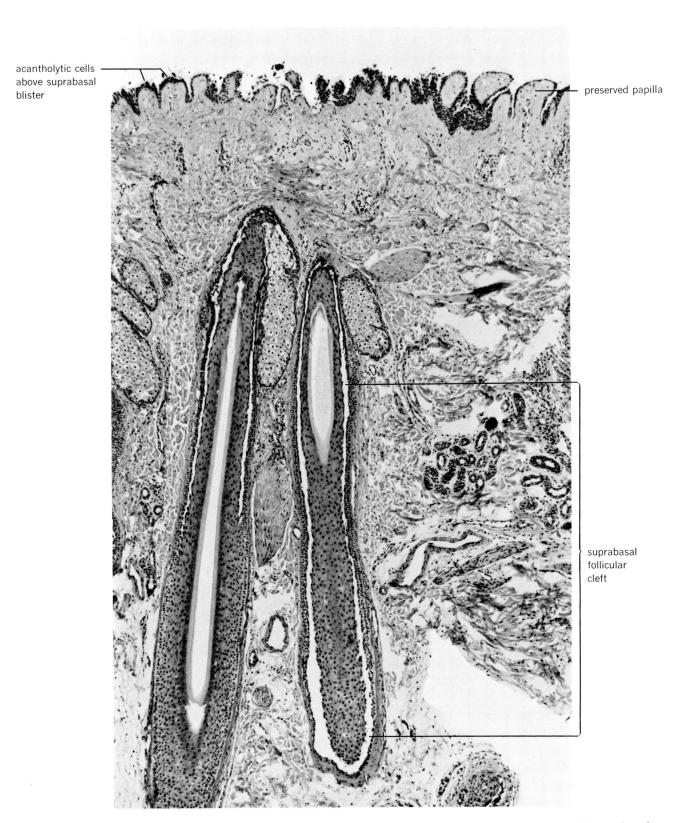

acantholytic cells
above suprabasal
blister

preserved papilla

suprabasal
follicular
cleft

FIG. 10-24. Pemphigus vulgaris. Note that separation extends to inferior portion of external root sheath. Often only a few acantholytic cells are seen above suprabasal clefts. (× 56.)

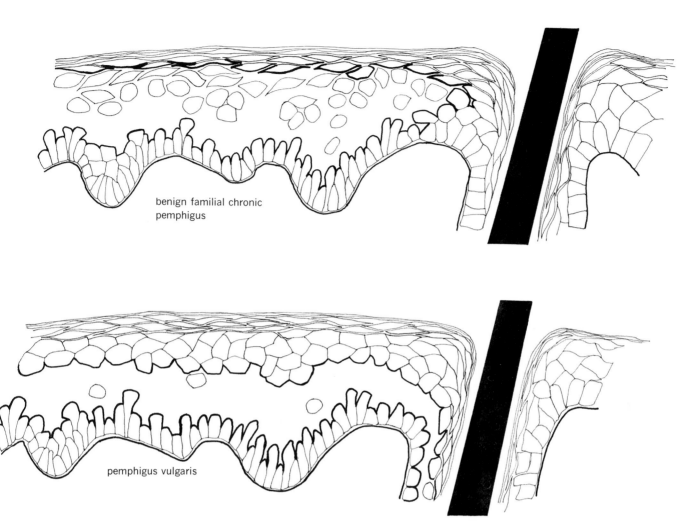

FIG. 10-25. Contrast in histologic patterns of benign familial chronic pemphigus (Hailey-Hailey disease) and pemphigus vulgaris.

When Civatte, in 1943, first noted acantholytic cells in pemphigus vulgaris, the rounded-up keratinocytes were thought to be markers specific for that disease. Now it is recognized that acantholytic cells occur in many other blistering (e.g., benign familial chronic pemphigus), clefting (e.g., keratosis follicularis), neoplastic (e.g., pseudoglandular squamous cell carcinoma), and hamartomatous (e.g., warty dyskeratoma) conditions. In the realm of intraepidermal blistering diseases, it must be acknowledged that pemphigus vulgaris at times may be indistinguishable on histologic grounds alone from benign familial chronic pemphigus and that superficial pemphigus may be impossible to differentiate from infectious processes like bullous impetigo and the staphylococcal scalded-skin syndrome in sections stained only by hematoxylin and eosin. In the clefting diseases, keratosis follicularis occasionally may be indistinguishable from transient acantholytic dermatosis. However, when the histologic features and the clinical picture are taken together, usually the diseases can be differentiated.

Pemphigus Vegetans (Fig. 10-26)

—Suprabasalar separations in the epidermis and its adnexa
—Intraepidermal abscesses composed of eosinophils
—Acantholytic cells above the suprabasalar clefts and within the eosinophilic abscesses
—Epidermal hyperplasia
—Scale-crusts
—Edema of the papillary dermis
—Superficial perivascular mixed inflammatory cell infiltrate of lymphocytes, histiocytes, eosinophils, and, sometimes, neutrophils.

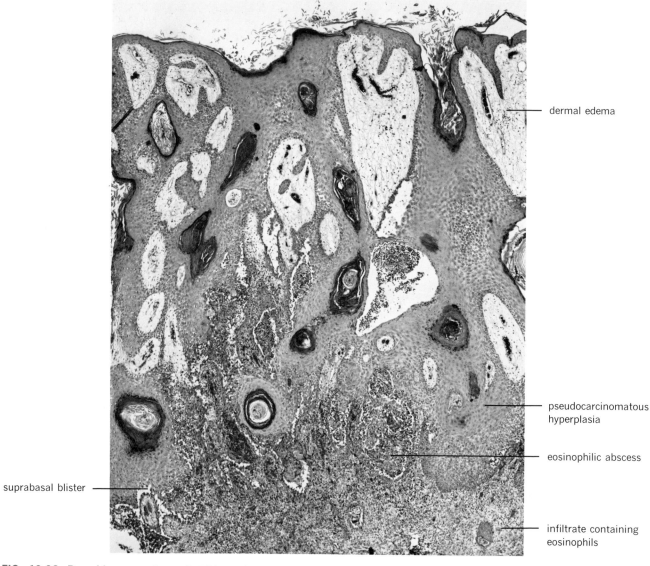

FIG. 10-26. Pemphigus vegetans. A, This variant preserves crucial diagnostic histologic features of pemphigus vulgaris: suprabasal blisters containing acantholytic cells. Distinctive additional attributes are numerous collections of eosinophils in exceedingly hyperplastic epidermis. (× 46.)

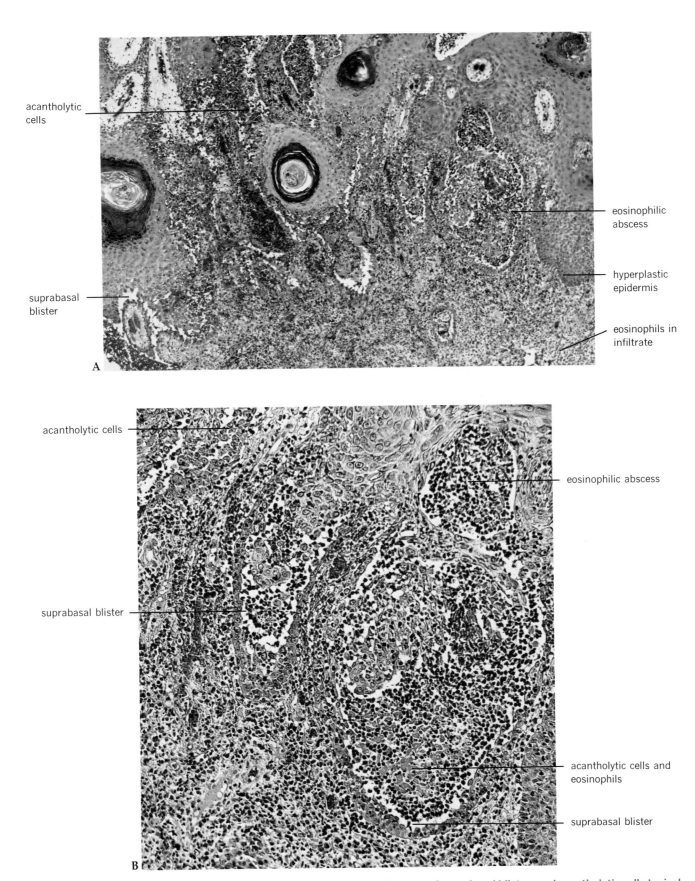

acantholytic
cells

eosinophilic
abscess

hyperplastic
epidermis

suprabasal
blister

eosinophils in
infiltrate

A

acantholytic cells

eosinophilic abscess

suprabasal blister

acantholytic cells and
eosinophils

suprabasal blister

B

FIG. 10-26. Pemphigus vegetans. B, Higher magnification shows combination of suprabasal blisters and acantholytic cells typical of pemphigus vulgaris with eosinophilic abscesses and hyperplastic epidermis that together are diagnostic of pemphigus vegetans. ($\times$ 84.) C, Still higher power view shows acantholytic cells and eosinophils above suprabasal separations. ($\times$ 163.)

Pemphigus vegetans, which probably represents a tumid variant of long-standing lesions of pemphigus vulgaris, is usually located in intertriginous sites. Clinically, the vegetative scale-crusts of pemphigus vegetans often occur in conjunction with typical lesions of pemphigus vulgaris. Histologically, pemphigus vegetans, like pemphigus vulgaris, has suprabasalar clefts containing acantholytic cells. Collections of eosinophils in an exceedingly hyperplastic epidermis are features that distinguish pemphigus vegetans from pemphigus vulgaris (Fig. 10-26A). The presence of eosinophilic abscesses, however, is not restricted to pemphigus vegetans but may be found in such disparate conditions as toxic erythema of the newborn and some examples of vesicular dermatophytosis. Immunofluorescent findings by both direct and indirect methods are identical in pemphigus vegetans and pemphigus vulgaris.

Benign Familial Chronic Pemphigus (Hailey-Hailey Disease) (Fig. 10-27)

—Suprabasalar blister
—Acantholytic cells involving at least the lower half of the overlying epidermis in some foci
—Epidermal hyperplasia
—Edema of the papillary dermis
—Superficial perivascular predominantly lymphohistiocytic infiltrate

Benign familial chronic pemphigus can usually be distinguished histologically from pemphigus vulgaris by three features (Fig. 10-25). As was mentioned in the discussion of pemphigus vulgaris, most of the epidermis above the blister in benign familial chronic pemphigus is involved in the acantholytic process, giving the epidermis the appearance of a crumbling brick wall, the bricks being acantholytic epidermal cells. In pemphigus vulgaris, most of the epidermis above the suprabasalar blister is intact, with only the lowermost cells of the spinous zone being acantholytic. In addition, in benign familial chronic pemphigus there is little or no involvement of adnexal structures (follicular and eccrine) by the acantholytic process in contrast to frequent adnexal involvement in pemphigus vulgaris. Finally, there is a tendency to epidermal hyperplasia in benign familial chronic pemphigus, but not in pemphigus vulgaris.

In some instances it may be exceedingly difficult to differentiate histologically between benign familial chronic pemphigus and pemphigus vulgaris, especially when there are only a few acan-

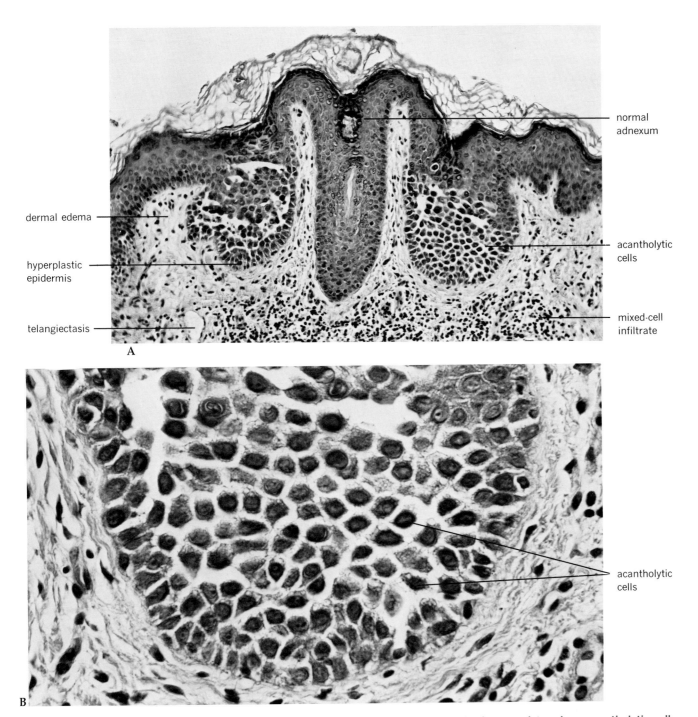

FIG. 10-27. Benign familial chronic pemphigus (Hailey-Hailey disease). Characteristic changes pictured are acantholytic cells within much of thickness of hyperplastic epidermis in some foci and tending to spare adnexal epithelial structures, intraepidermal vesiculation, edema of papillary dermis, and moderately dense superficial inflammatory-cell infiltrate. Note absence of inflammatory cells in zones of acantholysis, an indication that this is not spongiosis. (A, × 176; B, × 560.)

tholytic cells above the suprabasalar blister. In these cases a useful clue to the diagnosis of benign familial chronic pemphigus is the finding of a focus in which acantholytic cells involve most of the overlying epidermis (Fig. 10-28). Such foci may be confined to a single rete ridge. In such perplexing cases deeper sections should be cut through the specimen in search of diagnostic features.

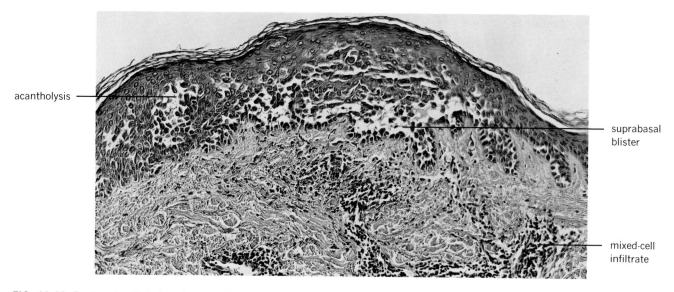

acantholysis

suprabasal blister

mixed-cell infiltrate

FIG. 10-28. Benign familial chronic pemphigus (Hailey-Hailey disease). Acantholytic cells throughout most of thickness of epidermis above a suprabasal blister is virtually diagnostic of this disease. (× 188.)

In addition to these histologic differences between benign familial chronic pemphigus and pemphigus vulgaris, the two diseases are wholly different by immunofluorescent criteria. In benign familial chronic pemphigus the direct and indirect tests are both negative, whereas in pemphigus vulgaris they are both usually positive for antibody to intercellular substance.

Clinically, the blisters of benign familial chronic pemphigus, like those of pemphigus vulgaris, are flaccid and can be extended laterally by downward pressure. Unlike the situation in pemphigus vulgaris, the sites of predilection for lesions of benign familial chronic pemphigus are the intertriginous regions, especially the axillary, inframammary, and inguinal. Furthermore, this disease, unlike pemphigus vulgaris, spares mucous membranes.

Keratosis Follicularis (Darier's Disease) (Fig. 10-29)

—Focal suprabasalar clefts
—Often short cords of basal cells beneath and perpendicular to the clefts
—Above the clefts, acantholytic, dyskeratotic cells in the spinous and granular zones ("corps ronds") and parakeratotic cornified layer ("grains")
—Focal vertical parakeratosis overlying the suprabasalar clefts
—Superficial perivascular lymphohistiocytic infiltrate

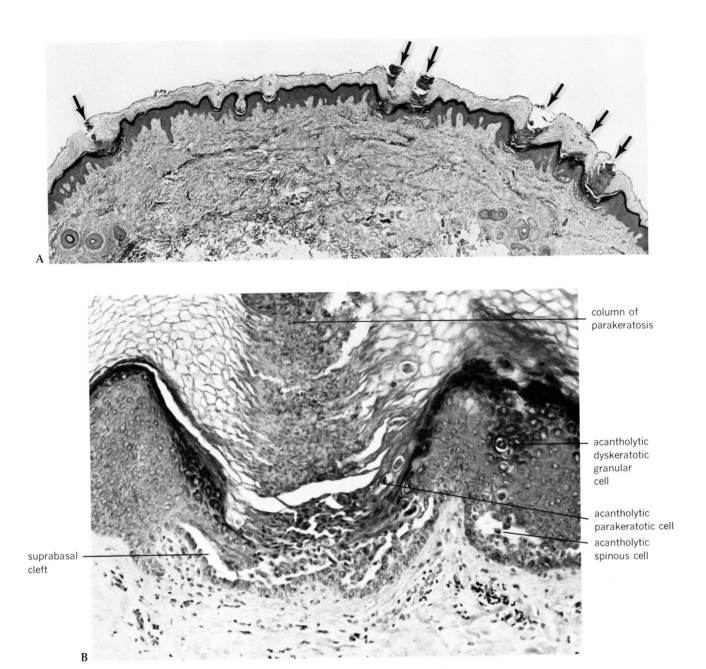

FIG. 10-29. Keratosis follicularis (Darier's disease). A, Under scanning magnification, multiple discrete zones of focal acantholytic dyskeratosis are seen. Arrows point to vertical columns of parakeratosis above suprabasal clefts that are responsible for the rough graterlike consistency to the clinical lesions of keratosis follicularis. (× 20.) B, Features illustrated are those of focal acantholytic dyskeratosis. Biopsy came from patient with Darier's disease, but identical histologic changes can be seen in systematized keratosis follicularis, transient acantholytic dermatosis (Grover's disease), solitary keratoses, and as an incidental finding in the epidermis above or to the side of another unrelated pathologic process. (× 220.)

The term *focal acantholytic dyskeratosis* describes the constellation of histologic findings common to Darier's disease and to other conditions of the skin such as systematized keratosis follicularis and Grover's disease that are histologically identical with, but clinically different from, Darier's disease (Fig. 10-30). Focal acantholytic dyskeratosis occurs in some cases of transient acantholytic dermatosis, systematized and zosteriform epidermal nevi, solitary

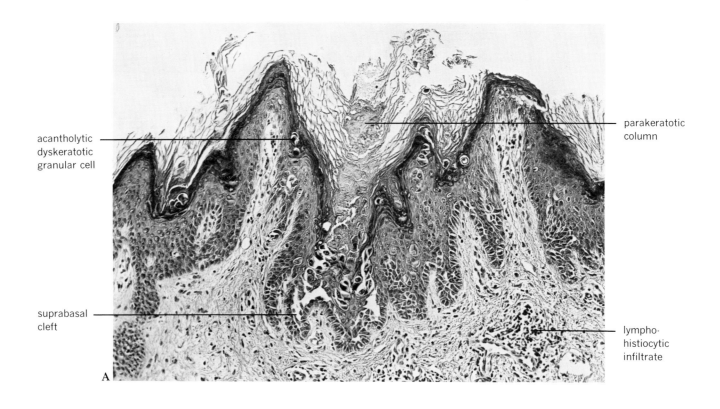

acantholytic
dyskeratotic
granular cell

parakeratotic
column

suprabasal
cleft

lympho-
histiocytic
infiltrate

A

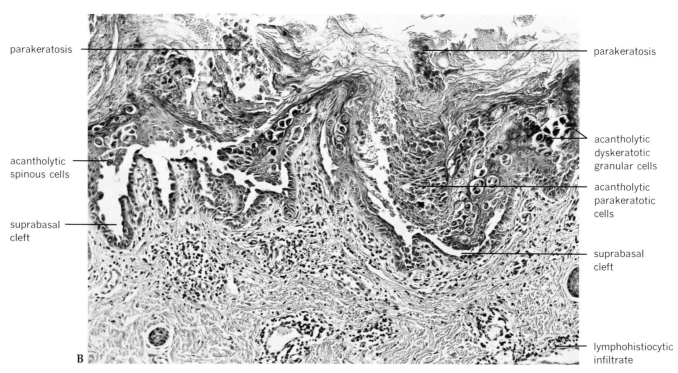

parakeratosis

parakeratosis

acantholytic
spinous cells

acantholytic
dyskeratotic
granular cells

acantholytic
parakeratotic
cells

suprabasal
cleft

suprabasal
cleft

lymphohistiocytic
infiltrate

B

FIG. 10-30. Focal acantholytic dyskeratosis. A, Crucial diagnostic features are suprabasal clefts above which there are acantho-lytic cells capped by a column of parakeratosis. (Acantholytic dyskeratotic cells in the granular zone are often called "corps ronds" and acantholytic parakeratotic cells "grains.") ($\times$ 173.) **B,** Two discrete zones of histologic changes illustrate one of many patterns of cutaneous epithelium such as epidermolytic hyperkeratosis and follicular mucinosis. ($\times$ 170.)

papules, and solitary follicular cysts (warty dyskeratoma, isolated dyskeratosis follicularis). Furthermore, the histologic changes of focal acantholytic dyskeratosis can be confined to a single rete ridge (or acrotrichium or acrosyringium), or be a histologic accompaniment to an unrelated neoplastic, hyperplastic, or inflammatory disease.

Focal acantholytic dyskeratosis is to Darier's disease what epidermolytic hyperkeratosis is to bullous congenital ichthyosiform erythroderma. Epidermolytic hyperkeratosis describes histologic changes that occur not only in the widespread congenital epidermal nevus (bullous congenital ichthyosiform erythroderma), but also in some linear systematized and zosteriform nevi (ichthyosis hystrix) and in solitary papules (isolated epidermolytic acanthoma), and as a microscopic curiosity lateral to other pathologic processes. In exceptional cases, focal acantholytic dyskeratosis and epidermolytic hyperkeratosis occur contiguous to one another in the same specimen. Epidermolytic hyperkeratosis has been discussed earlier in this chapter.

In a sense, Darier's disease (histologically focal acantholytic dyskeratosis) is a widespread epidermal nevus analogous to bullous congenital ichthyosiform erythroderma (histologically epidermolytic hyperkeratosis). Just as epidermolytic hyperkeratosis may be circumscribed clinically (e.g., ichthyosis hystrix), so, too, may focal acantholytic dyskeratosis (i.e., systematized keratosis follicularis) be circumscribed. When changes of acantholytic dyskeratosis occur in the lining of a follicular cyst, the lesion is termed warty dyskeratoma.

In Darier's disease, in contrast to pemphigus vulgaris and benign familial chronic pemphigus, the suprabasalar clefts are discrete, rather than confluent, and do not contain serum. Hence, keratosis follicularis is not a true vesicular disease. Clinically, there are no blisters in keratosis follicularis. The gross pathologic changes are rough-surfaced papules that feel like gravel and result from focal vertical parakeratosis. The keratotic papules tend to confluence and to plaque formation that is rough-surfaced and widespread. Keratosis follicularis often involves mucous membranes and nails, as well as the skin.

Sometimes lesions that are clinically and histologically typical of keratosis follicularis can be induced by sunlight, and then, instead of persisting indefinitely, as is usually the case in this disease, resolve spontaneously after a few weeks. Thus, there is a transient or an evanescent form of keratosis follicularis. Evanescent lesions of focal acantholytic dermatosis can thus occur in patients with typical keratosis follicularis as well as in those with transient acantholytic dermatosis.

Transient Acantholytic Dermatosis (Grover's Disease)

There are several histologic variants of transient acantholytic dermatosis, all of them having acantholytic cells in sharply circumscribed epidermal foci. One variant is similar, if not identical, histologically to keratosis follicularis (Fig. 10-31), whereas the others are histologically distinct. The "Darier's type" of transient acantholytic dermatosis may have less prominent parakeratosis than authentic keratosis follicularis and no cords of keratinocytes beneath the suprabasal cleft (Fig. 10-32). Although this type of transient acantholytic dermatosis bears a histologic resemblance to keratosis follicularis, it differs from it clinically by consisting of scattered discrete papules that are often smooth-surfaced, although they may be rough-topped, depending upon the extent of parakeratosis. Another distinction is that palmar-plantar, mucous-membrane, and nail involvement are not seen in transient acantholytic dermatosis.

A second histologic form of transient acantholytic dermatosis is the spongiotic type (Fig. 10-33). It is characterized by discrete intraepidermal spongiotic vesicles, some containing a few acantholytic cells, some suprabasalar clefts; edema of the papillary dermis; and a superficial perivascular mixed-cell infiltrate of lymphocytes, histiocytes, and varying numbers of eosinophils, plasma cells, and mast cells. This type of transient acantholytic dermatosis is unique because of spongiosis with acantholysis.

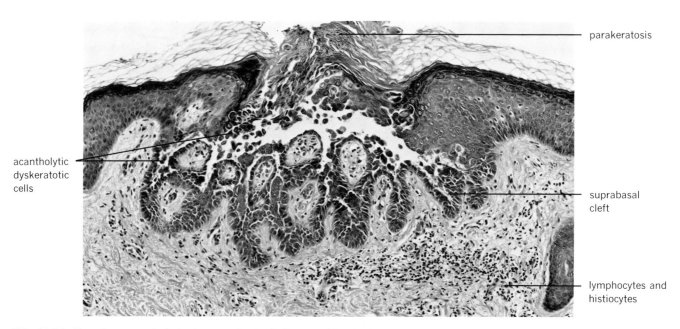

parakeratosis

acantholytic
dyskeratotic
cells

suprabasal
cleft

lymphocytes and
histiocytes

FIG. 10-31. Transient acantholytic dermatosis, Darier's type. Histologic change pictured, focal acantholytic dyskeratosis, can be seen in transient acantholytic dermatosis (Grover's disease), keratosis follicularis (Darier's disease), systematized epidermal nevi, solitary keratoses, and as incidental finding secondary to a variety of inflammatory and neoplastic processes. The lesion of Grover's disease pictured is indistinguishable histologically from Darier's disease. (× 170.)

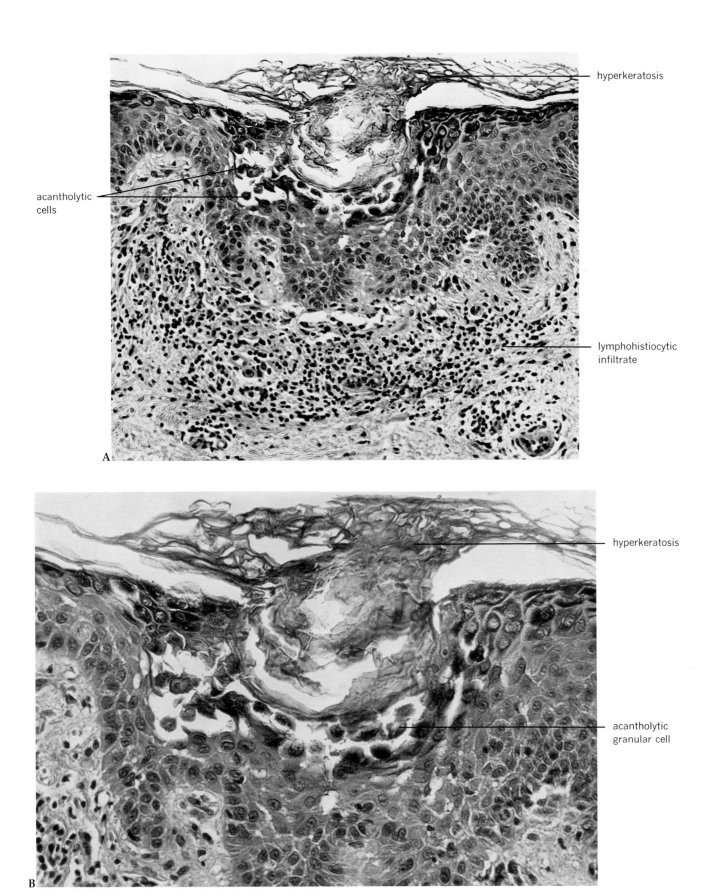

FIG. 10-32. Transient acantholytic dermatosis, Darier's type. Although changes of Grover's disease shown bear superficial resemblance to those of Darier's disease, they may sometimes be differentiated from it by absence of suprabasal cleft and of prominent focal vertical parakeratosis. (A, × 230; B, × 370.)

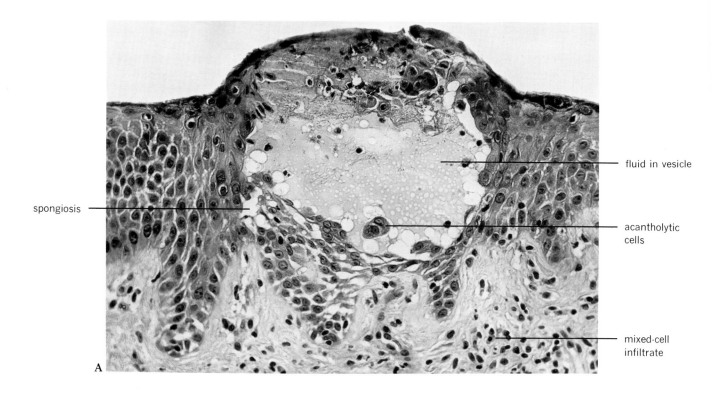

spongiosis

fluid in vesicle

acantholytic cells

mixed-cell infiltrate

A

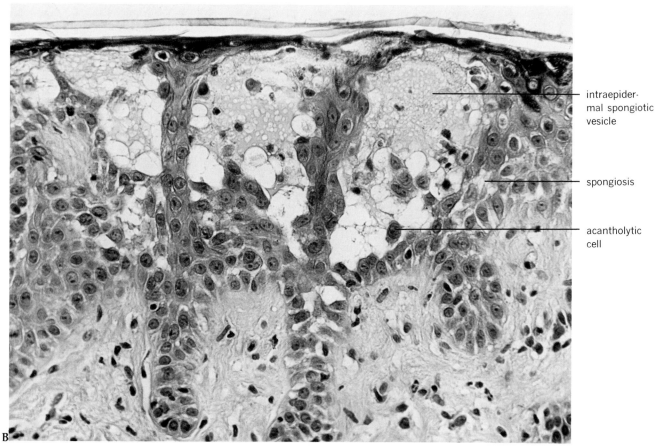

intraepidermal spongiotic vesicle

spongiosis

acantholytic cell

B

FIG. 10-33. Transient acantholytic dermatosis, spongiotic type. Tense well-circumscribed vesicle of Grover's disease shown contains acantholytic cells and is surrounded by spongiosis. (× 360.) B, Note acantholytic cells in spongiotic vesicles of Grover's disease unlike the finding in almost all other spongiotic vesicular dermatitides. The patient from whom this biopsy was taken had had the disease for more than 3 years (persistent acantholytic dermatosis). (× 400.)

A third histologic type of transient acantholytic dermatosis histologically resembles benign familial chronic phemphigus with acantholytic cells involving most levels of the epidermis (Fig. 10-34). Unlike the situation in benign familial chronic pemphigus, the acantholysis occurs in only a few discrete foci, and the epidermis is less hyperplastic.

The fourth histologic form of transient acantholytic dermatosis has features of pemphigus, superficial or deep types (Fig. 10-35). As in all variants of transient acantholytic dermatosis, the epider-

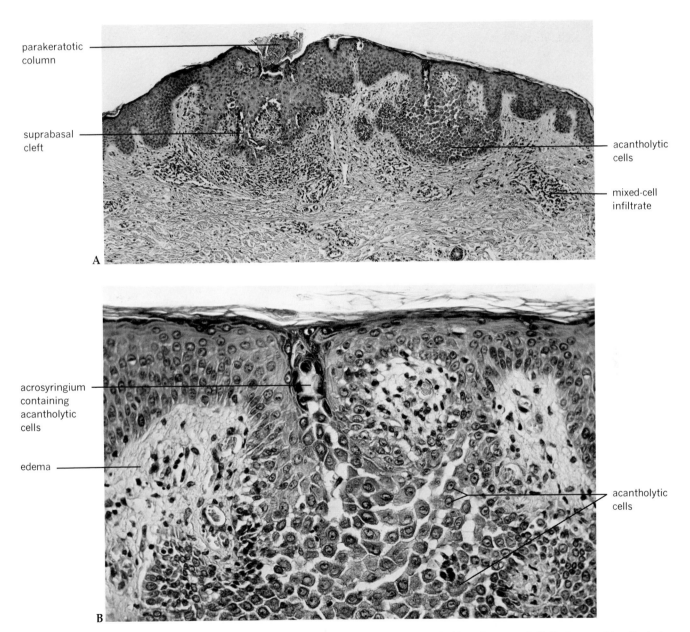

FIG. 10-34. Transient acantholytic dermatosis, Darier's and Hailey-Hailey types. A, Note focus on left that resembles Darier's disease (focal acantholytic dyskeratosis) and focus on right that simulates Hailey-Hailey disease (benign familial chronic pemphigus). The combination to two different histologic patterns with acantholytic cells in common is typical of Grover's disease. (× 80.) B, Higher power view shows that acantholytic process in this focus involves much of thickness of epidermis, a feature also of benign familial chronic pemphigus. (× 350.)

mal changes are sharply circumscribed, rather than confluent. Thus, there are discrete foci of suprabasalar clefts, above which there are a few acantholytic cells. Occasionally there are histologic features of superficial pemphigus (pemphigus foliaceus and erythematosus) as well as of deep pemphigus (pemphigus vulgaris) in biopsy specimens of transient acantholytic dermatosis.

A remarkable aspect of the histologic findings in transient acantholytic dermatosis is the wide variation in the appearance of the sections at different levels of the block on the same tissue

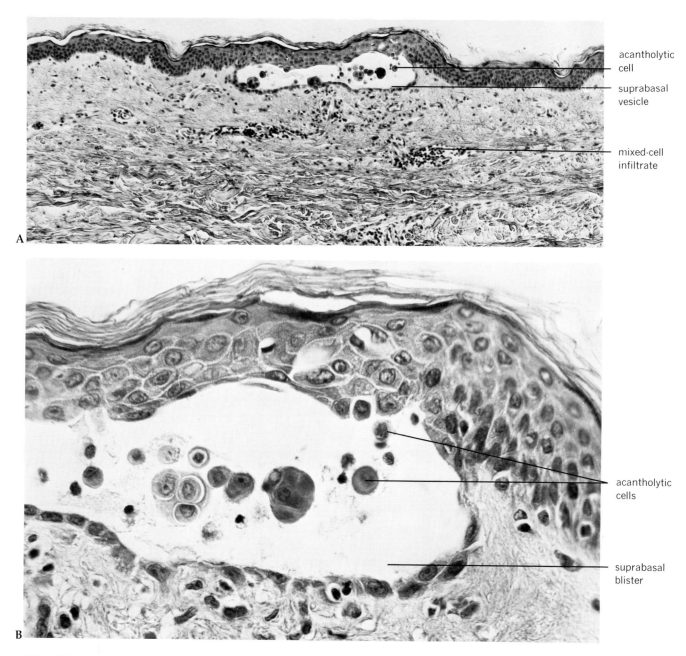

FIG. 10-35. Transient acantholytic dermatosis, pemphigus vulgaris type. Characteristic features illustrated are acantholytic cells within discrete intraepidermal blister. This type of Grover's disease resembles pemphigus vulgaris in miniature. (A, × 120; B, × 608.)

specimen. Within a few microns, all histologic variants of this disease can be seen (Fig. 10-36). Because the lesions are often pruritic, evidences of excoriations such as erosions, ulcerations, and scale-crusts may be present in the histologic sections.

The clinical features of transient acantholytic dermatosis are similar in each of the four histologic types: Darier, spongiotic, Hailey-Hailey, and pemphigus vulgaris. Only the Darier form of transient acantholytic dermatosis is ever marked by keratotic clinical lesions, the others being smooth-surfaced rather than scaly. Except for the Darier type, the eruption is generally disturbingly pruritic, the intensity of the pruritus being roughly proportioned to the numbers of eosinophils within the dermal infiltrate.

The eruption of transient acantholytic dermatosis is mainly distributed on the trunk and extremities of men and, less commonly, of women over the age of 40 years and frequently those who are over 60. Although the individual papules and papulovesicles wane within days, the disease itself usually persists for weeks or months before disappearing spontaneously and entirely. Occasionally this acantholytic disease is not transient, but persists for years (persistent acantholytic dermatosis). Immunofluorescent studies, both direct and indirect, are negative in transient acantholytic dermatosis.

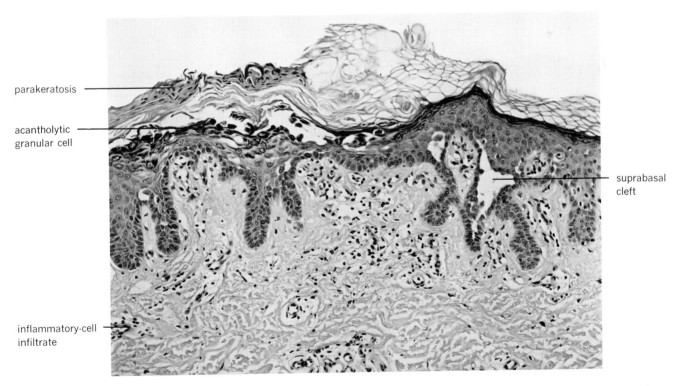

FIG. 10-36. Transient acantholytic dermatosis, mixed type. Note variation of histologic features. In this section there are features of forms of pemphigus and Darier's disease. (× 210.)

Intraspinous

Herpesvirus Infections (Herpes Simplex, Herpes Zoster, and Varicella) (Fig. 10-37)

—Intraepidermal vesicles containing acantholytic cells
—Multinucleated epithelial giant cells, some acantholytic, within the vesicle (Plate 4)
—Ballooned spinous cells with abundant, pale-staining cytoplasm
—Steel-gray nuclei with accentuation of the peripheral nucleoplasm
—Necrotic keratinocytes, some acantholytic
—Edema of the papillary dermis
—Dermal inflammatory-cell infiltrate varying in composition, density, and depth
—Extravasated erythrocytes in the papillary dermis

The earliest histologic changes in the epidermis of herpesvirus infections consist of pallor and swelling of the cytoplasm of the involved spinous cells, giving them the appearance of pale balloons. Concomitant with these cytoplasmic alterations, the nuclei develop a steel-gray hue and their peripheries become accentuated, a phenomenon termed "margination" of the nucleoplasm (Fig. 10-38). Shortly thereafter, multinucleated epithelial cells form within the epidermis, and eventually acantholytic changes supervene. Later, there are many multinucleated epidermal giant cells, acantholytic cells, and necrotic keratinocytes (Fig. 10-37). If necrosis supervenes early, multinucleated epithelial cells may not have time to form. Later, epidermal necrosis may be so severe that the characteristic nuclear changes of herpesvirus infections cannot be discerned. The diagnosis of herpesvirus infection can be suspected histologically in early lesions on the basis of the characteristic nuclear and cytoplasmic changes, even in the absence of multinucleated and acantholytic cells. The specific epithelial changes of herpesvirus infections can occur within the adnexal epithelium, as well as within the epidermis. Although the vesicles of herpesvirus infections always begin within the epidermis, sufficient pressure within such blisters can cause an intraepidermal "blow-out," and the result is subepidermal vesiculation (Fig. 10-39).

The dermal changes of the herpesvirus group are varied. There is often only a sparse to moderately dense lymphohistiocytic infiltrate around the dilated blood vesicles of the superficial plexus. However, in some cases of herpes simplex the infiltrate may be both dense and deep, sometimes extending diffusely throughout the entire dermis. An occasional dermal concomitant of lesions of herpes simplex and herpes zoster is leukocytoclastic

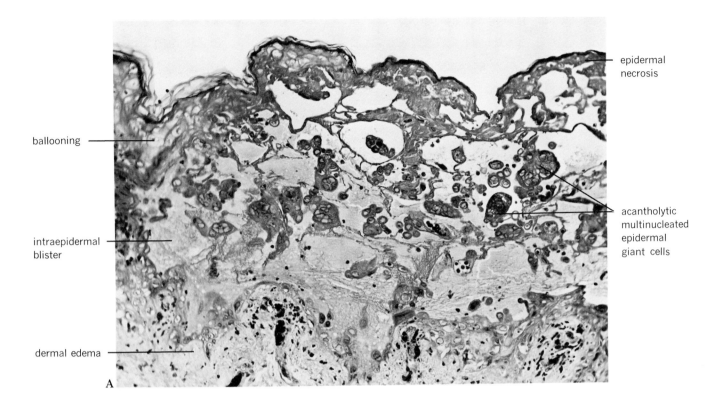

balloning

intraepidermal
blister

dermal edema

A

epidermal
necrosis

acantholytic
multinucleated
epidermal
giant cells

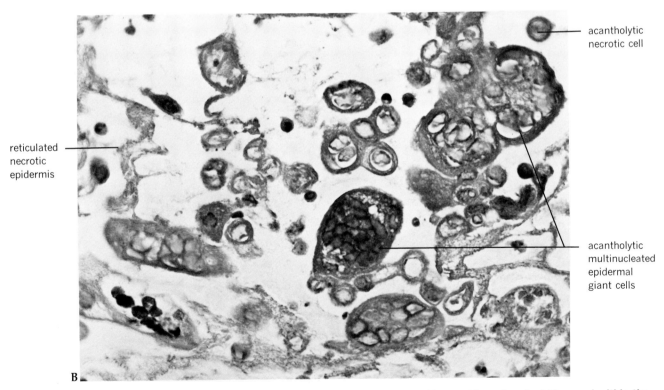

reticulated
necrotic
epidermis

B

acantholytic
necrotic cell

acantholytic
multinucleated
epidermal
giant cells

FIG. 10-37. Herpesvirus infection. The severe intracellular edema seen here caused intraepidermal vesiculation, and within the blister numerous acantholytic cells, some multinucleated and others necrotic, came loose. In later lesions necrosis may be so intensive that nuclei can no longer be identified and then the diagnosis cannot be made with certainty. A clue to herpetic cause, however, is the reticulated quality of the necrotic epidermis as is pictured here. (A, × 198; B, × 635.)

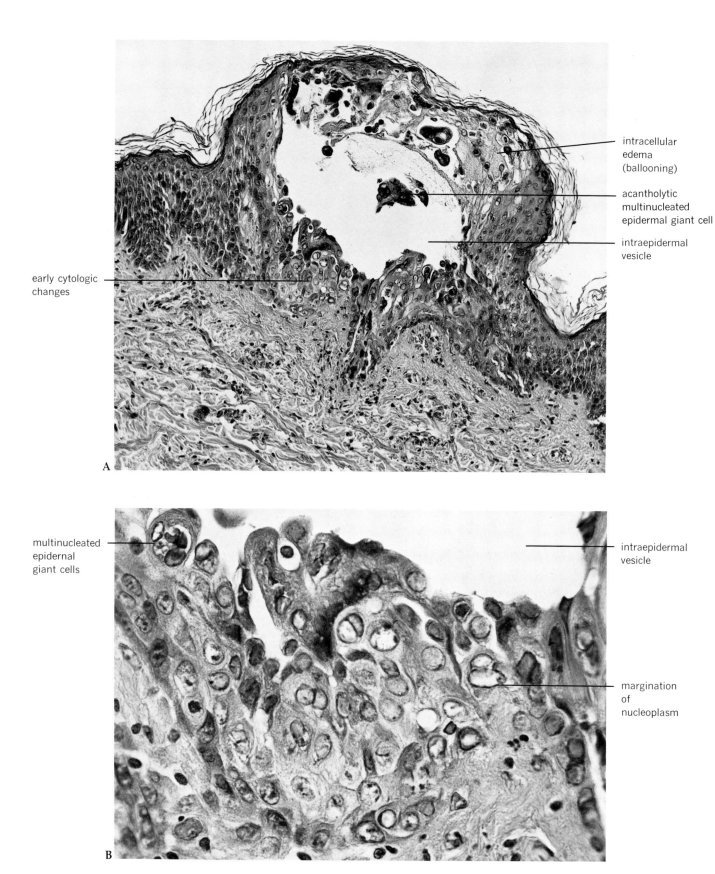

Labels on image A (clockwise from top right):
- intracellular edema (ballooning)
- acantholytic multinucleated epidermal giant cell
- intraepidermal vesicle
- early cytologic changes

Labels on image B:
- multinucleated epidernal giant cells
- intraepidermal vesicle
- margination of nucleoplasm

FIG. 10-38. Herpesvirus vesicle. A, Fresh vesicle shows earliest cytologic changes in epithelium—peripheral condensation of nucleoplasm in steel-gray colored nucleus combined with pale, swollen cytoplasm. The blister results from severe intracellular edema as illustrated. (× 166.) B, Higher magnification reveals accentuation of peripheral nucleoplasm and ballooning of cytoplasm. The nuclei are a steel-gray color and the cytoplasm is pale in sections stained by hematoxylin and eosin. (× 710.)

vasculitis with neutrophils, nuclear dust, and fibrin within and around the blood vessels of the superficial plexus. Numerous extravasated erythrocytes can be seen.

Clinically, herpes simplex, herpes zoster, and varicella are usually easily distinguished from one another. Herpes simplex presents tiny tense vesicles grouped atop edematous, red bases. The lesions of herpes simplex arise most commonly on the face, especially on the vermilion border of the lips, and on the genitals,

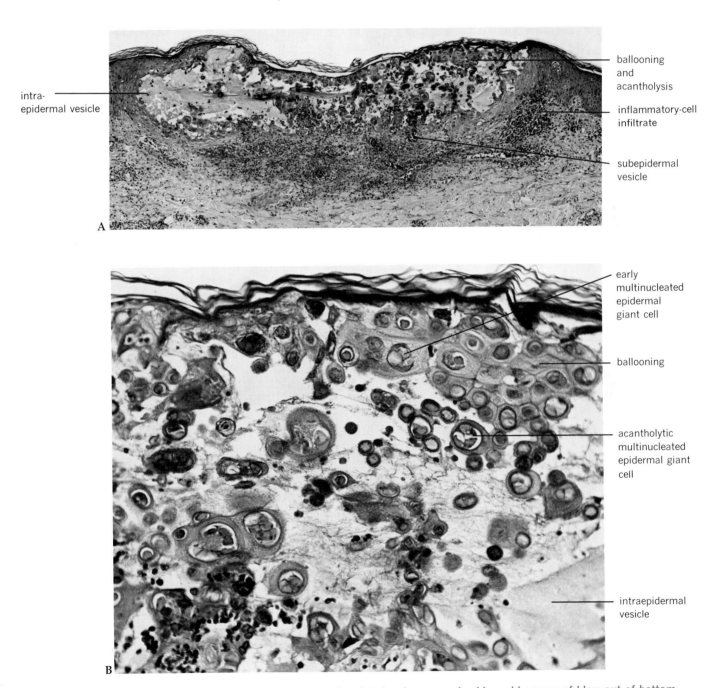

FIG. 10-39. Herpesvirus vesicular dermatitis. Intraepidermal vesicle has become subepidermal because of blow out of bottom of blister. Note also dense inflammatory-cell infiltrate in upper part of dermis, a common feature of herpetic infections in skin. (A, × 80; B, × 374.)

especially on the penis and vulva. The vesicles of herpes zoster are usually aligned along a dermatome, but rarely will the vesicles of herpes simplex have a similar distribution (zosteriform simplex). The vesicles of herpes zoster are often hemorrhagic. Varicella (chicken pox) consists of discrete "dewdrop" vesicles scattered principally on the trunk. All three diseases may ulcerate and resolve with scarring, in consequence of vasculitis, density and depth of the inflammatory-cell infiltrate, or excoriation.

Blister Beetle Dermatitis

Blister beetles, such as the Spanish fly (Cantharis vesicatoria), produce an oil, cantharidin, which causes vesicles or bullae within a few hours after contact with the skin. The blister forms within the spinous layer by intracellular edema and acantholysis. Necrotic keratinocytes can also be found in the affected epidermis.

Subcorneal

Pemphigus foliaceus, pemphigus erythematosus, and *fogo selvagem* (Portuguese, "wild fire") are sometimes referred to as "superficial pemphigus." These forms of pemphigus, the *staphylococcal scalded-skin syndrome,* and *bullous impetigo* will be discussed together because they are indistinguishable histologically in sections stained with hematoxylin and eosin. Each has characteristics in common with the others (Fig. 10-40).

—Blister formation in the subcorneal or granular region
—Acantholytic cells within the blister
—Varying numbers of neutrophils within the blister, which when numerous, produce a subcorneal pustule
—Mixed inflammatory-cell infiltrate of lymphocytes, histiocytes, neutrophils, and, sometimes, eosinophils around the blood vessels of the superficial plexus
—Edema of the papillary dermis

The numbers of acantholytic cells and of neutrophils within a blister of superficial pemphigus varies from few to many. If neutrophils are plentiful, it may be difficult to detect the acantholytic cells. In such instances, it may be impossible to distinguish histologically between superficial pemphigus and the subcorneal pustular dermatitides (see Subcorneal Pustular Dermatitis later in this chapter). The earliest histologic changes in superficial pemphigus are intercellular separations that resemble those of spongiosis but without associated intraepidermal inflammatory cells.

Clinically, the lesions of pemphigus foliaceus, pemphigus erythematosus, and fogo selvagem have characteristics in common, as would be expected in view of their similar histologic features. However, pemphigus erythematosus, so named because its distribution corresponds to that of lupus erythematosus, is often confined primarily to the face and V-area of the chest, whereas pemphigus foliaceus tends to involve the trunk and extremities, in addition to the face. Fogo selvagem is a superficial type of pemphigus seen in Brazil. The disease, which occurs in children and adolescents, as well as in adults, has clinical features

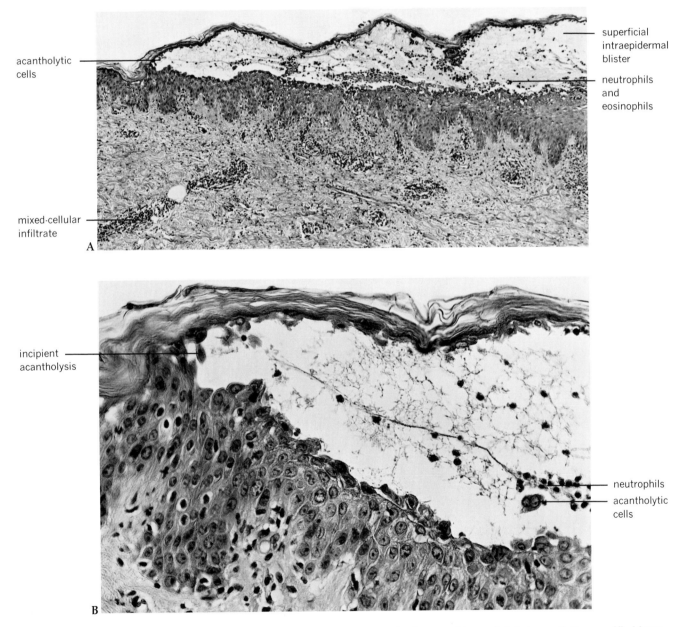

FIG. 10-40. Pemphigus, superficial type. A, Note blister in both the granular layer and immediately beneath the cornified layer. A few acantholytic cells and many polymorphonuclear leukocytes are present in the blister. (× 88.) B, A few acantholytic cells can be seen in blister. (× 407.)

of both pemphigus foliaceus and pemphigus erythematosus. The crusted, scaly lesions found in superficial pemphigus seem anomalous for a process that histologically is fundamentally bullous, but unlike the findings in pemphigus vulgaris, intact blisters are not usually seen in pemphigus foliaceus or in pemphigus erythematosus.

The immunofluorescent pattern of superficial pemphigus (foliaceus, erythematosus, and fogo selvagem) is the same as that of deep pemphigus (vulgaris and vegetans). In vivo bound and circulating antibodies are present which react with the intercellular substance of the epidermis. A unique feature of some cases of pemphigus erythematosus is the additional finding of antibodies in vivo bound at the basement-membrane zone. This finding can be demonstrated only by the direct immunofluorescent testing of involved skin.

The *staphylococcal scalded-skin syndrome* (Ritter) may be indistinguishable histologically from superficial pemphigus, especially when there are relatively few neutrophils within the epidermis and dermis. The inflammatory-cell infiltrate within the dermis is unusually sparse in the staphylococcal scalded-skin syndrome. A prodrome of conjunctivitis and/or rhinorrhea is common in this condition that affects infants or children, but rarely affects adults. The first cutaneous sign of the staphylococcal scalded-skin syndrome is erythema, especially on the face and in the flexural areas. In many youngsters, flaccid bullae then appear on the face and upper trunk. Both the erythema, which is sometimes tender or painful, and the bullae can be widespread. The erythematous lesions resolve with "potato-chip" desquamation, and the large flaccid bullae rupture, leaving denuded skin that is partially covered by detached epidermis resembling wet tissue paper.

The clinical appearance of "scalded skin" may be seen in several diseases besides the staphylococcal scalded skin syndrome, such as pemphigus neonatorum (bullous impetigo), severe erythema multiforme, toxic epidermal necrolysis, and thermal burns.

The staphylococcal scalded-skin syndrome is caused by a diffusible epidermolytic exotoxin produced usually by group 2 Staphylococcus aureus of phage-type 71. The bacteria are found principally in the eyes and nasopharynx. Although staphylococci can be cultured from the skin of patients with the scalded skin syndrome, they are isolated with difficulty from intact bullae.

A subcorneal blister also forms in *bullous impetigo*, a process caused by staphylococci and/or streptococci (Fig. 10-41). Older lesions of bullous impetigo are differentiated histologically from those of the staphylococcal scalded-skin syndrome only by the presence of numerous neutrophils within the blister, forming a

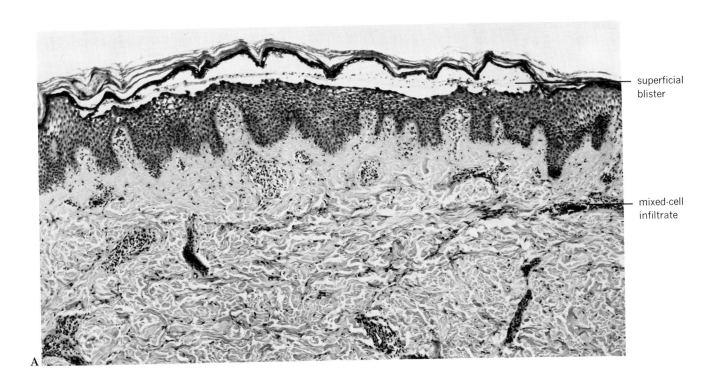

superficial
blister

mixed-cell
infiltrate

A

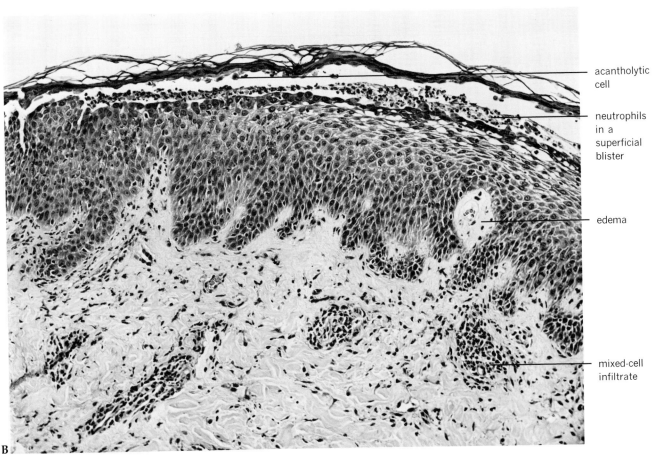

acantholytic
cell

neutrophils
in a
superficial
blister

edema

mixed-cell
infiltrate

B

FIG. 10-41. Bullous impetigo. A, Blister in granular zone and immediately beneath the cornified layer. (× 84.) B, Neutrophils and a few acantholytic cells are present within blister, just as in superficial types of pemphigus and in staphylococcal scalded skin syndrome. (× 175.)

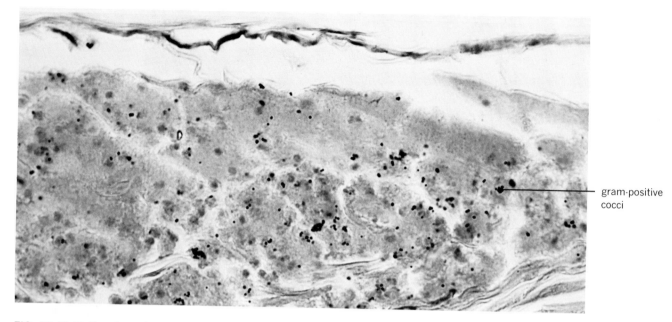

gram-positive
cocci

FIG. 10-41. Bullous impetigo. C, Gram's stain, especially the Brown-Brenn modification, makes it possible to identify causative organisms. (× 635.)

subcorneal pustule. In addition, unlike the situation in the staphylococcal scalded-skin syndrome, the causative bacteria can be grown easily from intact blisters of bullous impetigo and can be demonstrated there histologically with the Gram stain. (Fig. 10-41C). However, early lesions of bullous impetigo are indistinguishable from the other subcorneal blistering diseases when they are stained with hematoxylin and eosin.

The pustular lesions of *pyoderma gangrenosum* result from subcorneal collections of neutrophils. Pyoderma gangrenosum is discussed in Chapter 9.

Intragranular Vesicular Dermatitis

The histologic changes in *friction blisters* and in *Weber-Cockayne disease* are indistinguishable. Weber-Cockayne disease is a condition in which friction blisters occur readily, requiring less shearing force than is needed to produce blisters in normal skin.

—Blister in the granular zone or, less commonly, in the upper spinous zone
—Intracellular edema of spinous cells
—Slight inflammatory-cell infiltrate around the blood vessels of the superficial plexus

Blisters that result from friction can occur anywhere on the skin surface, but are most commonly located on acral sites, such as the palms and soles. Who has not experienced the development of a blister on the heel from wearing ill-fitting shoes or a blister on the hand from an imperfect grip on a baseball bat, tennis racquet, or a golf club? Weber-Cockayne disease, in which blisters never arise spontaneously, but only in response to friction, is inherited as an autosomal dominant trait. Although the bullae may appear in the first year or two of life, they often are not manifested until adulthood after prolonged trauma to the feet. These friction blisters may also form in the spinous zone.

Intrabasal Vesicular Dermatitis

Epidermolysis Bullosa Simplex (Fig. 10-42)

—Intrabasalar clefts in some foci
—Vacuolization within the epidermal cells to the sides of the blister
—Wholly subepidermal blister in other foci
—Well-preserved dermal papillae
—Little or no inflammatory-cell infiltrate

At first glance, the bulla of epidermolysis bullosa simplex appears subepidermal, but upon closer inspection it is sometimes possible to observe intrabasalar vacuolization and separation. This is usually best seen to the side of the fully formed bulla. To visualize these intrabasalar changes through the light microscope, it is necessary to do a biopsy of a lesion immediately after the skin has been traumatized, and before the development of a clinical blister. By the time that a clinical blister has arisen, the only vesiculobullous change that may be detected with the light microscope is subepidermal.

Epidermolysis bullosa simplex is inherited as an autosomal dominant trait and appears clinically at birth or shortly thereafter. It is probable that none of the bullae arise spontaneously but only secondary to trauma. Because the blistering process is actually intraepidermal with practically no inflammatory-cell infiltrate, it is to be expected that uncomplicated bullae will heal without any scarring.

Intraepidermal Vesiculopustular Dermatitis

A vesicle contains mostly serum, a pustule mostly neutrophils. Vesiculopustules have features of both and may represent a kind of neutrophilic spongiosis.

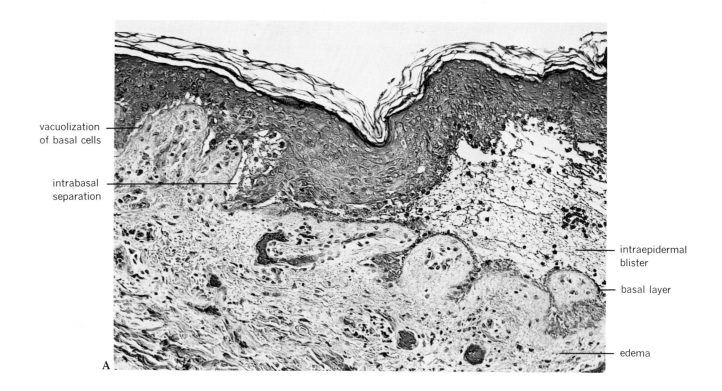

vacuolization of basal cells

intrabasal separation

intraepidermal blister

basal layer

edema

A

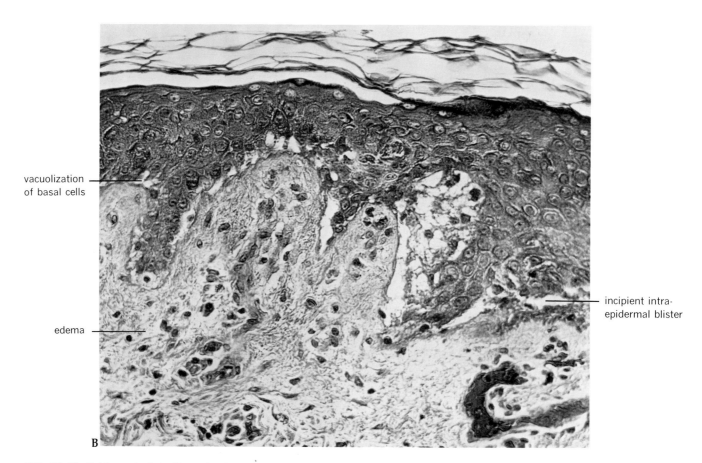

vacuolization of basal cells

edema

incipient intra-epidermal blister

B

FIG. 10-42. Epidermolysis bullosa simplex. A, Blister begins, as shown here, with formation of tiny vacuoles within basal-cell zone and progresses to intrabasal separation and eventual vesiculation. Note virtual absence of inflammatory cells within dermis. (× 238.) B, Higher magnification permits better visualization of early intraepidermal changes, vacuolization within basal layer. (× 400.)

The vesicles of *dermatophytic infections* often consist histologically of vesiculopustules (Fig. 10-43). Hyphae can be demonstrated within vesiculopustules and in the compact orthokeratotic cornified layer that roofs them. In the evolution of such lesions, the number of neutrophils may eventually increase to the extent that they become predominantly pustular.

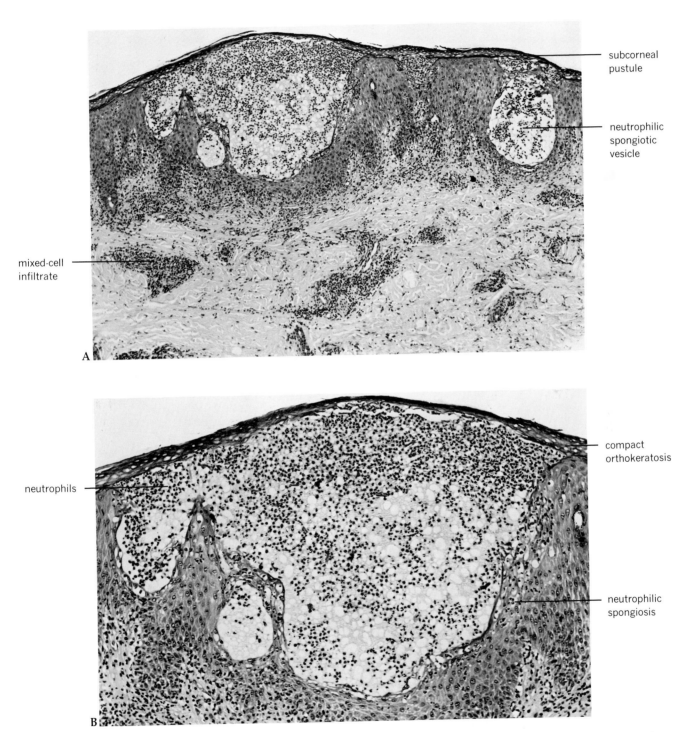

FIG. 10-43. Dermatophytosis, vesicular type. A, Biopsy reveals spongiotic vesicles containing many neutrophils and sometimes eosinophils. Numerous hyphae in cornified layer could be easily visualized with PAS stain. (A, × 78; B, × 162.)

Vesiculopustules, the result of neutrophilic spongiosis and ballooning, may be seen in *irritant contact dermatitis*. A clue to external irritation is the presence of necrotic keratinocytes within the epidermis.

Some pruritic *spongiotic vesicular dermatitides*, such as *allergic contact dermatitis* and *nummular dermatitis*, become impetiginized as a result of secondary infection occasioned by intense scratching (Fig. 10-44). The original lymphocytic spongiosis becomes vesiculopustular. In subacute stages of these diseases, the spongiotic psoriasiform character of the lesions is preserved, which is a strong indication of contact or nummular dermatitis.

Recalcitrant vesiculopustular dermatitis of the palms and soles is a resistant and recurrent condition that consists of well-circumscribed, tense, vesiculopustules within the spinous layer of the

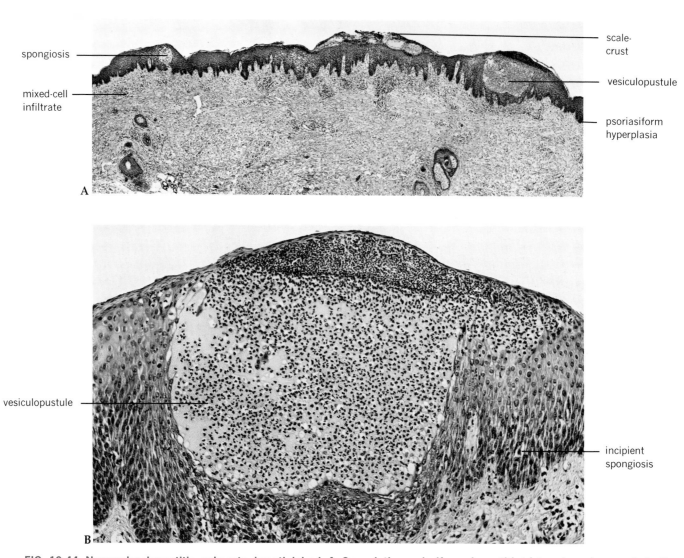

FIG. 10-44. Nummular dermatitis, subacute, impetiginized. A, Spongiotic psoriasiform dermatitis pictured can be seen in both subacute nummular and subacute allergic contact dermatitis. (× 28.) B, Vesiculopustule was produced by numerous neutrophils in spongiotic vesicle. (× 169.)

epidermis (Fig. 10-45). A sparse, mixed-cell infiltrate of lymphocytes, histiocytes, and neutrophils is situated around the blood vessels of the superficial plexus and within the papillary dermis. The earliest histologic change within the epidermis appears to be neutrophilic spongiosis. Although many cases are mistakenly diagnosed as localized pustular psoriasis (Barber), this condition of unknown cause is not related to pustular psoriasis, nor is it impetiginized allergic contact dermatitis or dermatophytosis. Other cases are equally wrongly termed pustular bacterid (Andrews). In fact, patients with recalcitrant vesiculopustular dermatitis of the palms and soles do not have lesions of psoriasis elsewhere nor internal foci of infection.

Persistent vesiculopustular dermatitis of childhood is a rare condition. It may occur in neonates, infants, or young children, up to about the ages of 3 or 4 years. The eruption is characterized by widespread tense vesicles scattered especially on the trunk and extremities. The hands and feet can sometimes be predominantly affected. This unusual condition usually poses a diagnostic conundrum for the primary physician and his consultants. The suggested diagnoses include vesicular lesions of papular urticaria and a bizarre viral eruption. However, even with hospitalization, the process persists, with new crops of tense vesicles developing continually. The process may last for many months and even for

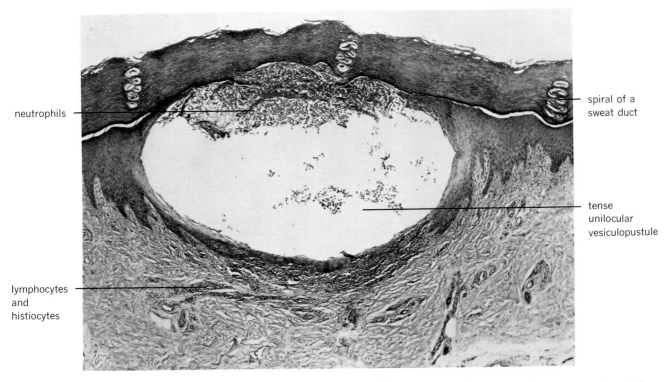

neutrophils

spiral of a sweat duct

tense unilocular vesiculopustule

lymphocytes and histiocytes

FIG. 10-45. Recalcitrant vesiculopustular dermatitis of the palms and soles. This specimen comes from recurrent pustular eruption of palms and soles that is exceedingly refractory to therapy. (× 59.)

more than a year. Unlike papular urticaria and most viral diseases, the histologic findings in this persistent vesiculopustular dermatitis of childhood are well-circumscribed tense vesiculopustules (Fig. 10-46).

Among the *reactions to fleabites* are vesicles which, on histologic examination, are seen to be vesiculopustules (Fig. 10-47). Like other reactions to arthropod assaults, the perivascular and interstitial dermal infiltrate is both superficial and deep, but, in contrast to them, neutrophils often dominate over eosinophils in reactions to fleabites. Fleas can also induce wholly pustular lesions.

Vesiculopustules and even frank pustules may develop in *leukocytoclastic and septic vasculitides* (Fig. 10-48). For example, a characteristic clinical feature of chronic gonococcemia is the acral distribution of a few vesiculopustules having gray roofs and surrounded by broad red areolae. Histologically, the epidermis associated with the vesiculopustule is largely necrotic, a consequence of thromboses in small blood vessels, accounting for the gray color of the lesion. Similar vesiculopustules appear in chronic meningococcemia and, episodically, in patients with leukocytoclastic vasculitis, usually when drug-induced.

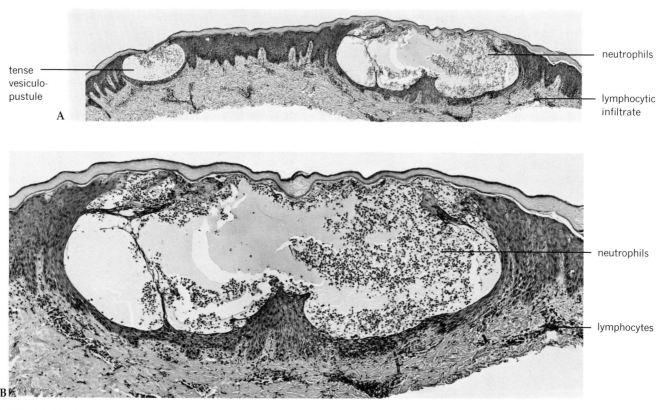

FIG. 10-46. Persistent vesiculopustular dermatitis of childhood. Well-circumscribed tense vesiculopustules pictured are from an infant with widespread vesiculopustular eruption on trunk and extremities, including the palms and soles. Histologically, these changes are indistinguishable from those of recalcitrant vesiculopustular dermatitis of palms and soles, a condition of adults that is confined wholly to the palms and soles. (A, × 36; B, × 74.)

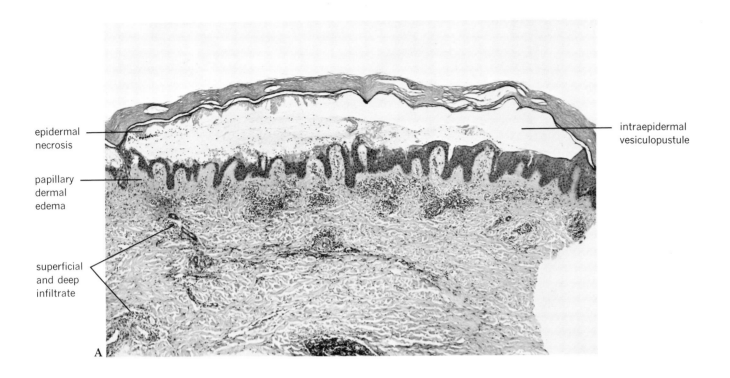

epidermal
necrosis

intraepidermal
vesiculopustule

papillary
dermal
edema

superficial
and deep
infiltrate

A

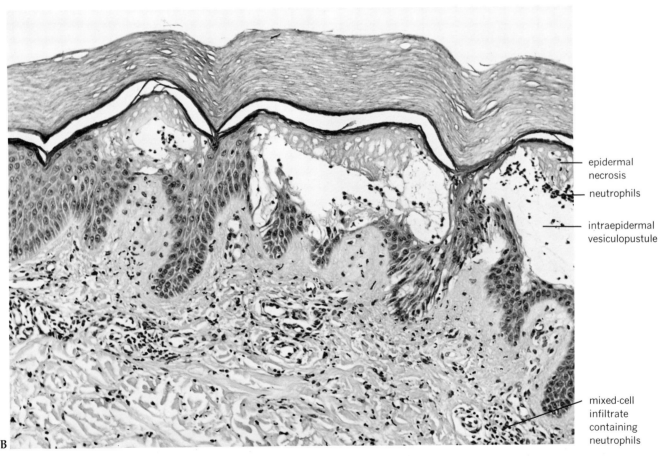

epidermal
necrosis

neutrophils

intraepidermal
vesiculopustule

mixed-cell
infiltrate
containing
neutrophils

B

FIG. 10-47. Fleabite reaction. Note intraepidermal vesiculopustules, epidermal necrosis, and superficial and deep perivascular and interstitial mixed-inflammatory-cell infiltrate containing neutrophils. (A, × 62; B, × 180.)

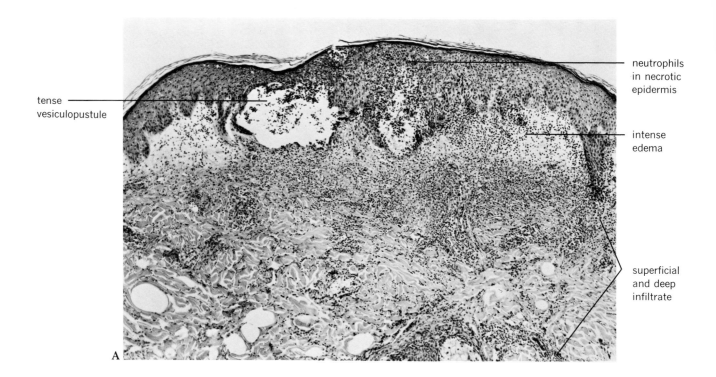

tense
vesiculopustule

neutrophils
in necrotic
epidermis

intense
edema

superficial
and deep
infiltrate

A

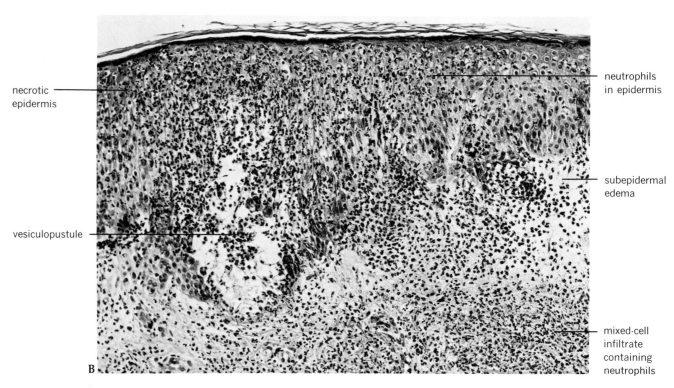

necrotic
epidermis

vesiculopustule

neutrophils
in epidermis

subepidermal
edema

mixed-cell
infiltrate
containing
neutrophils

B

FIG. 10-48. Gonococcemia. A, Tense intraepidermal vesiculopustules have perforated epidermis downward into dermis. Severe subepidermal edema may eventuate in subepidermal vesiculation. (× 86.) B, Common features of cutaneous lesions illustrated are dense infiltrate of neutrophils within necrotic epidermis and vesiculopustules. (× 216.)

Intraepidermal Pustular Dermatitis

Pustules form within the epidermis when neutrophils emerge from the capillaries in the papillary dermis and ascend. During their upward migration toward the skin surface, the neutrophils pass through the dermis, across the basement-membrane zone, and sequentially through the basal, spinous, granular, and cornified layers of the epidermis. The histologic appearance of a pustular dermatitis depends upon the moment in the evolution of the pustular process that a specimen is removed from the lesion and examined. At the earliest stage, before the clinical appearance of an obvious pustule, there may be no neutrophils within the epidermis. In an old, resolving pustule, a scale-crust containing neutrophils is situated atop the surface of the specimen. Between these extremes is a series of sequential changes that include a few neutrophils scattered in the spinous zone, a well-developed spongiform pustule, a sharply circumscribed subcorneal pustule, or a combination of these patterns.

The various morphologic descriptions for the distribution of neutrophils within the epidermis (e.g., intraspinous pustule, subcorneal pustule, intracorneal pustule) should be thought of as time-lapse photographic sequences in the pustular process. For example, if several biopsies are performed in a single patient with lesions of pustular psoriasis in different stages of development, some will show scale-crusts containing neutrophils, others subcorneal pustules, still others intraspinous spongiform pustules, and some practically no neutrophils within the epidermis. Thus, it is clearly an oversimplification to designate a dynamic process like pustular psoriasis merely as a spongiform pustular dermatitis. Every subcorneal pustular dermatitis must be spongiform at a previous stage.

Unilocular

Unilocular intraepidermal pustules may be found in fire ant dermatitis, pustular reactions to fleabites, keratotic-crusted scabies, and leukocytoclastic and septic vasculitis.

Fire Ant Dermatitis

Fire ant stings induce a tense unilocular intraepidermal pustule that may "blow-out" and result in a subepidermal pustule. Prominent degeneration of collagen occurs beneath the pustule at the site of the sting, often ending in fibrosis.

Pustular Reactions to Fleabites

Neutrophils are present to differing extents in vesicles, vesiculo-pustules, and pustules caused by fleabites. Some species of fleas consistently induce the formation of pustules.

Keratotic-crusted Scabies (Fig. 10-49)

Intraepidermal unilocular pustules may occur beneath the site of the mite (Sarcoptes scabiei) or its larvae and eggs. Whether the pustules in this keratotic, crusted form of scabies (Norwegian scabies) result in part from secondary bacterial infection of the scabietic lesion may only be surmised.

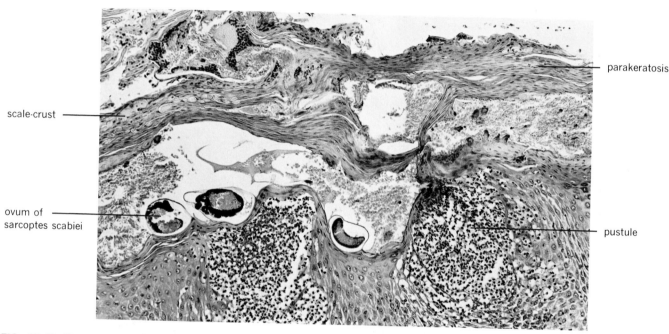

scale-crust

ovum of
sarcoptes scabiei

parakeratosis

pustule

FIG. 10-49. Keratotic-crusted scabies (Norwegian scabies), pustular lesion. Note the intraepidermal pustules near the eggs and the scale-crust. (× 175.)

Spongiform Pustular Dermatitis (Fig. 10-50)

Spongiform pustules are seen not only in psoriasis and its variants but also in infectious diseases such as pustular superficial fungus infections and rupial syphilis.

Pustular Psoriasis and Its Variants

Pustular psoriasis, acrodermatitis continua (dermatitis repens), impetigo herpetiformis, and keratoderma blenorrhagicum (and other variants of Reiter's disease such as balanitis circinata) are indistinguishable histologically, but can be differentiated from one another clinically. Each is characterized histologically by a spongiform pustule within the epidermis and a variably dense lymphohistiocytic infiltrate with neutrophils around widely dilated blood vessels of the superficial plexus. Scale-crusts containing collections of neutrophils in laminated array may be present. One hypothesis, with which I agree, proposes that these four spongiform pustules are all variants of psoriasis in different clinical guises.

Clinically, *pustular psoriasis* takes several forms, the three most common being pustular lesions on the palms and soles (Barber's type); an explosive widespread pustular disease that may involve mucous membranes and be debilitating (von Zumbusch's type); and crops of pustules within well-established, typical plaques of psoriasis. The spongiform pustule forms quickly and therefore the epidermis has no time to become hyperplastic as in plaque lesions of psoriasis.

Acrodermatitis continua (Hallopeau) and *dermatitis repens* (Crocker) are different names for the same clinical condition that involves the tips of the fingers with chronic redness, scaling, and pustulation. This conditition is said to follow trauma to the digit(s) as in Koebner's phenomenon.

Impetigo herpetiformis is a pustular eruption of pregnancy, disappearing at or shortly after term.

Keratoderma blenorrhagicum is a red, scaly, pustular eruption that occurs on the palms and soles as one manifestation of Reiter's disease. Other spongiform pustular lesions in patients with Reiter's disease may occur elsewhere on the skin surface and on

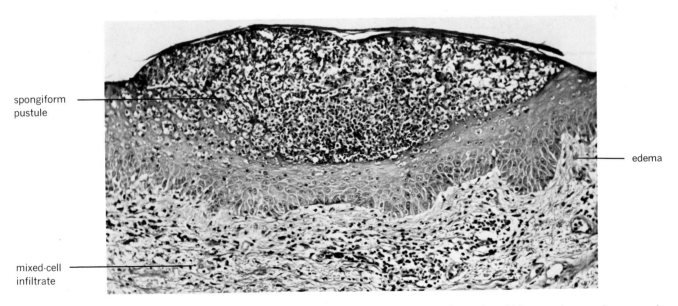

spongiform pustule

edema

mixed-cell infiltrate

FIG. 10-50. Spongiform pustular dermatitis, pustular psoriasis. Spongiform pustule pictured could be seen in any of presumed variants of psoriasis, including acrodermatitis continua, impetigo herpetiformis, keratoderma blenorrhagicum and subcorneal pustular dermatosis. ($\times$ 181.)

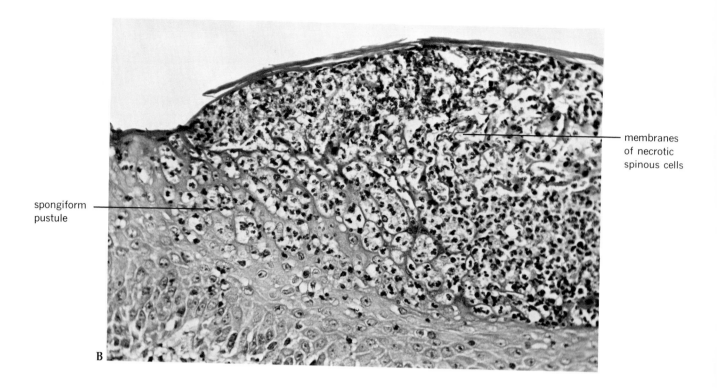

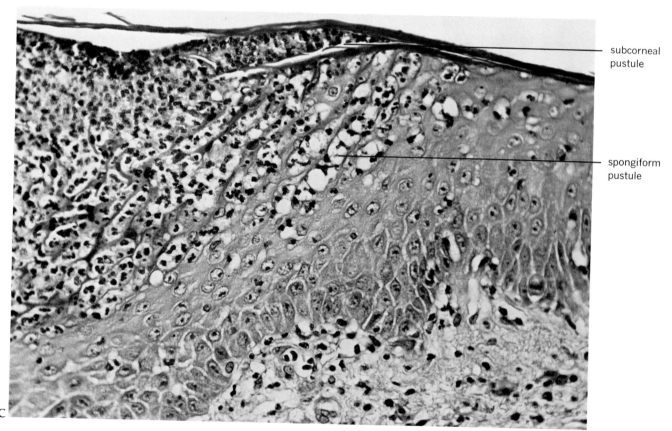

FIG. 10-50. Spongiform pustular dermatitis. B, Higher magnification of left side of pustule demonstrates numerous neutrophils among spinous cells, giving the appearance of a sponge. Note the netlike pattern formed by residual spinous cell membranes within whose interstices are scattered neutrophils. Spinous cells within pustule have mostly undergone necrosis. (× 396.) C, Higher magnification of right side of pustule illustrates ascent of neutrophils within epidermis and consequent development of spongiform, subcorneal, and intracorneal pustules. (× 396.) These are simply names for collections of neutrophils at different levels of the epidermis, and all three types of pustules can sometimes be seen together in the same specimen.

mucous membranes. Some of the cutaneous plaques closely resemble the lesions of psoriasis.

Geographic tongue is also a condition that consists histologically of spongiform pustules. It can appear as an isolated phenomenon on the tongue as well as a concomitant of widespread pustular psoriasis or Reiter's disease. It may be that geographic tongue occurring as an isolated abnormality is actually a manifestation of psoriatic diathesis just as in some persons with no skin lesions of psoriasis changes in the nails may be the sole expression of the disease. Oral lesions of lichen planus are frequently found in patients who never have cutaneous lesions of the disease and such may also be the relation of geographic tongue to psoriasis.

Rupial Secondary Syphilis (Fig. 10-51A, B)

The epidermal changes in *rupial secondary syphilis* are similar to those of the aforementioned spongiform pustular conditions (Fig. 10-51). However, this disease can be identified histologically

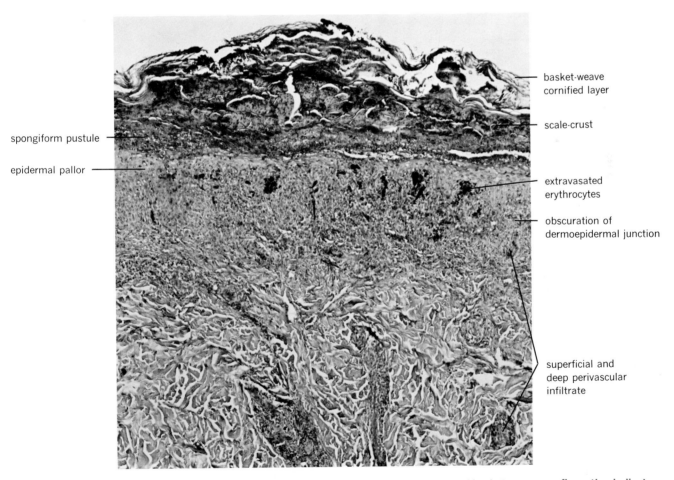

FIG. 10-51. Rupial secondary syphilis. A, Retention of original cornified layer with its normal basket-weave configuration indicates lesion is only several days old. Rupial features result from spongiform pustule and purulent scale-crust. ($\times$ 67.)

by other changes in the dermis consistent with commoner lesions of syphilis. In rupial syphilis, as in many forms of secondary syphilis, the epidermis is pale-staining and the perivascular inflammatory-cell infiltrate develops around the blood vessels of the deep, as well as the superficial, plexus. Furthermore, plasma cells are an invariable accompaniment of the inflammatory-cell infiltrate in rupial secondary syphilis.

Clinically, rupial syphilis, named for the filthy appearance of the lesions, consists of widespread, dirty-looking, scale-crusts on reddish-brown bases. The palms and soles are often involved.

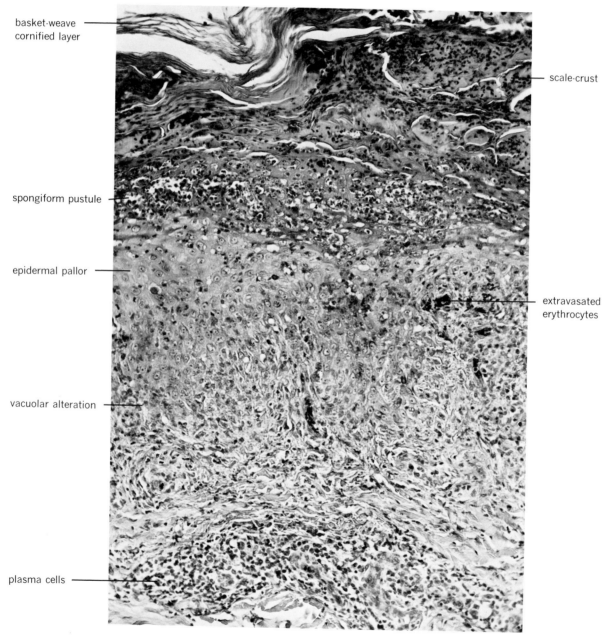

basket-weave cornified layer

scale-crust

spongiform pustule

epidermal pallor

extravasated erythrocytes

vacuolar alteration

plasma cells

FIG. 10-51. Rupial secondary syphilis. B, Spongiform pustule, pale epidermis, and plasma cells are diagnostic features. ($\times$ 363.)

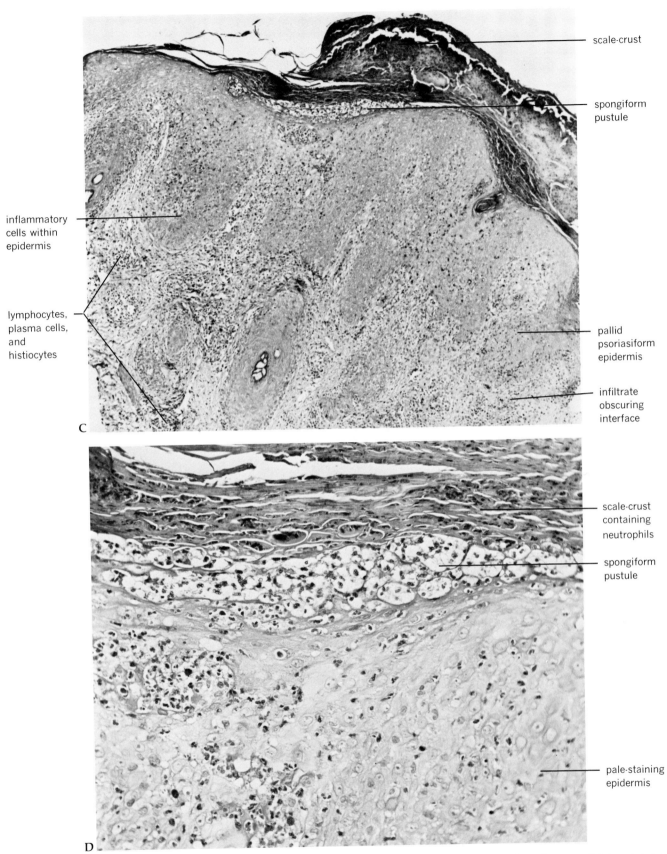

scale-crust

spongiform
pustule

inflammatory
cells within
epidermis

lymphocytes,
plasma cells,
and
histiocytes

pallid
psoriasiform
epidermis

infiltrate
obscuring
interface

C

scale-crust
containing
neutrophils

spongiform
pustule

pale-staining
epidermis

D

FIG. 10-51. Rupial secondary syphilis. C and D, Histologic features such as pale psoriasiform epidermis, superficial and deep perivascular infiltrate of mostly plasma cells and histiocytes, and obscuration of dermoepidermal junction by infiltrate indicate this is rupial syphilis, not pustular psoriasis or its variants. (C, × 58; D, × 620.)

Condyloma Latum (Fig. 10-52)

In condyloma latum, spongiform pustules form in the papillated and hyperplastic epidermis. The moist papulonodular lesions of this manifestation of secondary syphilis occur on mucous membranes and at mucocutaneous junctions, especially in the anogenital region.

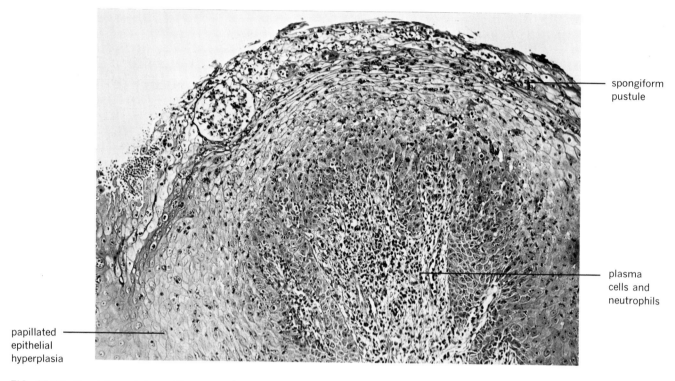

spongiform pustule

plasma cells and neutrophils

papillated epithelial hyperplasia

FIG. 10-52. Condyloma latum. Characteristics seen are many plasma cells within dermis and many neutrophils within papillated and hyperplastic epithelium. (× 186.)

Halogenodermas

The pustular lesions caused by halogens show spongiform pustules upon biopsy. Within the dermis there is a dense infiltrate composed largely of neutrophils, but there are also many eosinophils and atypical mononuclear cells.

Pyoderma Gangrenosum

Widespread tense pustules may appear in pyoderma gangrenosum in addition to the more typical ulcerated lesions. Microscopic examination of the pustules reveals them to be spongiform in character. Like all other spongiform pustules, those of pyoderma gangrenosum may evolve into subcorneal pustules. The dermis is marked by intense suppuration.

Dermatophytosis and candidiasis may be associated with spongiform pustules, and a careful search of the cornified layer should reveal the causative organisms. A PAS or silver methenamine stain will confirm the diagnosis.

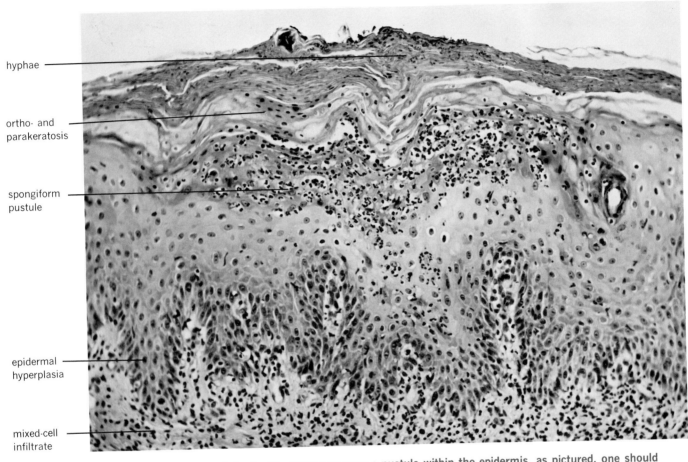

hyphae

ortho- and parakeratosis

spongiform pustule

epidermal hyperplasia

mixed-cell infiltrate

FIG. 10-53. Candidiasis, spongiform pustule. A, Whenever one sees a pustule within the epidermis, as pictured, one should look for monilial or dermatophytic hyphae within cornified cells of epidermis and adnexal epithelium. (× 187.)

Subcorneal Pustular Dermatitis

A number of diseases have in common an intraepidermal pustule situated immediately beneath the cornified layer that serves as its roof. A spongiform pustule may be continuous with the subcorneal one. Keratinocytes separated by acantholysis may be present within the pustule of any of the subcorneal pustular dermatitides. It may be impossible to distinguish among the subcorneal pustular group of diseases with the hematoxylin-eosin stain alone. However, the Gram stain reveals staphylococci within the subcorneal pustules of *impetigo* and *bullous impetigo* (Fig. 10-41C), and the PAS

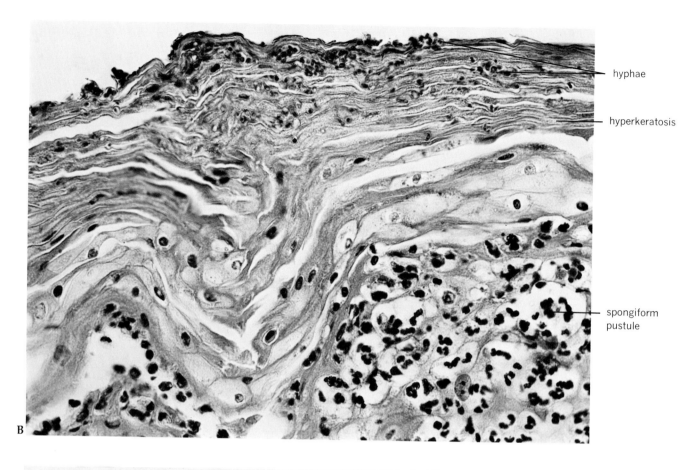

hyphae

hyperkeratosis

spongiform
pustule

B

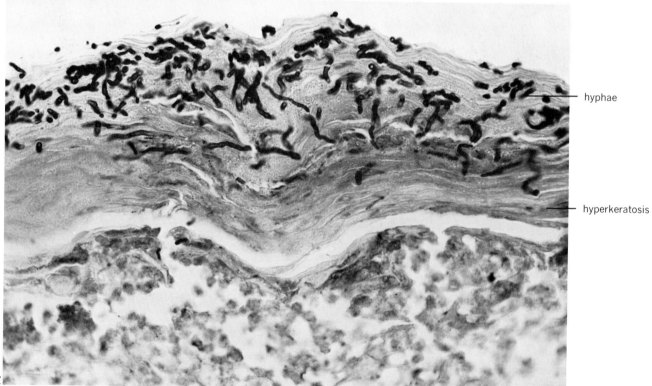

hyphae

hyperkeratosis

C

FIG. 10-53. Candidiasis, spongiform pustule. B, Numerous hyphae, some cut on end, can be seen in cornified layer above spongiform pustule in this higher magnification. (Hematoxylin and eosin stain; × 547.) C, Section stained with silver methenamine shows many characteristic hyphae of candida, in this instance Candida albicans, within thickened cornified layer. (× 565.)

or silver-methenamine stain demonstrates hyphae in the cornified layer and subcorneal pustules of *acute candidiasis* (Fig. 10-53) and *dermatophytosis.*

The three types of *superficial pemphigus* and the *staphylococcal scalded-skin syndrome* have been discussed previously in this chapter. The intraepidermal separation in both types of superficial pemphigus (foliaceus and erythematosus) occurs immediately beneath the cornified layer (subcorneal), within the granular zone, or in the upper portion of the spinous zone. Sometimes the separation can be in all three locales (Fig. 10-54). In addition to acantholytic cells within the blister there are often neutrophils and eosinophils. Histologic differentiation of superficial pemphigus from bullous impetigo often requires a special stain for bacteria, such as the Brown-Brenn modification of Gram's stain.

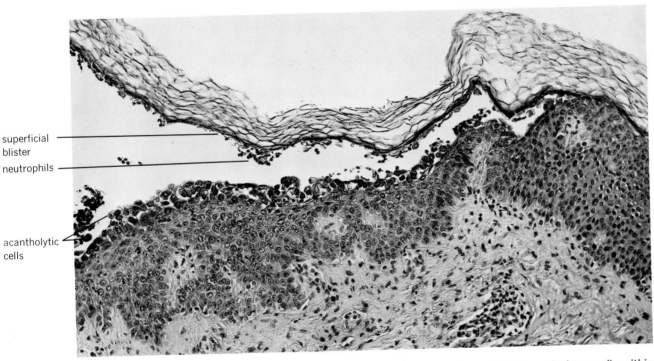

superficial blister

neutrophils

acantholytic cells

FIG. 10-54. Superficial pemphigus. Note intraepidermal separation immediately beneath cornified layer (subcorneal), within granular zone, and in upper portion of spinous zone. Acantholytic cells and neutrophils are also seen within the blister. (× 174.)

Subcorneal pustular dermatosis (Sneddon-Wilkinson disease) is a rare disease and consists of pustules that develop centrifugally, forming arcuate and annular configurations and leaving behind scaly and hyperpigmented sequellae. Erythema, the first detectable sign, continues to form a rim around each pustule. There are no unequivocal histologic markers for subcorneal pustular dermatosis, but the tense pustules occur mostly above, rather than below, the skin surface. (Fig. 10-55). It is likely that subcorneal pustular dermatosis, like impetigo herpetiformis, acrodermatitis continua, and keratoderma blenorrhagicum, is a form of pustular psoriasis.

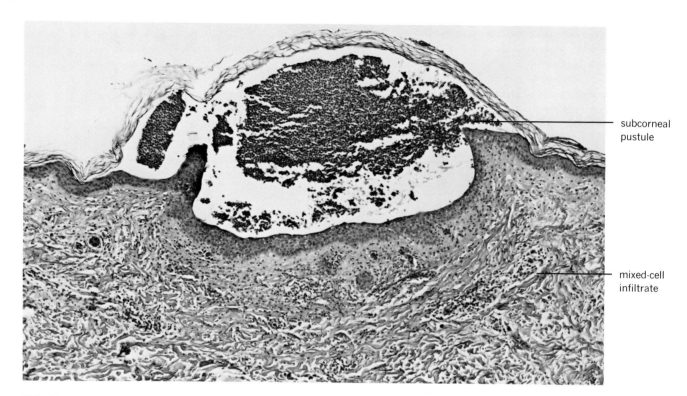

subcorneal
pustule

mixed-cell
infiltrate

FIG. 10-55. Subcorneal pustular dermatosis (Sneddon and Wilkinson). Note prominent elevation of tense pustule above skin surface rather than flaccid pustule as in superficial forms of pemphigus. (× 86.)

Miliaria crystallina is composed of tense, dewdrop-like vesicles on normal skin. Surprisingly enough, biopsy of these clear vesicles reveals neutrophils beneath their subcorneal roofs. (Fig. 10-56). The number of neutrophils is not sufficiently large, however, to produce a clinical pustule.

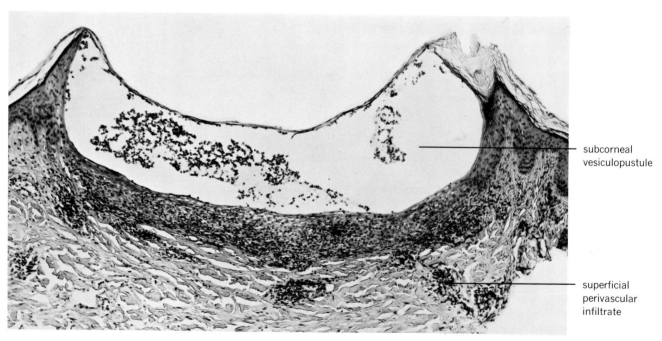

subcorneal
vesiculopustule

superficial
perivascular
infiltrate

FIG. 10-56. Miliaria crystallina. Although lesions appear clinically as tense dewdrop-like clear vesicles, they are seen histologically, as shown here, as vesiculopustules containing many neutrophils. (× 86.)

Impetigo and its variant, *bullous impetigo,* may be caused by either streptococci or staphylococci. Histologically, impetigo and old lesions of bullous impetigo contain a few acantholytic cells among the countless neutrophils in the subcorneal pustule, a feature that often makes differentiation difficult from some cases of superficial pemphigus (Fig. 41A, B). As neutrophils ascend from the dermis, they often form spongiform pustules before becoming subcorneal pustules (Fig. 10-57). Clinically, impetigo usually develops on the faces of children and consists of grouped pustules that resolve by formation of honey-colored crusts. Bullous impetigo is characterized by large, sharply circumscribed blisters that can become purulent. Early lesions of bullous impetigo are histologically identical with those of the staphylococcal scalded-skin syndrome and superficial pemphigus.

Superficial pyoderma is a common complication of *chronic granulomatous disease of childhood,* a condition associated with a severe defect in the capacity of peripheral leukocytes, both neutrophils and histiocytes, to kill bacteria of ordinarily low virulence. In addition to superficial skin lesions such as impetigo, recurrent and persistent suppurative granulomatous reactions to bacteria can develop in the skins of children with this fatal disease.

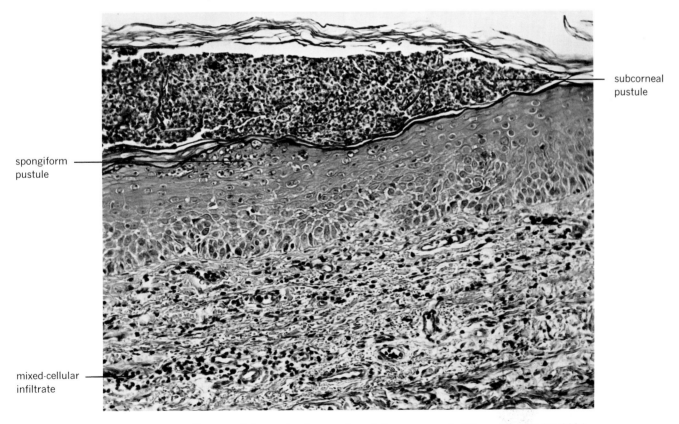

FIG. 10-57. Impetigo. Both spongiform pustules and subcorneal pustules are seen in this specimen. (× 220.)

Biopsy of papular lesions of *acute candidiasis* (Fig. 10-58) and *acute dermatophytosis* (Fig. 10-59) may reveal tiny subcorneal pustules. Rarely will eosinophils outnumber neutrophils and form intraepidermal eosinophilic abscesses. Candidiasis is a pustular disease that frequently involves intertriginous areas. Individual pustules ("satellite" pustules) at a distance from the major locus of involvement are a common feature. Zoophilic dermatophytes also produce vesiculopustules that can be arranged discretely or in groups. The finding of pustules within the epidermis should prompt a search for microorganisms, especially those of dermatophytosis and candidiasis, within the cornified layer of the epidermis. Hyphae are situated not only in the cornified layer but also in the pustules in the granular and spinous zones. Although the microorganisms can usually be spotted in sections stained with hematoxylin and eosin, they are better visualized when stained by PAS or silver methenamine.

Toxic erythema of the newborn passes through erythematous macular and papular stages before pustules develop. The pustules are actually subcorneal intrafollicular collections of eosinophils and a few neutrophils. Some pustules form around intraepidermal

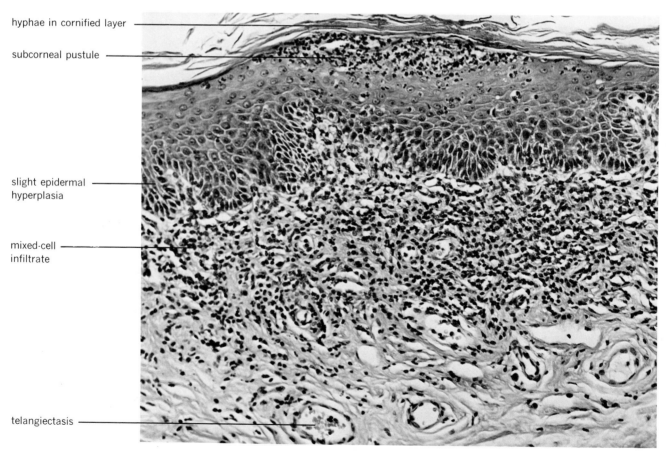

hyphae in cornified layer

subcorneal pustule

slight epidermal hyperplasia

mixed-cell infiltrate

telangiectasis

FIG. 10-58. Candidiasis, subcorneal pustule. Characteristic hyphae are seen in cornified layer immediately above collections of neutrophils within epidermis. ($\times$ 220.)

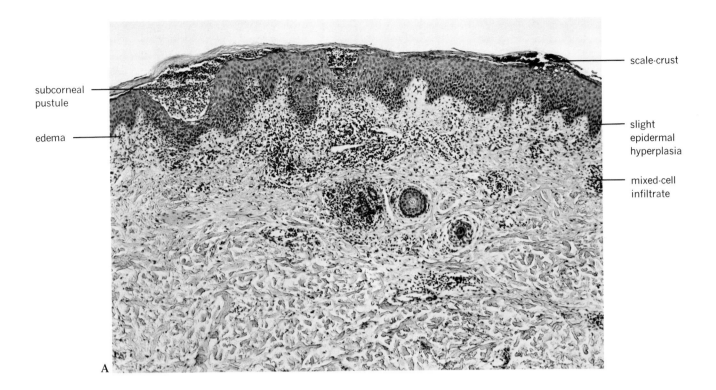

subcorneal pustule

edema

scale-crust

slight epidermal hyperplasia

mixed-cell infiltrate

A

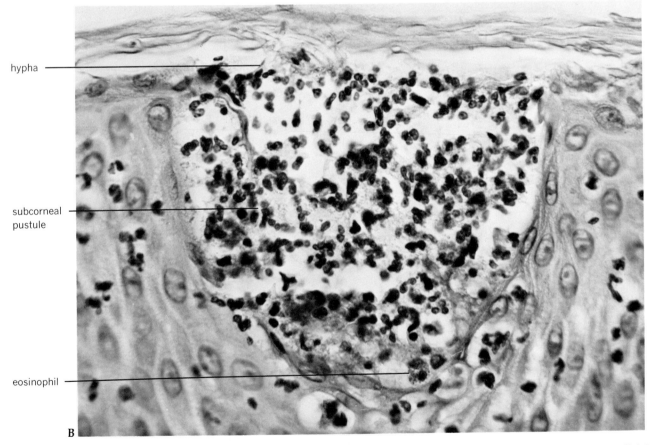

hypha

subcorneal pustule

eosinophil

B

FIG. 10-59. Dermatophytosis, pustular type. A, Well-circumscribed subcorneal pustules pictured are typical of pustular superficial fungal infections. (× 87.) B, Dermatophytic hypha is seen in cornified layer above subcorneal pustule. Special stains for fungi reveal them more readily than does this hematoxylin and eosin stain. Note eosinophils within subcorneal pustule, a not uncommon finding in pustular lesions caused by dermatophytes. (× 796.)

sweat ducts. A mixed-cell infiltrate of eosinophils predominantly collects around the blood vessels of the superficial plexus.

The presence of eosinophilic abscesses, rather than spongiotic foci, differentiates toxic erythema of the newborn from incontinentia pigmenti. The follicular location of the abscesses distinguishes it from pemphigus vegetans in which the eosinophilic abscesses are intraepidermal.

Toxic erythema is a common widespread eruption that spares the palms and soles in newborns. It appears within the first few days of life and disappears spontaneously, without sequelae, within a week. Eosinophils are present in increased numbers in the blood as well as in the skin.

Pyoderma gangrenosum, in addition to manifesting severe, rapidly advancing undermining ulcers, can be associated with widespread vesicles and vesiculopustules. The blistering lesions, upon biopsy, are noted to be subcorneal and/or spongiform pustules.

Pustular psoriasis (Fig. 10-60) and even florid lesions of *guttate psoriasis,* may consist of pustules seated immediately beneath the cornified layer. Other pustules within the very same specimen may be spongiform and still others may be lodged within parakeratotic foci (Fig. 10-61). Thus no type of histologic pustule is diagnostic for pustular psoriasis, but rather a range of types.

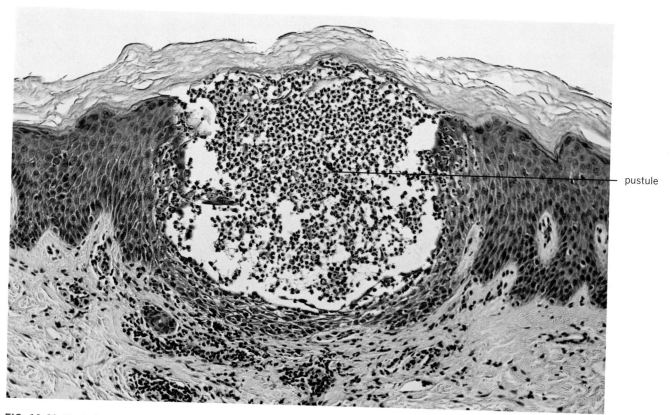

— pustule

FIG. 10-60. Pustular psoriasis. Sometimes well-circumscribed pustules with subcorneal and spongiform features such as the one pictured can develop. Note similarity to subcorneal pustular dermatosis. (× 186.)

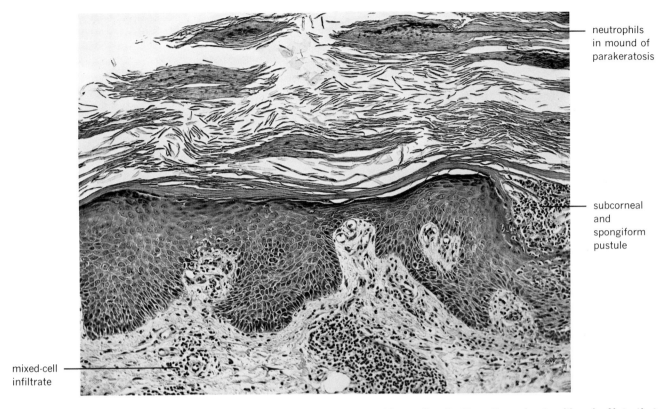

neutrophils
in mound of
parakeratosis

subcorneal
and
spongiform
pustule

mixed-cell
infiltrate

FIG. 10-61. Psoriasis, guttate lesion. Neutrophils are seen in dermis and in small collections throughout epidermis. Note that granular layer is mostly intact in this early lesion. (× 164.)

Intracorneal Pustular Dermatitis

Neutrophils in the cornified layer of any inflammatory condition of the skin are signs of active disease. For example, evolving lesions of psoriasis are accompanied by neutrophils staggered within the parakeratotic cornified layer. Resolving lesions of psoriasis have no neutrophils in this layer.

Psoriasis (Fig. 10-62)

Neutrophils participate in the early guttate lesions of psoriasis, as well as in those of pustular psoriasis. In guttate psoriatic lesions, neutrophils are sprinkled both solitarily and in small aggregates within all layers of the epidermis, especially near the summits of parakeratotic mounds. In the cornified layer of slightly older lesions, neutrophils are frequently intimately associated with laminated foci of parakeratosis. This association of parakeratotic cells and neutrophils in parakeratotic mounds and in laminated foci strongly suggests the diagnosis of psoriasis. The epidermis may not be hyperplastic in these early guttate and pustular lesions.

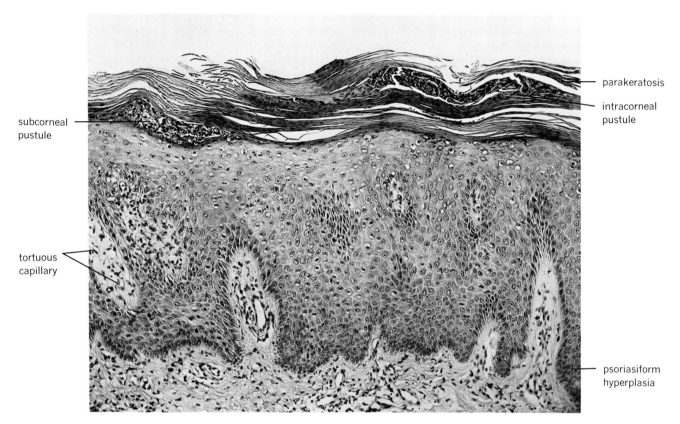

subcorneal
pustule

tortuous
capillary

parakeratosis

intracorneal
pustule

psoriasiform
hyperplasia

FIG. 10-62. Psoriasis, guttate lesion. Collections of neutrophils are seen in upper portion of epidermis, especially in the subcorneal and cornified regions. ($\times$ 160.)

Candidiasis, Subacute and Chronic, and Dermatophytosis, Subacute and Chronic (Fig. 10-63)

Intracorneal collections of neutrophils are also a feature of subacute and chronic stages of candidiasis and dermatophytosis. Whenever neutrophils are present within the cornified layer of a specimen that is not obviously psoriasis, a PAS or silver methenamine stain should be done in search of hyphae. The cornified layer of lesions of long-standing superficial fungal diseases is mostly compact and orthokeratotic, with relatively little parakeratosis. Hyphae are generally located in the orthokeratotic horn. The epidermis of these lesions often shows slight psoriasiform hyperplasia.

Neutrophils lodged within parakeratotic cells of the cornified layer ("neuts in the horn") are most commonly seen in eruptive (i.e., guttate) lesions of psoriasis, but also in evolving lesions of seborrheic dermatitis, pityriasis lichenoides et varioliformis acuta, and in some of secondary syphilis. Neutrophils within orthokeratotic cells of the cornified layer should prompt a search for fungi there, namely, dermatophytes and Candida.

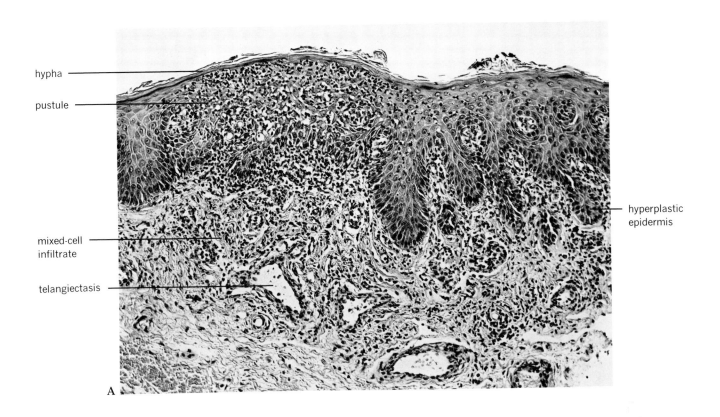

hypha —

pustule —

mixed-cell
infiltrate —

telangiectasis —

— hyperplastic
epidermis

A

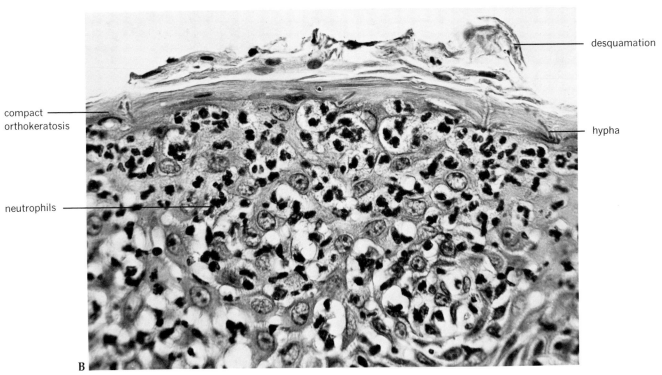

compact
orthokeratosis —

neutrophils —

— desquamation

— hypha

B

FIG. 10-63. **Candidiasis.** A, In the compact orthokeratotic cornified layer above spongiform, subcorneal, and intracorneal pustule, several hyphae can be spotted, even in this section stained by hematoxylin and eosin and of relatively low-power magnification (× 187.) B, At least four hyphae are visible in cornified layer of this higher magnification. The largely spongiform pustule pictured has ascended to become subcorneal and partially intracorneal. Eventually most of the neutrophils will be situated within the cornified layer. (× 747.)

Subepidermal Vesicular Dermatitis

Little or No Inflammatory-Cell Infiltrate

Epidermolysis bullosa
Junctional bullous epidermatosis (Herlitz's
syndrome, hereditary lethal epidermolysis
bullosa)
Dermolytic bullous dermatosis
Dominant type (hyperplastic dystrophic
epidermolysis bullosa)
Recessive type (polydysplastic dystrophic
epidermolysis bullosa)
Acquired type
Porphyria cutanea tarda
Pemphigoid, cell-poor type
Burns, second degree
Toxic epidermal necrolysis
Suction blister
Blisters secondary to hypoxemia and local
pressure
Gas gangrene
Subepidermal blisters over scars
Bullous amyloidosis
Autolysis

Lymphohistiocytic Infiltrate

Superficial perivascular
Vacuolar
Erythema multiforme
Toxic epiderman necrolysis
Lichen sclerosus et atrophicus

Lichenoid
Lichen planus, bullous type
Superficial and deep perivascular
Polymorphous light eruption

Eosinophils Prominent

Pemphigoid, cell-rich type
Herpes gestationis
Reactions to arthopods

Neutrophils Prominent

Dermatitis herpetiformis
Dermatitis herpetiformis-like drug eruption
Bullous disease of childhood
Bullous systemic lupus erythematosus
Leukocytoclastic vasculitis and septic
vasculitis
Cicatricial pemphigoid
Pemphigoid, rarely
Urticarial vesiculobullous allergic eruption
Erysipelas
Erythropoietic protoporphyria

Mast Cells Prominent

Bullous urticaria pigmentosa

Intradermal Blistering Diseases

Penicillamine-induced

Subepidermal Vesicular Dermatitis

11

THE SUBEPIDERMAL zone is seen through the electron microscope to consist of the basal-cell plasma membrane, intermembranous space, basal lamina, and anchoring collagen fibrils. Distinctions among the various subepidermal vesicular diseases can be made with the electron microscope on the basis of the level of separation of the constituents of the subepidermal zone. Unfortunately, these distinctions cannot be made with the light microscope. Nor are epidermal changes, histologically reviewed, usually helpful in distinguishing one subepidermal vesicular process from another. For example, necrotic keratinocytes can be seen in erythema multiforme, toxic epidermal necrolysis, graft-versus-host reactions, pityriasis lichenoides et varioliformis acuta, and bullous lichen planus. In fact, the epidermis may be completely necrotic in any long-standing subepidermal vesicular lesion. Thus, it is best to distinguish histologically among the subepidermal vesicular dermatitides on the basis of the composition and distribution of the inflammatory-cell infiltrates. When lymphocytes predominate, it is advantageous to determine whether the infiltrate is superficial or superficial and deep.

The pathologist must be alert to the pitfall of misinterpreting a subepidermal vesicle that is resolving with concomitant subjacent reepithelization as an intraepidermal vesicle. Cells from the follicular and eccrine epithelia spread out to cover the dermis, and these cells form the new epidermis (Fig. 11-1). Another hazard to be avoided is the misinterpretation of an intraepidermal vesicle that has burst as a primary subepidermal vesicle (Fig. 11-2).

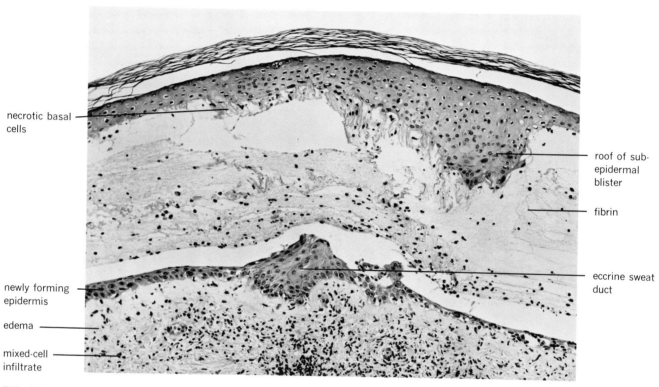

FIG. 11-1. Reepithelization beneath a subepidermal blister. This is not a primary intraepidermal blister because cells of newly forming epidermis have large nuclei typical of germinative cells. New epidermis derives, in large part, from adnexal epithelium and is seen here to be developing from an eccrine sweat duct. (× 175.)

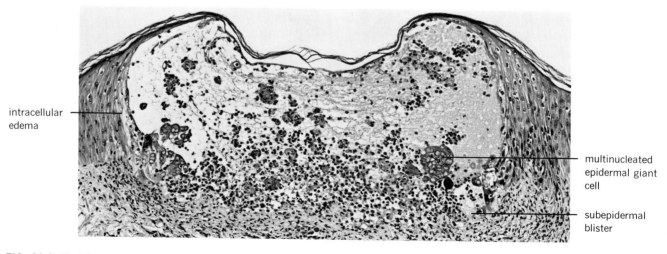

FIG. 11-2. Vesicle caused by herpesvirus as evidenced by numerous multinucleated epidermal giant cells. Tension became so great that blister fluid was forced into dermis, thereby converting intraepidermal vesicle into subepidermal one. (× 170.)

Little or No Inflammatory-cell Infiltrate (Fig. 11-3)

Subepidermal vesicular diseases in which there is little or no infiltration of inflammatory cells include epidermolysis bullosa, porphyria cutanea tarda, the cell-poor type of pemphigoid, and toxic epidermal necrolysis. The histologic pattern is also seen in lesions of second degree burns, suction blisters, gas gangrene, blisters secondary to hypoxia and local pressure, blisters over scars, bullous amyloidosis, and as one of the autolytic changes in the skin.

Often by examining the dermis, histologic distinctions can be made among the subepidermal blistering diseases that have little or no inflammatory-cell infiltrates. For example, extensive solar elastosis with papillae that have retained their shapes suggests porphyria cutanea tarda; necrosis of adnexal epithelium indicates blisters secondary to hypoxia and local pressure; and a few neutrophils and/or eosinophils in dermal papillae that are edematous and well preserved bespeak cell-poor pemphigoid.

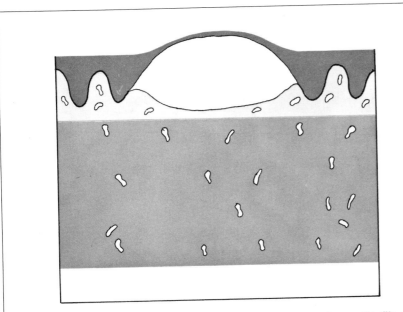

FIG. 11-3. Subepidermal blister with little or no inflammatory-cell infiltrate.

Epidermolysis Bullosa

Bullae and vesicles develop in a number of hereditary skin disorders classified as epidermolysis bullosa. Blisters may form at the dermoepidermal junction (junctional bullous epidermatosis) or below the epidermis (dermolytic bullous dermatosis). As a general rule, the deeper a blister forms beneath the plasma membranes of epidermal basal cells, the greater the likelihood of scarring.

Junctional Bullous Epidermatosis (Herlitz's Syndrome, Hereditary Lethal Epidermolysis Bullosa) (Fig. 11-4)

—Subepidermal blister
—Occasional necrotic basal keratinocytes
—Little or no inflammatory-cell infiltrate

The blister in junctional bullous epidermatosis has been shown electron-microscopically to form between the basal-cell plasma membrane and the basal lamina. This is also the location of the

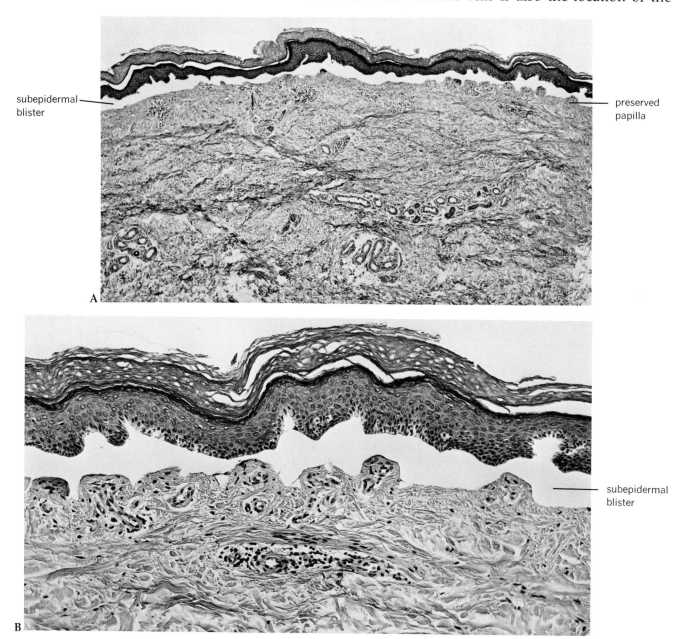

FIG. 11-4. Junctional bullous epidermatosis (Herlitz's syndrome). The subepidermal bulla not attended by an inflammatory-cell infiltrate is characteristic of junctional bullous epidermatosis. (A, × 52; B, × 169.)

subepidermal lysis in blisters caused by suction, liquid nitrogen, pemphigoid, and lichen planus.

The histologic pattern of junctional bullous epidermatosis somewhat resembles that of porphyria cutanea tarda in which there is also a subepidermal blister without much of an inflammatory-cell infiltrate. In porphyria cutanea tarda, however, there is nearly always solar elastosis which is not usually present in junctional bullous epidermatosis.

Junctional bullous epidermatosis is usually present at birth. Blisters form after slight injury to the skin and quickly progress to extensive erosions. The sites of predilection are the legs, buttocks, and perioral area where the lesions become C-shaped plaques on either side of the angles of the mouth. The erosions are often surmounted by vegetating crusts that result from secondary bacterial infection. Although these lesions heal slowly, they usually do not scar. Death normally occurs within months; some patients survive until young adulthood.

Dermolytic Bullous Dermatosis (Fig. 11-5)

—Subepidermal blister often containing erythrocytes
—Little or no inflammatory-cell infiltrate

Ultrastructural studies have demonstrated that the separation in all forms of dermolytic bullous dermatosis (dominant, recessive, and acquired) begins just below the basal lamina in the uppermost part of the papillary dermis. Anchoring collagen fibrils are absent in this region, suggesting that the process results from an abnormality of collagen. In actuality, the dermolytic types of epidermolysis bullosa are intradermal vesicular diseases.

The blisters in the *dominant type* of dermolytic bullous dermatosis (hyperplastic dystrophic epidermolysis bullosa, albopapuloid epidermolysis bullosa) appear secondary to trauma in infancy or early childhood. The hemorrhagic bullae occur principally on hands and feet, but may occur anywhere on the skin. The mucous membranes may also be involved by the blistering process.

The term *albopapuloid* refers to white hypertrophic scars that develop in some sites of previous blisters of the disease. There has been debate as to whether these hypertrophic scars always result from previous trauma and blister formation. Such controversy is as sterile as that of whether the pigment in incontinentia pigmenti always results from previous inflammation or whether keloids develop spontaneously. The albopapuloid lesions of dermolytic bullous dermatosis, the pigment in incontinentia pigmenti, and keloids are all end stages of previous inflammatory injuries.

As in the dominant and acquired types of dermolytic bullous dermatosis, the blister in the *recessive type* (polydysplastic dystrophic epidermolysis bullosa) occurs beneath the basal lamina in

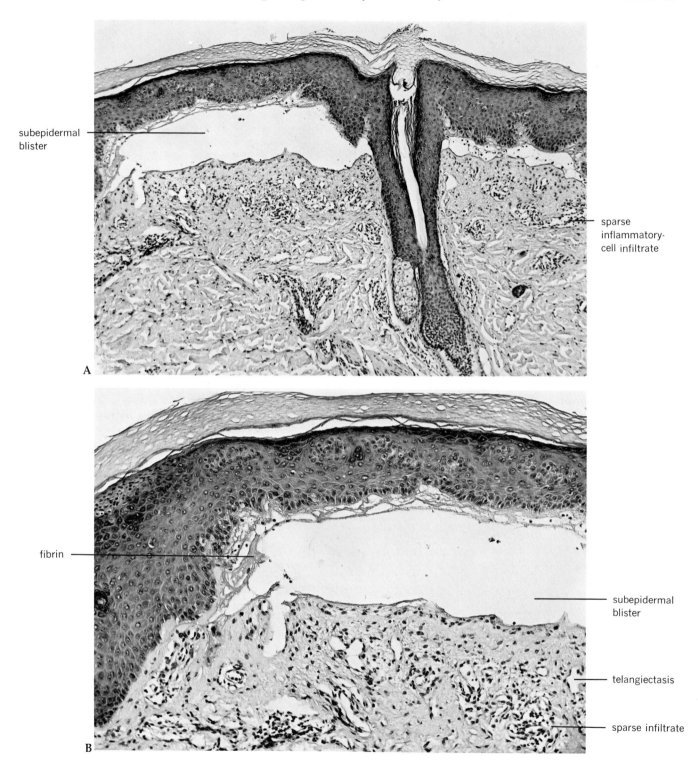

FIG. 11-5. Dermolytic bullous dermatosis. The subepidermal blister in dermolytic types of epidermolysis bullosa begins in the uppermost papillary dermis as shown here. Inflammatory cells may be absent or few as in this lesion. (A, × 92; B, × 175.)

the most superficial papillary dermis. The earliest histologic changes in recessive dermolytic bullous dermatosis are vacuoles that form at the dermoepidermal junction leading to a subepidermal cleft and eventually to a subepidermal blister.

Hemorrhagic blisters appear at birth, especially on the feet. The slightest trauma induces the blisters, which occur predominantly on the distal parts of the extremities. Repeated blistering and resultant scarring produce fusion of the digits, flexion deformity of the palms, and, eventually, hands that look as though permanently encased in mittens of atrophic skin. Such scarring results in contracture of other joints. Usually there is also mucous-membrane involvement, especially of the mouth, esophagus, and eyes. Scarring in these sites may lead to dysphagia and blindness. Scarring in hairy areas may produce alopecia. An occasional late complication of long-standing scars in recessive dermolytic bullous dermatosis is the development of squamous-cell carcinoma.

The electron microscope has shown the separation in the *acquired type* of dermolytic bullous dermatosis to be beneath the basal lamina in the most superficial portion of the papillary dermis (Fig. 11-6). This rare nonhereditary disease usually appears considerably after infancy, often in adulthood. The blisters, as in

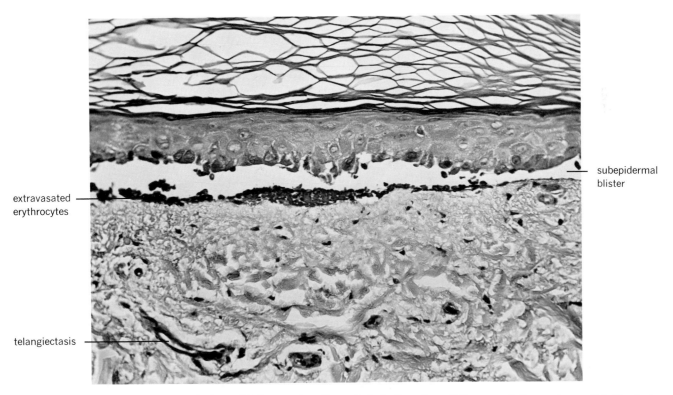

extravasated erythrocytes

subepidermal blister

telangiectasis

FIG. 11-6. Acquired epidermolysis bullosa. All forms of epidermolysis bullosa have little or no inflammatory-cell infiltrate in the dermis as illustrated. The subepidermal blister is often clinically hemorrhagic, the result of extravasated erythrocytes within the bulla as pictured here. ($\times$ 352.)

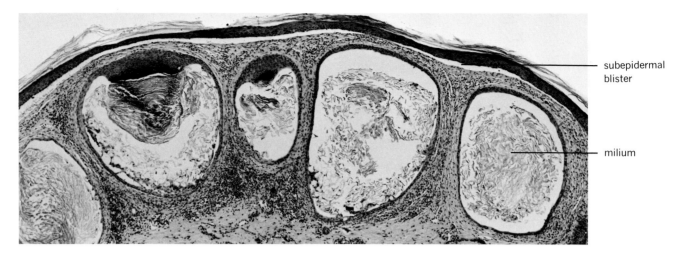

subepidermal blister

milium

FIG. 11-7. Milia secondary to healing of subepidermal blisters. A blister of epidermolysis bullosa has recurred above milia (infundibular cysts) that developed following a previous blister at this site. (× 52.)

other forms of epidermolysis bullosa, follow mechanical trauma and tend to involve the extremities, especially the acra.

In all forms of dystrophic epidermolysis bullosa, small adnexal cysts containing cornified cells (milia) may form at sites of previous blisters (Fig. 11-7). Most of these cysts are lined by follicular infundibular epithelium, but rarely are they lined by the upper portion of the eccrine sweat duct.

Porphyria Cutanea Tarda (Fig. 11-8)

—Subepidermal blister
—Little or no inflammatory-cell infiltrate or at most a sparse lymphohistiocytic infiltrate around the blood vessels of the superficial plexus
—Preservation of the dermal papillae
—Abundant solar elastotic material in the upper part of the dermis
—Erythrocytes often within the subepidermal blister (Fig. 11-9)

The histologic clues to the diagnosis of the vesiculobullous lesions of porphyria cutanea tarda are a subepidermal blister, practically no inflammatory-cell infiltrate, and abundant elastotic material. Any subepidermal blistering disease, however, can involve skin that has been injured by sunlight. Another, but uncommon, subtle clue to the histologic diagnosis of porphyria cutanea tarda is the occasional rim of homogeneous eosinophilic material that develops around some of the capillaries and venules in the upper dermis. Greater amounts of this material can also be seen in other forms of porphyria, such as erythropoietic protoporphyria. Similar-appearing material is also seen in lipoid proteinosis and, rarely, in chronic discoid lupus erythematosus.

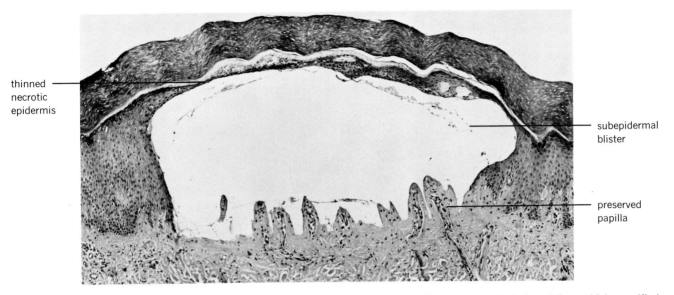

thinned necrotic epidermis

subepidermal blister

preserved papilla

FIG. 11-8. Porphyria cutanea tarda. Discrete subepidermal blister from side of finger, as can be inferred from thick cornified layer, shows preservation of dermal papillae but practically no inflammatory-cell infiltrate and is virtually diagnostic of porphyria cutanea tarda. (× 80.)

Porphyria cutanea tarda is an acquired disease that commonly occurs in people who have drunk large quantities of alcohol for many years, but also may develop in patients taking estrogens. Cutaneous signs of porphyria cutanea tarda, besides blisters, include ulcers, scars, and milia at sites of previous blisters; sclerodermoid changes, predominantly on the chest; hypermelanosis on the face; and hypertrichosis, especially lateral to the eyes. These patients often have abundant iron in the liver. The porphyrin abnormality is excessive production of uroporphyrin which causes photosensitivity. Its excretion via the kidneys causes a coral-red fluorescence when the urine is exposed to Wood's light. Similar fluorescence can be demonstrated in the skin lesions and also in the liver. In each instance it is due to porphyrin deposition.

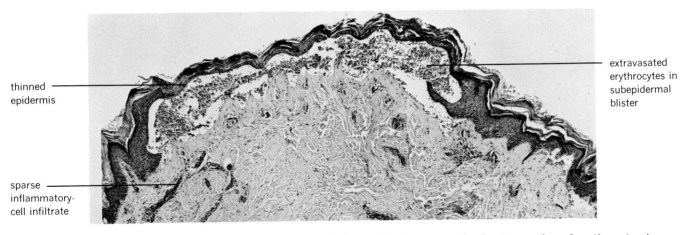

thinned epidermis

extravasated erythrocytes in subepidermal blister

sparse inflammatory-cell infiltrate

FIG. 11-9. Porphyria cutanea tarda. Blisters are often clinically hemorrhagic as a result of extravasation of erythrocytes in subepidermal vesicles and bullae as shown here. Note also thinned epidermis secondary to compression by blister fluid. Epidermal necrosis may also develop secondary to such tension. (× 63.)

Pemphigoid, Cell-poor Type (Fig. 11-10)

—Subepidermal blister
—Preservation of the pattern of epidermal rete and dermal papillae beneath the subepidermal space
—Edema of the papillary dermis
—Sparse mixed inflammatory-cell infiltrate of lymphocytes, histiocytes, neutrophils, and eosinophils around the vessels of the superficial plexus

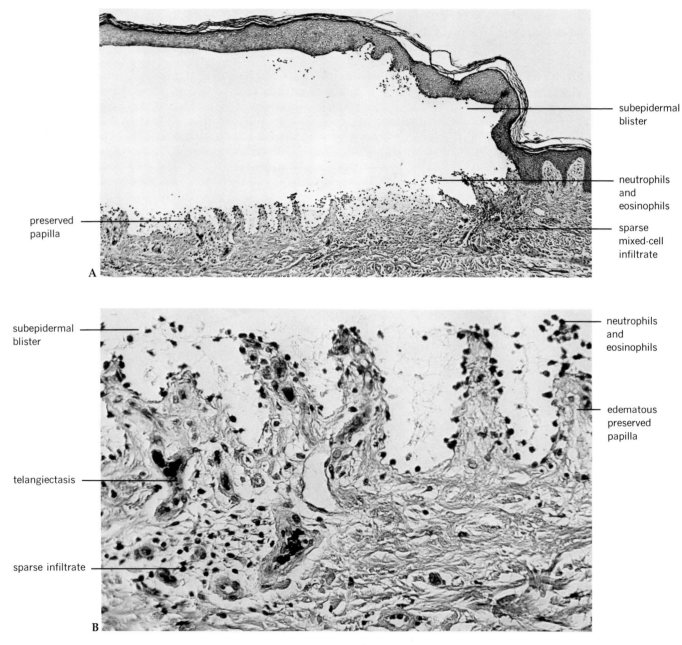

FIG. 11-10. Pemphigoid, cell-poor type. Sparse infiltrate consists mainly of neutrophils and eosinophils. Note that dermal papillae, although edematous, have preserved their configuration in floor of subepidermal blister. (A, × 82; B, × 400.)

Pemphigoid is a subepidermal vesicular dermatitis in which there are two inflammatory-cell patterns, namely cell-poor and cell-rich. Under scanning magnification, the cell-poor type of pemphigoid must be distinguished from the variants of epidermolysis bullosa and from porphyria cutanea tarda. However, even in the cell-poor type there are some inflammatory cells, almost always including a few eosinophils and neutrophils. Cell-rich pemphigoid is an exaggeration of the cell-poor type, having a moderately dense mixed inflammatory-cell infiltrate with numerous eosinophils and scarce neutrophils. Eosinophilic "abscesses" may form within the dermal papillae of cell-rich pemphigoid. These abscesses should not be mistaken for the neutrophilic abscesses in dermal papillae of dermatitis herpetiformis. Rarely, neutrophils can congregate within the papillae in pemphigoid, and then the histologic differentiation of pemphigoid from dermatitis herpetiformis may be difficult or impossible. Whether the lesions of pemphigoid are cell-poor or cell-rich does not seem to have prognostic significance vis-a-vis the course of the disease or its severity.

Clinically, pemphigoid begins with erythematous, edematous papules and plaques upon which vesicles and bullae develop. Biopsy of the urticarial lesions reveals edema of the papillary dermis and an infiltrate that varies in density. In some urticarial lesions, vacuoles can be seen at the dermoepidermal interface. In time, these vacuoles give rise to subepidermal clefts and, eventually, to subepidermal blisters. Solitary eosinophils can be present within the epidermis of the urticarial lesions, and occasionally foci of eosinophilic spongiosis can be seen in the papules and plaques of pemphigoid. Pemphigoid is usually a disease of older people.

Direct immunoflorescence of urticarial lesions and blisters of pemphigoid reveals immunoglobulin and complement at the dermoepidermal junction. Indirect immunofluorescent studies show circulating antibody to basement membrane material in most patients with this disease.

Burns, Second Degree (Fig. 11-11)

—Subepidermal blister
—Epidermal necrosis
—Intracellular and intercellular edema
—Sparse inflammatory-cell infiltrate in the papillary dermis composed of lymphocytes, histiocytes, and neutrophils

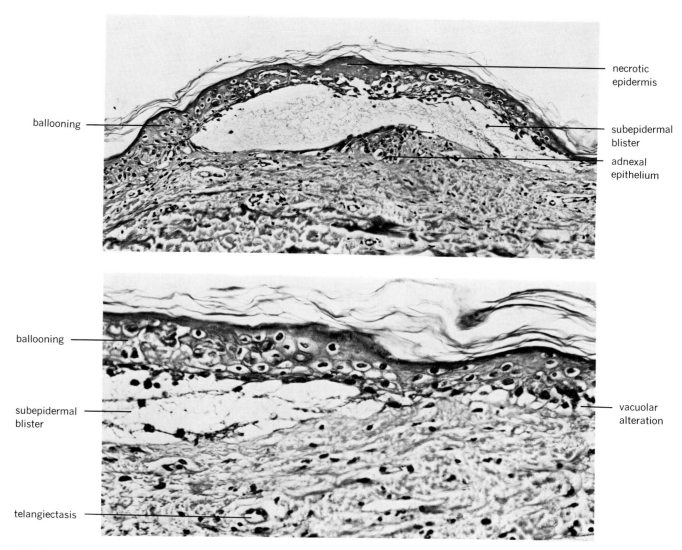

ballooning

necrotic
epidermis

subepidermal
blister

adnexal
epithelium

balloraphy

ballooning

subepidermal
blister

vacuolar
alteration

telangiectasis

FIG. 11-11. Chemical burn. A, Combination of intracellular edema within epidermal keratinocytes, necrosis of keratinocytes, subepidermal vesiculation, and absence of significant inflammatory-cell infiltrate indicates that damage to skin was from external source. Note beginnning of reepithelization at base of blister emerging from adnexal epithelium. (× 216.) B, Progression from vacuolar alteration to subepidermal vesiculation is better appreciated in this higher magnification. Note prominent ballooning of epidermal keratinocytes, a feature of external injuries to skin. (× 475.)

Burns can be classified according to severity, clinically and histologically. A biopsy of a first-degree burn shows only individually necrotic keratinocytes, extensive vasodilatation, and a sparse perivascular infiltrate of inflammatory cells. One from a second-degree burn shows intracellular and intercellular edema, variable epidermal necrosis, subepidermal vesiculation, and a sparse superficial perivascular lymphohistiocytic infiltrate with neutrophils. In a third-degree burn there will be ulceration with variable degrees of collagen degeneration, a mixed inflammatory-cell infiltrate, and necrosis of adnexal epithelial structures.

Burns can be induced by thermal, electrical, chemical, solar, or other electromagnetic damage. In most burns the blister forms subepidermally, but there are ballooning and spongiosis in the overlying necrotic epidermis. Necrosis is chemotactic for neutrophils that may be found within the necrotic epidermis of burn specimens. The cornified layer in burns usually maintains its normal basket-weave pattern, indicating that the damage has occurred suddenly.

Various dermatologic therapeutic modalities, for example, electrodesiccation, injure the skin. The epidermal damage caused by electrodesiccation is distinctive, revealing epidermal nuclei that are elongated and oriented perpendicular to the surface of the specimen (Fig. 11-12). In addition to the string-bean appearance of the nuclei, the cytoplasm on the undersurface of the basal cells is tufted, creating the impression of a fringe. Intracellular edema and intraepidermal vesiculation may be present also.

Phototoxic eruptions are merely exaggerated sunburns. Acute radiodermatitis has the histologic features of a second-degree burn. The histologic features of damage to the skin by congelation, such as induced by liquid nitrogen, are the same as those of low-grade thermal burns.

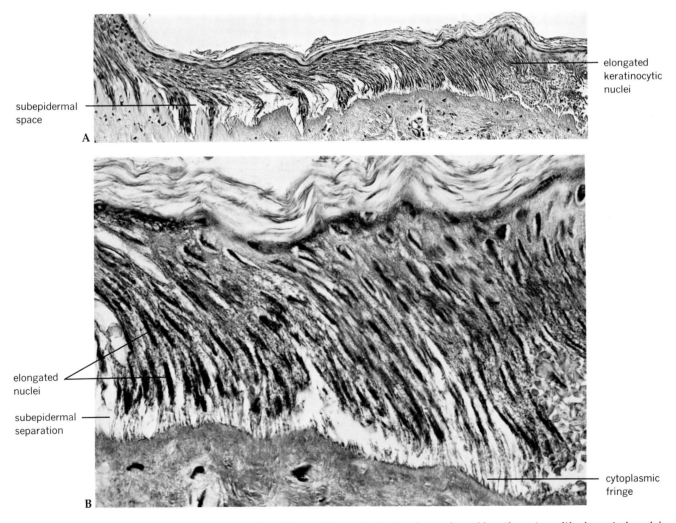

FIG. 11-12. Blister secondary to electrodesiccation. Changes illustrated, string-bean shaped keratinocytes with elongated nuclei and granular cytoplasms, are pathognomonic for injuries to epidermis from fulguration. Fringelike epidermis separates from dermis with consequent formation of clefts and sometimes blisters. (A, × 188; B × 752.)

Toxic Epidermal Necrolysis (Lyell)

Clinically and histologically, the lesions of toxic epidermal necrolysis resemble those of a burn. Because toxic epidermal necrolysis also has many features in common with erythema multiforme, to which it may be related, a more detailed description follows that of erythema multiforme later in this chapter.

Suction blister (Fig. 11-13)

—Subepidermal blister
—Pattern of dermal papillae preserved
—No or little inflammatory-cell infiltrate

The earliest histologic changes in suction blisters are vacuoles that appear at the dermoepidermal interface. These vacuoles soon become confluent and form subepidermal clefts that eventuate in subepidermal blisters. Electron microscopy has shown that the separation occurs between the plasma membrane of basal cells and the basal lamina as a result of detachment of hemidesmosomes.

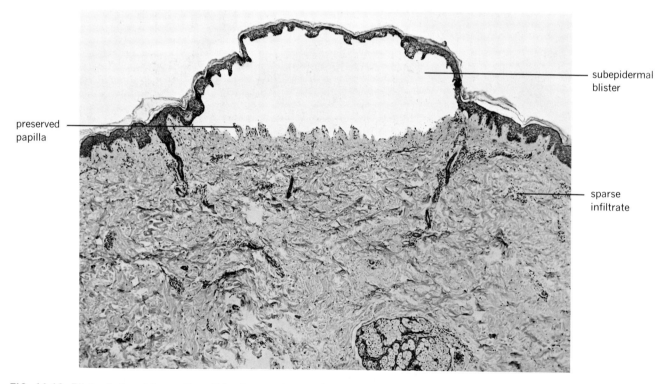

FIG. 11-13. Blister induced by suction. It is characterized by subepidermal separation that completely maintains structural integrity of dermal papillae and is associated with little or no inflammatory-cell infiltrate. (× 49.)

Blisters Secondary to Hypoxemia and Local Pressure (Fig. 11-14)

—Subepidermal blister
—Sparse inflammatory-cell infiltrate of lymphocytes, histiocytes, and neutrophils
—Adnexal necrosis of eccrine sweat glands and ducts especially, and also of follicular epithelium
—Occasional intraepidermal vesiculation, especially around intraepidermal adnexa

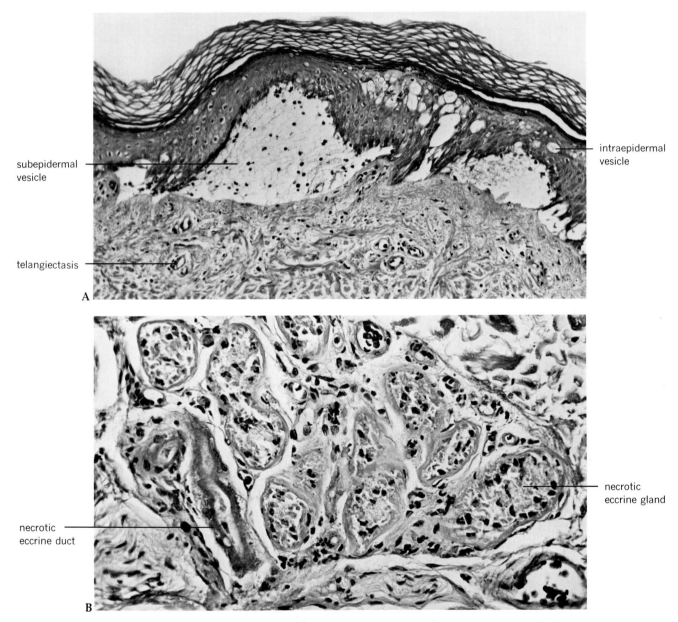

FIG. 11-14. Bulla secondary to barbiturate intoxication. A, Subepidermal vesiculation is combined with variable intraepidermal vesiculation and sparse inflammatory-cell infiltrate. (× 180.) B, Necrosis of sweat glands and other adnexal epithelia is virtually diagnostic of combined hypoxia and local pressure that occur in patients who are comatose as result of barbiturate overdosage. (× 400.)

Blisters secondary to hypoxemia and local pressure are often induced by drug overdosage (e.g., by barbiturates), carbon-monoxide intoxication, and central nervous system diseases. The outstanding histologic sign of hypoxia and local pressure is the presence of necrosis of adnexal epithelia, particularly the epithelium of the eccrine sweat gland. Commonly the sweat ducts and hair follicles are also necrotic, but the first epithelium to undergo necrosis is that of the eccrine sweat glands. The epidermis may also be necrotic.

Clinically, the lesions in barbiturate intoxication result from both hypoxia and external local pressure that is usually prolonged. The earliest lesions are erythematous patches and plaques at the sites of pressure on which vesicles and bullae of various sizes may develop.

Theories for the cause of these distinctive skin lesions range from friction alone to the toxic effect of a drug. Friction alone cannot be responsible because the separation in experimentally produced friction blisters occurs in the upper spinous or granular zone. The drug toxicity theory is unlikely because these lesions may develop in the absence of drug intake. The most satisfactory explanation is the combined effects of hypoxia and pressure.

Gas Gangrene (Fig. 11-15)

—Subepidermal vesicle, often containing erythrocytes
—Sweat gland necrosis occasionally
—Little or no inflammatory-cell infiltrate
—Holes, representing gas bubbles, in the dermis and subcutis

The gram-positive bacilli of Clostridium are abundant throughout the dermis and subcutis, including the walls of blood vessels, in specially stained histologic sections from skin lesions of gas gangrene. The basophilic-staining rods even can be seen by careful search of sections prepared with hematoxylin and eosin (Fig. 11-15B). A histologic sign of gas gangrene is the presence of holes of various sizes within the tissue in the dermis and subcutis, the result of gas production by the bacteria. A clinical clue to the diagnosis of gas gangrene is the "sparkling burgundy sign," i.e., bubbles within hemorrhagic blisters. The bullae arise on erythematous edematous skin in which crepitation from gas in the tissues can often be elicited. By the time that bullous lesions develop in this septic process, the patient is usually critically ill and in shock.

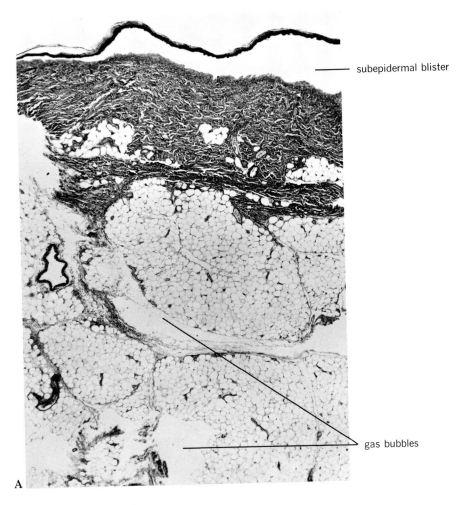

subepidermal blister

gas bubbles

A

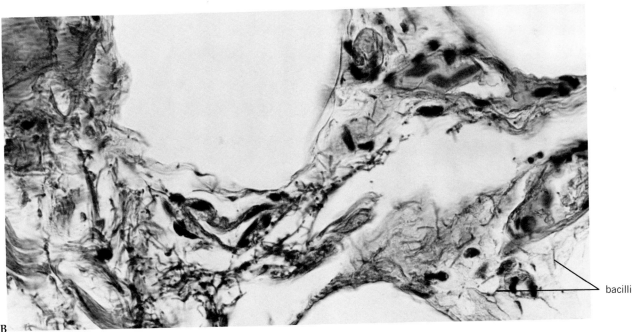

bacilli

B

FIG. 11-15. Gas gangrene. A, Histologic features pictured include pockets of gas in subcutaneous fat, subepidermal blister, and practically no inflammatory-cell infiltrate. When extravasated erythrocytes are present in bubbling subepidermal blister fluid, clinical appearance resembles sparkling burgundy. ($\times$ 24.) B, In section viewed with higher magnification, albeit stained merely with hematoxylin and eosin, numerous bacilli of Clostridia are recognizable throughout subcutis and in dermis. ($\times$ 794.)

Subepidermal Clefts or Blisters over Scars (Fig. 11-16)

—Subepidermal blister
—Scar in the papillary and, occasionally, the reticular dermis

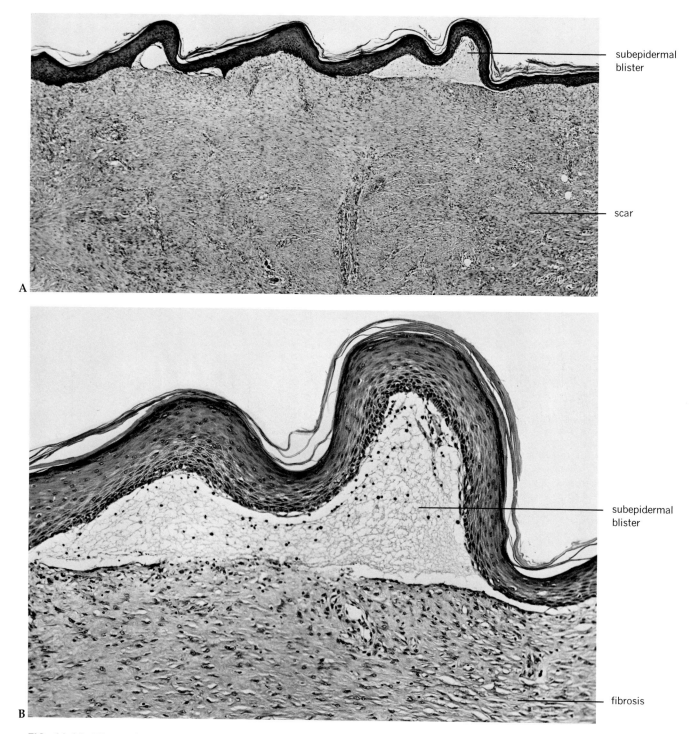

FIG. 11-16. Blister above a scar. Subepidermal blisters pictured are result of accumulation of fluid in subepidermal clefts. (A, × 31; B, × 128.)

Scarring in the papillary dermis sometimes results in faulty adhesion between the connective tissue and the overlying epidermis. Biopsy specimens of scars not uncommonly reveal subepidermal clefts that are an artifact of processing, much like the cleft that forms between an aggregate of basal-cell carcinoma and its surrounding stroma. In some instances, the subepidermal cleft that forms above a scar can fill with fluid, the result being a subepidermal blister that can sometimes be seen clinically. This phenomenon most commonly occurs in atrophic scars.

A distinction should be made between blisters that develop upon scars and scars that result from subepidermal blistering diseases such as porphyria cutanea tarda, dermolytic bullous dermatosis, and cicatricial pemphigoid. Histologically, the fibrosing dermatitis pictured in Figure 11-16 involves much of the reticular dermis, as well as the papillary dermis, and is a typical scar with fibrillary collagen and fibroblasts aligned parallel with and blood vessels oriented perpendicular to the skin surface. In clinical scarring that eventuates from subepidermal bullous diseases the fibrosis is confined to the papillary dermis and does not have the organized histologic pattern of a scar.

Bullous Amyloidosis

—Subepidermal blister, usually containing erythrocytes
—Homogeneous eosinophilic globules throughout the dermis, especially in the upper part and around blood vessels
—Variable numbers of lymphocytes and plasma cells in foci throughout the dermis

Bullous amyloidosis is rare and occurs only in primary systemic amyloidosis, especially above amyloid deposits in the skin of the eyelids, but also elsewhere. Blisters are not associated with the common forms of cutaneous amyloidosis, the macular and papular (lichenoid) types, or with the amyloid which is deposited incidentally in a variety of inflammatory, hamartomatous, and neoplastic diseases of the skin.

Amyloid in the skin is easily recognized in sections stained by hematoxylin and eosin as globules of homogeneous eosinophilic material. The identity of amyloid can be confirmed by its capacity to stain metachromatically red with crystal violet, its dichroism (i.e., doubly refractile quality and apple-green color) when sections stained by Congo red are viewed with polarizing lens, and its fluorescence when sections stained by thioflavin T are examined with ultraviolet light.

Autolysis (Fig. 11-17)

Among the postmortem changes in skin is the artifact of dermo-epidermal separation which at first glance resembles a subepidermal blister. In fact, there is no blister, as is evidenced by the absence of serum or blood cells in the subepidermal space. The collagen tends to be basophilic in sections stained by hematoxylin and eosin. Autolytic changes in the skin occur independent of the cause of death and of the presence or absence of skin disease.

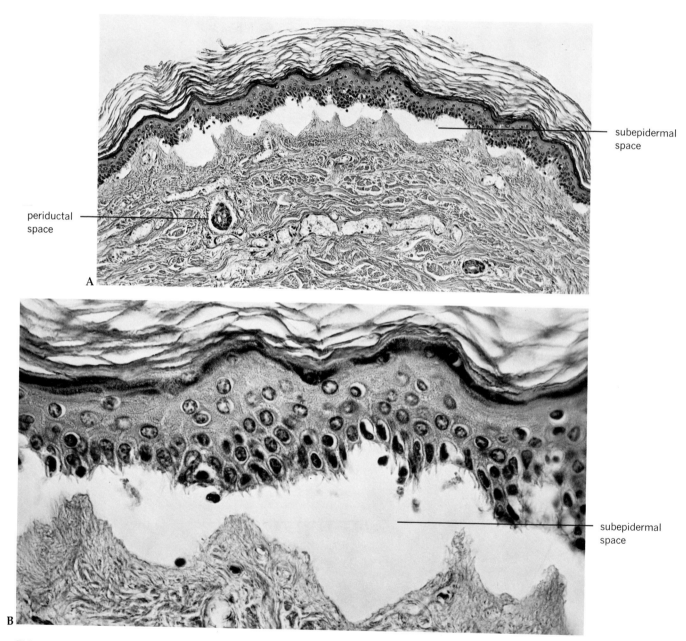

FIG. 11-17. Subepidermal separation caused by autolysis. A common postmortem finding shown here is separation of cutaneous epithelial structures from dermis. That these changes are a postmortem event and not related to blister formation in vivo is suggested by absence of serum or fibrin from spaces (unlike blisters in the living), separation between eccrine sweat duct and dermis, and absence of inflammatory cells in upper part of dermis. (A, × 180; B, × 624.)

The subepidermal vesicular diseases with changes at the dermo-epidermal interface may be further subdivided as superficial (Fig. 11-18) or superficial and deep perivascular. The changes at the interface in superficial perivascular forms of subepidermal vesicular dermatitis are either vacuolar or lichenoid. Vacuoles and only a scant infiltrate of lymphocytes and histiocytes are seen in erythema multiforme and toxic epidermal necrolysis. A somewhat bandlike infiltrate of lymphocytes and histiocytes is characteristic of lichen planus.

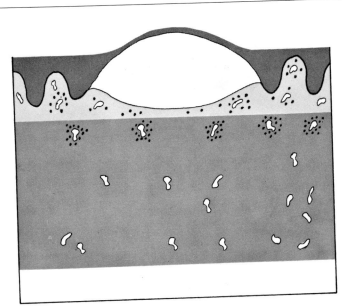

FIG. 11-18. Subepidermal blister with superficial perivascular dermatitis.

Erythema Multiforme (Fig. 11-19; Plate 6)

—Subepidermal blister
—Necrotic keratinocytes at the dermoepidermal junction, usually scattered throughout the epidermis, and, sometimes, confluent epidermal necrosis
—Intracellular and intercellular edema, rarely intraepidermal vesiculation
—Edema of the papillary dermis
—Extravasated erythrocytes in the papillary dermis
—Lymphohistiocytic infiltrate around the dilated vessels of the superficial plexus

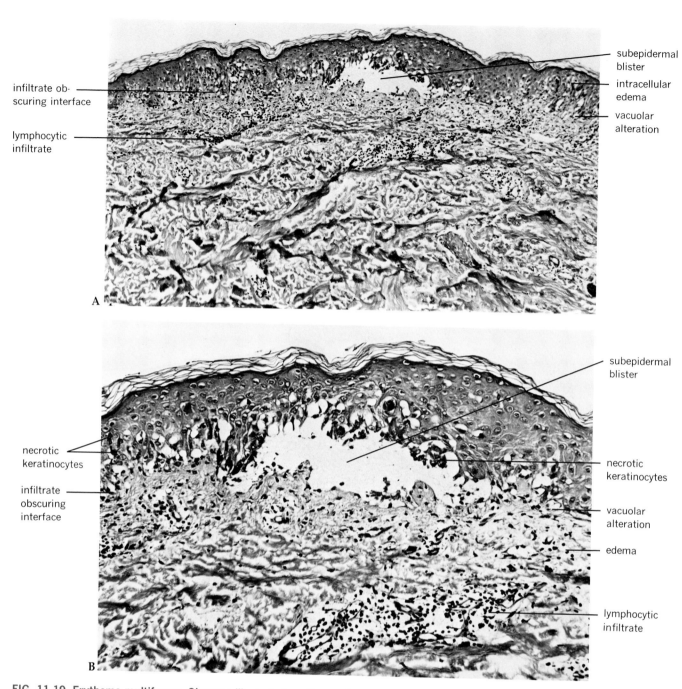

FIG. 11-19. Erythema multiforme. Changes illustrated are those of relatively early lesion in which subepidermal blister is forming. Note superficiality of predominantly lymphocytic perivascular infiltrate, scattered individual necrotic keratinocytes within epidermis, and extensive vacuolar alteration at dermoepidermal junction, a forerunner of subepidermal vesiculation. (A, × 86; B, × 255.)

The blister in erythema multiforme is usually subepidermal, but sometimes intracellular and intercellular edemas will produce intraepidermal vesiculation, in combination with, or even in the absence of, subepidermal vesiculation (Figs. 11-20, 11-21). The intraepidermal location results from ballooning and spongiosis, and the subepidermal from vacuolar alteration at the dermoepidermal junction (Plate 6).

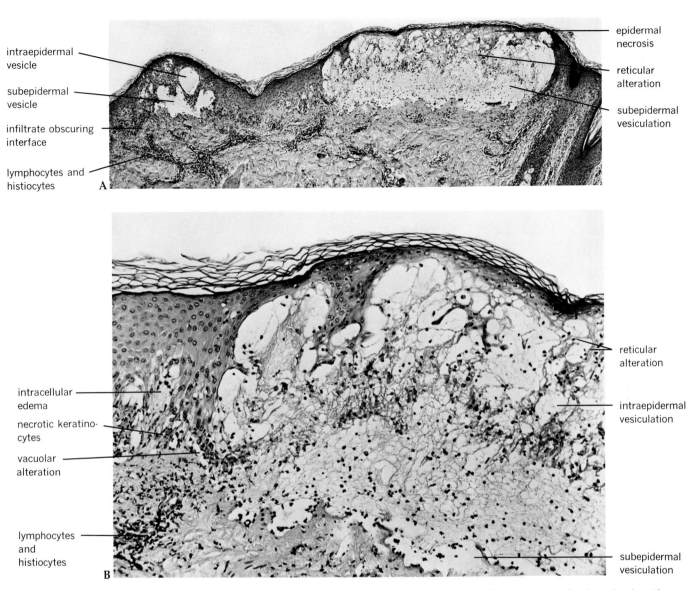

FIG. 11-20. Erythema multiforme. A, Intraepidermal and subepidermal blisters are pictured. Note that superficial predominantly lymphocytic infiltrate is moderately dense in contrast to that of toxic epidermal necrolysis wherein it is sparse. (× 44.) B, In this higher magnification changes in epidermis and at dermoepidermal interface, so critical to diagnosis, are better seen. Note necrotic keratinocytes, vacuolar alteration progressing to subepidermal vesiculation, and ballooning that eventuates in intraepidermal vesiculation. (× 175.)

There has been considerable confusion about the histologic features of erythema multiforme. The major reason for this is that until the late 1940's, pemphigoid was considered to be chronic bullous erythema multiforme. Even today, many cases of pemphigoid are misdiagnosed clinically as bullous erythema multiforme. Pathologists, receiving biopsy specimens from lesions of pemphigoid misdiagnosed clinically as bullous erythema multiforme, conclude mistakenly that erythema multiforme has histologic features in common with pemphigoid. Another source of error in the histologic diagnosis of erythema multiforme is that some clinicians regard many nonscaly annular and erythematous

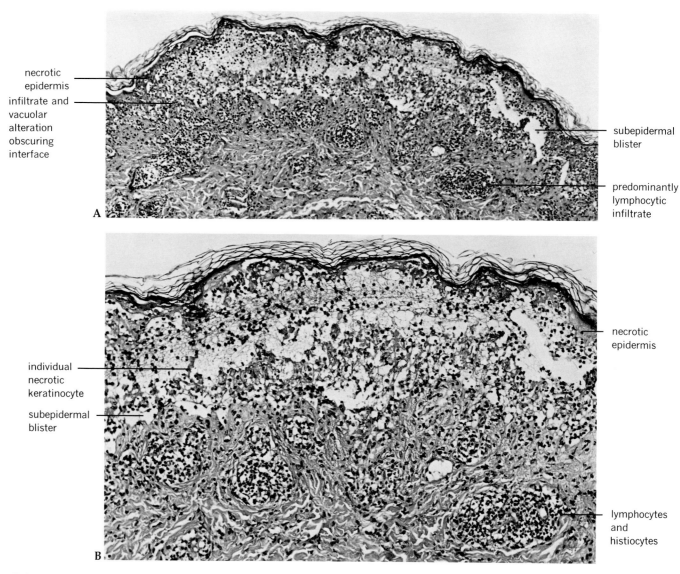

necrotic epidermis

infiltrate and vacuolar alteration obscuring interface

subepidermal blister

predominantly lymphocytic infiltrate

individual necrotic keratinocyte

subepidermal blister

necrotic epidermis

lymphocytes and histiocytes

FIG. 11-21. Erythema multiforme. A, Blister shown is subepidermal, the result of extensive vacuolar alteration and consequent dermoepidermal separation. In addition, there is a suggestion of intraepidermal vesiculation secondary to severe intracellular and intercellular edema. (× 91.) B, In this higher magnification one can see predominantly lymphocytic infiltrate that obscures dermoepidermal junction, intraepidermal and subepidermal vesiculation, and numerous necrotic keratinocytes. (× 179.)

diseases as erythema multiforme. Hence, urticarial and urticarial vesiculobullous drug eruptions, gyrate erythemas, and the urticarial stage of pemphigoid are termed erythema multiforme by them. In fact, erythema multiforme has a distinctive histologic appearance regardless of the precipitating cause. The crucial histologic features are a superficial perivascular lymphohistiocytic infiltrate with noticeable vacuolar alteration of the dermoepidermal interface and necrotic keratinocytes within the epidermis. In older lesions the entire affected epidermis may be necrotic.

In the histologic differential diagnosis of erythema multiforme, toxic epidermal necrolysis must be considered. It may well be that these two diseases are related, if not identical. The acute graft-versus-host reaction has many of the histologic features of erythema multiforme.

Clinically, erythema multiforme almost always involves mucous membranes, as well as skin, and its classic presentation includes concentrically ringed iris and target lesions. Lesions of erythema multiforme begin as erythematous macules that quickly become edematous, often purpuric, papules. Upon these lesions, vesicles and bullae subsequently develop. The acral parts are the sites of predilection for erythema multiforme, but the disease may be widespread. Iris and target lesions are not absolutely essential for the clinical diagnosis of erythema multiforme.

Toxic Epidermal Necrolysis (Lyell) (Fig. 11-22)

—Subepidermal blister
—Individually necrotic keratinocytes and, eventually, confluent epidermal necrosis
—Sparse lymphohistiocytic infiltrate around the dilated blood vessels of the superficial vascular plexus

Clinically and histologically, toxic epidermal necrolysis appears to be closely related to erythema multiforme. Clinical features of both may appear concurrently in the same patient. Both

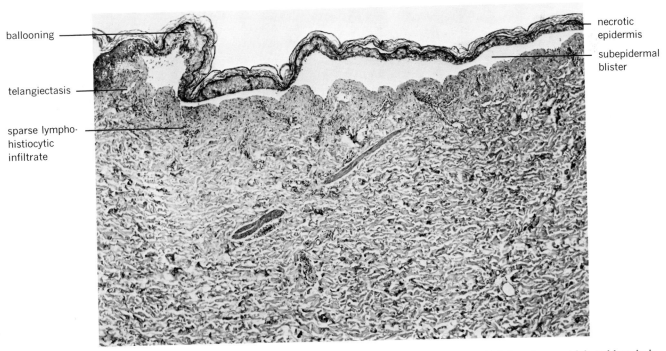

ballooning

telangiectasis

sparse lympho-histiocytic infiltrate

necrotic epidermis

subepidermal blister

FIG. 11-22. Toxic epidermal necrolysis. A, Characteristic features pictured are subepidermal blister above which epidermis is necrotic and beneath which there is only sparse superficial perivascular lymphohistiocytic infiltrate. (× 50.)

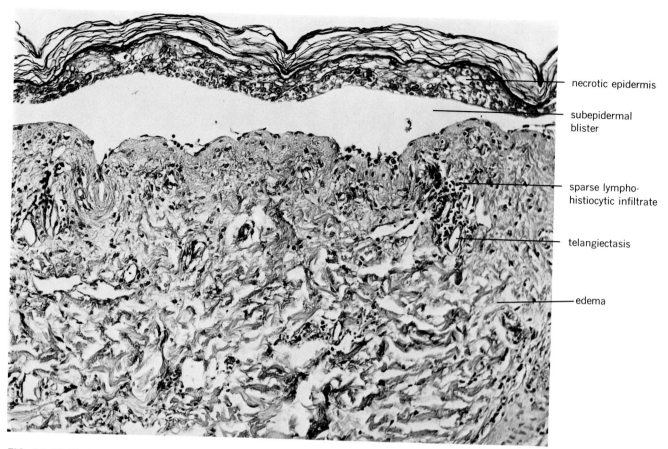

necrotic epidermis

subepidermal blister

sparse lympho-histiocytic infiltrate

telangiectasis

edema

FIG. 11-22. Toxic epidermal necrolysis. B, In this higher magnification, ballooning and necrosis of keratinocytes and dermal infiltrate of lymphocytes and histiocytes are seen to resemble closely those of erythema multiforme, but superficial infiltrate is sparse as shown here and not moderately dense as in erythema multiforme. (× 175.)

are characterized histologically by necrotic keratinocytes within the epidermis, vacuolar alteration at the dermoepidermal junction, subepidermal vesiculation, and a superficial perivascular lymphohistiocytic infiltrate. As a rule, the inflammatory-cell infiltrate is more dense in erythema multiforme than in toxic epidermal necrolysis. In rare instances eosinophils may be present in the infiltrate of toxic epidermal necrolysis. Clinically, many patients with toxic epidermal necrolysis have flaccid blisters that resemble sheets of scalded skin. As in erythema multiforme, a specific cause cannot always be determined for toxic epidermal necrolysis. A drug is most commonly incriminated in those instances of both diseases in which a cause is identified.

Toxic epidermal necrolysis is a subepidermal vesicular disease, in contrast with the staphylococcal scalded-skin syndrome (Ritter) that is histologically similar to bullous impetigo and to superficial pemphigus, i.e., the blister forms high in the epidermis. Severe erythema multiforme should be used synonymously with Lyell's disease, and staphylococcal scalded-skin syndrome, with Ritter's disease.

—Subepidermal blister, usually containing erythrocytes
—Thin epidermis
—Compact orthokeratosis, often with adnexal plugging by cornified cells
—Sclerosis or edema of the thickened papillary dermis
—Telangiectases within the papillary dermis
—Moderately dense, predominantly lymphocytic infiltrate around the dilated blood vessels immediately beneath the thickened, sclerotic or edematous papillary dermis

Lichen sclerosus et atrophicus is usually not associated with blisters. Typical lesions are white, sclerotic patches and plaques with erythematous borders. Histologically, a nearly constant feature of the sclerotic lesions of lichen sclerosus is vacuolar alteration at the dermoepidermal junction that results in blisters. Sometimes subepidermal clefts are seen. In exceptional cases, especially of the vulva, erythrocytes pour out of the telangiectatic vessels in the sclerotic papillary dermis and spill into the subepidermal cleft, producing a hemorrhagic blister. This phenomenon is restricted almost wholly to long-standing sclerotic lesions of lichen sclerosus on the vulva.

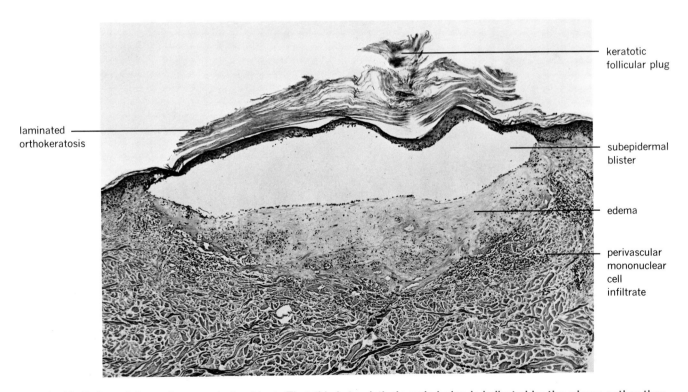

FIG. 11-23. Bullous lichen sclerosus et atrophicus. That this is a relatively early lesion is indicated by the edema, rather than sclerosis, of upper part of dermis, and primarily perivascular, rather than lichenoid, infiltrate. (× 66.)

Lichenoid
Lichen Planus, Bullous Type (Fig. 11-24)

—Subepidermal blister
—Irregular epidermal hyperplasia
—Hypergranulosis
—Compact orthokeratosis
—Moderately dense bandlike lymphohistiocytic infiltrate in the papillary dermis with similar cells around the blood vessels of the superficial vascular plexus

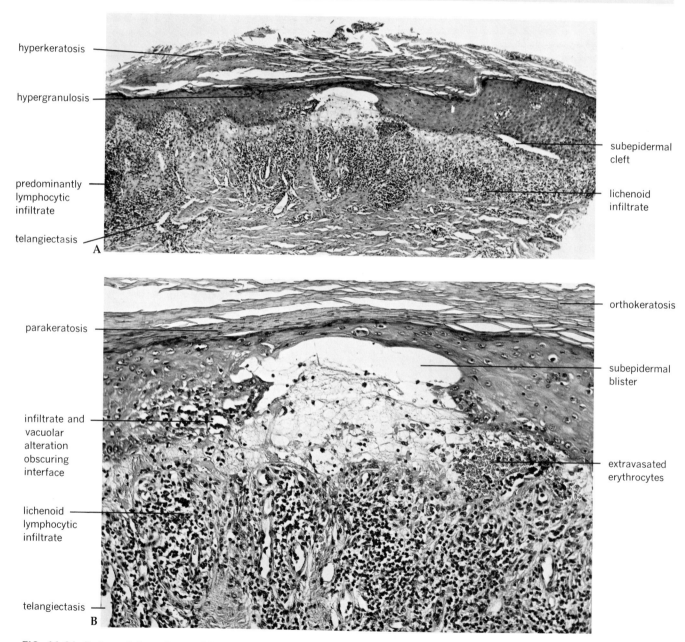

FIG. 11-24. Bullous lichen planus. Blister shown developed atop moderately well-developed papule of lichen planus as is told by dense bandlike infiltrate in thickened papillary dermis and by epidermal hyperplasia. (A, × 62; B, × 200.)

Lichen planus is a common dermatitis, yet the bullous form of the disease is singularly uncommon. Histologically, the blister is simply an exaggeration of the prominent vacuolar alteration that typically occurs in lichen planus. In some instances this vacuolar alteration gives rise to small clefts at the dermoepidermal junction. These clefts in association with numerous dyskeratotic cells are commonly seen in lichen planus. The clefts have been called Max Joseph spaces, and the dyskeratotic cells called Civatte bodies. Clefts occur not only in lesions of lichen planus but in lesions of other diseases with extensive vacuolar alteration of cells at the dermoepidermal junction, such as erythema multiforme and lichen sclerosus et atrophicus.

Although the blister of lichen planus may occur in association with the typical histologic features of lichen planus, it may also be accompanied by only a moderately dense superficial perivascular lymphohistiocytic infiltrate with no bandlike configuration and relatively little epidermal hyperplasia. In these instances, the blister probably occurs in relatively early lesions (Fig. 11-25) rather than in long-standing ones with fully developed histologic findings of lichen planus. Sometimes, however, subtle epidermal changes such as focal hypergranulosis suggestive of lichen planus

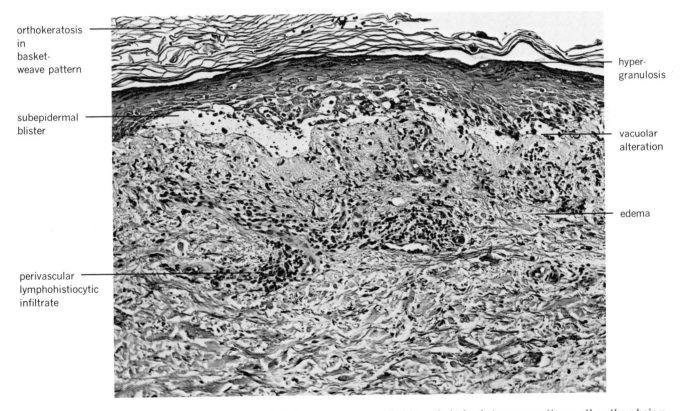

orthokeratosis in basket-weave pattern

hypergranulosis

subepidermal blister

vacuolar alteration

edema

perivascular lymphohistiocytic infiltrate

FIG. 11-25. Bullous lichen planus. This is an early lesion because cornified layer is in basket-weave pattern rather than being compact, epidermis shows but slight hypergranulosis and hyperplasia, and inflammatory-cell infiltrate is mostly perivascular rather than lichenoid. ($\times$ 200.)

occur at the sides of the blister (Fig. 11-26). Clinically, blisters with dense lichenoid infiltrates develop atop typical lesions of lichen planus, whereas those with sparse inflammatory-cell infiltrates arise on apparently normal skin.

A rare bullous variant of lichen planus is associated with ulcerative lesions in the mouth and on the feet, permanent loss of toenails, and scarring alopecia of the scalp. The ulcers on the soles are often disabling in "erosive" lichen planus.

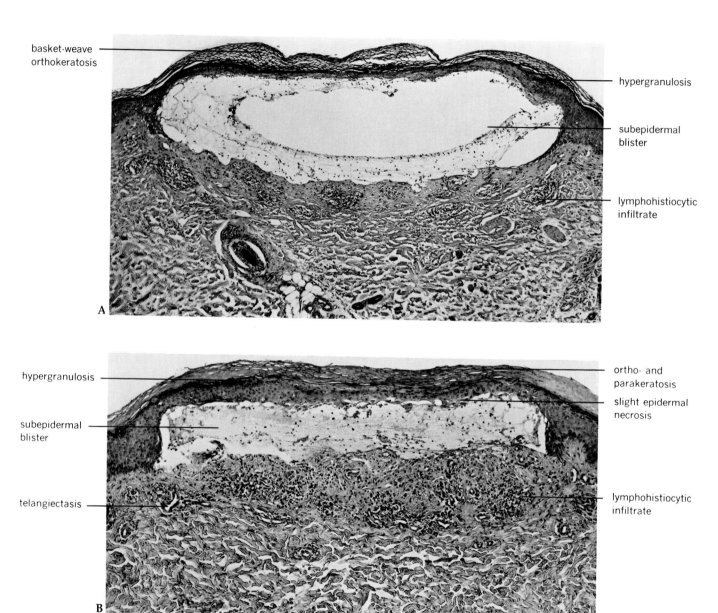

FIG. 11-26. Bullous lichen planus. A, Some lesions, such as the one pictured, erupt rapidly and not necessarily from a pre-existing papule and are characterized by superficial perivascular lymphohistiocytic infiltrates rather than bandlike infiltrates, subepidermal blisters that may contain some neutrophils, and partially necrotic epidermis. An important clue to correct diagnosis is presence of focal hypergranulosis. Note that cornified layer has a basket-weave configuration rather than compact one as is usually the case in long-standing lesions of lichen planus. (× 61.) B, Blister shown developed from early papule of lichen planus in which perivascular infiltrate had become slightly bandlike and cornified layer compact and hyperkeratotic. Focal hypergranulosis is an important hint that the condition is actually lichen planus. (× 92.)

—Subepidermal blister
—Severe edema of the papillary dermis
—Superficial and deep perivascular, predominantly lymphohistiocytic infiltrate
—Extravasated erythrocytes in the edematous papillary dermis

The histologic features of polymorphous light eruption are diagnostic when there is a moderately dense, predominantly lymphocytic infiltrate around both vascular plexuses associated with edema of the papillary dermis wherein there may be extravasated erythrocytes. In the early papular phase of polymorphous light eruption, the massive edema of the papillary dermis separates the collagen fibrils from one another so that they have a cobweblike quality. If enough fluid accumulates in the papillary dermis, the epidermis is entirely lifted from its connective tissue moorings, and a subepidermal blister results (Fig. 11-28). This is an unusual happening in polymorphous light eruption.

Polymorphous light eruption is differentiated histologically from discoid lupus erythematosus by the absence of thinned epidermis, vacuolar alteration, and a thickened basement membrane and by the presence of edema rather than mucin in the upper part of the dermis.

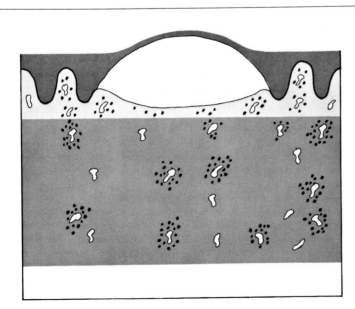

FIG. 11-27. Subepidermal blister with superficial and deep perivascular infiltrate.

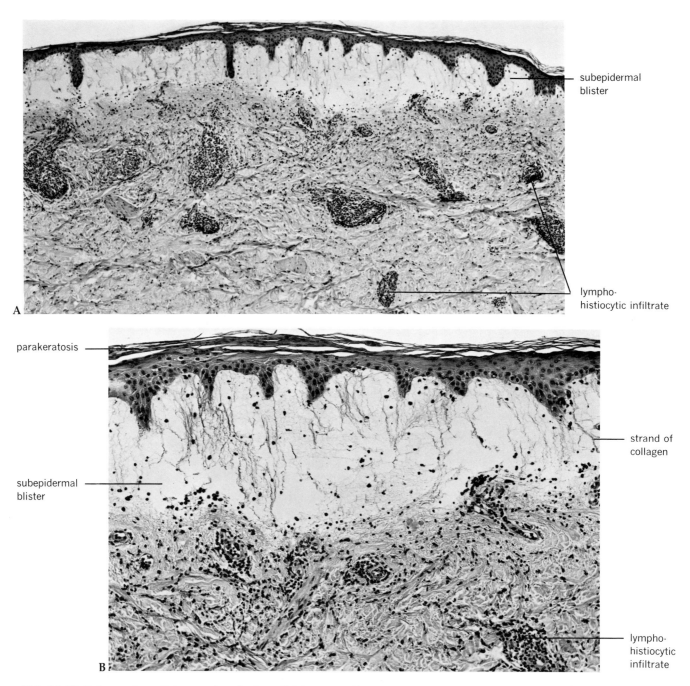

FIG. 11-28. Polymorphous light eruption. A, Superficial and deep perivascular predominantly lymphocytic infiltrate as pictured is common denominator for all lesions, and papillary dermis may have no to massive edema. Subepidermal blister formed as result of severe edema. (× 62.) B, In higher magnification transition between massive subepidermal edema and subepidermal vesiculation is distinguishable. As long as gossamer threads of collagen connect epidermis to dermis, lesion is considered to be edematous rather than vesicular. As soon as collagen ties are broken, as shown in some foci, lesion is considered to be vesicular. (× 178.)

Many different types of polymorphous light eruption, including "eczematous," purpuric, urticarial, and plaque have been described. In fact, polymorphous light eruption is one process, with a consistent histologic picture, that clinically shows edematous papules that may become confluent to form plaques. Vesicles develop rarely. Spongiosis is exceptional in my experience.

Eosinophils Prominent

Pemphigoid, Cell-rich Type (Fig. 11-29; Plate 6)

—Subepidermal blister containing eosinophils and neutrophils
—Well-preserved dermal papillae beneath the blister (Fig. 11-30)
—Edema of the papillary dermis
—Moderately dense lymphohistiocytic infiltrate with numerous eosinophils around the vessels of the superficial plexus and scattered throughout the papillary dermis. A few neutrophils may be present.

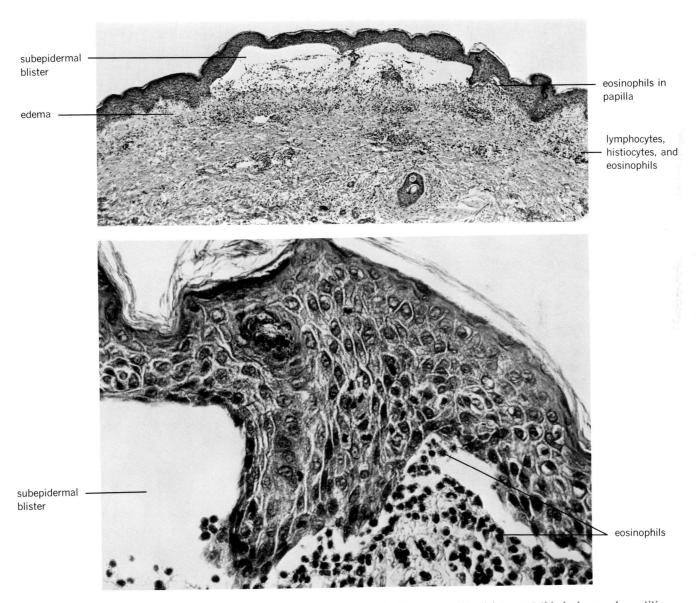

FIG. 11-29. Pemphigoid, cell-rich type. A, With scanning power magnification one could misinterpret this lesion as dermatitis herpetiformis. However, in that disease, papillary abscesses truly consist of neutrophils, whereas in this section abscesses are composed of eosinophils which almost always outnumber neutrophils. (× 58.) B, In this higher magnification an eosinophilic abscess typical of pemphigoid is present in dermal papilla and in subepidermal vesicle. (× 525.)

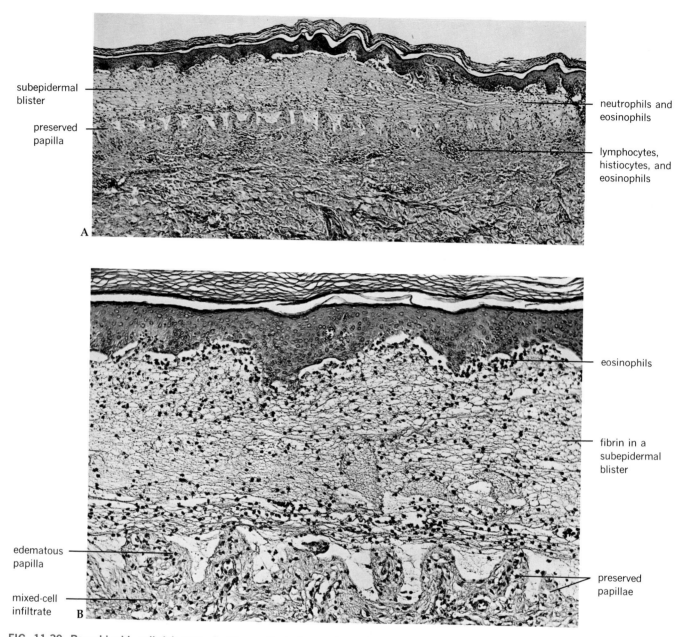

subepidermal blister

preserved papilla

neutrophils and eosinophils

lymphocytes, histiocytes, and eosinophils

eosinophils

fibrin in a subepidermal blister

edematous papilla

mixed-cell infiltrate

preserved papillae

A

B

FIG. 11-30. Pemphigoid, cell-rich type. A, Diagnostic features pictured are subepidermal vesiculation, preservation of dermal papillae, and perivascular and interstitial infiltrate replete with eosinophils. (× 45.) B, As illustrated in this higher magnification pemphigoid usually can be differentiated from dermatitis herpetiformis because there are more eosinophils than neutrophils within papillary dermis and blister and dermal papillae tend to line up like tombstones, an appearance sometimes referred to as festooning. (× 169.)

The eosinophil is the most important cell for the histologic diagnosis of the cell-rich type of pemphigoid. Eosinophils are usually numerous in pemphigoid, and in their absence the diagnosis is made with difficulty. Even in the early papular and plaque stages of pemphigoid, eosinophils are numerous within the papillary dermis (Fig. 11-31) and can be scattered within the epidermis, sometimes in spongiotic foci. Although neutrophils may also be present within the dermis of the cell-rich type of pemphigoid, they are almost always less numerous than the eosinophils and are located predominantly in the blister fluid rather than within the dermis. Pemphigoid is partly differentiated histologically from dermatitis herpetiformis by the large numbers of eosinophils, rather than neutrophils, in the papillary dermis. Eosinophils may be seen in the papillae and subepidermal blisters of dermatitis herpetiformis, but almost always, except in old lesions, they are outnumbered by neutrophils.

Pemphigoid, both cell-poor and cell-rich types, is a disease of older people. Its early lesions are urticarial papules and plaques with varied shapes, some arcuate, others annular, some serpiginous and others gyrate. In some patients, urticarial lesions may be the only manifestation of the disease; thus the term pemphigoid is more apt than is bullous pemphigoid. The urticarial stage of pemphigoid may be misinterpreted clinically as erythema multiforme. In pemphigoid, however, the lesions are usually not purpuric as they are in erythema multiforme, and, if annular, they do not consist of concentric rings. The blisters of pemphigoid vary from small tense vesicles to massive bullae and usually arise on preexisting papules and plaques. Usually the mucous membranes are not involved. Furthermore, pemphigoid does not favor the acral regions, as does erythema multiforme. Rarely can the lesions of pemphigoid be localized to one region of the body.

Antibodies to the basement-membrane zone can be demonstrated by both direct and indirect immunofluorescence in pemphigoid, but not in erythema multiforme.

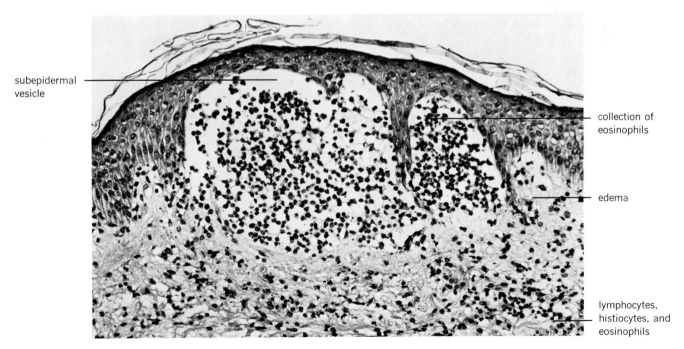

subepidermal vesicle

collection of eosinophils

edema

lymphocytes, histiocytes, and eosinophils

FIG. 11-31. Pemphigoid, cell-rich type. Many eosinophils may be seen in papillae and in subepidermal vesicles. Such features are not to be confused with those of dermatitis herpetiformis in which neutrophils collect in papillae and vesicles. ($\times$ 232.)

Herpes Gestationis (Fig. 11-32)

—Subepidermal blister
—Occasional spongiotic intraepidermal vesicles
—Necrotic keratinocytes in the basal-cell zone
—Vacuolar alteration at the dermoepidermal junction
—Edema of the papillary dermis forming teardrop-shaped papillae
—Superficial and sometimes deep perivascular lymphohistiocytic infiltrate with numerous eosinophils and rare neutrophils
—Eosinophilic "abscesses" at summits of dermal papillae

Herpes gestationis is an intensely pruritic disease that may begin at any time during pregnancy, but usually develops during the second trimester. It resolves spontaneously postpartum and almost always recurs in subsequent pregnancies. The vesiculo-bullous lesions of herpes gestationis rarely develop in newborns of affected mothers. The disease in these infants is similar clinically, histologically, and immunologically to that in adults. The lesions regress in a few weeks after birth and do not recur.

Clinically and histologically, herpes gestationis resembles pemphigoid. There are widespread erythematous, edematous papules and plaques, some surmounted by vesicles and bullae. Herpes gestationis differs from pemphigoid clinically by its rings of tense vesicles that extend at the periphery and heal in the center. Herpes gestationis may be a variant of pemphigoid in pregnancy.

Histologically, the urticarial lesions of herpes gestationis are characterized by a moderately dense, perivascular, mixed inflammatory-cell infiltrate of lymphocytes, histiocytes, and eosinophils around the vessels of the superficial (and sometimes the deep) dermal plexus, papillary dermal edema, spongiosis, and focal necrosis of the basal cells over the tips of the dermal papillae. Eosinophils may be found within the epidermis, particularly in spongiotic foci. In some instances, neutrophils are present in the infiltrate, but only in small numbers. Severe edema of the papillary dermis can result in bulbous, teardrop-shaped dermal papillae (Fig. 11-32). Sections cut to the side of these papillae can give the illusion of intraepidermal vesicles. This possible misinterpretation can be avoided by the examination of serial sections that reveal subepidermal edema and vesiculation. The tendency to form teardrop-shaped edematous dermal papillae containing eosinophilic "abscesses" beneath necrotic basal keratinocytes is greater in herpes gestationis than in pemphigoid.

Direct immunofluorescence of lesions of herpes gestationis reveals the third component of complement to be deposited at the dermoepidermal junction in a linear pattern, sometimes in association with C1q, properdin, and IgG. Indirect immunofluorescence has usually been negative for antibodies in the basement membrane in herpes gestationis, but complement-binding factor and circulating IgG have been demonstrated.

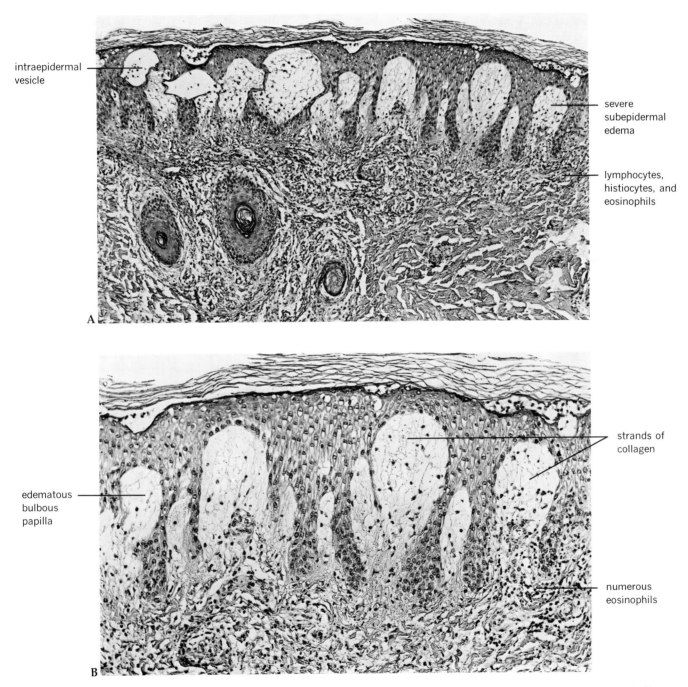

FIG. 11-32. Herpes gestationis. A, The blister results primarily from intense edema of papillary dermis as illustrated. Note bulbous (teardrop) shape of edematous papillae. Concurrent intraepidermal vesicles may also form as shown. Eosinophils are a constant histologic feature of this disease. ($\times$ 92.) B, Note gossamer strands of collagen still connected to epidermis, an indication that this is severe edema rather than subepidermal vesiculation. Changes pictured closely resemble those of early urticarial lesions of pemphigoid in which there are also many eosinophils in infiltrate in addition to edema of papillary dermis. ($\times$ 175.)

Reactions to Arthropods (Fig. 11-33)

The tense vesicle that results from a reaction to an insect bite is usually intraepidermal, but sometimes there is such severe subepidermal edema that a subepidermal vesicle also develops. Eosinophils are typically scattered among collagen bundles throughout the dermis and, occasionally, in the subcutaneous fat.

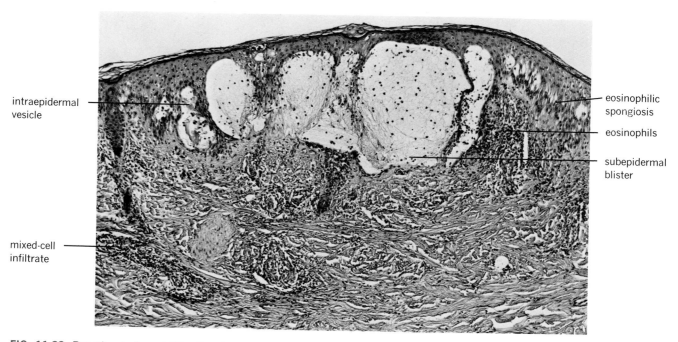

FIG. 11-33. Reaction to insect bite. Developing subepidermal blister pictured resulted from confluence of fluid of spongiosis and contents of tense intraepidermal vesicles. A clue to diagnosis of reaction to arthropod assault is presence of eosinophils in perivascular and interstitial inflammatory-cell infiltrate. (× 96.)

Neutrophils Prominent

Dermatitis Herpetiformis (Fig. 11-34; Plate 6)

—Subepidermal blister
—Neutrophils, band forms, and nuclear dust at the tips of the dermal papillae
—Basophilia of the collagen in the dermal papillae
—Edema of the papillary dermis
—Superficial perivascular lymphohistiocytic infiltrate with neutrophils
—Eosinophils within the papillary dermis of later lesions
—Fibrin, often, in the subepidermal space
—Rarely acantholytic keratinocytes singly and in groups at the base of the epidermis
—Necrotic basal cells often

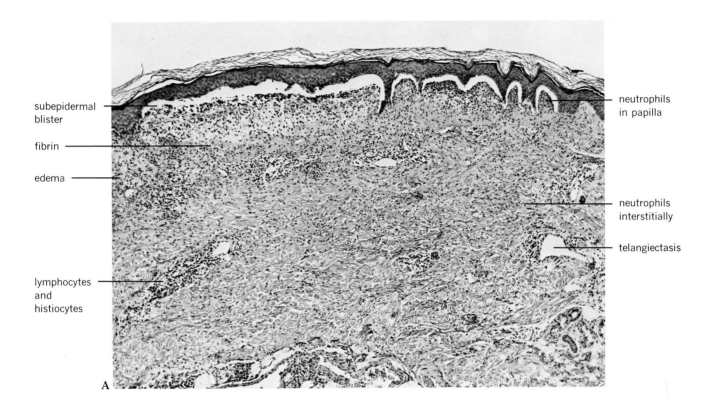

subepidermal
blister

fibrin

edema

lymphocytes
and
histiocytes

neutrophils
in papilla

neutrophils
interstitially

telangiectasis

A

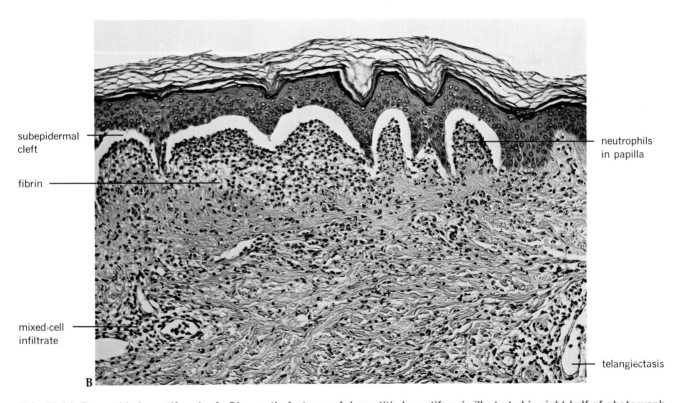

subepidermal
cleft

fibrin

mixed-cell
infiltrate

neutrophils
in papilla

telangiectasis

B

FIG. 11-34. Dermatitis herpetiformis. A, Diagnostic features of dermatitis herpetiformis illustrated in right half of photograph are numerous neutrophils at tips of dermal papillae. Subepidermal blister on left is not in itself diagnostic of dermatitis herpetiformis. The blister and changes in adjacent papillae are diagnostic. (× 80.) B, Higher magnification shows diagnostic features to better advantage, namely, many neutrophils within tips of dermal papillae and within early subepidermal vesicle where fibrin has formed. (× 197.)

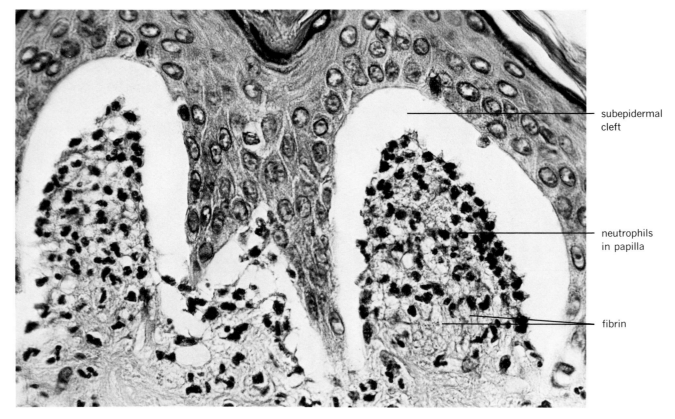

FIG. 11-34. Dermatitis herpetiformis. C, Still higher magnification shows neutrophils, nuclear debris, and occasional neutrophil band forms, as well as fibrin within elongated dermal papillae and subepidermal clefts. Collagen in vicinity of these papillae has basophilic hue in sections stained by hematoxylin and eosin. (× 676.)

The critical cell for the diagnosis of dermatitis herpetiformis is the neutrophil (Fig. 11-35) just as the eosinophil is the critical cell for the diagnosis of cell-rich pemphigoid. Eosinophils are late arrivals on the inflammatory-cell scene of dermatitis herpetiformis, usually appearing 24 to 48 hours after the appearance of neutrophils. Thus, the diagnostic change in dermatitis herpetiformis is the presence of neutrophilic abscesses at the tips of the dermal papillae associated with elongated nuclear forms (presumably bands), nuclear dust, and basophilia of the collagen in the papillary dermis (Fig. 11-36). The papillary abscesses often occur at the sides of the blister rather than beneath it (Fig. 11-37).

It is difficult to root out fictions in dermatopathology and elsewhere. For decades, and even now, it was written in standard textbooks that eosinophils, rather than neutrophils, are the telling cells for the diagnosis of dermatitis herpetiformis, that erythema multiforme is either a dermal or epidermal disease rather than being both dermal and epidermal, and that pityriasis lichenoides et varioliformis acuta is a vasculitis rather than a superficial and deep perivascular dermatitis. The reader is encouraged to look critically at these pages and at histologic sections and come to his own conclusions.

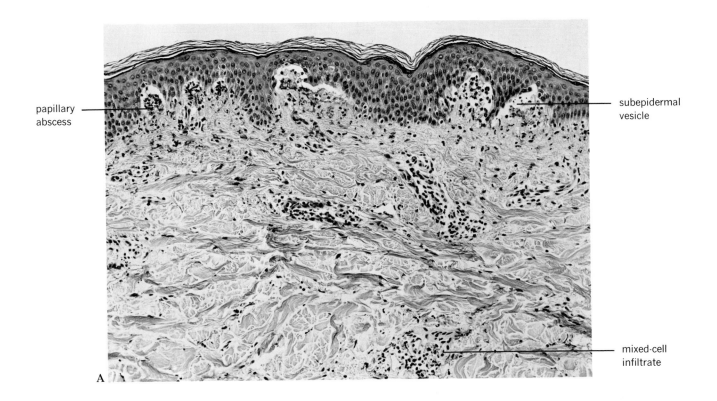

papillary
abscess

subepidermal
vesicle

mixed-cell
infiltrate

A

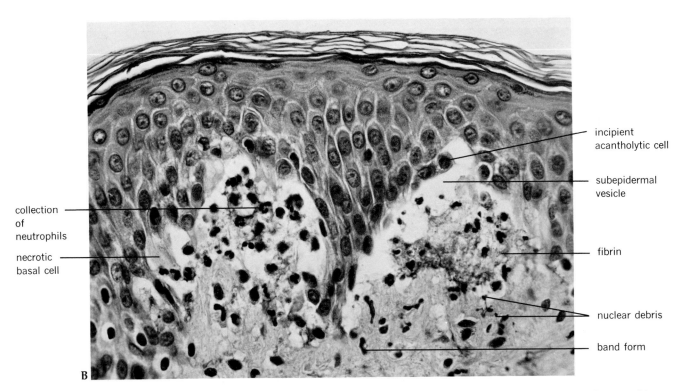

incipient
acantholytic cell

subepidermal
vesicle

collection
of
neutrophils

fibrin

necrotic
basal cell

nuclear debris

band form

B

FIG. 11-35. Dermatitis herpetiformis. A, Early changes shown include superficial and middermal perivascular infiltrate of lymphocytes, histiocytes, and neutrophils as well as variably sized collections of neutrophils within edematous dermal papillae and in subepidermal clefts or vesicles. (× 197.) B, Critical features for histologic diagnosis are pictured: neutrophils, band forms, and nuclear debris at tips of dermal papillae and in subepidermal space. Acantholytic epidermal cells and fibrin are also frequently present in the vesicle. (× 705.)

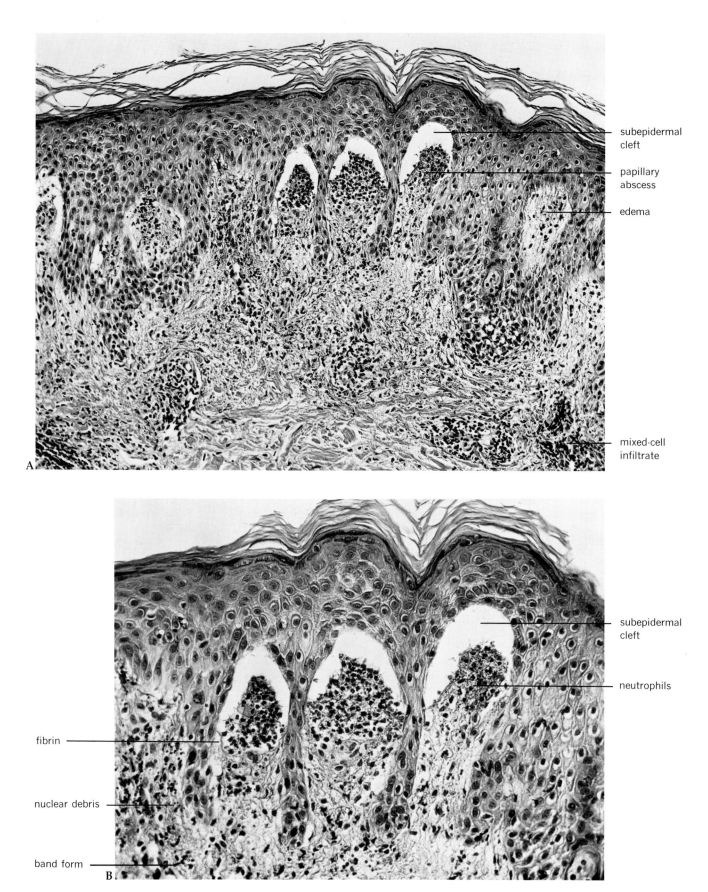

subepidermal
cleft

papillary
abscess

edema

mixed-cell
infiltrate

subepidermal
cleft

neutrophils

fibrin

nuclear debris

band form

FIG. 11-36. Dermatitis herpetiformis. Neutrophils are present in varying numbers in every papillae pictured in this specimen. There are also nuclear debris, neutrophilic bands, fibrin, basophilia of the collagen, and edema. (A, × 180; B, × 340.)

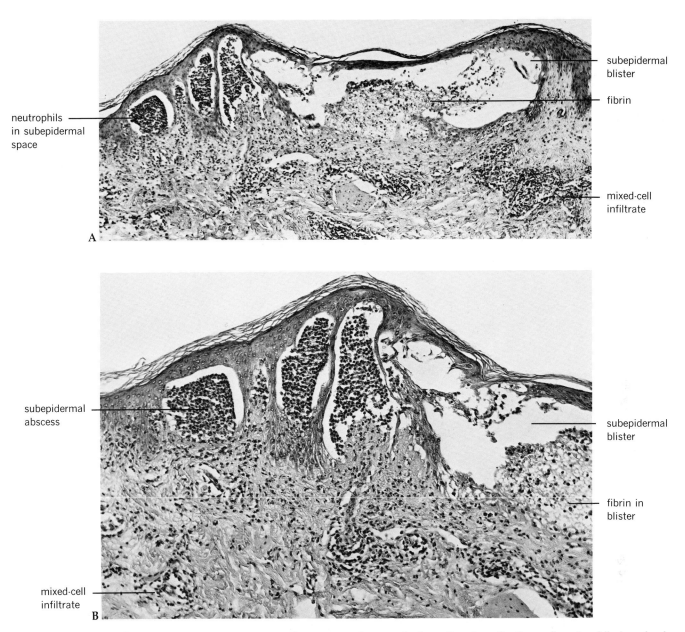

neutrophils in subepidermal space

subepidermal blister

fibrin

mixed-cell infiltrate

A

subepidermal abscess

subepidermal blister

fibrin in blister

mixed-cell infiltrate

B

FIG. 11-37. Dermatitis herpetiformis. A, Diagnostic features can be seen in four discrete collections of neutrophils in subepidermal spaces and dermal papillae to left of subepidermal blister. These crucial changes are usually found beside the blister rather than beneath it. ($\times$ 100.) B, Abscess in middle appears to be intraepidermal, but that is an illusion caused by tangential sectioning through subepidermal space. ($\times$ 176.)

Dermatitis herpetiformis is one subepidermal vesicular disease in which acantholysis sometimes occurs (Fig. 11-38). Acantholysis is almost always associated with intraepidermal vesicle and pustule formation like that occurring in superficial and deep forms of pemphigus, benign familial chronic pemphigus (Hailey-Hailey disease) and the subcorneal pustular dermatitides. In dermatitis herpetiformis, acantholytic epidermal cells can be found immediately above papillary abscesses. Also, very rarely, abscesses form within the epidermis, as well as in the dermal papillae of dermatitis herpetiformis (Fig. 11-39).

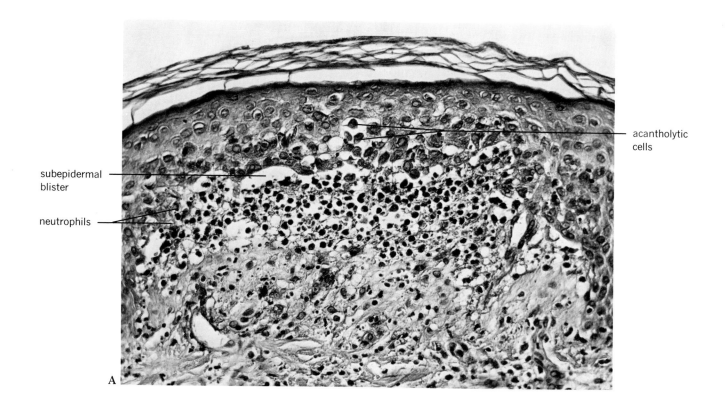

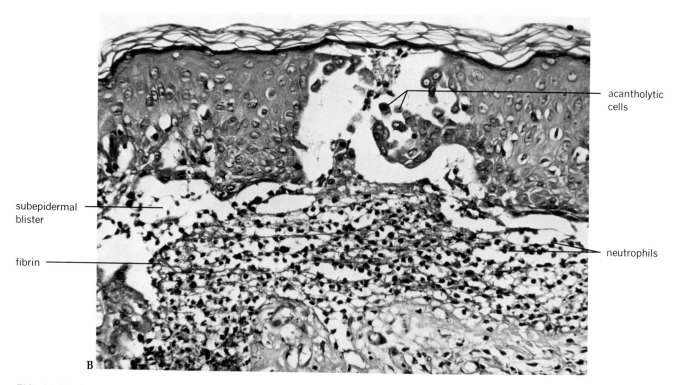

FIG. 11-38. **Dermatitis herpetiformis.** Several acantholytic cells may be seen in epidermis above subepidermal collections of neutrophils in these sections. Release of lysosomal enzymes by numerous neutrophils beneath epidermis is probably responsible for induction of acantholysis. (A, × 405; B, × 405.)

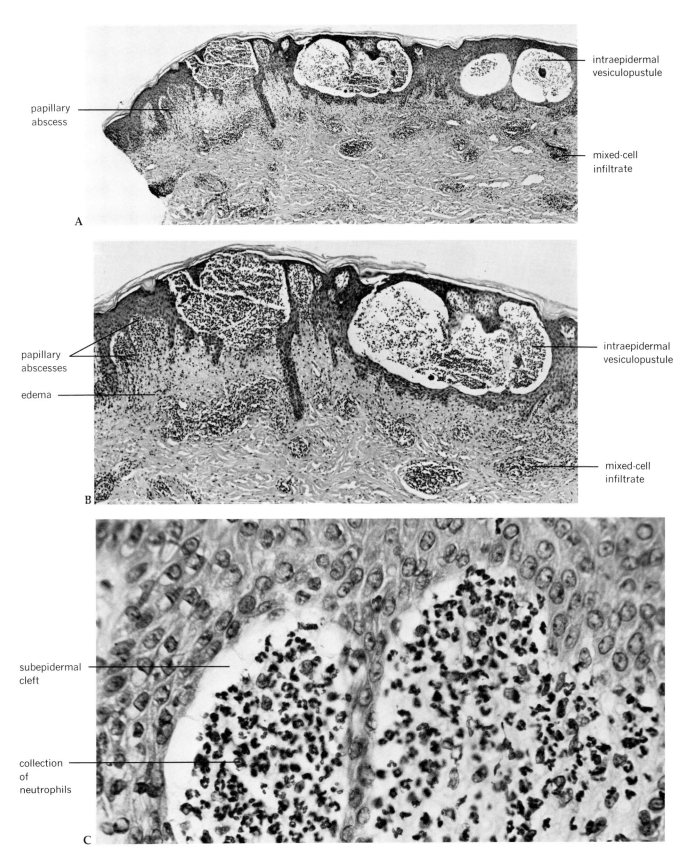

FIG. 11-39. Dermatitis herpetiformis. At first glance with scanning power magnification, this appears to be an intraepidermal vesiculopustular dermatitis. More careful scrutiny, however, even with this low magnification, reveals dermal papillae on left replete with neutrophils, a sign of dermatitis herpetiformis. Intraepidermal changes pictured are unusual and rare. Dermatitis herpetiformis is usually characterized by subepidermal vesiculation only. (A, × 47; B, × 92; C, × 574.)

Dermatitis herpetiformis usually develops in young adults but may occur in children and in middle-aged people. It is very rare in black people. The clinical lesions are urticarial papules, papulo-vesicles, and vesicles usually arranged symmetrically on the scapulae, sacrum, and extensor surfaces of the arms and legs. The scalp is commonly involved, but the mucous membranes rarely. The lesions are pruritic, and erosions and ulcerations are therefore common clinical features. Sometimes it is difficult to find undisturbed papules and vesicles because they have been scratched. In exceptional instances, dermatitis herpetiformis may be wholly urticarial or bullous, rather than papular and vesicular. The histologic changes in the papillary dermis in all lesions of dermatitis herpetiformis—papules, vesicles, and bullae—are similar.

Approximately two thirds of all patients with dermatitis herpetiformis have an associated abnormality of the small intestine that resembles that of celiac disease or of sprue. Histologically, the villi are flattened but return to normal when a gluten-free diet is practiced. In most instances, however, the skin lesions of dermatitis herpetiformis respond slowly, if at all, to a gluten-free diet.

Direct immunofluorescent studies in dermatitis herpetiformis show deposits of IgA, properdin, and the third component of complement at the tips of the dermal papillae contiguous to the lesions. Indirect immunofluorescent tests are negative.

Dermatitis Herpetiformis-like Drug Eruption (Fig. 11-40)

The term *dermatitis herpetiformis-like* in this context refers to the histologic appearance, rather than to the clinical features, of this bullous drug eruption. Clinically, it does not resemble dermatitis herpetiformis at all. It consists of bullae rather than vesicles. Moreover the bullae are randomly distributed rather than herpetiform and do not have a decided predilection for the scalp, scapulae, sacrum, and extensor surfaces of the extremities.

Histologically, there are innumerable neutrophils in the dermal papillae, the collagen of which stains basophilically with hematoxylin and eosin. Above the neutrophil-laden dermal papillae, large subepidermal blisters form. One clue to the recognition of the dermatitis herpetiformis-like drug eruption, as contrasted with true dermatitis herpetiformis, is the tendency in the drug eruption of the neutrophils to fill many contiguous papillae diffusely, whereas in idiopathic dermatitis herpetiformis, fewer contiguous papillae, and even isolated papillae, tend to be involved. Drugs are capable of inducing various inflammatory reactions in the skin, among them the changes of dermatitis herpetiformis.

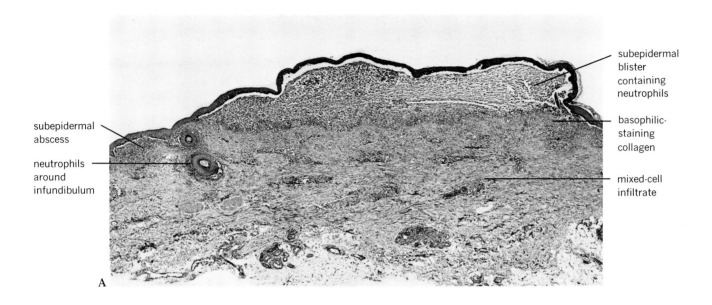

subepidermal
blister
containing
neutrophils

basophilic-
staining
collagen

subepidermal
abscess

neutrophils
around
infundibulum

mixed-cell
infiltrate

A

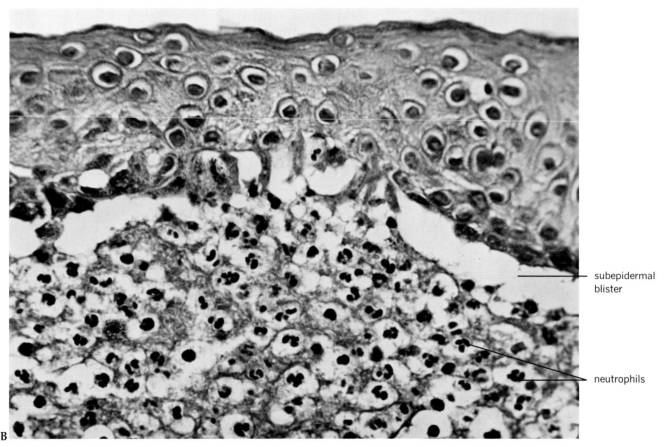

subepidermal
blister

neutrophils

B

FIG. 11-40. Dermatitis herpetiformis-like drug eruption. Histologic changes shown are indistinguishable from those of dermatitis herpetiformis. Clinically the patient did not have lesions of dermatitis herpetiformis but had large bullae, especially in intertriginous regions, and severe blistering of mucous membranes. The patient was taking many medications, and when they were stopped the eruption gradually resolved. One helpful hint that the histologic features are not those of authentic dermatitis herpetiformis is absence of scattered neutrophils or abscesses of them in dermal papillae to sides of large blister. (A, × 35; B, × 842.)

Bullous Disease of Childhood (Fig. 11-41)

—Subepidermal blister
—Neutrophils scattered in the papillary dermis
—Superficial perivascular lymphohistiocytic infiltrate with neutrophils
  and rare eosinophils

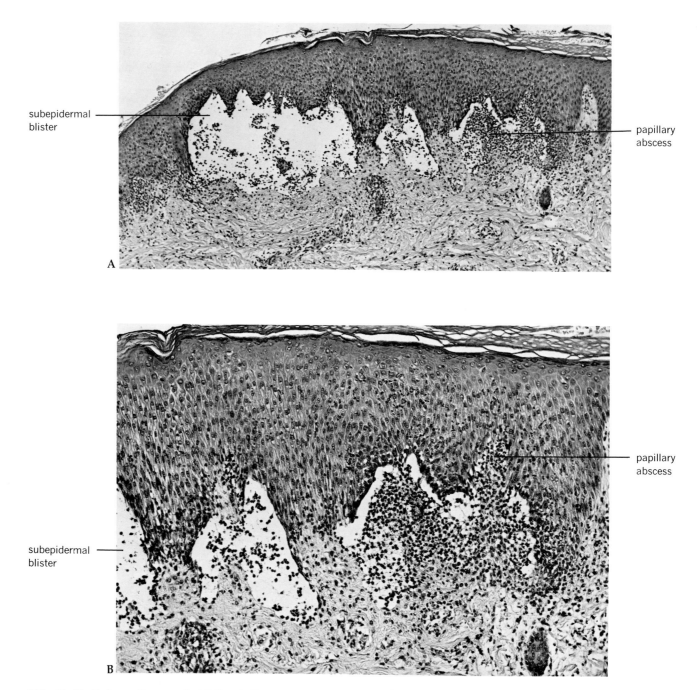

FIG. 11-41. Bullous disease of childhood. Note close resemblance to dermatitis herpetiformis. Blister is subepidermal and numerous neutrophils have collected at tips of dermal papillae and in vesicles above them. (A, × 84; B, × 174.)

Histologically, bullous disease of childhood more closely resembles dermatitis herpetiformis than it does any other blistering disease. Clinically, however, this bullous disease of preschool children is quite distinctive, consisting predominantly of bullae with relatively few urticarial lesions. The large, tense, clear blisters often assume arcuate and annular shapes and tend to involve the genital region, extremities, and trunk, although the face and scalp may also be affected. There is no clinical resemblance to typical dermatitis herpetiformis.

Direct immunofluorescence of sections from the lesions of bullous disease of childhood, from the skin adjacent to the lesions, and from uninvolved skin demonstrates linear deposition of IgA, IgG, and C3 at the dermoepidermal junction. No circulating antibodies to skin components have yet been detected.

Whether bullous disease of childhood is a distinct pathologic process or a variant of dermatitis herpetiformis has not yet been determined. Many chronic vesiculobullous diseases that are usually found in adults also occur in children, such as dermatitis herpetiformis, pemphigoid, and pemphigus. On the other hand, diseases such as syphilis that have no vesicles or bullae when they occur in adults may be blistering in infants.

Bullous Systemic Lupus Erythematosus (Fig. 11-42)

—Subepidermal blister
—LE cells and hematoxylin bodies in the blister fluid sometimes
—Neutrophils and nuclear dust at the tips of the dermal papillae
—Superficial or superficial and deep perivascular lymphohistiocytic infiltrate with neutrophils
—Abundant mucin among collagen bundles, especially in the upper half of the dermis

Bullous systemic lupus erythematosus, an uncommon phenomenon, is sometimes difficult to differentiate histologically from dermatitis herpetiformis, especially in the early papular lesions. The blisters in both diseases are subepidermal and are associated with neutrophilic abscesses in the papillary dermis. Features helpful in distinguishing bullous systemic lupus erythematosus from dermatitis herpetiformis are the superficial and deep perivascular infiltrations and abundant mucin in the dermis of lupus erythematosus. The deposition of mucin is probably the single most important distinguishing feature. Clinically, the lesions of bullous systemic lupus erythematosus usually occur on the exposed parts of the face, chest, back, and hands. A thoroughly

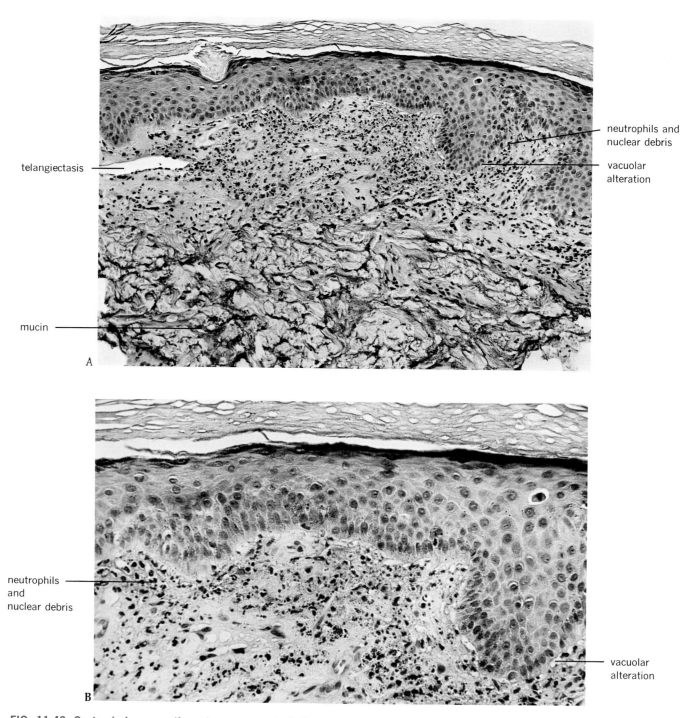

telangiectasis

mucin

A

neutrophils and
nuclear debris

vacuolar
alteration

neutrophils
and
nuclear debris

vacuolar
alteration

B

FIG. 11-42. Systemic lupus erythematosus, an early bullous lesion. A, Note resemblance of blisters to those of dermatitis herpetiformis because of numerous neutrophils and abundant nuclear debris in papillary dermis. A clue critical to correct diagnosis is puddles of mucin throughout dermis as shown here. (× 200.) B, Higher magnification illustrates better the vacuolar alteration at dermoepidermal junction that progresses to dermoepidermal separation and finally subepidermal vesiculation. (× 467.)

unusual presentation is bullae appearing on preexisting lesions of discoid lupus erythematosus (Fig. 11-43). In addition to the characteristic histologic features of discoid lupus erythematosus, there is an infiltrate of neutrophils in the papillary dermis with a subepidermal blister above. Histologic study of lesions of discoid lupus erythematosus gives no clue to whether the patient has internal-organ disease, i.e., systemic lupus erythematosus. By contrast, bullous lesions of lupus erythematosus that histologically simulate dermatitis herpetiformis show a high correlation with visceral involvement.

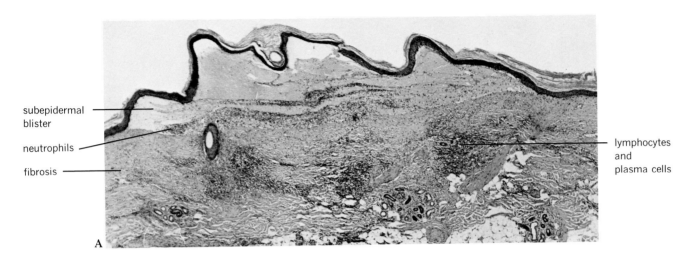

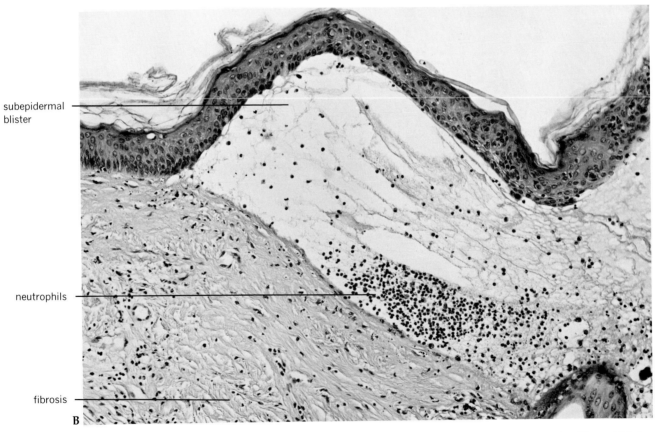

FIG. 11-43. Bullous systemic lupus erythematosus. The feature pictured that suggests the diagnosis is a subepidermal blister containing neutrophils. An unusual happenstance in this specimen is superimposition of bullous changes upon those of chronic discoid lupus erythematosus identified by dense superficial and deep perivascular infiltrate of lymphocytes, histiocytes, and plasma cells coupled with fibrosis in upper part of dermis. Clinically, patient had systemic lupus erythematosus together with widespread lesions of discoid lupus erythematosus and a few bullae atop discoid plaques. (A, × 37; B, × 180.)

Leukocytoclastic Vasculitis and Septic Vasculitis (Fig. 11-44)

—Subepidermal blister
—Occasionally, intraepidermal vesiculation
—Some epidermal necrosis
—Dense infiltrate of neutrophils in the papillary dermis, often with prominent nuclear dust
—Superficial and deep infiltrate of neutrophils, nuclear dust, eosinophils (in leukocytoclastic vasculitis), and some lymphocytes and histiocytes, within and around blood-vessel walls
—Fibrin in blood-vessel walls of the superficial and/or deep plexuses in leukocytoclastic vasculitis; thrombi in lumina of septic vasculitis

Vesicular leukocytoclastic vasculitis and septic vasculitis must be differentiated histologically from dermatitis herpetiformis and bullous systemic lupus erythematosus, each of which may have a dense infiltrate of neutrophils within the papillary dermis. The significant histologic features of leukocytoclastic vasculitis and septic vasculitis that distinguish them from dermatitis herpetiformis and systemic lupus erythematosus are neutrophils and fibrin in the walls of dermal capillaries and venules in leukocytoclastic vasculitis and thrombi in septic vasculitis. Leukocytoclastic

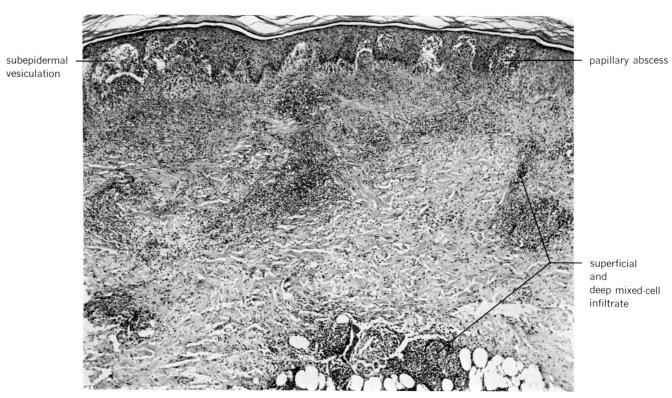

subepidermal vesiculation

papillary abscess

superficial and deep mixed-cell infiltrate

FIG. 11-44. Cutaneous changes in gonococcemia. A, Collections of neutrophils in dermal papillae simulate those of dermatitis herpetiformis. Septic vasculitis can usually be differentiated from dermatitis herpetiformis by presence of thrombi within small dermal blood vessels and from leukocytoclastic vasculitis by absence of fibrin within walls of dermal blood vessels. (× 59.)

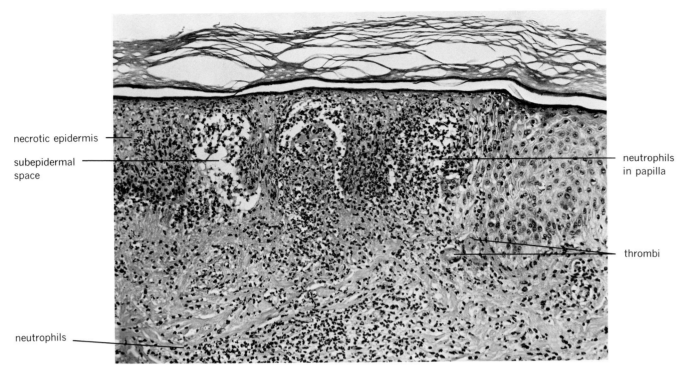

necrotic epidermis

subepidermal space

neutrophils

neutrophils in papilla

thrombi

FIG. 11-44. Cutaneous changes in gonococcemia. B, Thrombi, numerous neutrophils within epidermis and dermis, and prominent epidermal necrosis are diagnostic clues. Blisters in vasculitis may be either intradermal or subepidermal, and sometimes both varieties occur. (× 185.)

vasculitis may, however, occur as one manifestation of systemic lupus erythematosus.

Clinically, leukocytoclastic vasculitis is usually associated with urticarial papules that soon become purpuric. Early lesions of septic vasculitis are generally petechiae, ecchymoses, and vesiculopustules. When vesicles and bullae occur in leukocytoclastic and septic vasculitis, they are also usually purpuric.

Cicatricial Pemphigoid (Fig. 11-45)

—Subepithelial blister
—Neutrophils in the papillary dermis and lamina propria, as well as in the blister fluid
—Superficial perivascular lymphohistiocytic infiltrate with neutrophils and rare eosinophils

Neutrophils are prominent in the subepithelial blistering process known as cicatricial pemphigoid. It predominantly affects mucous membranes, but can also involve the skin. The lesions often heal with scarring. A serious consequence of conjunctival scarring is blindness. The title *benign mucous membrane pemphigoid*

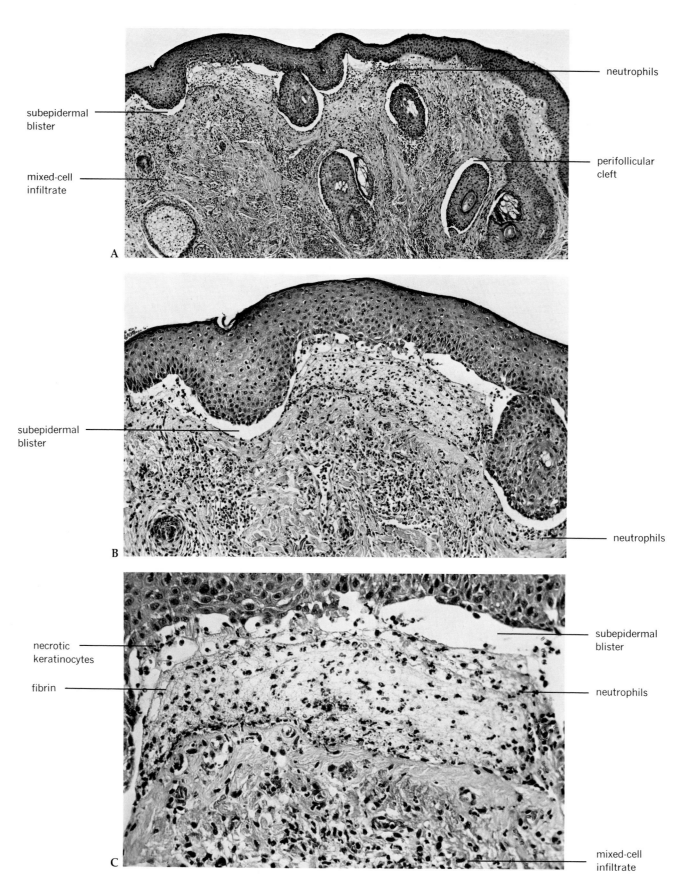

FIG. 11-45. Cicatricial pemphigoid. The subepidermal blister may extend down along epithelial structures of adnexa, such as of hair follicles pictured here in tangential sections. Infiltrate in papillary dermis invariably consists mostly of neutrophils, unlike that of pemphigoid in which eosinophils usually predominate. (A, × 76; B, × 170; C, × 340.)

does not convey the devastating consequences of the mucosal changes; furthermore, because both skin and mucous membrane are affected, the title should not simply be mucous membrane pemphigoid. A more accurate designation for the disease is scarring pemphigoid or cicatricial pemphigoid.

Because of immunofluorescent data that indicate similarities between cicatricial pemphigoid and pemphigoid, it has been argued that these two diseases are really one pathologic process. Clinically and histologically, however, there are notable differences between them. Pemphigoid usually does not involve mucous membranes, whereas cicatricial pemphigoid usually does. Pemphigoid practically never scars, whereas cicatricial pemphigoid often does. Histologically, eosinophils are the dominant cells in pemphigoid, especially of the cell-rich type, whereas neutrophils are the dominant cells in cicatricial pemphigoid. For these reasons, it is premature to conclude that cicatricial pemphigoid is simply a variant of pemphigoid. The histologic features of bullous disease of the scalp are indistinguishable from those of cicatricial pemphigoid.

Pemphigoid, Rarely

—Subepidermal blister
—Neutrophils scattered in the papillary dermis
—Lymphohistiocytic infiltrate with neutrophils around the vessels of the superficial plexus
—Edema of the papillary dermis

Eosinophils, rather than neutrophils, are usually the most prominent cells in pemphigoid. In exceptional instances of pemphigoid proven by immunofluorescence, neutrophils may be more numerous than eosinophils. The neutrophils are found scattered throughout the papillary dermis and grouped at the tips of the dermal papillae. The composite histologic picture in these cases of pemphigoid may be indistinguishable from that of dermatitis herpetiformis.

Although the predominance of neutrophils over eosinophils in pemphigoid is exceptional, other exceptional findings also occur now and then in other vesiculobullous diseases. For example, an inflammatory-cell infiltrate may actually be present in epidermolysis bullosa, the blister in erythema multiforme may be wholly intraepidermal, and epithelial structures of adnexa may be affected by the acantholytic process in benign familial chronic pemphigus.

Urticarial Vesiculobullous Allergic Eruption (Fig. 11-46)

—Subepidermal blister
—Edema of the papillary dermis
—Superficial and mid-dermal perivascular mixed cell infiltrate of neutrophils and eosinophils, as well as lymphocytes, histiocytes, and mast cells
—Extravasated erythrocytes often

The urticarial vesiculobullous reaction is an exaggeration of the urticarial allergic eruption that usually develops secondary to drug ingestion or injection. Urticarial allergic eruptions are common; the vesiculobullous variant is rare. Because the urticarial component is often annular, this condition is frequently misdiagnosed clinically as erythema multiforme. The urticarial allergic eruption (nonvesicular and vesicular types) is differentiated clinically from erythema multiforme by absence of mucous membrane lesions and of true iris and target lesions (concentric rings). Histologically, urticarial allergic eruptions, unlike erythema multiforme, have neutrophils and eosinophils and lack necrotic keratinocytes within the epidermis.

The blister in urticarial allergic eruption develops secondary to severe edema of the papillary dermis. Curiously, despite edema of

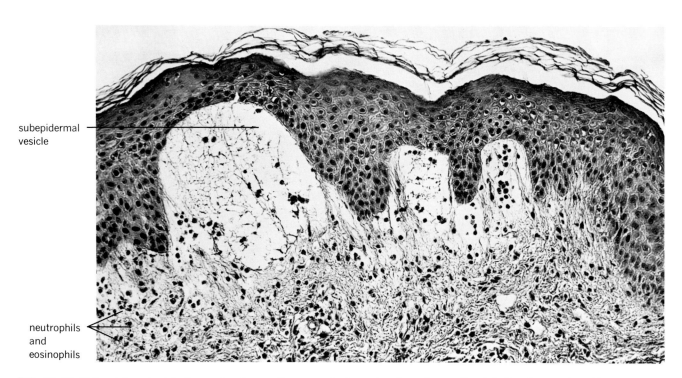

FIG. 11-46. Urticarial vesiculobullous allergic eruption, a vesicular extension of an urticarial allergic eruption. Mixed inflammatory-cell infiltrate contains many neutrophils and eosinophils that are distributed interstitially as well as perivascularly. Intense edema in dermal papillae has progressed to subepidermal vesiculation. (× 209.)

the papillary dermis, actual subepidermal vesiculation occurs rarely in urticarial allergic eruptions. However, massive edema of the papillary dermis inevitably leads to subepidermal vesiculation such as in polymorphous light eruption and erysipelas.

Erysipelas (Fig. 11-47)

—Subepidermal blister, often containing erythrocytes
—Edema of the papillary dermis
—Sparse, predominantly neutrophilic, infiltrate around the vessels of the superficial and deep vascular plexuses and among collagen bundles

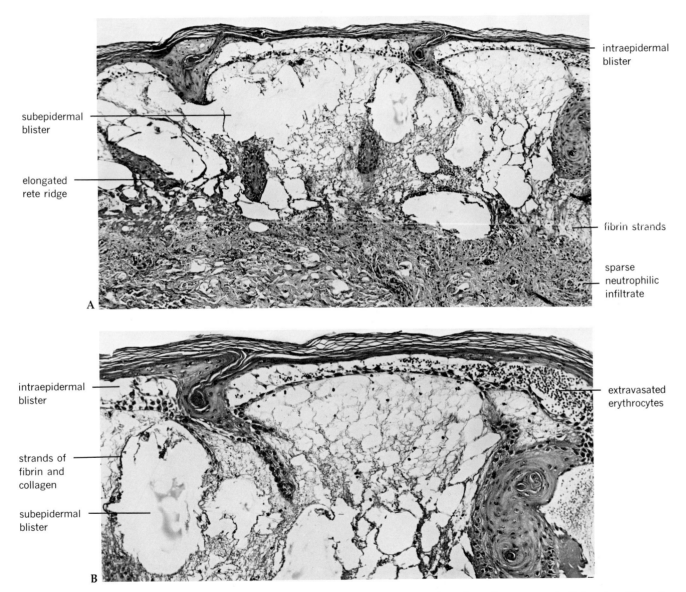

FIG. 11-47. Erysipelas. Blisters are in main subepidermal and secondary to massive edema in upper part of dermis, although concomitant intraepidermal vesiculation may also occur as pictured. Rete ridges remain in contact with dermis despite extensive edema, infiltrate of neutrophils is sparse, and extravasated erythrocytes are numerous. (A, × 80; B, × 175.)

The essential histologic features of erysipelas are those of a phlegmonous dermatitis, in which neutrophils are present around the vessels of both plexuses and among collagen bundles. The tense plaques of erysipelas result from massive edema of the papillary dermis that may progress to true blister formation. Before such subepidermal vesiculation occurs, the epidermal retia are almost completely detached from the papillary dermis by edema so that they appear to tiptoe across the edematous papillae. The histologic distinction between edema of the papillary dermis and subepidermal vesiculation is that in the former, some collagen fibrils remain contiguous with the epidermis, whereas in the latter, total separation of the dermis from the epidermis occurs. In some conditions, such as erysipelas, subepidermal vesiculation results from severe edema of the papillary dermis.

In contrast to erysipelas, which is a phlegmonous dermatitis with subepidermal vesiculation, erysipeloid is a suppurative dermatitis with intraepidermal pustulation.

Mast Cells Prominent

Bullous Urticaria Pigmentosa

Bullous urticaria pigmentosa is a rare subepidermal vesiculobullous disease that develops in newborns and infants who usually also have papular and nodular lesions of urticaria pigmentosa. Rarely will tense blisters be the only manifestation of the disease. A dense, diffuse infiltrate of mast cells is present within the dermis beneath the blister. The blistering aspect of the disease wanes and usually disappears completely within a year.

Intradermal Blistering Diseases

Penicillamine-induced (Fig. 11-48)

The blisters induced by penacillamine are situated in the upper dermis and are often hemorrhagic. Penicillamine has lathyrogenic activity which may be responsible for the defect in collagen that subsequently leads to intradermal blister formation. Clinically, the bullae resemble polyethylene bags.

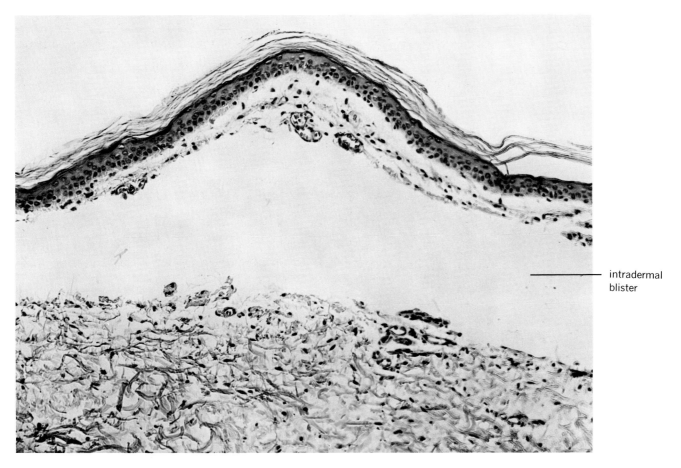

intradermal
blister

FIG. 11-48. Blister induced by penicillamine. The effects of penicillamine may so alter collagen in upper part of dermis that an intradermal blister develops as pictured here. (× 204.)

Folliculitis and Perifolliculitis

Perifolliculitis

Predominantly lymphocytic infiltrate
  Keratosis pilaris, lichen spinulosus
  Folliculitis ulerythematosa reticulata
  Lichen planopilaris
  Discoid lupus erythematosus
  Scurvy
Predominantly histiocytic (granulomatous) in-
    filtrate
  Rosacea and perioral dermatitis, papular
    stage
  Acneiform secondary syphilis

Folliculitis

Suppurative and suppurative-granulomatous
    folliculitis
  Superficial infectious folliculitis
    Bacterial infections (impetigo Bockhart)
    Fungal infections
      Dermatophytosis
      Candidiasis
    Viral infections
      Herpes simplex
      Herpes zoster
      Varicella
    Spirochetal infections
      Secondary syphilis
  Superficial noninfectious folliculitis
    Acne vulgaris
    Rosacea and perioral dermatitis
    Halogenodermas
    Chemical and mechanical injuries
    Pseudofolliculitis

Deep papulonodular infectious folliculitis
  Furuncle
  Carbuncle
  Sycosis
  Folliculitis decalvans
  Majocchi's granuloma
  Tinea barbae
  Favus
  Kerion
Deep papulonodular noninfectious folliculitis
  Acne vulgaris (papulonodular, "cystic,"
    conglobate, and keloidal)
  Hidradenitis suppurativa
  Dissecting cellulitis of the scalp
  Rosacea and perioral dermatitis
  Perforating folliculitis
  Kyrle's disease
  Elastosis perforans serpiginosa
  Halogenodermas
Spongiotic folliculitis
  Infundibulofolliculitis
  Atopic dermatitis
  Fox-Fordyce disease
Nonscarring inflammatory alopecias
  Alopecia areata
  Trichotillomania and traction alopecia
  Follicular mucinosis
  Secondary syphilis
Scarring inflammatory alopecias
  Scleroderma
  Necrobiosis lipoidica
  Physical and chemical injuries
  Sarcoidosis
  Lichen planopilaris
  Discoid lupus erythematosus

Folliculitis

and

Perifolliculitis

12

PERIFOLLICULITIS signifies inflammatory cells around the blood vessels of the perifollicular connective tissue (Fig. 12-1), and folliculitis denotes the presence of inflammatory cells within the follicular epithelium (Fig. 12-2). Both perifolliculitis, such as discoid lupus erythematosus and lichen planopilaris, and folliculitis, such as that caused by bacteria and fungi, can result in destruction of hair follicles and consequently in permanent alopecia.

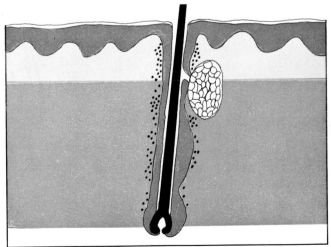

FIG. 12-1. Perifolliculitis.

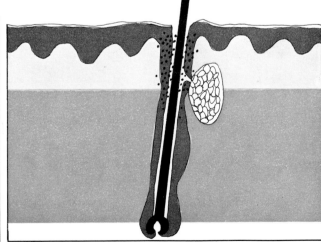

FIG. 12-2. Folliculitis.

641

Hair follicles vary in size and shape on different parts of the body (Fig. 12-3). They are small and slender on the cheeks and nose, but long and broad on the scalp (Fig. 12-4). The hair bulb extends for only a short distance below the sebaceous gland on the cheeks, but reaches into the subcutaneous fat on the scalp. The sebaceous glands associated with follicles containing puny hairs on the face, scalp, and back are large (sebaceous follicles) (Fig. 12-5), but on the leg are minuscule. There are also regional variations in the size and shape of the hair follicle infundibulum. Vellus follicles have short infundibula compared with the much longer infundibula of sebaceous follicles (Fig. 12-5).

Infundibular and epidermal epithelium are indistinguishable histologically. The similarities between these continuous epithelial structures include the basket-weave configuration of their cornified cells (Fig. 12-6). Abnormal cornification of the infundibulum may occur in the absence of folliculitis or perifolliculitis. Comedones (Fig. 12-7A, B) and tiny infundibular cysts (milia) (Fig. 12-7C, D), both containing orthokeratotic cells in laminated array, are examples of abnormal infundibular cornification without an inflammatory-cell infiltrate. In other noninflammatory conditions, such as porokeratosis, the infundibula may be widened and plugged partially or completely by parakeratotic cells (Fig. 12-8). A superficial perivascular lymphohistiocytic infiltrate may accompany parakeratotic infundibular plugs, as in keratosis follicularis (Darier's disease) (Fig. 12-9), orthokeratotic plugs as in lichen

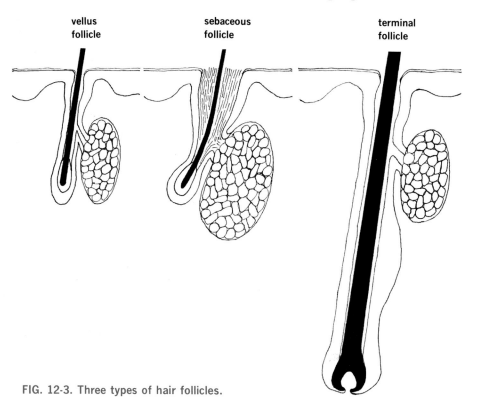

FIG. 12-3. Three types of hair follicles.

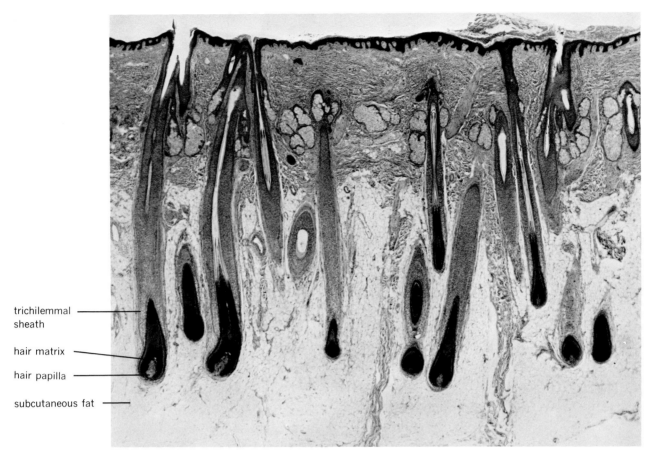

trichilemmal sheath —

hair matrix —

hair papilla —

subcutaneous fat —

FIG. 12-4. Normal scalp. Numerous bulbs of growing (anagen) hair follicles are rooted deep in subcutaneous fat. (× 19.)

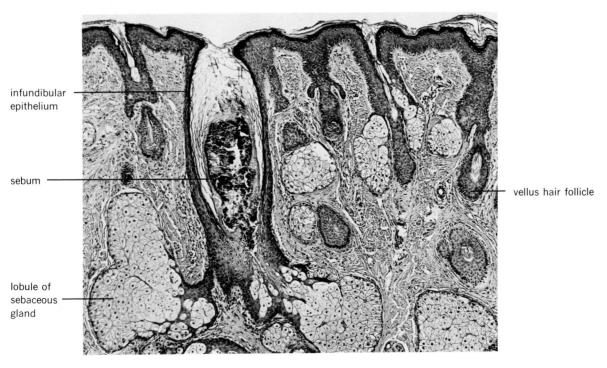

infundibular epithelium —

sebum —

lobule of sebaceous gland —

— vellus hair follicle

FIG. 12-5. Sebaceous follicle and vellus follicles. The sebaceous follicle shown is characterized by a long infundibulum into which feed several sebaceous ducts connected to large lobules of a sebaceous gland. In contrast, the follicles of vellus hairs have relatively short infundibula, fewer associated sebaceous ducts, and smaller lobules of sebaceous glands. (× 71.)

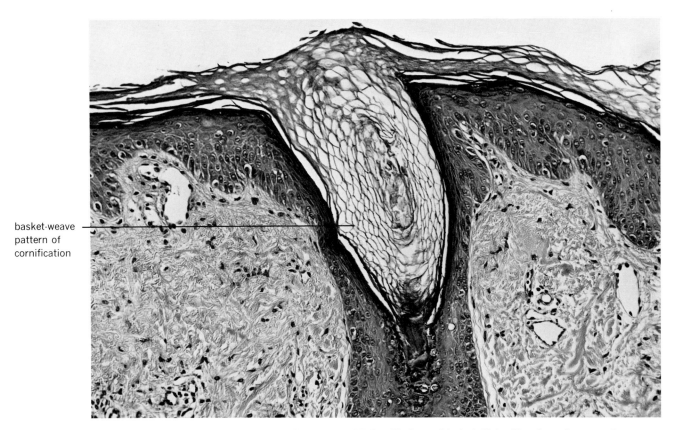

FIG. 12-6. Normal follicular infundibulum. Cornified cells in normal infundibulum of hair follicle, like those in normal stratum corneum, are arranged in basket-weave pattern. (× 220.)

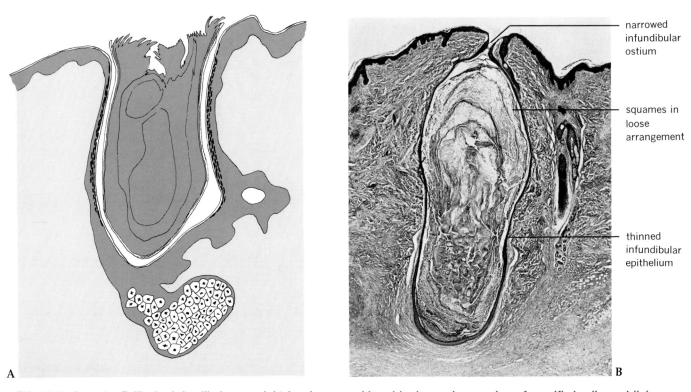

A

B

FIG. 12-7. Comedo. Follicular infundibulum on right has become widened by increasing number of cornified cells, and lining epithelium has become thinned. Note that infundibular ostium, although narrowed, remains structurally, though not functionally, patent. Sebaceous gland formerly associated with this infundibulum withered and disappeared. A, Drawing of open comedo. B, Photomicrograph of closed comedo. (× 22.)

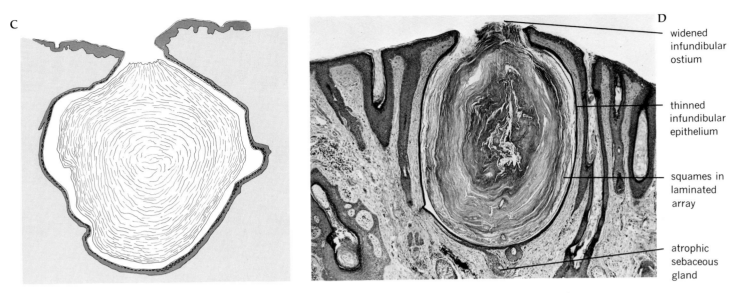

C

D

widened
infundibular
ostium

thinned
infundibular
epithelium

squames in
laminated
array

atrophic
sebaceous
gland

FIG. 12-7. Milium involving infundibular portion of hair follicle. C, Drawing. D, Photomicrograph. As the increasing number of laminated squames pushes outward, lining epithelium becomes thinned, infundibar ostium widened, and sebaceous gland shrunken. (× 83.)

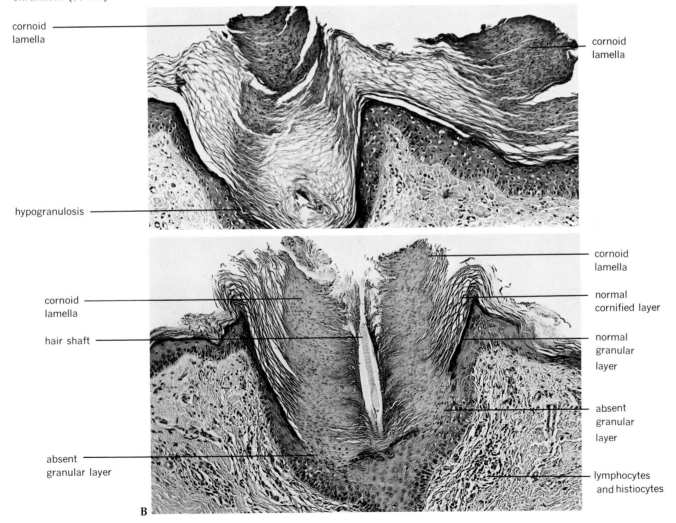

cornoid
lamella

cornoid
lamella

hypogranulosis

cornoid
lamella

normal
cornified layer

cornoid
lamella

normal
granular
layer

hair shaft

absent
granular
layer

absent
granular layer

lymphocytes
and histiocytes

B

FIG. 12-8. Porokeratosis, disseminated superficial type. A, Note cornoid lamellae (columns of parakeratosis) characteristic of all forms of porokeratosis in both follicular and epidermal epithelium. (× 179.) B, Two cornoid lamellae are seen on either side of thin hair shaft within an expanded infundibulum. Note loss of granular layer beneath cornoid lamellae. (× 171.)

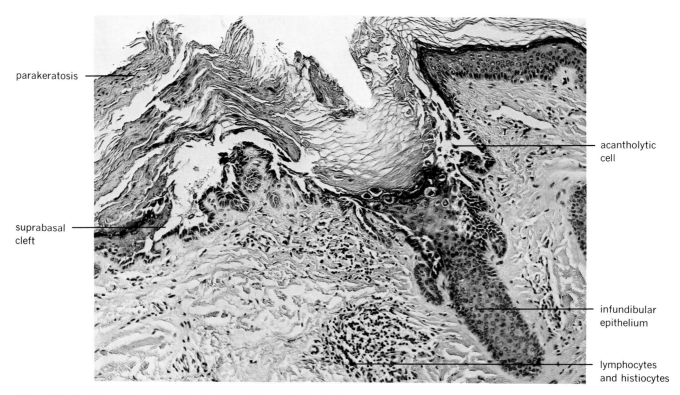

parakeratosis

acantholytic
cell

suprabasal
cleft

infundibular
epithelium

lymphocytes
and histiocytes

FIG. 12-9. Focal acantholytic dyskeratosis involving follicular infundibulum and epidermis. Characteristic changes are suprabasal clefts, acantholytic cells in spinous, granular, and cornified layers, and parakeratosis. (× 169.)

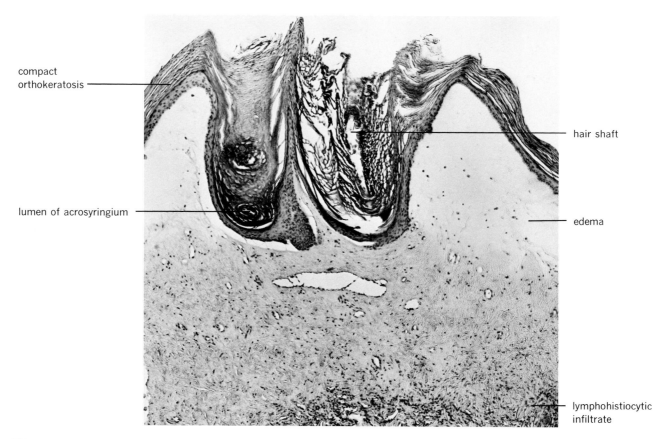

compact
orthokeratosis

hair shaft

lumen of acrosyringium

edema

lymphohistiocytic
infiltrate

FIG. 12-10. Keratotic plugs within adnexal ostia of eccrine sweat duct and hair follicle accompanied by superficial lymphohistiocytic infiltrate in lichen sclerosus et atrophicus. (× 72.)

sclerosus et atrophicus (Fig. 12-10), and alternating orthokeratotic and parakeratotic plugs in pityriasis rubra pilaris (Fig. 12-11).

Sometimes numerous organisms of Pityrosporon orbiculare or ovale, or both, are seen within the infundibula of folliculitides and perifolliculitides. Pityrospora are normal inhabitants of the follicular infundibula and their presence in great numbers in folliculitis and perifolliculitis is probably coincidental rather than causal of inflammation. Pityrospora are no more likely to be a cause of folliculitis than is the mite, Demodex folliculorum (Fig. 12-12).

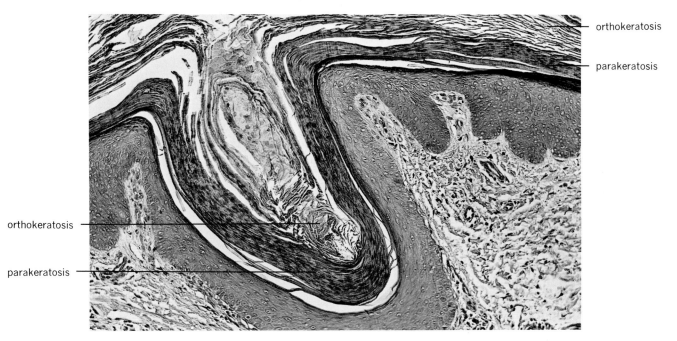

FIG. 12-11. Pityriasis rubra pilaris. Characteristic feature pictured is alternation of orthokeratosis and parakeratosis in cornified layers of epidermis and infundibulum of hair follicle. Plugging of dilated infundibula by cornified cells is inconstant. (× 200.)

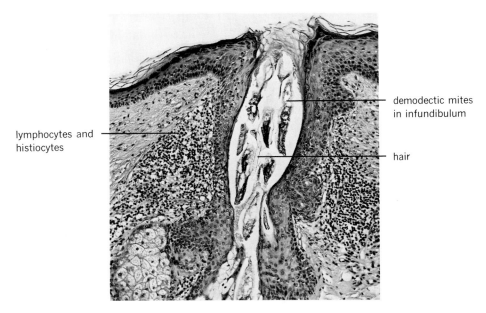

FIG. 12-12. Demodectic mites and perifolliculitis. Demodectic mites are seen within an infundibulum surrounded by inflammatory cells. In my opinion the inflammatory process is incidental and not in response to the mites. (× 165.)

Perifolliculitis (Fig. 12-13)

The inflammatory cells around the blood vessels of the perifollicular connective tissues are predominantly lymphocytes in keratosis pilaris, lichen spinulosus, folliculitis ulerythematosa reticulata, lichen planopilaris, discoid lupus erythematosus, and scurvy. Histiocytes predominate in rosacea, perioral dermatitis, and acneiform secondary syphilis.

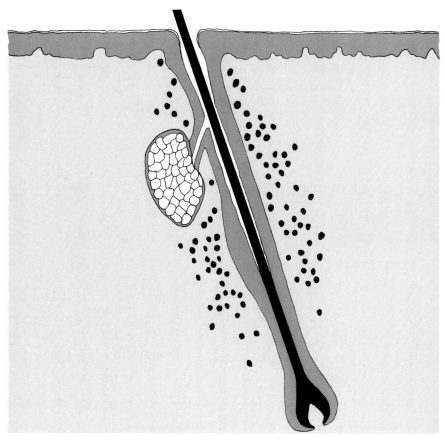

FIG. 12-13. Perifolliculitis.

Predominantly Lymphocytic Infiltrate

Keratosis Pilaris, Lichen Spinulosus (Fig. 12-14)

—Laminate orthokeratotic cells (with parakeratotic cells occasionally) within widened infundibula
—Conical cornified infundibular plugs protruding slightly above the skin surface (Fig. 12-14B)
—Sparse peri-infundibular and superficial perivascular lymphohistiocytic infiltrate

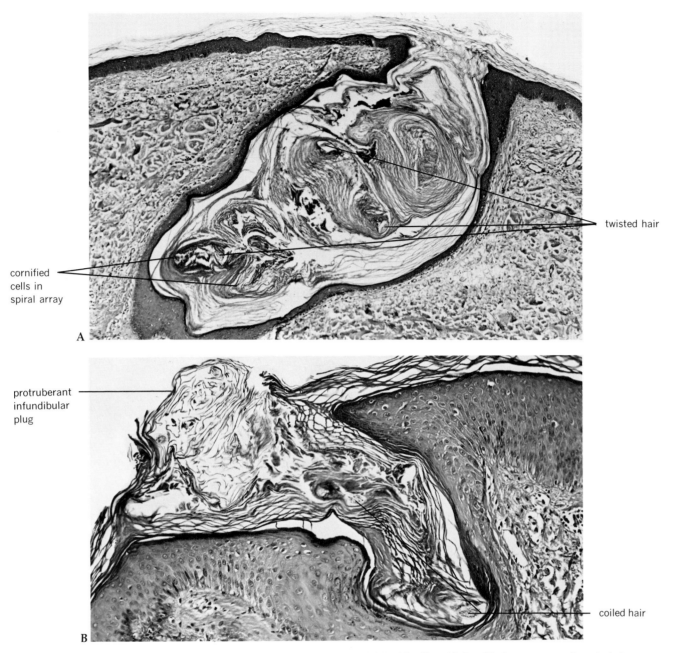

cornified
cells in
spiral array

twisted hair

A

protruberant
infundibular
plug

coiled hair

B

FIG. 12-14. Keratosis pilaris. A, Hair shaft and other cornified cells within this dilated infundibulum are seen to spiral. In some instances, as illustrated, there is virtually no inflammatory-cell infiltrate. ($\times$ 94.) B, Dilated infundibulum containing coiled hair around which also swirl an increasing number of cornified cells which protrude above surface of skin. ($\times$ 98.)

Histologically and clinically, individual lesions of keratosis pilaris and lichen spinulosus are indistinguishable. The two conditions differ only in the distribution of the keratotic papules. In keratosis pilaris, discrete keratotic lesions, scattered extensively, principally on the arms and legs, may be surrounded by a subtle rim of erythema. In lichen spinulosus, the keratotic papules are grouped, especially on the neck, trunk, buttocks, and extensor surfaces of the arms. There is a greater incidence of keratosis pilaris in persons with ichthyosis vulgaris and atopic dermatitis. (Fig. 12-15).

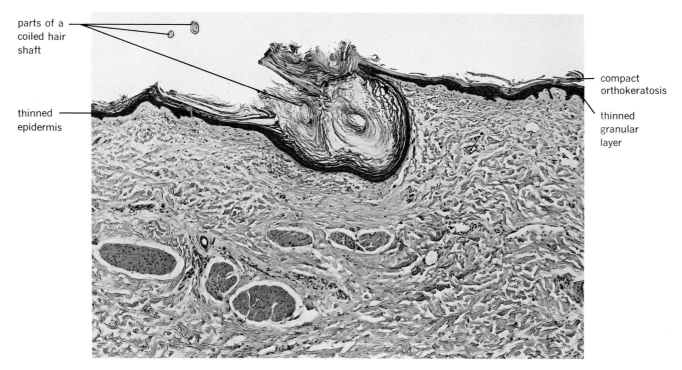

parts of a
coiled hair
shaft

compact
orthokeratosis

thinned
epidermis

thinned
granular
layer

FIG. 12-15. Keratosis pilaris in association with ichthyosis vulgaris. Widened infundibulum plugged by cornified cells and containing coiled hair is typical. Compact laminated orthokeratosis, diminished or absent granular layer, and thinned epidermis with reduced epidermal rete ridges are histologic features of common form of ichthyosis. (× 76.)

The nutmeg-grater roughness of the lesions of both keratosis pilaris and lichen spinulosus results from the extension of the cornified infundibular plugs above the skin surface (Fig. 12-14B). The inflammatory-cell infiltrate is so slight and the blood vessels so little dilated that there often is hardly any clinical sign of inflammation in either condition. Sometimes there is no inflammatory-cell infiltrate whatsoever. Rarely will the keratotic plug penetrate the infundibular epithelium into the dermis, inducing a suppurative granulomatous folliculitis and perifolliculitis.

Folliculitis Ulerythematosa Reticulata

Folliculitis ulerythematosa reticulata begins in childhood and occurs bilaterally and symmetrically on the sides of the forehead and the cheeks. Often it is associated with keratosis pilaris or lichen spinulosus on the lateral aspects of the arms and legs. Folliculitis ulerythematosa reticulata resembles lichen spinulosus, but clinically there is greater erythema and the keratotic follicular plugs do not usually extend above the skin surface. Histologically there is a denser lymphohistiocytic infiltrate. With time, the infundibular plugs are lost, and the residual patulous ostia resemble those of pitted acne.

—Dense, bandlike predominantly lymphocytic infiltrate along the length of the hair follicle, partly obscuring it
—Vacuolar alteration at the follicular epithelial-connective tissue junction
—Infundibular plugging by orthokeratotic cells
—Fibrotic tracts in older lesions at sites of former hair follicles

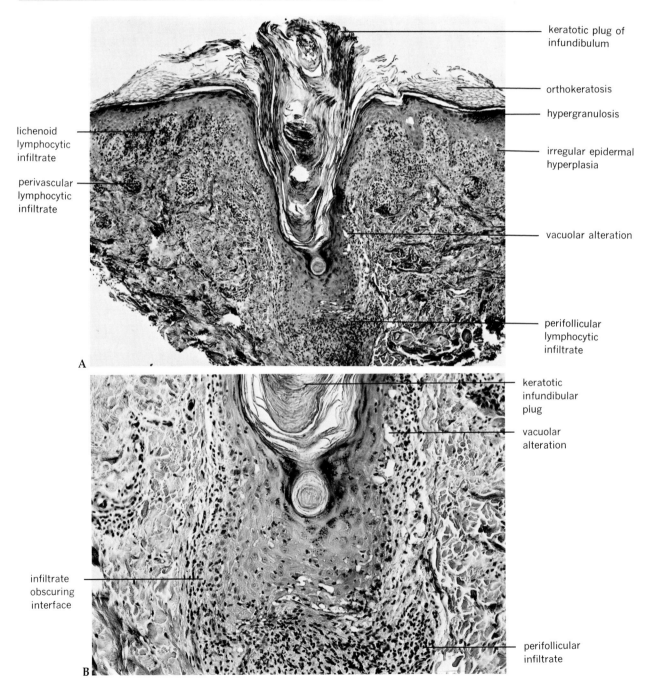

FIG. 12-16. Lichen planopilaris. Characteristic bandlike infiltrate is seen at interface between epidermis and dermis and between follicular epithelium and dermis. Focal hypergranulosis is important diagnostic clue. (A, × 76; B, × 187.)

In lichen planopilaris the characteristic histologic features of lichen planus are present, especially at the interface between the follicular epithelium and the surrounding periadnexal dermis, rather than primarily at the dermoepidermal junction (Fig. 12-17). The bandlike lymphohistiocytic infiltrate consistently involves not only the infundibular portion of the hair follicle but often the isthmic and inferior parts as well (Fig. 12-68). Sometimes the linearly arranged collections of lymphocytes seem to extend downward along the follicle from the undersurface of the infundibulum. When the process is long-standing, as is often the case, the hair follicles are replaced by linear fibrotic tracts.

Clinically, lichen planopilaris is characterized by keratotic follicular papules that often have a somewhat violaceous hue. Although most commonly involving the scalp, these keratotic follicular papules can occur anywhere on the skin surface. They may or may not be associated with typical skin or mucous-membrane lesions of lichen planus. The scalp lesions of lichen planopilaris often culminate in alopecia marked by irregularly shaped white atrophic patches. Because the alopecic areas of the end-stage lichen planopilaris bear some resemblance to alopecia areata, the condition was known formerly as pseudopelade, *pelade* being the French word for alopecia areata. The eponymon for lichen planopilaris is the Graham Little syndrome.

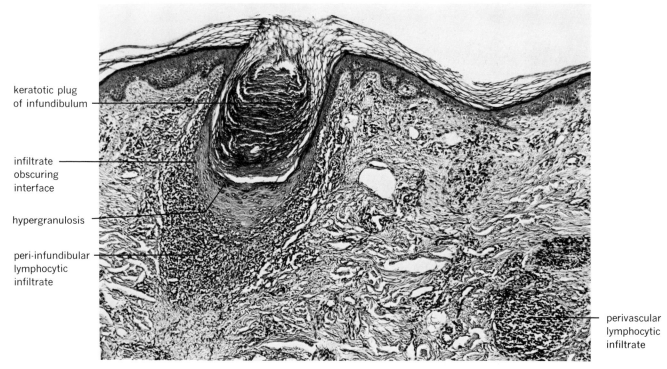

keratotic plug of infundibulum

infiltrate obscuring interface

hypergranulosis

peri-infundibular lymphocytic infiltrate

perivascular lymphocytic infiltrate

FIG. 12-17. Lichen planopilaris. Bandlike infiltrate envelops follicular epithelium rather than being distributed beneath epidermis. Other features confined to the follicle in this lesion, rather than to the epidermis, are orthokeratosis, hypergranulosis, and obscuration of interface between infundibulum and dermis by infiltrate. (A, × 87; B, × 181.)

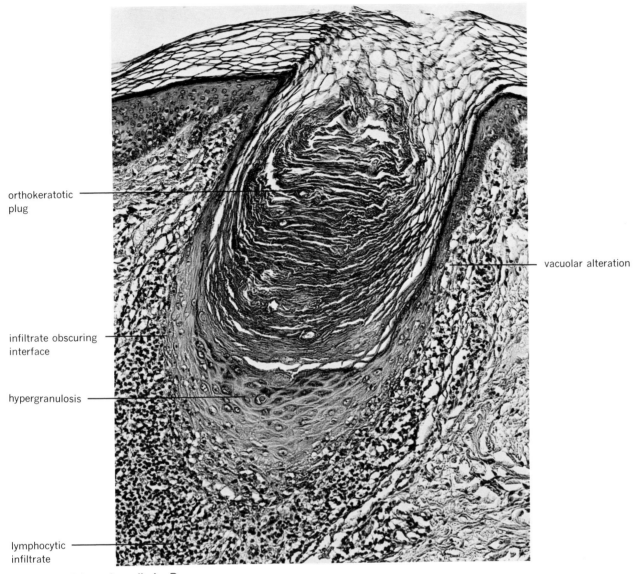

orthokeratotic plug

infiltrate obscuring interface

hypergranulosis

lymphocytic infiltrate

vacuolar alteration

FIG. 12-17. Lichen planopilaris. B.

Discoid Lupus Erythematosus (Fig. 12-18)

—Dense, bandlike predominantly lymphocytic infiltrate along the length of the hair follicle, partly obscuring it

—Vacuolar alteration at the follicular epithelial-connective tissue junction

—Infundibular plugs of orthokeratotic cells

—Fibrotic tracts in older lesions at sites of former hair follicles

—Dense, predominantly lymphocytic infiltrate around the blood vessels of the superficial and deep plexuses

—Mucin in the dermis of acute and subacute lesions

—Vacuolar alteration at the dermoepidermal junction

—Thickened epidermal and follicular basement membrane in some lesions

—Thinned and/or alternately thickened epidermis

—Compact orthokeratosis

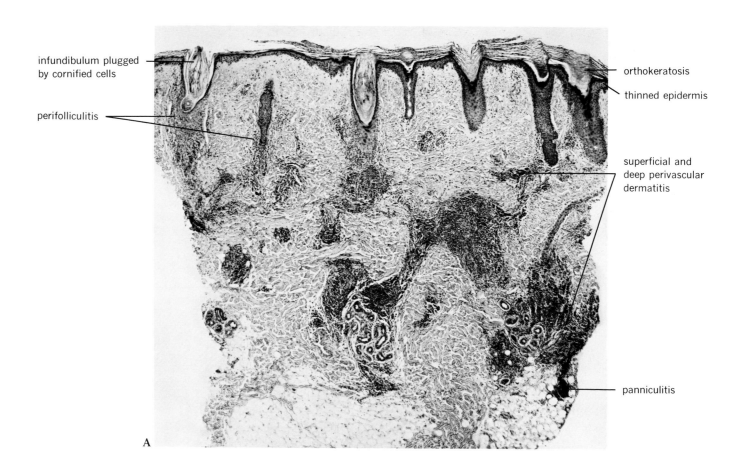

infundibulum plugged by cornified cells

perifolliculitis

orthokeratosis

thinned epidermis

superficial and deep perivascular dermatitis

panniculitis

A

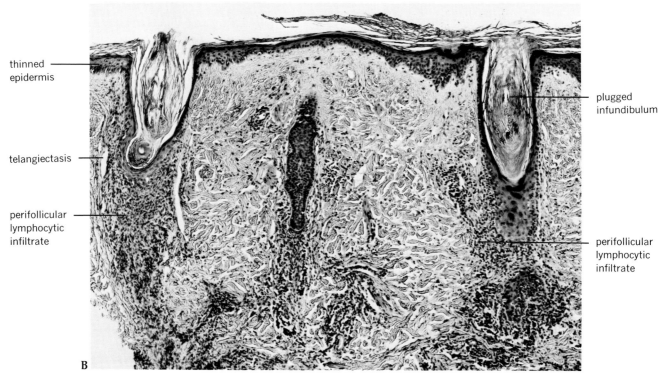

thinned epidermis

telangiectasis

perifollicular lymphocytic infiltrate

plugged infundibulum

perifollicular lymphocytic infiltrate

B

FIG. 12-18. Discoid lupus erythematosus, perifollicular infiltrate. A, Thinned epidermis, deep as well as superficial perivascular inflammatory-cell infiltrate, and extension of infiltrate into subcutaneous fat differentiate this specimen from one in lichen planopilaris. ($\times$ 38.) B, In higher magnification, perifollicular predominantly lymphocytic infiltrate may be seen to affect each hair follicle, and both epidermal and infundibular epithelia are thinned. ($\times$ 92.)

Because discoid lupus erythematosus has been discussed in general in Chapter 7, the present comments will focus on the follicular aspects of the disease. Regardless of the stage of discoid lupus erythematosus, whether acute or chronic, there are changes in the epidermis and the dermoepidermal interface. These include vacuolar alteration, basement-membrane thickening, hypoplasia and hyperplasia of the epidermis, and orthokeratosis. In acute and subacute discoid lupus erythematosus, the dense predominantly lymphocytic perifollicular infiltrate occurs in concert with a similar infiltrate around the blood vessels of the superficial and deep vascular plexuses. The dilated infundibula are plugged by orthokeratotic cells. Clinical concomitants of these histologic findings are red, indurated plaques, frequently dotted by patulous infundibular orifices, some being occluded by "carpet-tack scales."

In scars of chronic discoid lupus erythematosus, there is fibrosis at sites of former hair follicles and sclerosis in the upper dermis (Fig. 12-19). The hair erector muscles are often spared from destruction. Little inflammatory-cell infiltrate may be present in these "burned-out" lesions, although numerous melanophages and widely dilated capillaries and venules may be found in the upper dermis. The clue to the diagnosis of chronic discoid lupus erythematosus is a thickened basement membrane. The clinical correlates of these findings are hairless atrophic scars, variously colored by postinflammatory pigmentary changes and showing telangiectases.

It is sometimes difficult to differentiate the perifollicular inflammatory changes of discoid lupus erythematosus from those of lichen planopilaris. However, in discoid lupus erythematosus the most critical alterations are usually at both the junction between the epidermis and the dermis, as well as between the follicular epithelium and the periadnexal connective tissue (Fig. 12-18). In lichen planopilaris, the dermoepidermal interface usually is mostly spared. Furthermore, in chronic discoid lupus erythematosus the follicular and epidermal basement membranes are usually thickened, whereas in the lichen planopilaris they are not.

Scurvy (Fig. 12-20)

—Peri-infundibular lymphohistiocytic infiltrate
—Extravasated erythrocytes in the peri-infundibular region
—Orthokeratotic infundibular plugs
—Superficial perivascular lymphohistiocytic infiltrate with siderophages

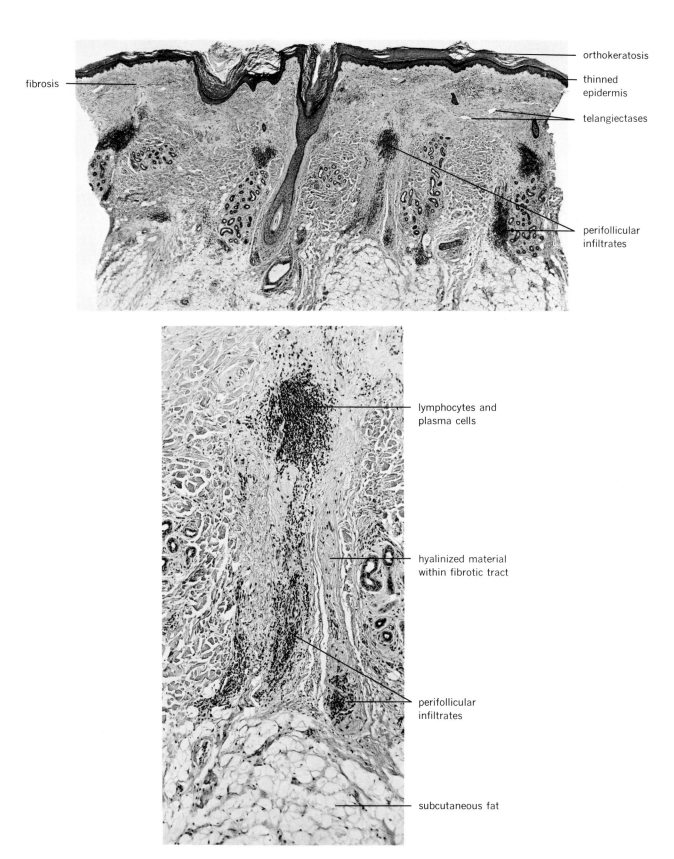

fibrosis

orthokeratosis

thinned
epidermis

telangiectases

perifollicular
infiltrates

lymphocytes and
plasma cells

hyalinized material
within fibrotic tract

perifollicular
infiltrates

subcutaneous fat

FIG. 12-19. Alopecia in discoid lupus erythematosus. A, Lone hair follicle remains in specimen from scalp of patient. Moderately dense infiltrates of mononuclear cells (lymphocytes and plasma cells) are concentrated at sites of former hair follicles whose remnants are fibrotic tracts. (× 28.) B, In higher magnification, two fibrotic tracts and accompanying predominantly lymphocytic infiltration are seen in greater detail. Careful scrutiny reveals remnants of follicular glassy membranes that have been caught within fibrotic processes. (× 72.)

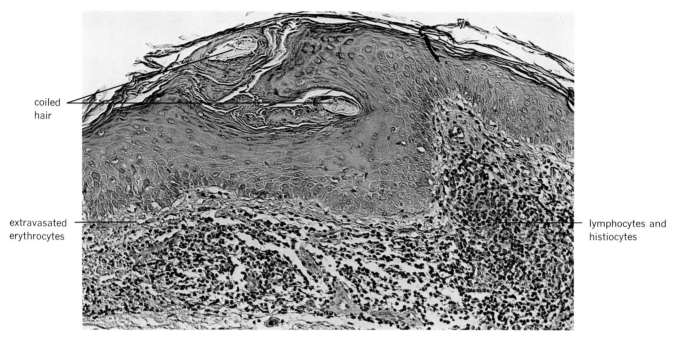

coiled hair

extravasated erythrocytes

lymphocytes and histiocytes

FIG. 12-20. Scurvy. Dilated infundibulum pictured is plugged by cornified cells surrounding coiled hair, and the follicle, in turn, is surrounded by moderately dense inflammatory-cell infiltrate and extravasated erythrocytes. (× 220.)

Scurvy, now a rare condition, is characterized histologically by a dilated infundibulum plugged by cornified cells surrounding a hair coiled in its follicle (Fig. 12-21). Spiraled hairs are common findings in scurvy and other severe nutritional deficiencies. The reason for this phenomenon is not known. A moderately dense inflammatory-cell infiltrate and extravasated erythrocytes will also be seen. These characteristic findings are reflected clinically as corkscrew hairs, follicular keratoses, and perifollicular purpura. In some patients spiraled hairs occur in the absence of perifollicular purpura.

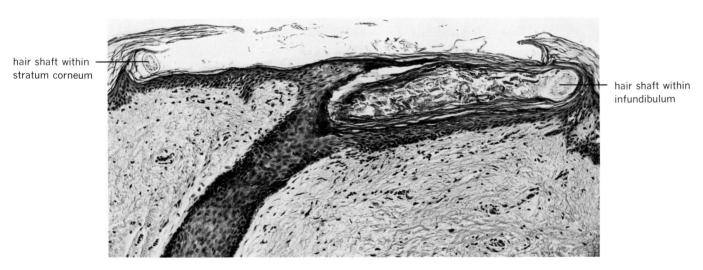

hair shaft within stratum corneum

hair shaft within infundibulum

FIG. 12-21. Coiled hair in scurvy. Two cross sections marked "hair shaft" are of single spiraled hair from patient with scurvy. The fact of its singularity may be inferred from the finding of only one hair in the infundibulum. (× 155.)

Predominantly Histiocytic (Granulomatous) Infiltrate

Rosacea and Perioral Dermatitis, Papular Stage (Fig. 12-22)

—Peri-infundibular epithelioid tubercles surrounded by lymphocytes and plasma cells
—Epithelioid tubercles also randomly distributed in the upper dermis
—Sometimes necrosis within the epithelioid tubercles
—Telangiectases

Papular lesions of rosacea, formerly termed acne rosacea, are clinical counterparts of granulomatous folliculitis and perifolliculitis. When the follicular nature of the process cannot be recognized either because follicles have been destroyed or because particular sections do not show follicles, rosacea must be differentiated from sarcoidosis, lupus vulgaris, and other diseases characterized by epithelioid tubercles. The tuberculoid granulomas of rosacea and perioral dermatitis are differentiated from other granulomatous dermatitides by the predominantly perifollicular location of the epithelioid tubercles and by the prominent telangiectases. Early papular lesions of either rosacea or perioral dermatitis may not be diagnostic histologically, consisting as they do merely of superficial perivascular lymphohistiocytic infiltrates and telangiectases. Later granulomatous papules are sometimes known as rosacea-like tuberculid (Lewandowsky).

Rosacea and perioral dermatitis are related conditions that occur separately or together and result from inflammatory-cell reactions in and around follicular infundibula. Histologically,

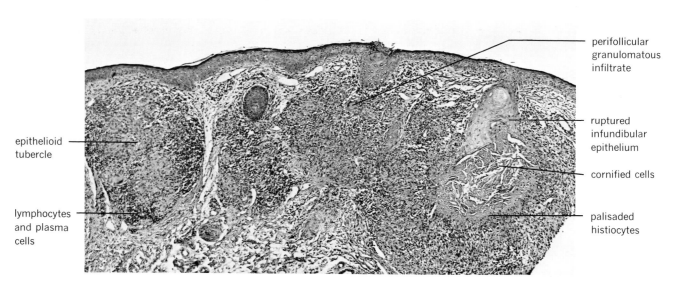

FIG. 12-22. Rosacea. A, Several foci of granulomatous inflammation pictured are each closely associated with infundibula of hair follicles. (× 68.)

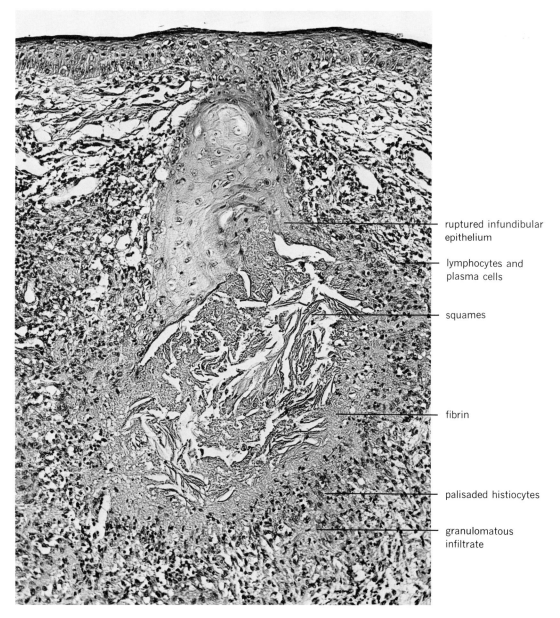

ruptured infundibular
epithelium

lymphocytes and
plasma cells

squames

fibrin

palisaded histiocytes

granulomatous
infiltrate

FIG. 12-22. Rosacea. B, In this higher magnification, part of the process and progress of rosacea can be seen to be related to rupture of follicular infundibulum with consequent granulomatous folliculitis. (× 176.)

except for the rhinophyma of rosacea, the two diseases are indistinguishable. Although rosacea and perioral dermatitis have clinical lesions in common—pustules, papules, and telangiectases—they are distributed differently. Rosacea tends to affect the middle of the face, whereas perioral dermatitis is usually restricted to the region around the mouth and lower eyelids. Rosacea occurs in middle-aged men and women with about equal frequency, but perioral dermatitis is almost wholly a disease of younger women. Rosacea may be associated with a keratitis, blepharitis, and conjunctivitis; perioral dermatitis is not. Prolonged topical use of fluorinated corticosteroids may induce lesions of both rosacea and perioral dermatitis.

Acneiform Secondary Syphilis

—Predominantly histiocytic infiltrate with lymphocytes and plasma cells around the follicular units, especially the infundibula
—Epithelioid tubercles occasionally, some with multinucleated histiocytes
—Infundibular plugging by orthokeratotic cells
—Superficial and deep perivascular infiltrate of histiocytes, lymphocytes, and plasma cells
—Focal parakeratosis

Clinically, the follicular papules of secondary syphilis must be differentiated from other acneiform processes. Often the patient will have concurrent lesions in areas such as palms and soles, which have no follicles. Mucosal lesions and adenopathy are common concomitants of secondary syphilis. Diagnosis is established by serologic test and absolutely by demonstrating the spirochetes by dark-field examination or special silver stains on histologic sections.

Folliculitis

In contrast with perifolliculitis, in which the inflammatory-cell infiltrate consists primarily of lymphocytes and histiocytes, folliculitis is usually composed initially of a predominantly neutrophilic infiltrate. These cells emanate from the blood vessels of the peri-infundibular connective tissue and move into the hair follicles. In superficial folliculitis the neutrophils are confined to the infundibulum, especially to its upper part (Fig. 12-23). Clinically, the lesions of superficial folliculitis are painless follicular pustules that heal without scars. When neutrophils fill the entire infundibulum and extend into either the isthmic or inferior portion of the hair follicle and to the surrounding dermis, a deep folliculitis results (Fig. 12-24). Clinically, deep folliculitides are not always pustules, but are commonly composed of papules and nodules. When pustules are found in deep folliculitides, they are almost always situated atop areas of redness and induration. As a rule, the lesions of deep folliculitis are painful and heal with scars. Calcification and ossification can also be sequelae of long-standing deep folliculitis.

In addition to the depth of the inflammatory-cell infiltrate within the follicle and the extent of dermal involvement, the chronicity of the process is another factor that determines whether folliculitis will cause scarring. Many suppurative folliculitides are short-lived and resolve with no clinical residua. Others are long-standing, progressing from suppuration to granulomas and eventually to fibrosis. The clinical concomitants of this progression include pustules, papules, nodules, and finally alopecic scars.

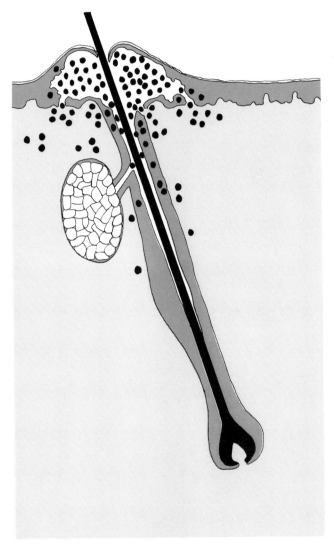

FIG. 12-23. Superficial folliculitis.

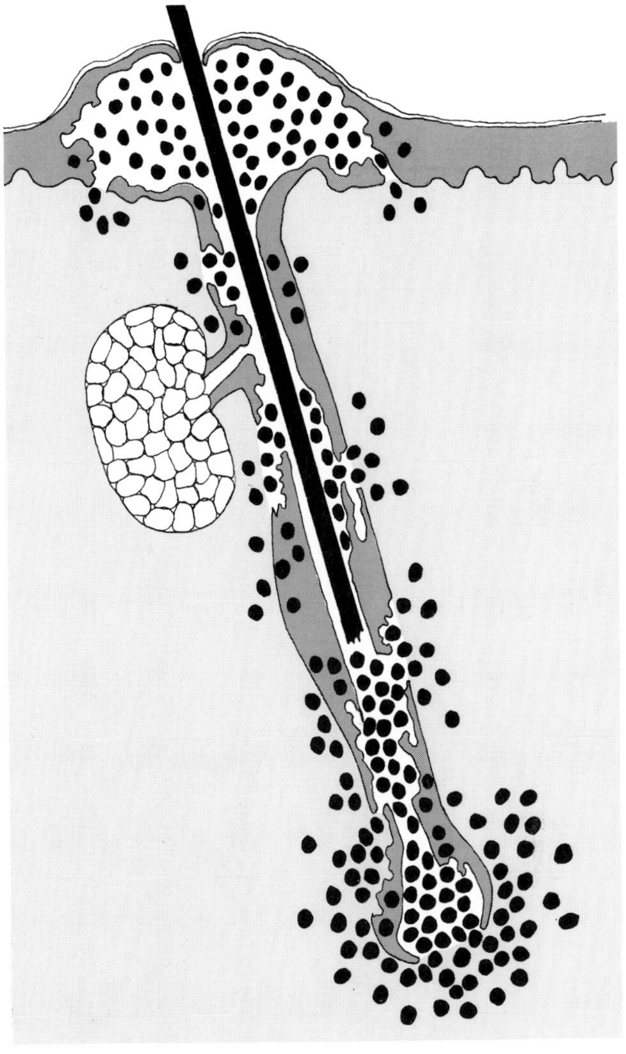

FIG. 12-24. Deep folliculitis.

Suppurative and Suppurative-Granulomatous Folliculitis

Folliculitis may be classified as suppurative folliculitis and suppurative-granulomatous folliculitis because any suppurative folliculitis, if persistent, may become granulomatous (Fig. 12-25). These disorders may be subdivided into superficial folliculitis and deep folliculitis on an anatomic basis and further divided according to cause, that is, infectious or noninfectious.

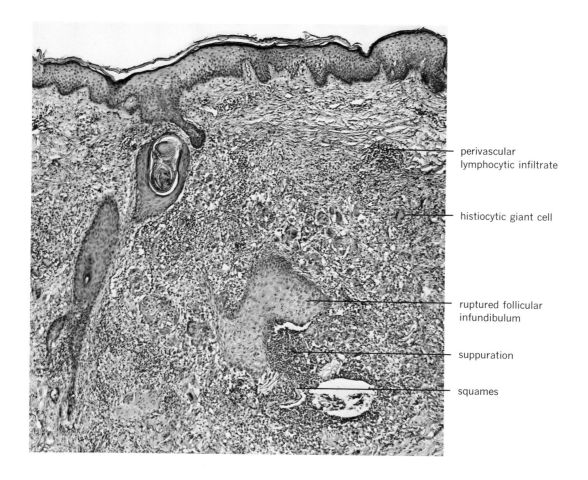

perivascular
lymphocytic infiltrate

histiocytic giant cell

ruptured follicular
infundibulum

suppuration

squames

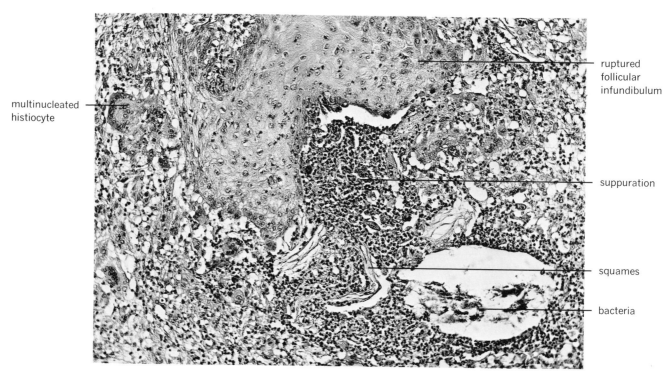

multinucleated
histiocyte

ruptured
follicular
infundibulum

suppuration

squames

bacteria

FIG. 12-25. Suppurative granulomatous dermatitis secondary to rupture of a follicular infundibulum. Follicular contents, especially cornified cells (squames), have been expelled to dermis. Initial response to this extrusion of foreign material is prompt mobilization of neutrophils (suppuration) followed by appearance of histiocytes, many of which become multinucleated (bespeaking granulomatous inflammation). (A, × 59; B, × 176.)

Infectious and noninfectious superficial folliculitides are virtually indistinguishable from one another with low power (scanning) magnification (Fig. 12-26). Both show neutrophils in varying quantities within the follicular infundibulum, and both may be associated with rupture of the follicle at different levels of the infundibulum (Fig. 12-27). A sparse, superficial, mixed inflammatory-cell infiltrate of lymphocytes, histiocytes, neutrophils, and occasionally eosinophils and plasma cells may be seen around the vessels of the superficial plexus. With higher magnification, differentiation may sometimes be made among them, even in preparations stained with hematoxylin and eosin. For example, careful search within the pustule may reveal numerous bacteria, suggesting superficial staphylococcal folliculitis (impetigo of Bockhart). Scouring of the cornified elements of the follicle, such as the internal root sheath, hair shaft, and infundibular horn may reveal hyphae and/or spores, suggesting a dermatophytic or yeast folliculitis. Special stains, such as the Gram for bacteria and the PAS for fungi, will confirm these observations. Often, even after special stains have been applied, no cause can be ascertained for a suppurative folliculitis.

Superficial Infectious Folliculitis

Clinically, superficial *staphylococcal folliculitis* (*impetigo of Bockhart*) consists of pustules that develop in clusters, especially on the scalp and extremities of children. These pustules usually heal within several days, and only rarely will they persist to become furuncles. Superficial *dermatophytic folliculitis* (*ringworm*) is usually due to zoophilic fungi and presents as tiny follicular pustules surmounting an indurated erythematous plaque. *Tinea capitis*, except for kerion, is not usually pustular, but is scaly and only slightly erythematous. *Candida folliculitis* also appears as small follicular pustules. Satellite lesions of candidiasis are also often follicular.

Only rarely will the typical changes of herpesvirus infection in *herpes simplex*, *herpes zoster*, and *varicella* involve the follicular infundibula and associated sebaceous glands (Fig. 12-28). If sufficiently destructive of the follicular epithelium, herpesvirus infections may result in permanent hair loss.

The early changes caused by the herpesvirus in follicular epithelium, like those in epidermal epithelium, are subtle and consist of steel gray nuclei with peripheral concentration of the nucleoplasm within ballooned cytoplasm. It is not necessary to see multinucleated epithelial giant cells to make a certain diagnosis of infection by the herpesvirus.

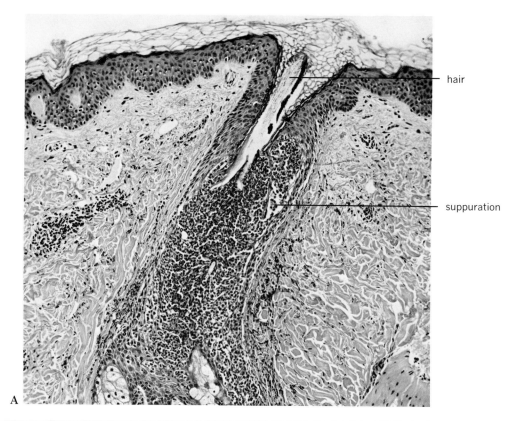

hair

suppuration

A

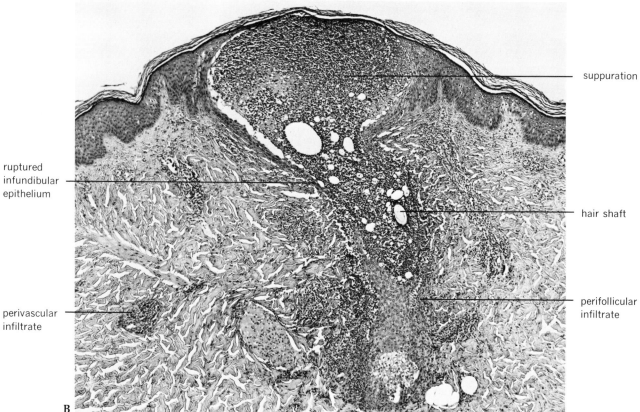

suppuration

ruptured
infundibular
epithelium

hair shaft

perivascular
infiltrate

perifollicular
infiltrate

B

FIG. 12-26. Suppurative folliculitis. A, Often no microbial or other cause can be demonstrated as in example pictured. (× 122.) B, Collection of pus has progressed from within infundibulum, into infundibular epithelium, and through it into dermis. Histologic changes shown are those of superficial suppurative folliculitis, but special stains were negative for infectious agents, and the cause of this process was not resolved. (× 67.)

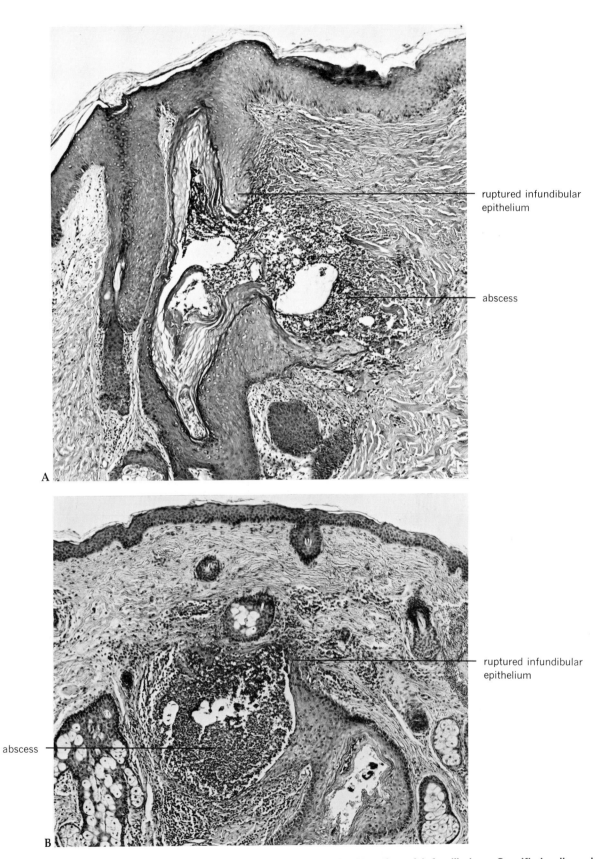

FIG. 12-27. Suppurative folliculitis. A, Follicle has ruptured at level of midportion of infundibulum. Cornified cells, sebum, bacteria, and yeasts have been discharged into dermis with resultant suppuration. (× 80.) B, Follicle ruptured at base of infundibulum near entrance of duct of sebaceous gland. As a consequence of spewing of infundibular contents into dermis, an abscess has formed. (× 82.)

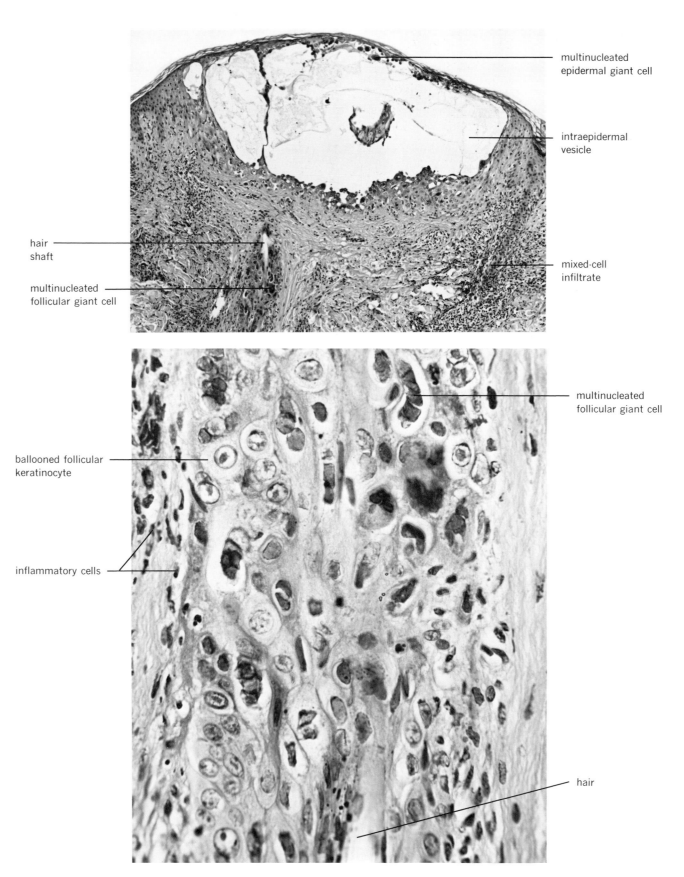

FIG. 12-28. Folliculitis caused by herpesvirus. In addition to vesicular changes within epidermis induced by herpesvirus, follicular epithelium may also show pathognomonic features of multinucleated epithelial giant cells, margination of nucleoplasm, and ballooning of cytoplasm. (A, × 76; B, × 590.)

Labels on figure:
- multinucleated epidermal giant cell
- intraepidermal vesicle
- hair shaft
- multinucleated follicular giant cell
- mixed-cell infiltrate
- multinucleated follicular giant cell
- ballooned follicular keratinocyte
- inflammatory cells
- hair

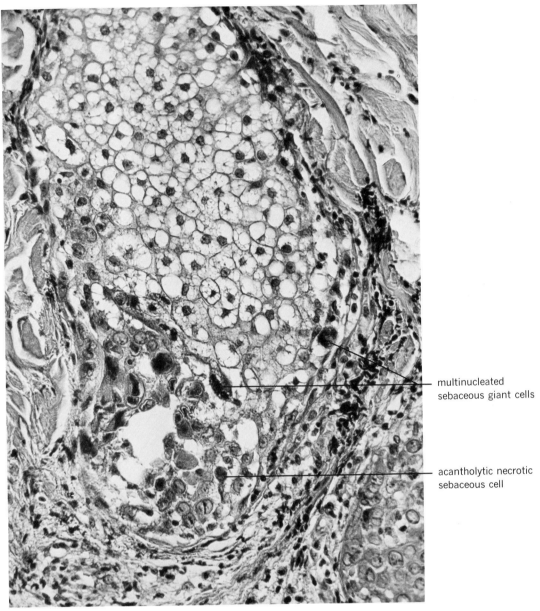

multinucleated
sebaceous giant cells

acantholytic necrotic
sebaceous cell

FIG. 12-28. C, Herpesvirus infection of sebaceous epithelium. The characteristic cytologic feature of infection by herpesvirus, multinucleated epithelial giant cells, is evident within sebaceous gland. (× 331.)

Cutaneous syphilis is characterized histologically and clinically by a broad range of pathologic patterns, among them the suppurative as manifested in follicular secondary syphilis, condyloma latum, and rupial syphilis (Fig. 12-29). Spirochetes in pustular lesions are more readily demonstrated by silver stain than in any other cutaneous form of secondary syphilis. The spirochetes are more easily found in epidermal and in follicular epithelia than in the dermis. A rule that applies, not only to syphilis but to infectious diseases in general, is that organisms are found readily in suppurative foci and practically never in wholly granulomatous ones.

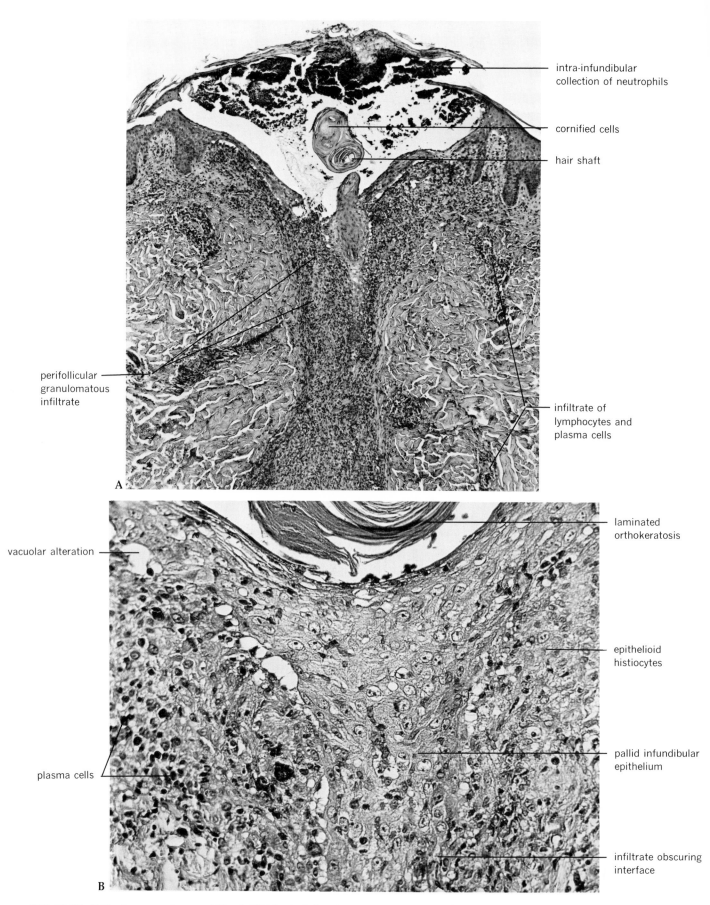

intra-infundibular
collection of neutrophils

cornified cells

hair shaft

perifollicular
granulomatous
infiltrate

infiltrate of
lymphocytes and
plasma cells

vacuolar alteration

laminated
orthokeratosis

epithelioid
histiocytes

pallid infundibular
epithelium

plasma cells

infiltrate obscuring
interface

FIG. 12-29. Follicular secondary syphilis. A, Within the infundibulum of this follicle from patient with secondary syphilis is a fresh infiltrate of neutrophils, whereas a more long-standing infiltrate composed mostly of histiocytes is seen along the length of the follicle. Plasma cells are also present in the dermal infiltrate. (× 65.) B, In higher magnification, plasma cells can be seen more clearly. Other changes are pallor of epithelial cells and tendency of infiltrate to obscure junction between follicular epithelium and dermis. (× 392.)

It is not always possible to distinguish histologically among the noninfectious superficial folliculitides, even if special stains are employed (Fig. 12-30). Pustular lesions of acne vulgaris, rosacea and perioral dermatitis, halogenodermas (Fig. 12-31), and chemical and mechanical folliculitides are all characterized by collections of neutrophils within the follicular infundibulum. However, in acne vulgaris and in acne secondary to chlorinated hydrocarbons, there are comedones, as well as collections of neutrophils, within the infundibula, whereas in acne due to systemic corticosteroids no comedones are usually seen. When a superficial folliculitis is thought to be noninfectious, after special stains have failed to reveal organisms, a note should be appended to the diagnosis of suppurative folliculitis, superficial, to include the histologic differential diagnosis. In these instances the clinical history and course of the disease are critical to establishing the correct diagnosis.

The pustules of *acne vulgaris* occur primarily on the face, shoulders, upper part of the chest, and back of adolescents. They are associated with comedones and, in more severe cases, with nodules, some of which may discharge pus. The pustular stage of *rosacea* and *perioral dermatitis* is distinguished clinically from acne vulgaris by the absence of comedones and the presence usually of telangiectases. Rosacea tends to involve the middle of the face, whereas perioral dermatitis is primarily confined to the lower third of the face. *Acneiform pustular lesions due to systemic corticosteroids* are not usually associated with clinical comedo formation. *Halogenodermas* can be differentiated from acne vulgaris and from rosacea by the tendency of the pustules to be more widespread, often involving the extremities. The pustules of *chemical and mechanical folliculitides* arise only in the areas where the offending materials have been applied. An example is the superficial folliculitis occurring on the thighs and legs of automobile mechanics, whose trousers, often tight-fitting, are smeared with various machine and cutting oils. Comedones generally precede pustules in oil-induced acne.

Toxic erythema of the newborn is a common widespread eruption characterized histologically by subcorneal and intrafollicular predominantly eosinophilic "abscesses" that are manifested clinically as follicular pustules (see Chapter 10). Some neutrophils may accompany the eosinophils.

A condition that simulates folliculitis (*pseudofolliculitis*) occurs primarily in the beards of black people who have spiraled hairs. The condition results from the penetration of the dermis by the

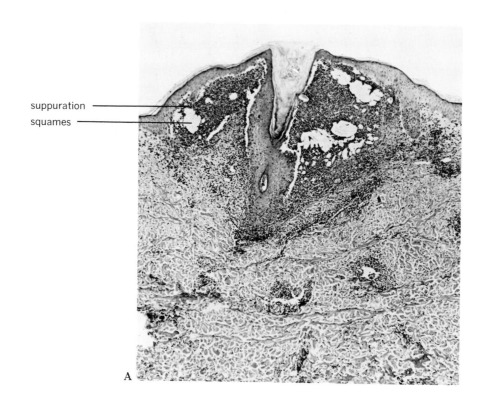

suppuration

squames

A

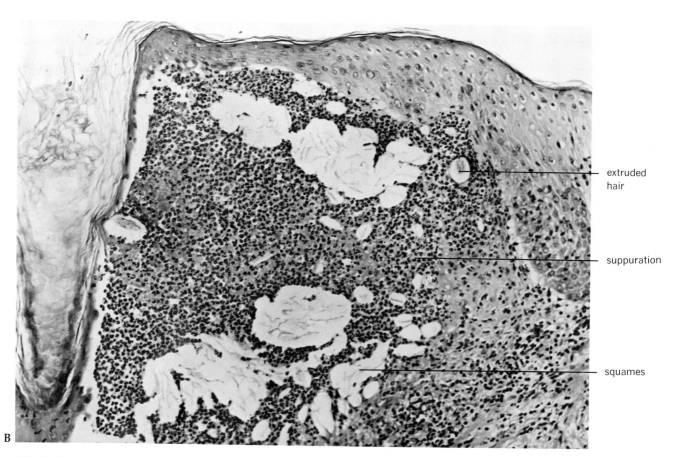

extruded
hair

suppuration

squames

B

FIG. 12-30. Suppurative folliculitis. Individual cornified cells and fragments of hair were extruded from the follicular infundibulum with resultant acute inflammatory response that is suppurative. No cause could be determined, even with the use of special stains. (A, × 51; B, × 209.)

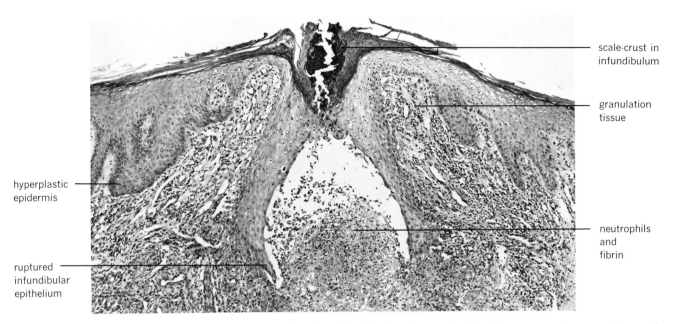

FIG. 12-31. Halogenoderma. In this reaction to iodides the infundibulum has ruptured with consequent suppuration and formation of granulation tissue. (× 83.)

sharp tips of shaved hairs, either directly through the wall of the hair follicle (Fig. 12-32) or more commonly by emerging from the follicular orifice and curving backward from above the skin surface to reenter the skin. In both circumstances the hair acts as a foreign body, eliciting first neutrophils, which form abscesses, and later granulomas and fibrosis. Bacteriologically, these pustules are

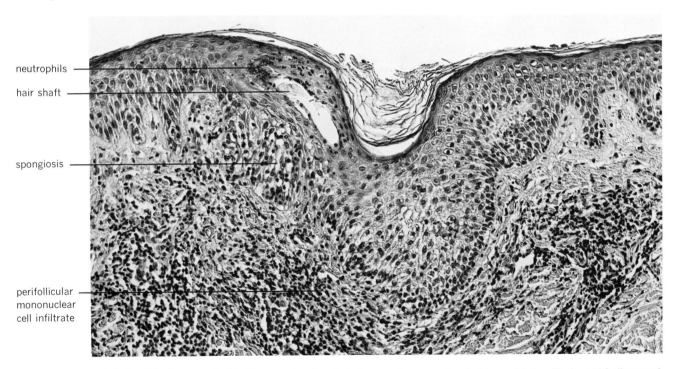

FIG. 12-32. Pseudofolliculitis (ingrown hair). Sharp ends of curly hairs may become directed toward infundibular epithelium and penetrate into dermis instead of emerging through ostium of infundibulum. Cellular infiltrate in adjacent papillary dermis and epidermis is the inflammatory response. (× 196.)

either sterile or contain bacteria of the normal skin flora, namely, coagulase-negative Staphylococci and Corynebacterium acnes. A variant of pseudofolliculitis occurs when a coiled hair springs through the natural container provided by infundibular epithelium and enters the dermis (Fig. 12-33). An inflammatory response to this cornified foreign object ensues. Similar to the phenomenon of pseudofolliculitis of the beard is pseudofolliculitis of the finger webs that occurs in barbers secondary to implantation of human hairs. The histologic response to the introduction of hair into the dermis is the same in all pseudofolliculitides.

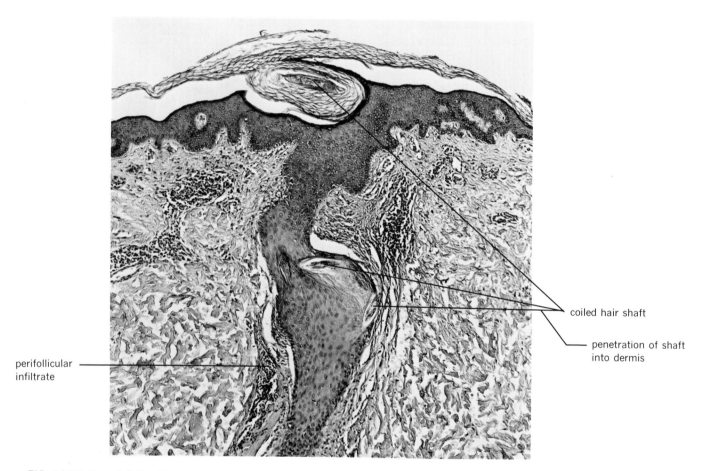

perifollicular
infiltrate

coiled hair shaft

penetration of shaft
into dermis

FIG. 12-33. Pseudofolliculitis. Coiled hair shaft has sprung through infundibular epithelium and now lies partially naked in the dermis. Shortly, neutrophils will accumulate around the cornified foreign body. (× 86.)

Deep Papulonodular Infectious Folliculitis

Deep folliculitis may begin as superficial folliculitis. The suppuration often extends through the follicular wall into the surrounding dermis where it may move downward along the follicle or from the outset involves most, if not the entire length, of the follicular unit. Thus all of the previously discussed superficial folliculitides may become deep folliculitides. As with the superficial types, the deep types may be infectious or noninfectious. Deep infectious folliculitides may be further subdivided as bacterial or dermatophytic.

When the superficial infection of the follicular infundibulum by Staphylococcus aureus (*impetigo of Bockhart*) extends to the hair follicle beneath the infundibulum, a *furuncle* results (Fig. 12-34). Furuncles may arise, however, without preceding superficial folliculitis. Multiple, intercommunicating furuncles constitute a *carbuncle*, a deep staphylococcal infection of a group of hair follicles (Fig. 12-35). Deep infection by Staphylococcus aureus of the entire length of the hair follicles of the beard is termed *sycosis*. *Folliculitis decalvans* is staphylococcal scarring alopecia of the scalp. Thus the terms *furuncle, carbuncle, sycosis,* and *folliculitis decalvans* are different names for variants of the same pathologic process, a deep staphylococcal folliculitis that often results in scarring. During the suppurative phase of deep staphylococcal folliculitis, the bacteria may often be demonstrated with a Gram stain. Later, during the suppurative granulomatous and the granulomatous and fibrosing stages, the organisms are difficult, if not impossible to find. A rare form of deep folliculitis is caused by gram-negative bacteria.

Majocchi's granuloma describes a deep suppurative and granulomatous dermatophytic folliculitis, usually appearing as papules, nodules, and plaques, especially on the shaved legs of women.

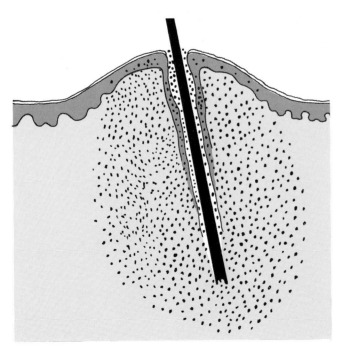

FIG. 12-34. A furuncle.

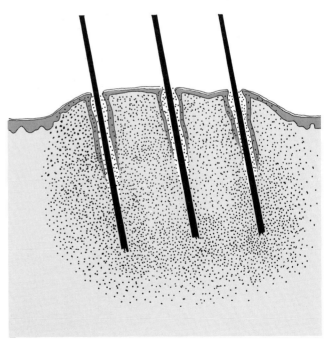

FIG. 12-35. A carbuncle.

Even in sections stained with hematoxylin and eosin, hyphae can usually be identified within the cornified cells of the epidermis and the follicle. PAS stain should be done on all suspicious sections. The earliest histologic findings in Majocchi's granuloma are numerous hyphae within the cornified cells of the hair follicles (Fig. 12-36). Soon suppurative folliculitis ensues, the follicular epithelium ruptures (Fig. 12-37), and follicular contents (including dermatophytic hyphae in cornified cells, especially of hair shafts) are spewed into the dermis (Fig. 12-38). Granulomatous inflammation develops after suppurative inflammation in response to these foreign materials. If the inflammatory reaction is sufficiently intense and destructive, the lesions heal with fibrosis. Clinically, Majocchi's granuloma differs from a superficial dermatophytic folliculitis by being papular and nodular, rather than pustular.

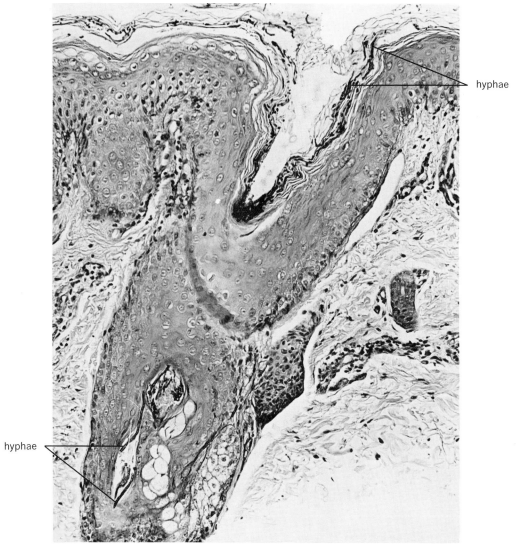

FIG. 12-36. Dermatophytosis. A, Dermatophytic infection of the follicular infundibulum in this section stained by PAS is forerunner of Majocchi's granuloma. Note numerous hyphae within cornified layer of epidermis and infundibulum (× 196.)

Tinea barbae is a deep suppurative folliculitis of the beard, usually caused by Trichophyton mentagrophytes. Because the fungus elements extend all the way down the fully cornified hair shaft to the level of the matrix, the intrafollicular abscesses also extend deep. Usually, the abscess ruptures through the outer root sheath into the dermis, where hyphae, spores, and squames are also expelled. Suppuration is followed by granulomatous inflammation and eventual fibrosis. Clinically, the follicular pustules of tinea barbae evolve into inflamed nodules that slowly resolve with alopecic scars.

Favus is a severe suppurative granulomatous folliculitis usually caused by Trichophyton schoenleinii. Organisms are easily identified in routine and special stains. This chronic infection results in scarring and permanent hair loss.

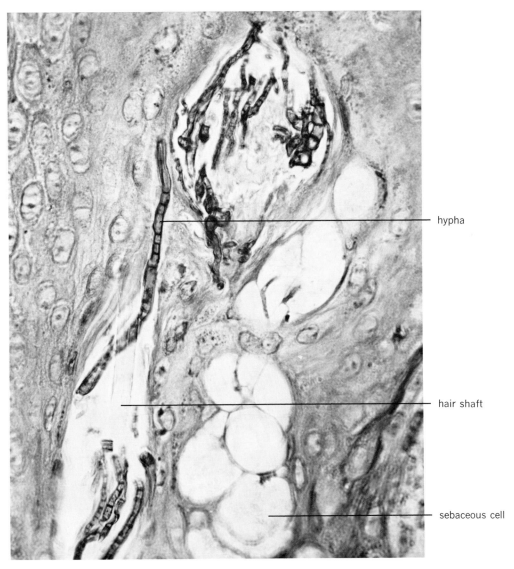

FIG. 12-36. Dermatophytosis. B, Septate hyphae are shown clogging lowest portion of infundibulum near its junction with sebaceous gland. ($\times$ 766.)

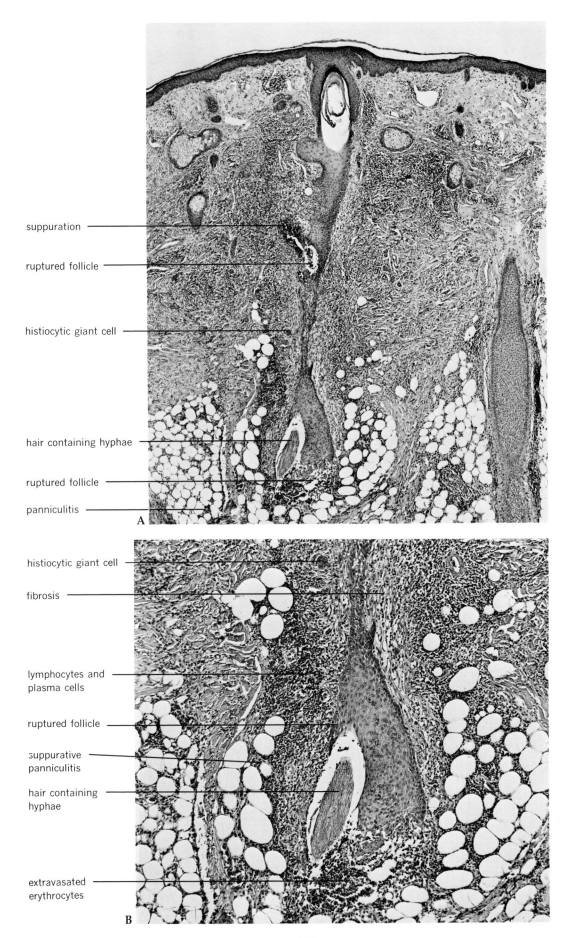

suppuration —

ruptured follicle —

histiocytic giant cell —

hair containing hyphae —

ruptured follicle —

panniculitis —

A

histiocytic giant cell —

fibrosis —

lymphocytes and
plasma cells —

ruptured follicle —

suppurative
panniculitis —

hair containing
hyphae —

extravasated
erythrocytes —

B

FIG. 12-37. Majocchi's granuloma. Legend on page 677.

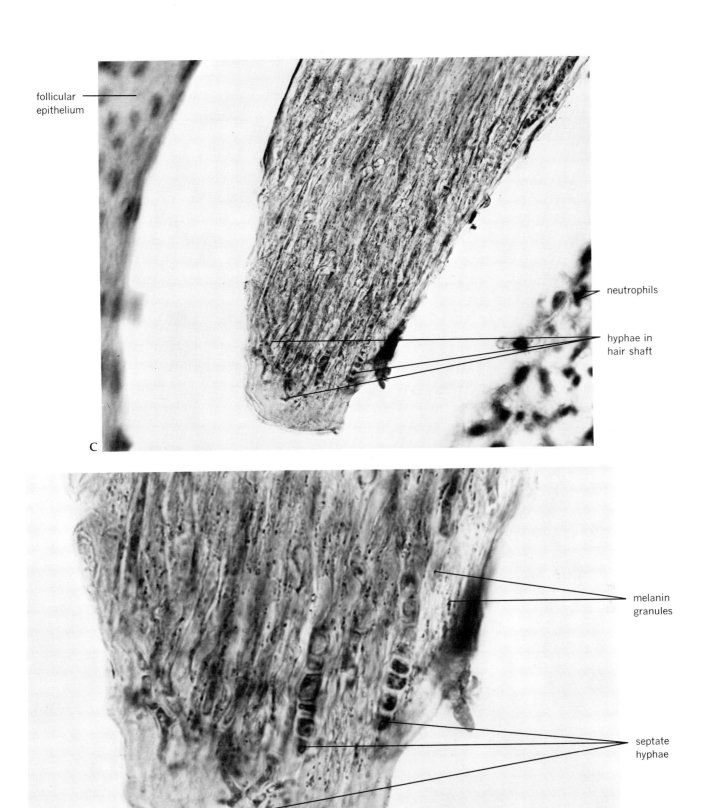

follicular epithelium

neutrophils

hyphae in hair shaft

melanin granules

septate hyphae

hair shaft

C

D

FIG. 12-37. Majocchi's granuloma. The entire sequence of histopathologic changes—infection of cornified cells of hair follicle (including infundibular horn, internal root sheath, and hair shaft) by dermatophytic fungi, rupture of follicular epithelium, discharge of its contents into dermis, suppuration, granulomatous inflammation, and fibrosis—is seen in these photomicrographs. (A, × 35; B, × 76; Fig. 12-37. C, × 706; D, × 1700.)

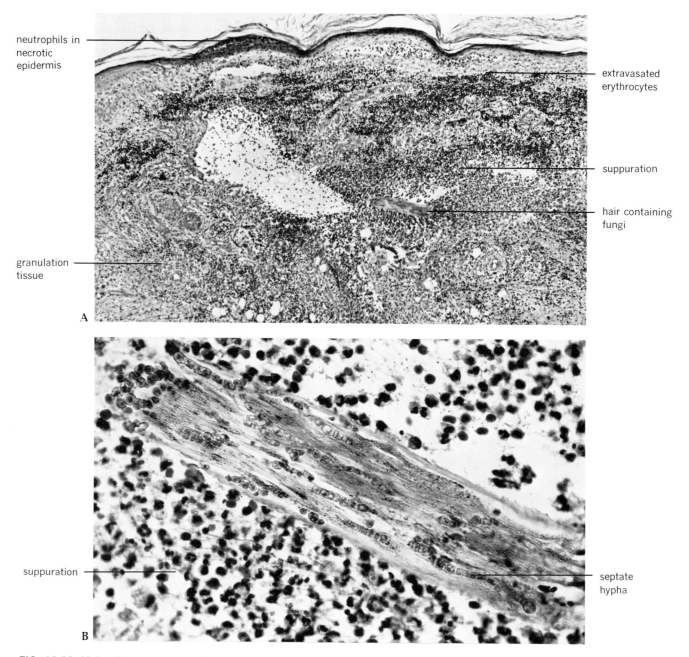

neutrophils in
necrotic
epidermis

extravasated
erythrocytes

suppuration

hair containing
fungi

granulation
tissue

A

suppuration

septate
hypha

B

FIG. 12-38. Majocchi's granuloma. A, Suppuration and granulation tissue are responses to foreign bodies spewed into dermis when hair follicles containing hyphae in cornified cells ruptured. (× 88.) B, Within abscess is hair shaft containing many septate hyphae. (× 740.)

A *kerion* is a deep suppurative folliculitis induced by dermatophytes, especially Microsporum canis and Trichophyton verrucosum in the United States. Unlike in favus, fungi are difficult to demonstrate histologically in a kerion because of the extensive inflammatory-cell infiltrate. These boggy lesions occurring primarily on the scalp, but also on the bearded part of the face and the eyebrows, last for weeks or months and frequently resolve with scarring. Like the lesions of conglobate acne, kerion progresses from follicular abscess to sinus formation and scarring alopecia.

Histologically, the findings in the conglobate form of acne vulgaris (Fig. 12-39), dissecting cellulitis of the scalp (perifolliculitis capitis abscedens et suffodiens), and *hidradenitis suppurativa* (Fig. 12-40) are similar. These are deep folliculitides that proceed to abscess formation (Fig. 12-41), coupled with attempts at re-epithelization of the follicular unit (Fig. 12-42), eventual sinus formation, and finally fibrosis within which hair shafts are trapped (Fig. 12-43). The same can be said for pilonidal sinus. Clinically, all three conditions (i.e., conglobate acne, dissecting cellulitis, and hidradenitis suppurativa) appear as burrowing abscesses that culminate in irregular disfiguring scars that may be either atrophic or keloidal. The term *hidradenitis* is a misnomer because it implies that the process is primarily an inflammation of the apocrine glands, whereas in fact it is a deep folliculitis that secondarily extends to involve the glands and other structures that are deep in the skin.

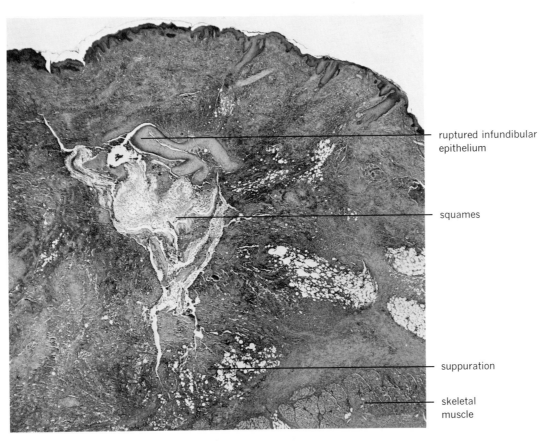

ruptured infundibular epithelium

squames

suppuration

skeletal muscle

FIG. 12-39. Acne conglobata. Subsequent to rupture of infundibular cyst shown, contents of cyst were extruded into dermis and subcutaneous fat with consequent suppuration, granulomatous inflammation, and eventual fibrosis. Note that inflammatory process extends deep into muscle at base of this section. Histologic changes pictured are similar to those of dissecting cellulitis of scalp and hidradenitis suppurativa. (× 14.)

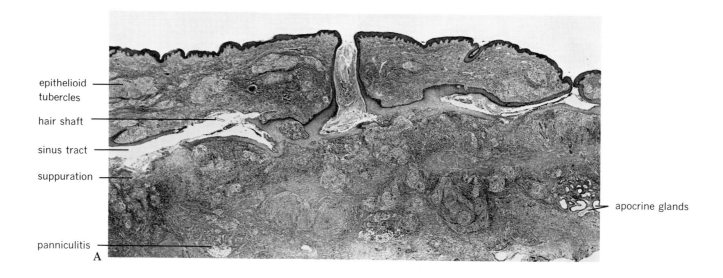

epithelioid tubercles

hair shaft

sinus tract

suppuration

apocrine glands

panniculitis

A

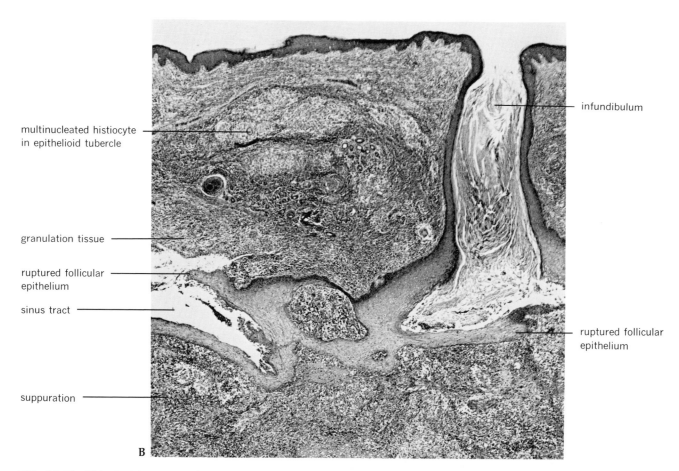

infundibulum

multinucleated histiocyte in epithelioid tubercle

granulation tissue

ruptured follicular epithelium

sinus tract

ruptured follicular epithelium

suppuration

B

FIG. 12-40. Hidradenitis suppurativa. A, Initial events are rupture of follicular infundibula with suppurative inflammation followed, in time, by formation of sinus tracts, granulomatous inflammation, and fibrosis. Apocrine glands at base of this lesion are affected only secondarily, evidence that this is fundamentally an inflammatory disease of hair follicles. The changes pictured are similar to those of conglobate acne, dissecting cellulitis of the scalp, and pilonidal sinus. (× 8.) **B,** Higher magnification shows to better advantage ruptured follicular infundibulum and resultant suppuration, granulomatous inflammation, and hyperplasia of infundibular epithelium. Convoluted epithelial sinuses represent faulty attempts by infundibular epithelium to encompass spewed follicular contents and to restore integrity of hair follicle. (× 34.)

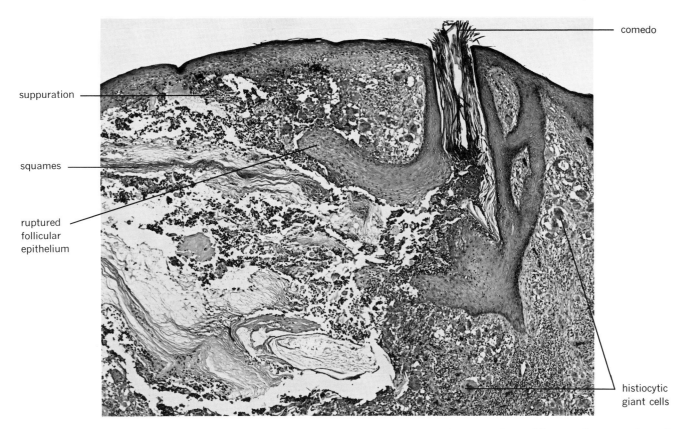

comedo

suppuration

squames

ruptured
follicular
epithelium

histiocytic
giant cells

FIG. 12-41. Cystic acne, acute and subacute stages (folliculitis and suppurative granulomatous dermatitis secondary to rupture of an infundibular cyst). Rupture of infundibular cyst pictured was followed by extrusion of its contents, especially cornified cells (squames), into dermis with subsequent suppuration and granulomatous inflammation. ($\times$ 63.)

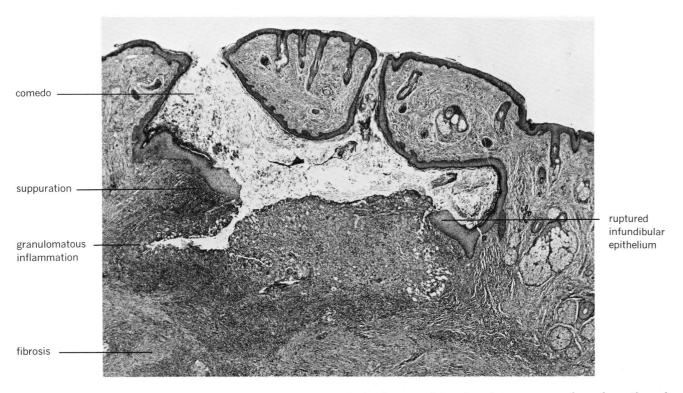

comedo

suppuration

granulomatous
inflammation

fibrosis

ruptured
infundibular
epithelium

FIG. 12-42. Cystic acne, subacute and chronic stages. Histologic changes pictured capture sequence from formation of comedones and infundibular cysts, through rupture of cysts, suppuration, and granulomatous inflammation to fibrosis. ($\times$ 27.)

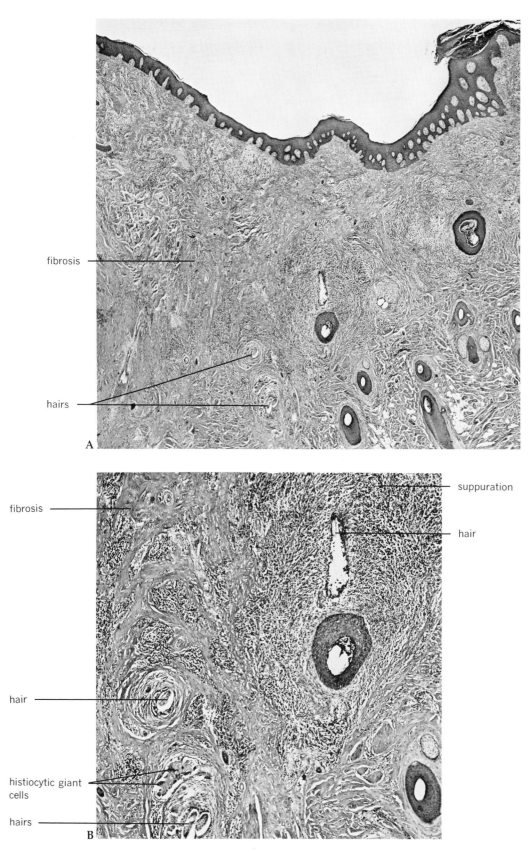

FIG. 12-43. Cystic acne, chronic stage (acne keloidalis). A, Note hair shafts, not within hair follicles, but surrounded by granulomatous inflammation and extensive fibrosis which are late phenomena in process of acne. Note dell in skin surface which would be seen clinically as a depressed scar. (× 17.) B, Higher magnification shows sequence of acne from suppuration around naked hair shafts to granulomatous inflammation around them to eventual fibrosis. (× 39.)

Rosacea, which is fundamentally an inflammatory disease of the infundibula of hair follicles, and its circumscribed variant, *perioral dermatitis*, are characterized clinically by various lesions including erythema, telangiectases, inflammatory papules, nodules, and pustules or any combination of these lesions. Pustular rosacea is a superficial suppurative folliculitis (Fig. 12-44), whereas the papulonodular form of rosacea is a deep suppurative folliculitis that progresses to granulomatous folliculitis and fibrosis (Fig. 12-45).

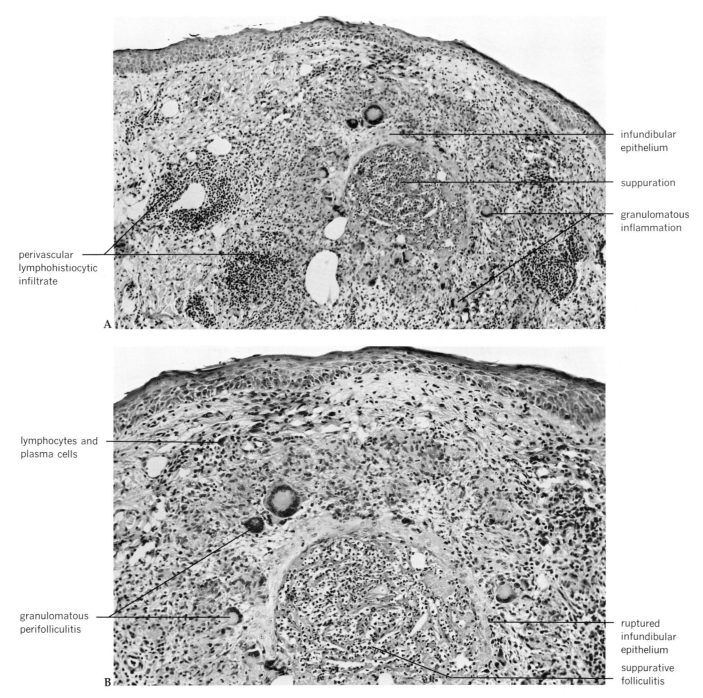

FIG. 12-44. Rosacea, early lesion. Suppuration and granulomatous inflammation and other histologic features may be indistinguishable from those of perioral dermatitis. (A, × 100; B, × 187.)

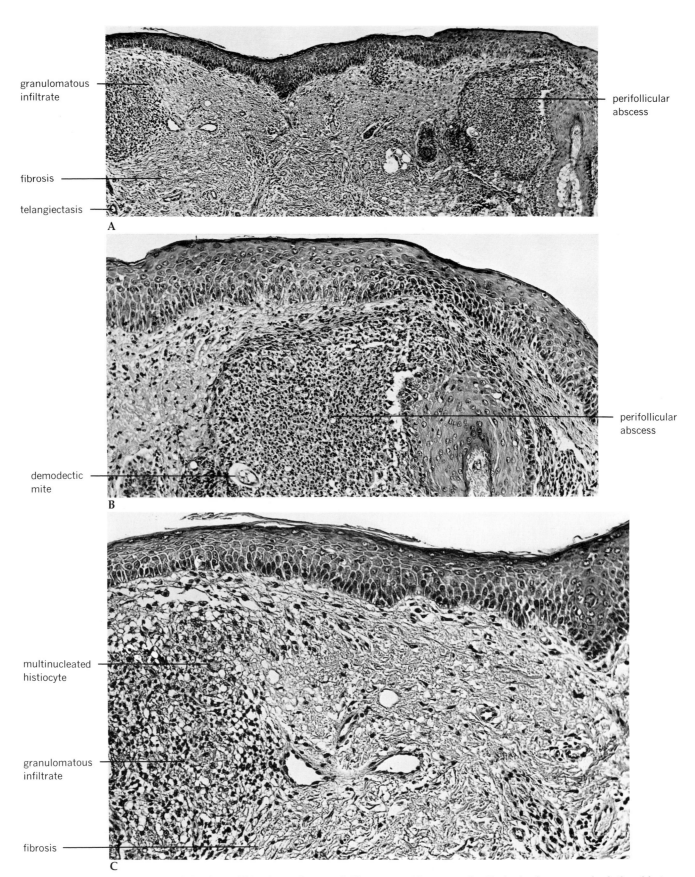

granulomatous infiltrate

perifollicular abscess

fibrosis

telangiectasis

A

perifollicular abscess

demodectic mite

B

multinucleated histiocyte

granulomatous infiltrate

fibrosis

C

FIG. 12-45. Rosacea, papulonodular form. This photomicrograph illustrates wide range of pathologic changes and relationship to abnormalities of hair follicle. On right an abscess contiguous to follicular infundibulum (presumably secondary to leakage of infundibular contents into dermis) is sign of acute stage; on left granulomatous infiltration is sign of subacute stage; and finally, in between are signs of chronicity—fibrosis and telangiectases. (A, × 84; B, × 194; C, × 194.)

Epithelioid tubercles, some with central necrosis, are surrounded by lymphocytes and plasma cells, causing some lesions of rosacea to resemble tuberculosis histologically (thus the misinterpretation of rosacea as rosacea-like tuberculid of Lewandowsky). The epithelioid tubercles are responsible for the papular appearance of some lesions of rosacea. These comments about rosacea apply equally to perioral dermatitis. In addition to the difference in locations of the lesions, rosacea differs from perioral dermatitis in another respect, namely, its association with rhinophyma, a condition that causes bulbous enlargement of the nose, incorrectly and unfairly called "rummy nose." Rhinophyma is due to massive sebaceous-gland hyperplasia associated with infundibular cysts of various sizes that leak their contents or rupture, inducing suppuration and eventually granulomatous dermatitis and scarring. Rosacea, unlike acne vulgaris, has no comedo component.

Perforating folliculitis and *Kyrle's disease* (hyperkeratosis follicularis et parafollicularis in cutem penetrans) have widely dilated infundibula filled with orthokeratotic and parakeratotic cells (Figs. 12-46, 12-47). Sometimes neutrophils are also present within the

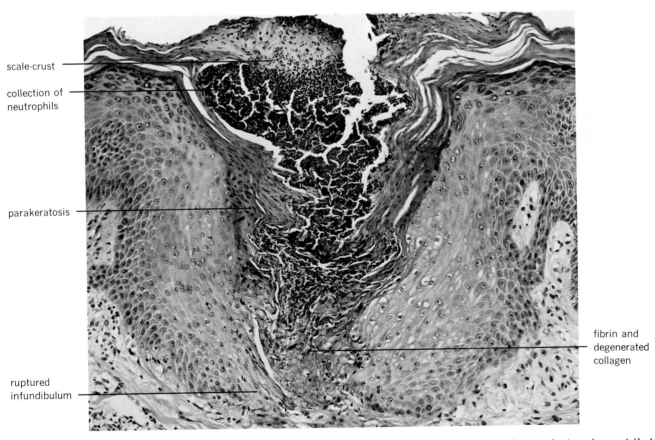

FIG. 12-46. Perforating folliculitis. Widely dilated infundibulum of this ruptured follicle is plugged by purulent scale-crust that extends directly into dermis. The cause or mechanism is not demonstrable by histologic techniques. (× 158.)

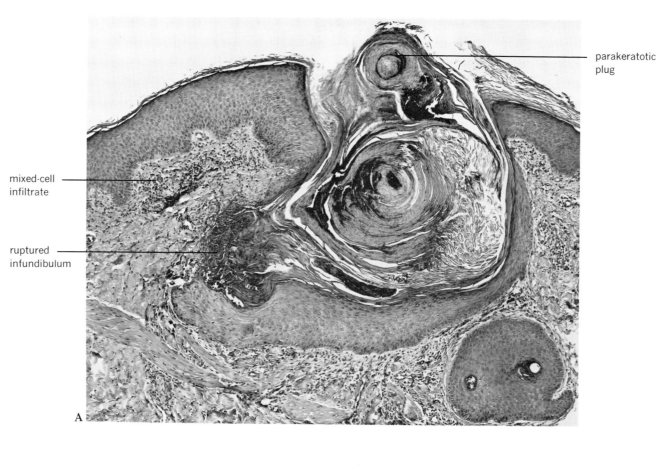

parakeratotic
plug

mixed-cell
infiltrate

ruptured
infundibulum

A

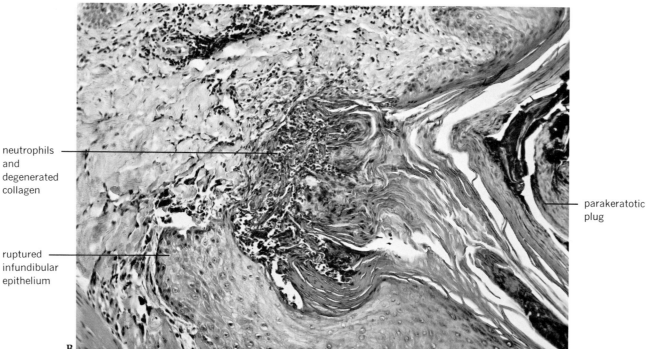

neutrophils
and
degenerated
collagen

parakeratotic
plug

ruptured
infundibular
epithelium

B

FIG. 12-47. Kyrle's disease. A, Huge plug of parakeratotic cells has caused infundibulum to dilate and to rupture with consequent degeneration of adjacent collagen and chemotactic attraction of neutrophils. (× 76.) B, Higher magnification reveals certain similarities between Kyrle's disease and elastosis perforans serpiginosa (Fig. 12-48), namely, rupture of base of infundibulum with neutrophils, degenerated collagen, and sometimes a few eosinophilic, opalescent elastic fibers at site of rupture. Prominent hyperkeratosis within infundibulum differentiates this disease from elastosis perforans serpiginosa. (× 187.)

infundibulum. The cornified plug penetrates through the infundibular epithelium into the dermis where initially there is a collection of neutrophils that later are joined by lymphocytes, histiocytes, and multinucleated histiocytes (giant cells). Clinically, both conditions are characterized by follicular keratotic papules.

Perforating folliculitis is a common phenomenon and, in some instances, may represent nothing more than severe keratosis pilaris in which the cornified plug has penetrated through the infundibular epithelium. Other instances of perforating folliculitis are simply fulminant folliculitides with discharge of purulent infundibular contents through the follicular epithelium into the dermis. Although the break can occur anywhere in the infundibulum from beneath the ostium to immediately above the entrance of the sebaceous duct, neutrophils previously harbored tend to extend down along the hair follicle. Eosinophilic-staining elastic fibers are sometimes intermixed with neutrophils at the junction of the ruptured infundibulum and the dermis.

Kyrle's disease is extremely rare and consists clinically of large reddish-brown keratotic papules, especially on the extremities of diabetics. The large keratotic papules of Kyrle's disease are composed of confluent scale-crusts that emerge from contiguous follicular infundibula. The pathologic findings in Kyrle's disease are simply exaggerations of those in perforating folliculitis.

Perforating folliculitis and Kyrle's disease must be differentiated from *reactive perforating collagenosis,* in which umbilicated papules arise at sites of external trauma in genetically disposed individuals. Histologically, the central umbilication is plugged by a column of degenerated collagen in the papillary dermis, by parakeratotic cells, and by remnants of inflammatory cells. The vertical column extends from the papillary dermis, through the epidermis, and up to the skin surface. One explanation of the events in reactive perforating collagenosis is that, in response to trauma, the collagen in the papillary dermis degenerates and this basophilic-staining mass is then eliminated from the skin by extrusion upward and outward. Reactive perforating collagenosis is not a follicular process.

Elastosis perforans serpiginosa (perforating elastosis) has a distinctive histologic appearance. The follicular infundibulum is widely dilated and plugged by cornified cells that penetrate through the epithelium into the dermis (Fig. 12-48). A collection of neutrophils is present in the dermis at its junction with the ruptured infundibulum. The neutrophils extend through the epithelial channel into the infundibulum where they intermingle with nuclear dust, necrotic cells, and eosinophilic, opalescent elastic fibers (Fig. 12-49). The aberrant elastic fibers are easily visualized in

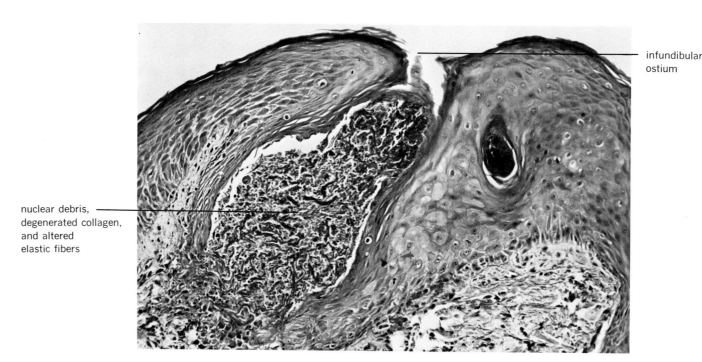

infundibular
ostium

nuclear debris,
degenerated collagen,
and altered
elastic fibers

FIG. 12-48. Elastosis perforans serpiginosa. Diagnostic features pictured within ruptured infundibulum are neutrophils, degenerated collagen, and numerous eosinophilic, opalescent, thickened elastic fibers. Follicular ostium in an instance like this may be mistakenly interpreted to be a perforation of epidermis rather than that of a preexisting follicular infundibulum. (× 209.)

sections stained with hematoxylin and eosin, but they are more readily demonstrated with elastic tissue stains. These unusual intrafollicular elastic fibers, coupled with increased numbers of elastic fibers in the papillary dermis, are the features that distinguish elastosis perforans serpiginosa from perforating folliculitis (Fig. 12-50), Kyrle's disease, and other folliculitides in which there is also rupture of the infundibular epithelium. The finding of altered elastic fibers alone in relationship to the infundibulum is not diagnostic of elastosis perforans serpiginosa; they can be seen in any suppurative folliculitis. Although the pathologic process in elastosis perforans serpiginosa usually involves follicular infundibula, occasionally the epidermis may be the critical site.

Clinically, elastosis perforans serpiginosa presents keratotic follicular papules arranged in arcuate, annular, or serpiginous fashion, especially on the neck, face, or upper extremities of males. It tends to be associated with other connective tissue abnormalities such as the Ehlers-Danlos syndrome, Marfan's syndrome, or osteogenesis imperfecta and with Down's syndrome in which it may be widespread. In pseudoxanthoma elasticum, there is perforation of the distinctive "steel-wool" elastic fibers through the epidermis, but no elastosis perforans serpiginosa.

A halogenoderma, especially bromoderma, may begin as a superficial folliculitis, evolve into a deep folliculitis, and resolve with fibrosis (Fig. 12-51).

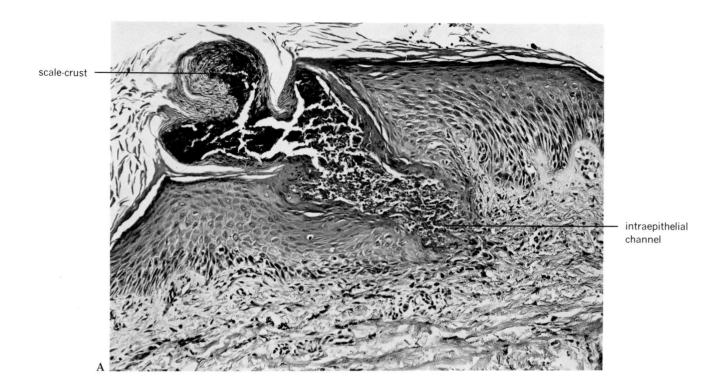

scale-crust

intraepithelial channel

A

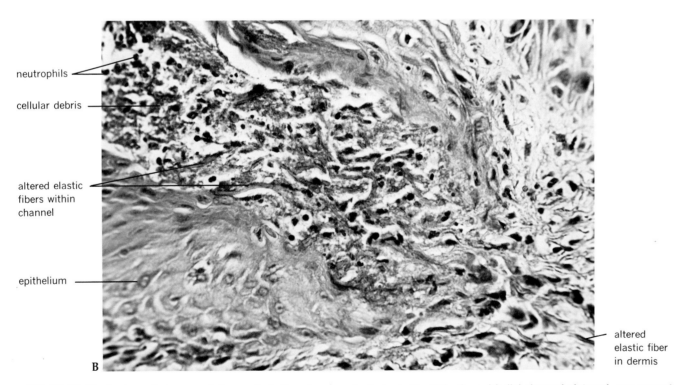

neutrophils

cellular debris

altered elastic fibers within channel

epithelium

altered elastic fiber in dermis

B

FIG. 12-49. Elastosis perforans serpiginosa. A, In the absence of a hair shaft within the epithelial channel pictured, one cannot identify it with certainty as a follicular infundibulum, despite its suggestive funnel-shaped configuration. The alternative interpretation is that a channel unassociated with a hair follicle has formed in epidermis. ($\times$ 211.) B, In this higher magnification diagnostic histologic changes may be better appreciated, namely, altered elastic fibers in upper part of dermis and within epithelial channel where neutrophils and cellular debris are intermingled. ($\times$ 624.)

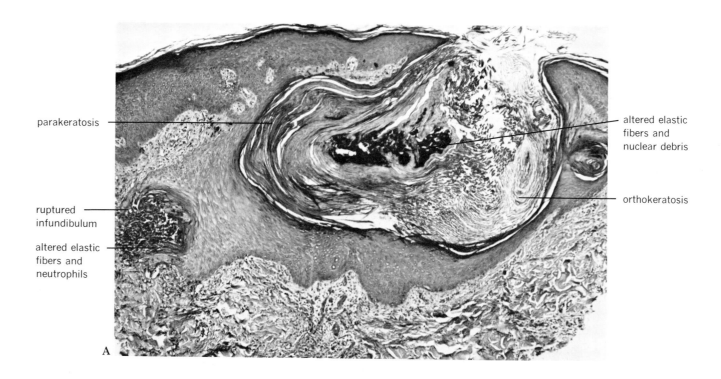

parakeratosis

altered elastic
fibers and
nuclear debris

ruptured
infundibulum

altered elastic
fibers and
neutrophils

orthokeratosis

A

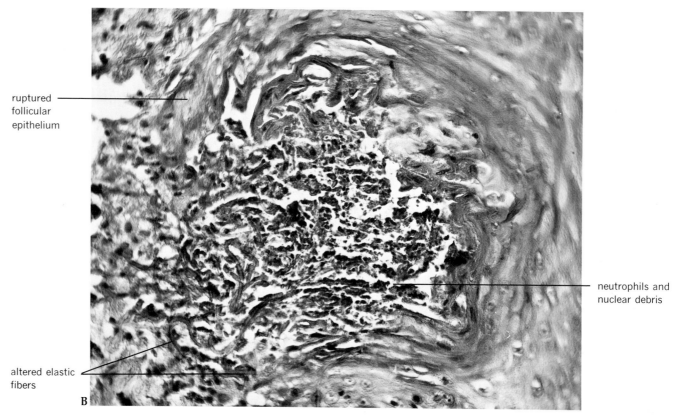

ruptured
follicular
epithelium

neutrophils and
nuclear debris

altered elastic
fibers

B

FIG. 12-50. Elastosis perforans serpiginosa or perforating folliculitis? Infundibulum of lesion is widened and plugged by orthokeratotic and parakeratotic cells, altered elastic fibers, neutrophils, and cellular debris. Collection of altered elastic fibers and neutrophils appears to be engulfed by tongs of epithelium from ruptured infundibulum. These are features of perforating folliculitis, the diagnosis I favor because of extensive hyperkeratosis within widened follicular infundibulum. Patient had no clinical signs of elastosis perforans serpiginosa. (A, × 79; B, × 374.)

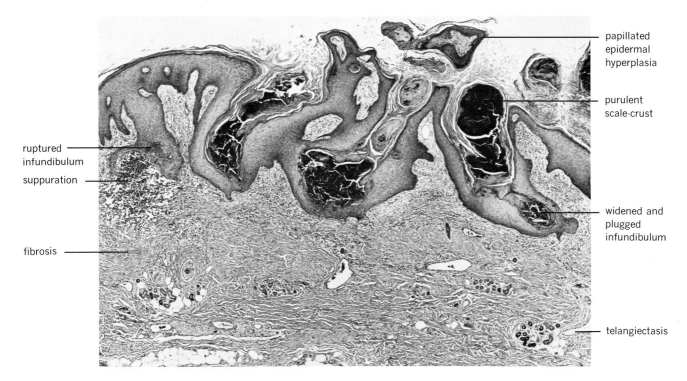

FIG. 12-51. Bromoderma. The changes pictured, stereotypic of all halogenodermas, are those of suppurative folliculitis, which, if deep enough and enduring, may proceed to fibrosis. Portions of five affected infundibula are shown in this photomicrograph. (× 38.)

Spongiotic Folliculitis

In infundibulofolliculitis, atopic dermatitis, and Fox-Fordyce disease there are small spongiotic foci within follicular infundibula associated with a very sparse superficial perivascular lympho-histiocytic infiltrate. Clinically, *infundibulofolliculitis* consists of innumerable, pinpoint skin-colored follicular papules especially on the trunk and proximal portions of the upper extremities of black people, each papule representing an infundibulum altered by very slight spongiosis (Fig. 12-52).

The spongiotic folliculitis of *atopic dermatitis* is seen only in the follicular papules associated with that disease (Figs. 12-53). More commonly, the manifestations of atopic dermatitis are flexural erosions, ulcerations, and lichen simplex chronicus, changes due to scratching and prolonged rubbing of pruritic skin. Whether the spongiotic changes within the infundibula of follicular papules are directly related to the atopic state and whether there are, in fact, any recognizably characteristic pathologic changes in atopic dermatitis, has yet to be determined with certainty. The spongiotic changes are probably not related to the mechanism of the disease. Unfortunately, most biopsy specimens submitted with the clinical diagnosis of atopic dermatitis show histologic signs of scratching and rubbing only.

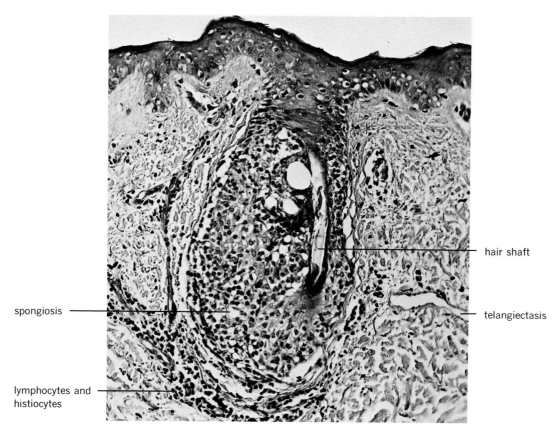

hair shaft

spongiosis

telangiectasis

lymphocytes and
histiocytes

FIG. 12-52. Infundibulofolliculitis. Slight spongiotic changes in infundibulum illustrated would be seen clinically as a tiny follicular papule in skin of black person. (× 204.)

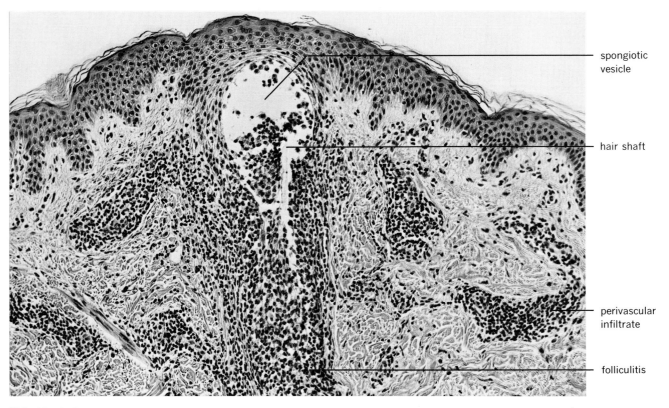

spongiotic
vesicle

hair shaft

perivascular
infiltrate

folliculitis

FIG. 12-53. Atopic dermatitis, follicular papule. Spongiosis involving infundibulum is well illustrated in early lesion. (× 186.)

The spongiosis in *Fox-Fordyce disease* occurs at the site in the infundibulum where the apocrine duct enters it (Fig. 12-54). The infundibula are widely dilated by plugs of orthokeratotic cells that extend above the skin surface. These plugs impart the clinical appearance of grouped, conical, skin-colored, follicular papules, whose sites of predilection are the axillary, periumbilical, and pubic regions. The disease most commonly develops in girls shortly after puberty.

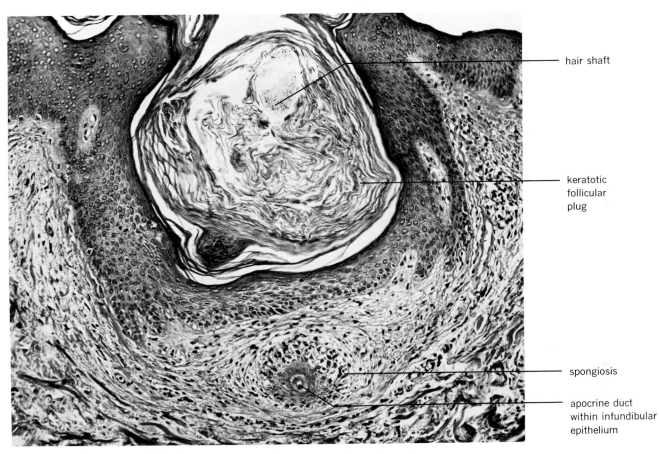

FIG. 12-54. Fox-Fordyce disease. Histologic features illustrated are keratotic follicular plug and spongiosis around apocrine duct at its junction with infundibular epithelium. (× 165.)

Nonscarring Inflammatory Alopecias

The types of alopecia are many, but the known causes and mechanisms of hair loss are few. Although the diagnosis of alopecia can often be made clinically, in numerous instances the histologic features are critical to precise identification. In order for clinical and histologic scrutiny of the diseased scalp to be meaningful, the examiner must be fully conversant with the normal anatomy. Microscopic judgments about pathologic processes involving the hair follicles should take into account the presence or absence of an inflammatory-cell infiltrate, the character and location of the infiltrate, the presence or absence of fibrosis, the extent and location of the fibrosis, the status of the follicles vis-a-vis the anagen-catagen-telogen cycle, microorganisms being causal, and the condition of the hair shaft itself.

The frequent therapeutic failures in the management of scalp diseases have dampened the dermatologist's interest in pursuing a histologic confirmatory diagnosis. Knowledge of the follicular and dermal changes can yield important diagnostic, therapeutic, and prognostic information. To ensure a meaningful interpretation by

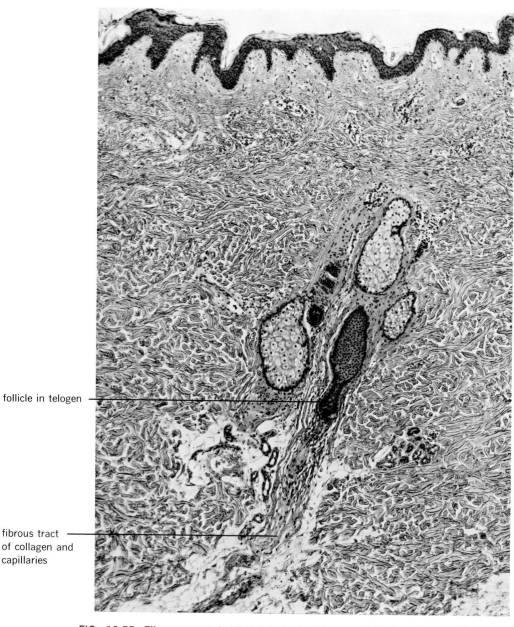

follicle in telogen

fibrous tract of collagen and capillaries

FIG. 12-55. Fibrous tract behind follicle in telogen. Delicate collagen fibrils and elongated dilated capillaries shown here arranged in a tract have formed normally in path of hair follicle as it ascended into position of telogen phase of hair cycle. (× 68.)

the pathologist, fusiform surgical biopsies should be no smaller than 1 cm in length and should include subcutaneous tissue.

A distinction must be made between the fibrous tracts that form behind hair follicles as they ascend into telogen as occurs normally and in nonscarring alopecias such as telogen effluvium and common (androgenic) baldness (Fig. 12-55), and the fibrotic tracts that completely replace hair follicles in some scarring alopecias (Fig. 12-56). A fibrous tract consists of delicate fibrillary collagen, whereas a fibrotic tract is composed of coarse, usually sclerotic collagen.

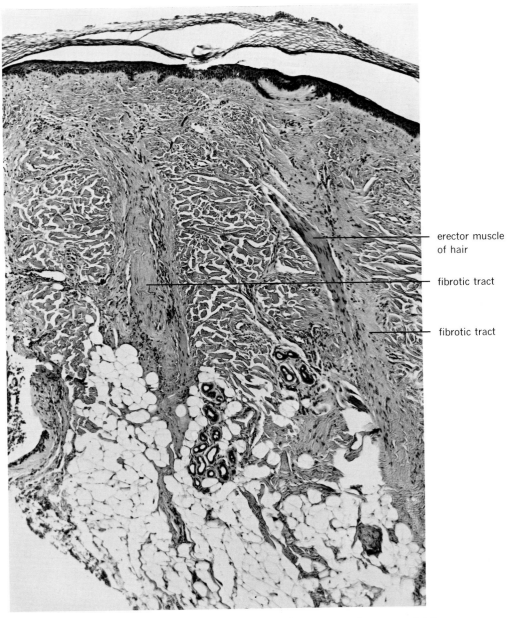

erector muscle of hair

fibrotic tract

fibrotic tract

FIG. 12-56. Fibrotic tracts replacing hair follicles. Fibrotic tracts have completely replaced follicles, resulting in permanent scarred alopecia. Note that muscles of arrectores pilorum remain after follicular epithelial elements have been destroyed. (× 68.)

Alopecia areata (Fig. 12-57)

—Predominantly lymphocytic infiltrate around blood vessels in the hair papillae and around the hair bulbs and vascular plexuses
—Increased numbers of catagen and telogen hairs
—Fibrous tracts in path of telogen hairs
—Widely dilated capillaries, apparently increased in number, in the regions of the original hair papillae
—Melanophages at the original sites of the hair papillae
—Increased numbers of mast cells around blood vessels in fibrous tracts and among collagen bundles throughout the dermis
—Few normal hair follicles amid involuting and resting ones

Early lesions of alopecia areata are characterized by a predominantly lymphocytic infiltrate around the dilated capillaries and venules in the vicinity of hair bulbs (Fig. 12-58). The lymphocytes have been likened to a swarm of bees (Fig. 12-58B). Many hair follicles will be in catagen and telogen (Fig. 12-59). The involvement of hair follicles by the pathologic process is consonant with the clinical findings in which hairs are lost completely in circumscribed areas. This feature is in contrast to trichotillomania in which some follicles in a histologic section are spared because the patient usually does not tamper with every single hair in a particular locus, but pulls, tugs, and twists hairs randomly.

Late lesions show only whorls of sclerosis in the deep reticular dermis, tombstones of former follicles (Fig. 12-60). Masses of melanin are often present within these discrete sclerotic "onion-skin" residues. The sclerotic whorls probably represent a combination of entrapped thickened glassy membranes of catagen hairs and perifollicular fibrous sheaths.

The fibrous tracts seen in alopecia areata are an expected finding in the wake of telogen hair follicles (Fig. 12-61). These fibrous tracts do not signify permanent hair loss as do the fibrotic tracts that are associated with some scarring alopecias, such as in lichen planopilaris and chronic discoid lupus erythematosus. The presence of sclerotic whorls, however, signifies permanent hair loss in alopecia areata.

In alopecia areata there is a sudden cessation of hair-matrix activity during anagen. This stoppage predisposes to eventual breakage of the hair shaft. By the time the shaft actually breaks, the follicle has begun to taper toward the base as a result of transformation into catagen or telogen. The term *exclamation-point hair* has been applied to these tapered club hairs that remain.

Alopecia areata takes the clinical forms of hair loss confined to sharply circumscribed, smooth, white, round-to-oval patches;

alopecia totalis is complete loss of scalp hair, and alopecia universalis is complete loss of hair everywhere. The most active areas, as gauged by the density of the lymphocytic infiltrate, are at the periphery of the patches. In some patients the hair loss is permanent as when sclerotic whorls have developed at former sites of papillae and hair bulbs. In others there often is spontaneous and

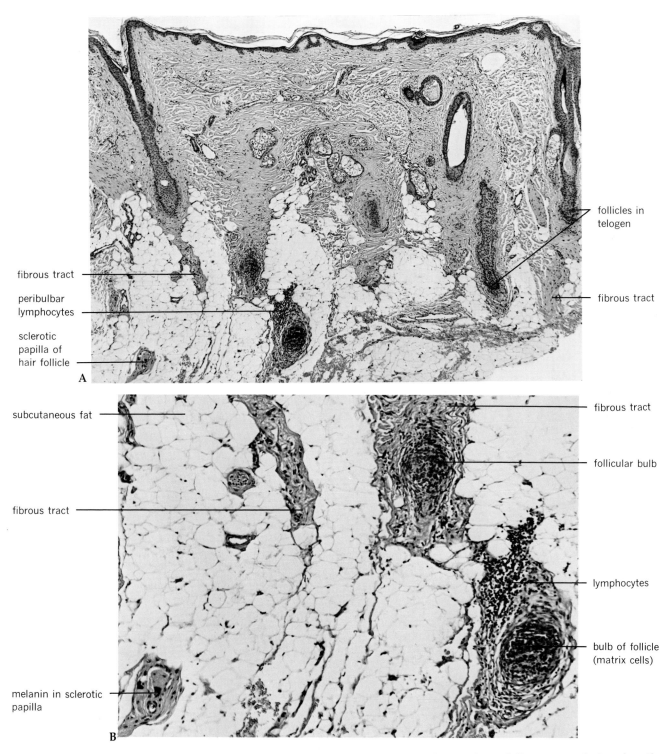

fibrous tract

peribulbar lymphocytes

sclerotic papilla of hair follicle

A

follicles in telogen

fibrous tract

subcutaneous fat

fibrous tract

melanin in sclerotic papilla

B

fibrous tract

follicular bulb

lymphocytes

bulb of follicle (matrix cells)

FIG. 12-57. Alopecia areata, subacute lesion. In this stage there are some features of acute phase of disease, namely, lymphocytic infiltrates in regions of follicular papillae and bulbs, as well as features that bespeak chronicity such as sclerosis of papillae. Note that several follicles are in telogen and are marked by fibrous tracts. (A, × 57; B, × 123.)

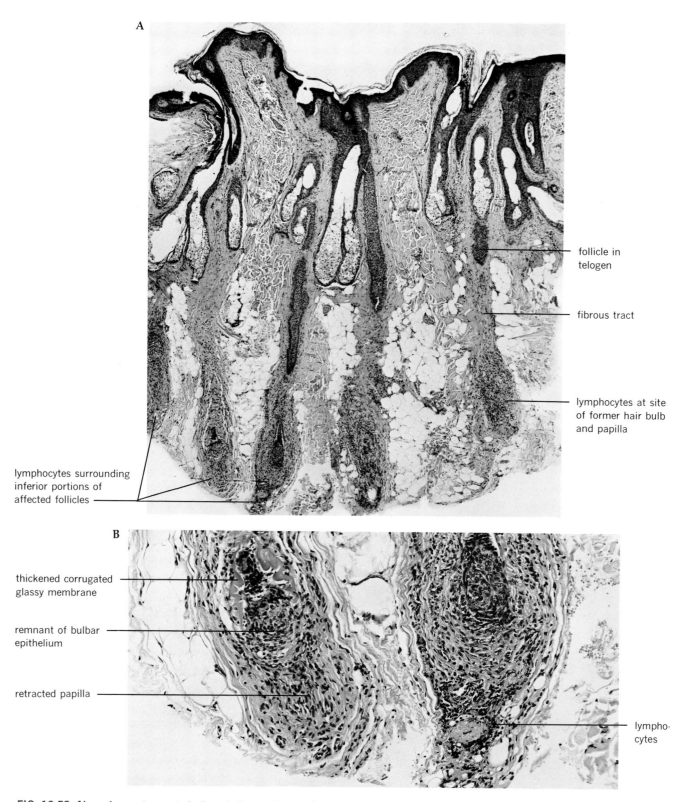

A

follicle in
telogen

fibrous tract

lymphocytes at site
of former hair bulb
and papilla

lymphocytes surrounding
inferior portions of
affected follicles

B

thickened corrugated
glassy membrane

remnant of bulbar
epithelium

retracted papilla

lympho-
cytes

FIG. 12-58. Alopecia areata, acute lesion. A, Predominantly lymphocytic infiltrate surrounds bulbs and papillae of each hair follicle shown in this biopsy specimen from relatively early lesion. Note that every follicle is affected by pathologic process. (× 43.) B, Follicle on left has entered catagen as can be judged by thickened, corrugated, glassy membrane. Follicle on right is probably also in catagen because bulbar epithelium has withered, although no characteristic thickening of glassy membrane is seen. (× 167.)

complete return of the hairs, although in some the terminal hairs are replaced by vellus ones. Hair regrowth is not always accompanied by restoration of pigment. Patches of white hairs may be found among the normally pigmented ones. In addition to abnormalities of the hair follicles in alopecia areata, there can be pits and ridges in the nails and vitiligo of the skin.

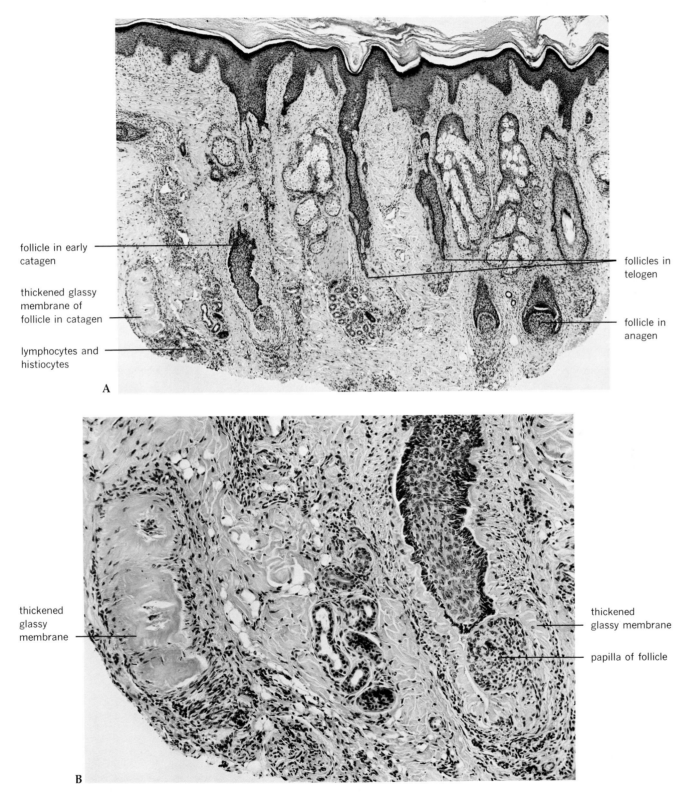

follicle in early catagen

thickened glassy membrane of follicle in catagen

lymphocytes and histiocytes

follicles in telogen

follicle in anagen

A

thickened glassy membrane

thickened glassy membrane

papilla of follicle

B

FIG. 12-59. Alopecia areata, subacute lesion. A, All of hair follicles pictured are degenerating or are about to degenerate. (× 53.) B, Both follicles pictured are in catagen phase of the hair cycle as is told by their thickened, corrugated, glassy (hyaline) membranes. (× 167.)

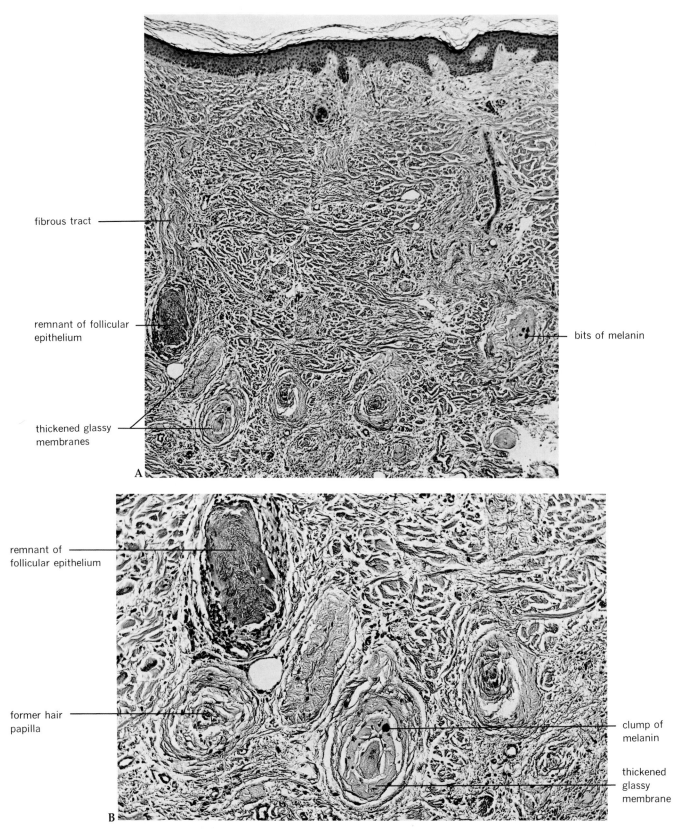

FIG. 12-60. Alopecia areata, chronic lesion. A, Few or no remnants of follicular epithelium are left. Telltale signs of former hair follicles are merely sclerotic hair papillae surrounded by thickened, corrugated, glassy membranes. The absence of any inflammatory-cell infiltrate is another indication of chronicity of this process. (× 70.) B and C, In these higher magnifications sclerotic papillae and thickened glassy membranes are better visualized. Note that the process is confined to regions of hair follicles and that surrounding dermis is unaffected. (B, × 176; C, × 353.)

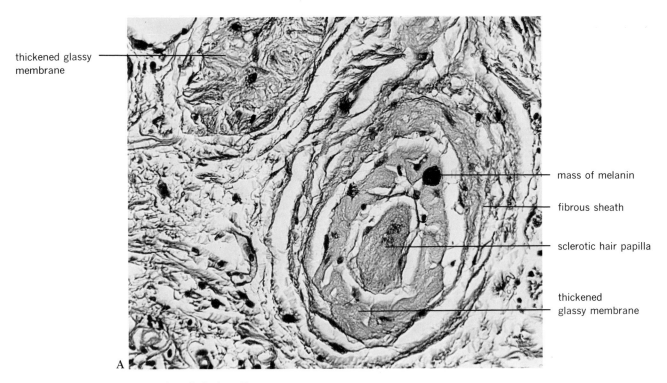

thickened glassy
membrane

mass of melanin

fibrous sheath

sclerotic hair papilla

thickened
glassy membrane

A

FIG. 12-60. Alopecia areata, chronic lesion. C

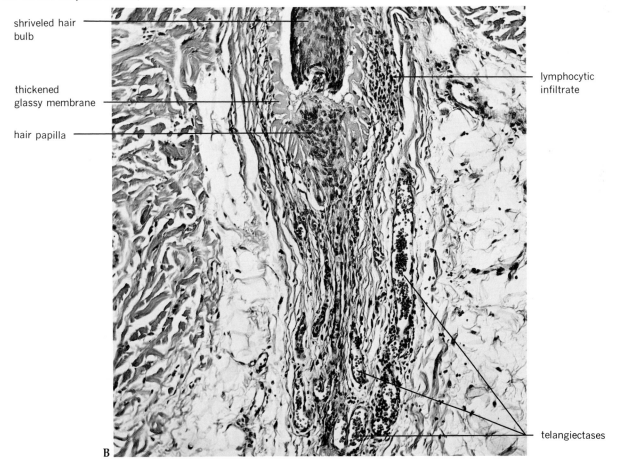

shriveled hair
bulb

thickened
glassy membrane

hair papilla

lymphocytic
infiltrate

telangiectases

B

FIG. 12-61. Alopecia areata, fibrous tract. Histologic changes typical of early stage of alopecia areata are sparse lymphocytic infiltrate and telangiectases in wake of ascending catagen hair. Characteristic marker of catagen follicle is thickened convoluted glassy membrane surrounding effete hair bulb. (× 169.)

Trichotillomania and Traction Alopecia (Fig. 12-62)

—Sparse perivascular lymphohistiocytic infiltrate throughout the dermis
—Increased numbers of catagen and telogen hairs
—Some normal hair follicles amid the involuting and resting ones
—Melanophages at the original sites of hair papillae
—Separation of hair follicle epithelium from surrounding connective tissue
—Everted trichilemmal sheaths, occasionally
—Crumpled, plicated, hair shafts (trichomalacia) within some follicles
—Small collections of extravasated erythrocytes within and around some follicles
—No hairs in some follicles
—Perifollicular fibrosis, occasionally
—Fibrotic tracts replace hair follicles in long-standing cases

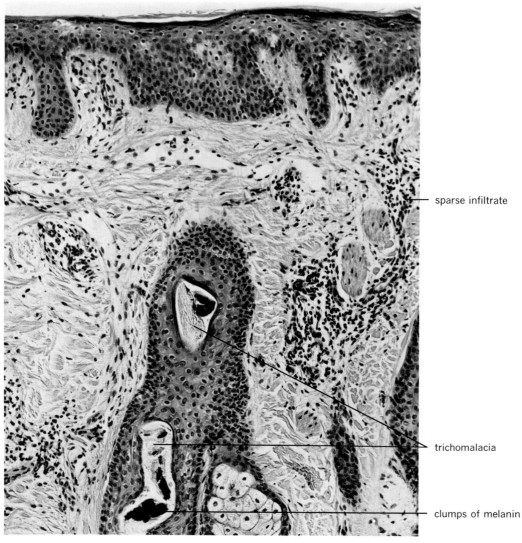

sparse infiltrate

trichomalacia

clumps of melanin

FIG. 12-62. Trichotillomania. (A, × 176.) Refer to B and C on pages 703 and 704.

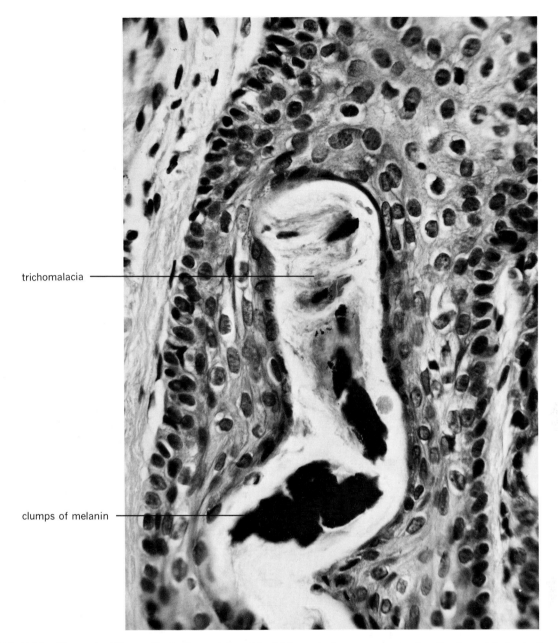

trichomalacia

clumps of melanin

FIG. 12-62. Trichotillomania. Diagnostic feature pictured is trichomalacia, appearance of softening of hair shaft, caused by twisting, turning, and pulling it. Morphologic signs are focal dissolution of hair shafts and irregular clumps of melanin within them. B, (× 593.)

The crucial features for histologic diagnosis of trichotillomania and traction alopecia are increased numbers of catagen and telogen hairs in a dermis containing a meager inflammatory-cell infiltrate. Catagen hairs are easily recognized by their thickened, corrugated glassy membranes. The relative numbers of catagen, telogen, and anagen hair follicles depend upon the time elapsed between plucking hairs and biopsy. If the biopsy is obtained days after hairs have been plucked, several follicles will be in catagen and practically none in telogen. If the biopsy is taken some weeks after plucking, no hairs will be in catagen but several will be in telogen.

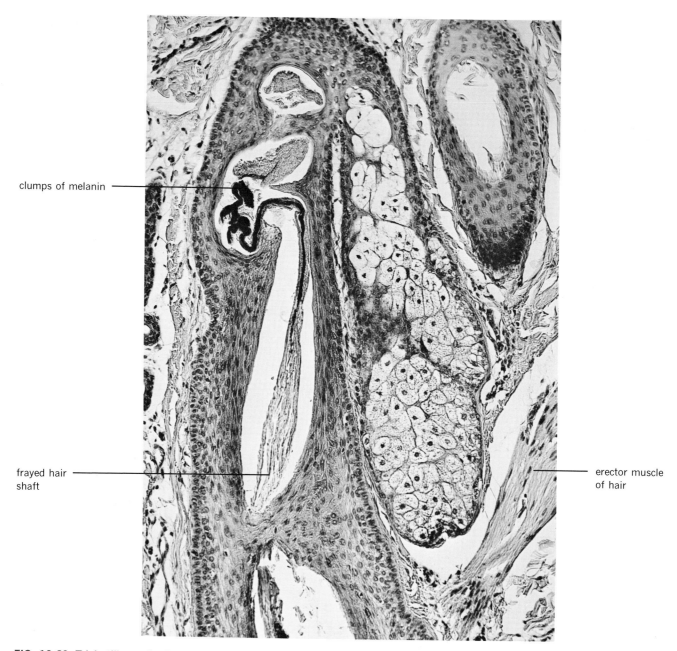

clumps of melanin

frayed hair shaft

erector muscle of hair

FIG. 12-62. Trichotillomania. C, Note fraying of hair shaft and clumping of pigment. (× 180.)

Clinically, trichotillomania is a hair-pulling and plucking habit that results in irregularly-shaped, poorly-circumscribed, partially alopecic patches. The broken-off hairs vary in length and are intermingled with normal hairs. When the habit is corrected, the hairs grow normally. Prolonged traction on the hair can result in permanent alopecia, seen histologically as fibrotic tracts at sites of former follicles. Scarring occurs both at sites of former follicles and in the interfollicular dermis when hot oil burns the scalp secondary to attempts to straighten hair by use of hot combs and petrolatum.

—Mucin within trichilemmal sheaths, sebaceous glands, and possibly the interfollicular epidermis
—Mixed inflammatory-cell infiltrate of lymphocytes, plasma cells, histiocytes, histiocytic giant cells, and eosinophils of varying density around the dermal blood vessels, among collagen bundles, and within the affected follicles (Fig. 12-64)

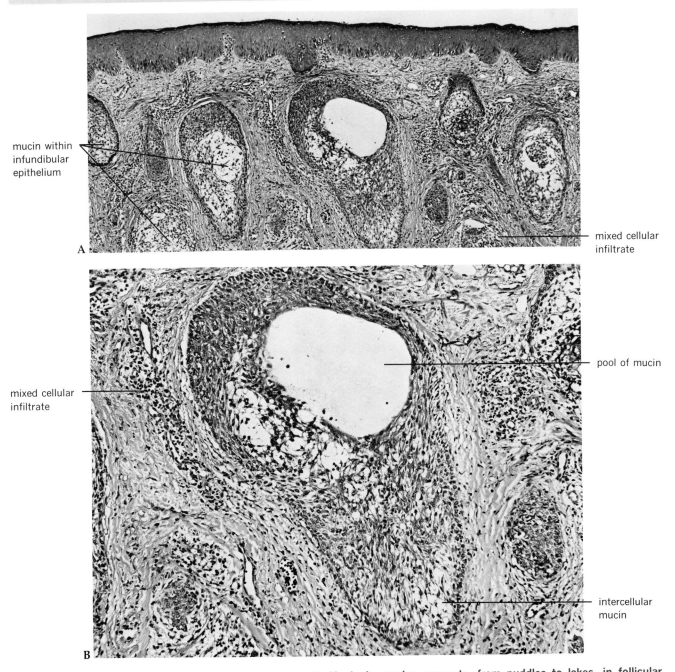

mucin within infundibular epithelium

mixed cellular infiltrate

A

mixed cellular infiltrate

pool of mucin

intercellular mucin

B

FIG. 12-63. Follicular mucinosis in alopecia mucinosa. A, Mucin in varying amounts, from puddles to lakes, in follicular infundibula denotes primary form because no signs of another pathologic process such as mycosis fungoides are present. (× 80.) B, Note mixed inflammatory-cell infiltrate accompanying primary form and inflammatory cells in follicles with mucin deposits. (× 165.)

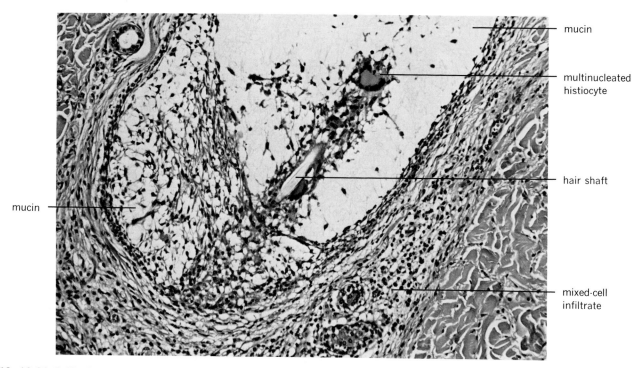

mucin

multinucleated
histiocyte

hair shaft

mixed-cell
infiltrate

mucin

FIG. 12-64. Follicular mucinosis. In addition to abundant mucin within follicular epithelium, an infiltrate of inflammatory cells is seen within dermis and involved follicles. Occasionally histiocytic giant cells as pictured may be present in involved follicles. (× 198.)

The acid mucopolysaccharide in follicular mucinosis is hyaluronic acid, presumably manufactured by the follicular epithelium rather than by fibroblasts. Follicular mucinosis may occur as a primary process, sui generis, as slightly pink, indurated, alopecic plaques composed of numerous closely set follicular papules (alopecia mucinosa). This primary type of follicular mucinosis develops most commonly in children and young adults and is a wholly benign inflammatory process.

Mucin deposition within pilosebaceous epithelium is also seen occasionally as a secondary phenomenon in plaques of malignant lymphoma, especially of mycosis fungoides, and other diseases such as angiolymphoid hyperplasia with eosinophils. Deposition of follicular mucin in the lesions of these diseases is a histologic concomitant of the underlying pathologic process and seems to be entirely unrelated biologically to primary follicular mucinosis.

Follicular mucinosis is but one of many examples of morphologic expressions of altered epithelial metabolism in the skin. In this sense follicular mucinosis is analogous to epidermolytic hyperkeratosis, focal acantholytic dyskeratosis, and cornoid lamellation. I think that confusion would be avoided if the term *follicular mucinosis* was used only histologically, e.g., follicular mucinosis in diseases like alopecia mucinosa, mycosis fungoides, and angiolymphoid hyperplasia.

—Perifollicular lymphohistiocytic infiltrate with plasma cells
—Mononuclear-cell infiltrate with plasma cells around blood vessels throughout the dermis
—Similar infiltrate may obscure dermoepidermal junction of the hyperplastic epidermis
—Increased numbers of telogen and catagen hairs

The patchy irregular hair loss in secondary syphilis is often aptly described as "moth-eaten."

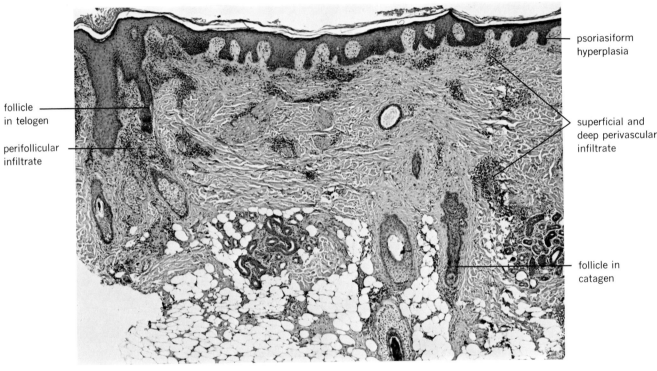

FIG. 12-65. Alopecia of secondary syphilis. Histologic features seen are hair follicles in catagen and telogen and perivascular infiltrate of histiocytes, lymphocytes, and plasma cells throughout dermis and even in subcutaneous fat. Note that infiltrates of inflammatory cells are present around papillae of hair follicles, probably factors in eventual alopecia. (× 56.)

Scarring Inflammatory Alopecias

There are two major types of scarring alopecia. One consists of scarring only in the region of the hair follicle, as in lichen planopilaris, and is seen histologically as linear fibrotic tracts that replace the follicles. The other consists of diffuse scarring throughout the dermis, as occurs following deep ulcers caused by burns, acute radiodermatitis, or following inflammatory processes such as necrobiosis lipoidica.

Scleroderma (Fig. 12-66)

In scleroderma there is initial involvement of the dermis and the subcutaneous fat by a predominantly mononuclear-cell infiltrate (see Chapter 7). With time, severe sclerosis occurs in both the dermis and the subcutis causing obliteration of adnexal epithelium, especially the pilosebaceous units. The sclerotic changes wrought throughout the dermis slowly strangle the hair follicles, but the muscles, elements of the arrectores pilorum, are more resistant and remain intact after the follicles have been destroyed (Fig. 12-66). The result is permanent scarring alopecia.

Scarring alopecia can occur in all forms of scleroderma—morphea, guttate, linear (including en coup de sabre), facial hemiatrophy (Romberg's syndrome), acrosclerosis, and diffuse.

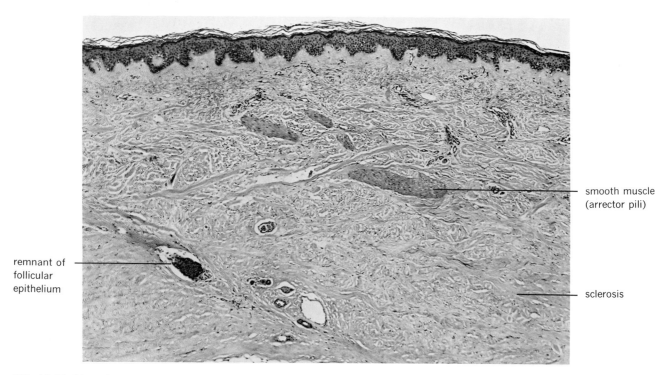

FIG. 12-66. Alopecia caused by scleroderma. Remnant of hair follicle is seen at left. Note that smooth muscle of arrector pili is intact. (× 67.)

Necrobiosis Lipoidica (Fig. 12-67)

Like scleroderma, necrobiosis lipoidica is a chronic progressive inflammatory disease that eventuates in sclerosis of the dermis and subcutaneous fat (see Chapter 9). Hair follicles are destroyed by the sclerosing process. Clinically the shiny atrophic patches of necrobiosis lipoidica are devoid of hairs.

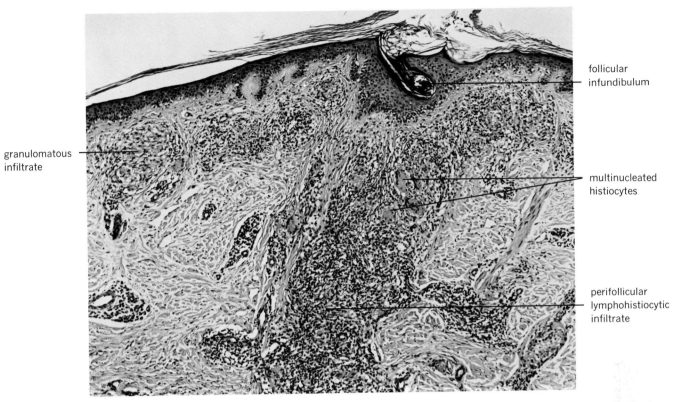

granulomatous infiltrate

follicular infundibulum

multinucleated histiocytes

perifollicular lymphohistiocytic infiltrate

FIG. 12-67. Hair loss caused by necrobiosis lipoidica. Broad band of granulomatous infiltration aligned almost perpendicular to surface of specimen is actually along axis of former hair follicle as may be inferred from remaining infundibulum. Granulomatous band will be replaced in time by fibrotic cord, a sign of permanent alopecia. (× 90.)

Physical and Chemical Injuries

Acids, alkalis, electromagnetic radiation, physical trauma, heat, or cold may cause injuries that produce ulcers and heal with scars in which hair follicles are destroyed. The deeper the ulcer, the more likely will scarring alopecia result.

Sarcoidosis

Rarely, the granulomatous inflammation of sarcoidosis resolves with extensive scarring and permanent alopecia as consequences. In active lesions there is a dense nodular granulomatous infiltrate of epithelioid tubercles in the dermis and sometimes in the subcutaneous fat. The inflammatory-cell infiltrate often impinges on the epidermis and on hair follicles. Clinically, papules and nodules coalesce to form a plaque extending centrifigually and leaving behind a hairless, atrophic, irregularly-shaped scar. The clinical alopecia of sarcoid occurs predominantly in middle-aged black women who generally have other cutaneous lesions of sarcoidosis. (Sarcoidosis is considered more extensively in Chapter 9.)

Lichen Planopilaris (Fig. 12-68)

Lichen planopilaris has been discussed earlier in this chapter. The predominantly lymphocytic infiltrate usually is disposed primarily around the hair follicles rather than at the dermoepidermal junction. In some cases, however, the superficial bandlike lymphohistiocytic infiltrate characteristic of lichen planus is also seen. In time the follicle degenerates, and an elongated fibrotic tract replaces it (Fig. 12-69). Fibrotic tracts at sites of former hair follicles signify a scarring alopecia. In short, lichen planopilaris is simply lichen planus affecting the regions of the hair follicles.

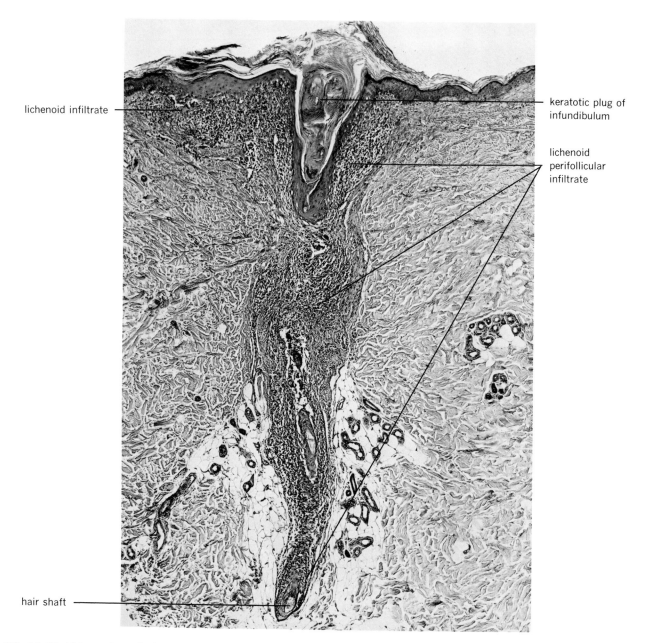

lichenoid infiltrate

keratotic plug of
infundibulum

lichenoid
perifollicular
infiltrate

hair shaft

FIG. 12-68. Lichen planopilaris. A, Dense, predominantly lymphocytic bandlike infiltrate extends along entire length of hair follicle. (× 54.)

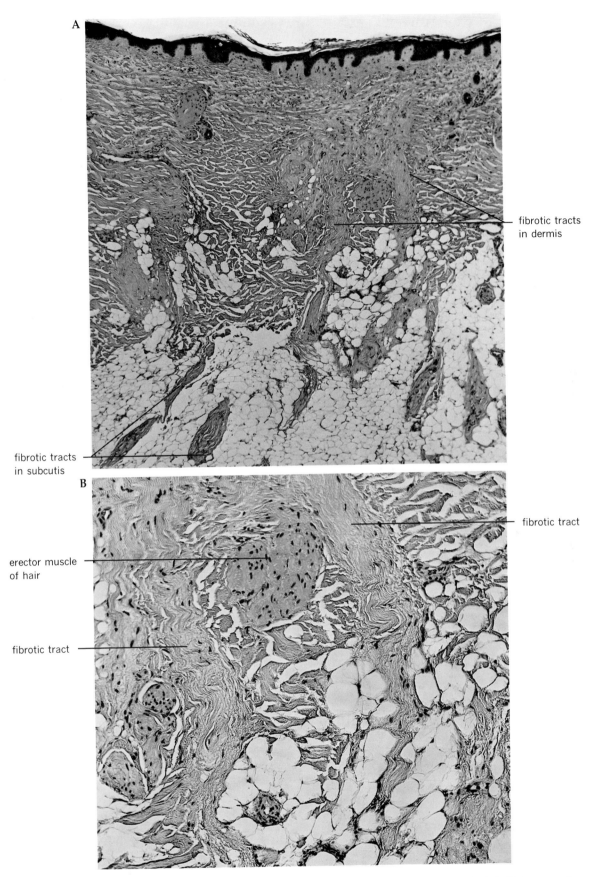

A

fibrotic tracts
in dermis

fibrotic tracts
in subcutis

B

fibrotic tract

erector muscle
of hair

fibrotic tract

FIG. 12-69. End stage of lichen planopilaris (pseudopelade). A, Six fibrotic tracts mark where hair follicles were in subcutis. (× 65.) B, Higher power shows vertically oriented fibrotic tracts in dermis and subcutis. (× 165.)

Discoid Lupus Erythematosus (Fig. 12-70) See Chapter 7.

Discoid lupus erythematosus is marked initially by a perifolliculitis and is discussed under that heading in this chapter and also in Chapter 7.

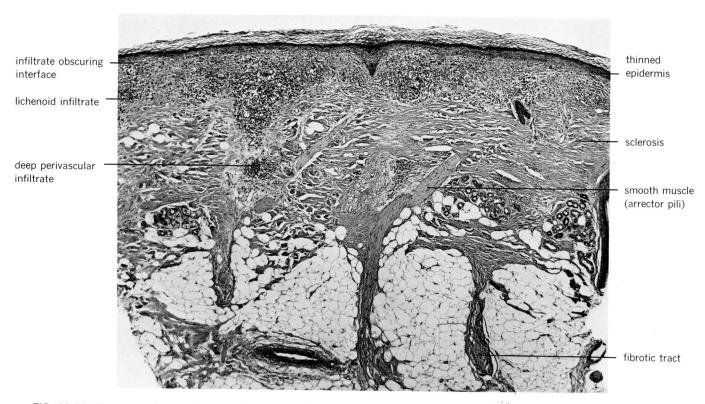

infiltrate obscuring interface

lichenoid infiltrate

deep perivascular infiltrate

thinned epidermis

sclerosis

smooth muscle (arrector pili)

fibrotic tract

FIG. 12-70. Alopecia of discoid lupus erythematosus. A, Vertically oriented fibrotic tracts are in subcutis at sites of former hair follicles. Muscle elements of arrectores pilorum persist despite destruction of hair follicles. Histologic features differentiating this section from one of lichen planopilaris are extensive lichenoid infiltrate, perivascular infiltrate involving deep plexus, sclerotic dermis, and thinned epidermis. (× 47.)

Alopecias have traditionally been classified clinically as scarring (as in chronic discoid lupus erythematosus) and nonscarring (as in alopecia areata). Perhaps it would be more helpful for prognosis and treatment to speak also of permanent and temporary alopecias. For example, all of the scarring alopecias are permanent, but sometimes so-called nonscarring alopecias are eventually scarring ones histologically and therefore permanent. Such is the case in long-standing lesions of alopecia areata (and alopecias totalis and universalis) which histologically shows whorls of sclerotic collagen, scars of sorts, at sites of former hair bulbs and papillae. Persistent traction on hairs is followed by development of thin fibrotic tracts along the paths where follicles formerly resided, and the resultant alopecia is therefore permanent. Although common (androgenic) alopecia is accompanied by neither sclerosis nor fibrosis, it is nevertheless irrevocably permanent and I can attest to that personally!

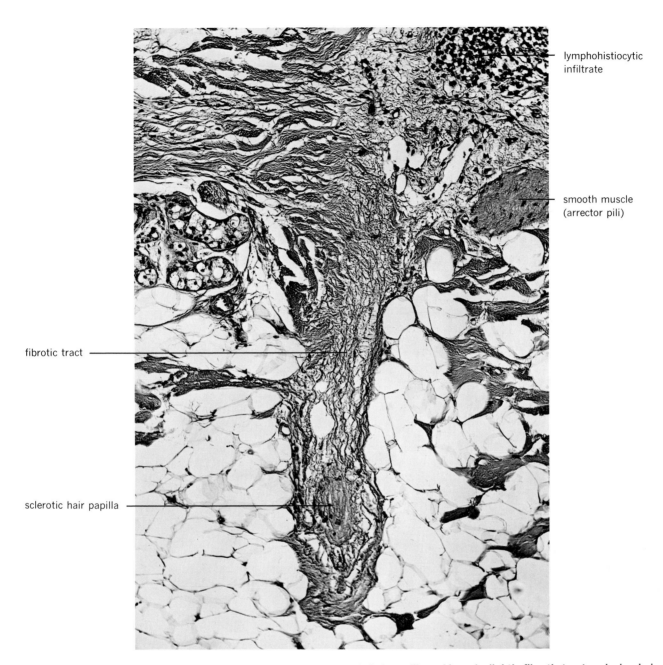

lymphohistiocytic
infiltrate

smooth muscle
(arrector pili)

fibrotic tract

sclerotic hair papilla

FIG. 12-70. B, Indications that alopecia will be permanent are sclerotic hair papilla and broad, slightly fibrotic tract replacing hair follicle, of which no epithelial remnant remains. (× 172.)

Fibrosing Dermatitis

Antecedents to Fibrosis

    Injuries to the skin surface
      Ulcer
      Chondrodermatitis nodularis helicis
      Pressure papules from prostheses
    Vascular proliferations
      Granulation tissue
      Pyogenic granuloma

Fibroses

    Hypertrophic fibroses
      Scar, hypertrophic
      Keloid
      Dermatofibroma
      Chronic lymphedema
    Atrophic fibroses
      Scar, atrophic
      Striae distensae
      Macular atrophies
      Acrodermatitis chronica atrophicans

    Poikiloderma
    Disseminated superficial porokeratosis
    Lichen planus, atrophic

Scleroses

    Hypertrophic scleroses
      Scleroderma
    Atrophic scleroses
      Lichen sclerosus et atrophicus
      Chronic radiodermatitis
      Necrobiosis lipoidica
      Chronic discoid lupus erythematosus

Fibrohistiocytic Proliferations

    Granuloma faciale, juxta-articular nodes, xan-
      thomas
    Histiocytoma
    Histoid leprosy
    Xanthogranulomas, juvenile and adult

Fibrosing
Dermatitis

13

Fɪʙʀᴏsɪs bespeaks the resolving stage of an intense or insidious inflammatory process (Fig. 13-1), but most inflammatory reactions in skin do not resolve with fibrosis. Generally, superficial perivascular and superficial and deep perivascular dermatitides resolve spontaneously with no permanent structural alteration. Fibrosis results mainly as a consequence of collagen destruction. Following destruction of normal collagen, fibroblasts attempt to repair the defect, but they practically never completely restore the original state of the dermis. However, fibrosis that is recognizable histologically does not necessarily produce a visible clinical scar. For example, dermabrasion confined to the level of the papillary dermis results in microscopic, but not clinical, scarring. Destruction of collagen follows a wide variety of injuries like physical trauma, thermal and chemical burns, and chronic inflammatory processes from infections and causes unknown.

Elastic fibers are invariably significantly reduced in number or altered in character in fibrotic and sclerotic conditions. Therefore, elastic-tissue stains are helpful in assessing these dermatitides.

Sclerosis of the papillary dermis produces lesions that are visibly white clinically, such as in lichen sclerosus et atrophicus and malignant atrophic papulosis. In other sclerosing diseases, such as chronic discoid lupus erythematosus, lesions may be either hypopigmented or hyperpigmented, depending upon the amount of melanin that remains or is further produced within the epidermis and the amount that is lost into the papillary dermis. Some

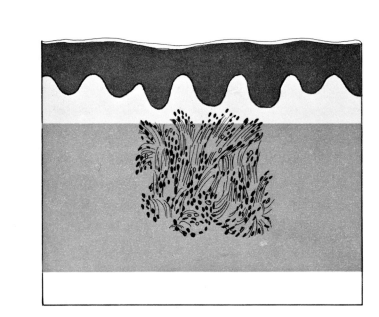

FIG. 13-1. Pattern of fibrosing dermatitis.

fibrosing processes, such as dermatofibroma, are hyperpigmented because of an increase in the quantity of melanin within the epidermis. A yellowish hue is imparted to skin lesions with sclerosis of the reticular dermis, as in morphea, and additionally by lipid deposits in the sclerotic dermis of necrobiosis lipoidica.

Many diseases that resolve with sclerosis of the papillary dermis may eventuate in malignant neoplasms, especially in squamous cell carcinomas and basal cell carcinomas, and even malignant melanomas. Chief among these sclerotic forerunners of malignancy are the long-standing lesions of radiation dermatitis, lupus vulgaris, syphilitic gumma, discoid lupus erythematosus, epidermolysis bullosa (recessive type), lichen sclerosus et atrophicus (lesions on the genitalia and in the perineum), granuloma inguinale, draining sinus tracts, porokeratosis (all types), acrodermatitis chronica atrophicans, and vaccination and burn scars.

This chapter deals with some preliminary stages in inflammatory processes preceding fibrosis, such as ulceration and granulation tissue, and concentrates on the end stages that are fibrosis and sclerosis.

Antecedents to Fibrosis

Some injuries to the skin surface, such as ulcerations, are the antecedents to fibrosis. An intermediate stage in the inflammatory response between ulceration and fibrosis is granulation tissue.

In assessing injuries to the skin surface a distinction must be made between an ulcer and an erosion. An *ulcer* in skin involves at least loss of the entire epidermis and some of the dermis. Some ulcers extend into the papillary dermis and others into the reticular dermis and beyond, depending upon the severity of the injury. Ulcers are invariably covered by scale-crusts that are often hemorrhagic. In addition to the parakeratotic cells, serum, and inflammatory cells, bacteria may be present within the crust. An infiltrate of neutrophils, lymphocytes, and histiocytes, some containing melanin, occurs around blood vessels beneath an ulcer.

An *erosion* is partial or full-thickness loss of the epidermis that does not affect the dermis. The most common cause of erosions in skin is scratching, the reflex response of patients to severe pruritus. Histologically, erosions are well-circumscribed defects within the epidermis covered by scale-crusts. A sparse inflammatory-cell infiltrate is present beneath an erosion.

Theoretically, erosions should not be associated with scarring because they do not damage the collagen of the papillary dermis. Subepidermal blisters that become unroofed are erosions and in the case of pemphigoid, for example, lesions heal usually without scarring, an indication that there has been little or no damage to the collagen in the papillary dermis. By contrast, the subepidermal blisters of the recessive dystrophic type of epidermolysis bullosa frequently heal with scarring. In this disease the collagen in the papillary dermis is irreparably injured. The same may be said for the subepidermal blistering diseases porphyria cutanea tarda and cicatricial pemphigoid. In each of these conditions there is fibrosis of the papillary dermis and diminution of the normal undulations between epidermal rete ridges and dermal papillae.

Ulcer (Fig. 13-2)

—Loss of the entire epidermis, focally or diffusely
—Epidermal hyperplasia, often atypical, at ulcer margin
—Varying loss of the dermis ranging to complete
—Scale-crust, usually hemorrhagic, overlying ulcer
—Mixed inflammatory-cell infiltrate primarily beneath the ulcer
—Fibrosis, if ulcer sufficiently deep

Whether fibrosis supervenes in an ulcer depends upon the amount and depth of damage to the dermal collagen. Ulcers that cause damage to collagen in the upper part of the papillary dermis only do not usually culminate in scarring, whereas all ulcerations that extend into the reticular dermis inexorably proceed to fibrosis and consequently to clinical scars.

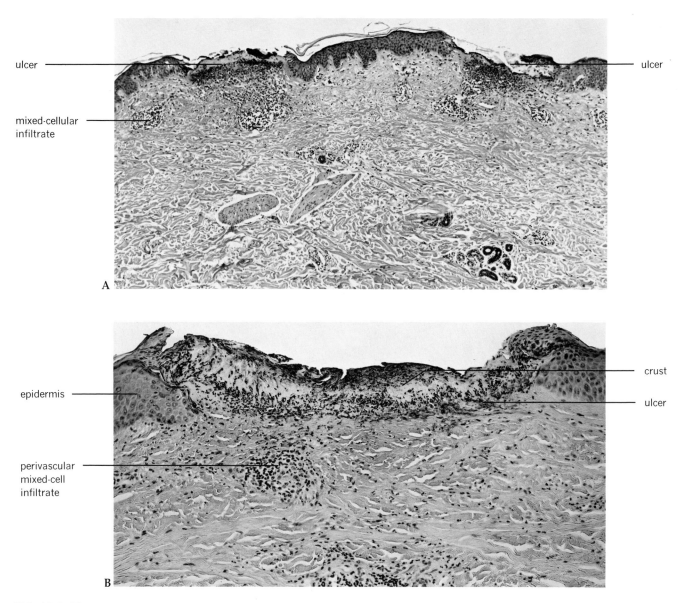

ulcer

mixed-cellular
infiltrate

A

epidermis

perivascular
mixed-cell
infiltrate

B

ulcer

crust

ulcer

FIG. 13-2. Ulcers produced by excoriations. A, Two well-circumscribed, shallow, ragged ulcers pictured are typical of those produced by vigorous scratching. (× 65.) B, Higher magnification of ulcer produced by admitted vigorous scratching. No other cause for the ulcer, such as thrombosis, necrotizing vasculitis, or blister formation can be discerned in this picture. (× 172.)

Chondrodermatitis Nodularis Helicis (Fig. 13-3)

—Erosion or ulceration
—Fibrin beneath the ulcer (Fig. 13-4)
—Sclerosis beneath the fibrin (Fig. 13-5)
—Granulation tissue or highly vascularized connective tissue lateral to the zones of fibrin and sclerosis
—Perichondrial fibrosis or sclerosis
—Variable degeneration of cartilage
—Re-epithelized epidermis often covered by moundlike hyperkeratosis

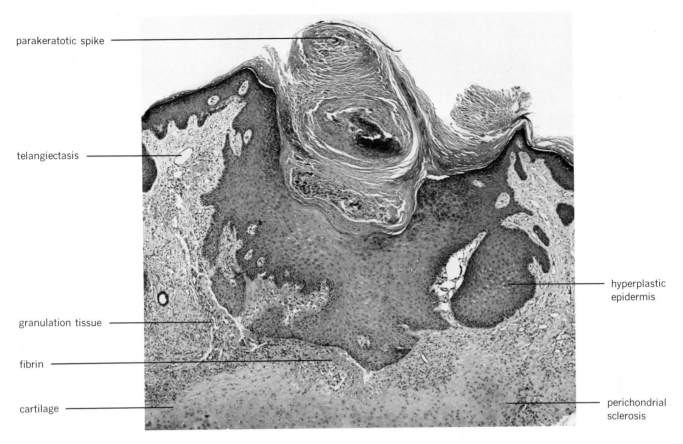

parakeratotic spike

telangiectasis

granulation tissue

fibrin

cartilage

hyperplastic epidermis

perichondrial sclerosis

FIG. 13-3. Chondrodermatitis nodularis helicis. Cornified excrescence shown emanating from a cup-shaped depression in hyperplastic epidermis is characteristic feature. Horny plug acts like a carpenter's nail which is driven into cartilage of ear and induces, sequentially, ulceration, granulation tissue with fibrin, and perichondrial fibrosis. Similar horny growths extend from skin of comparable lesions such as pressure papules from prostheses and surfers' knots. (× 54.)

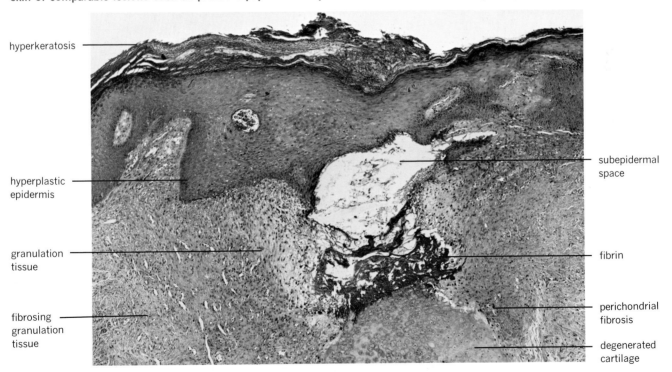

hyperkeratosis

hyperplastic epidermis

granulation tissue

fibrosing granulation tissue

subepidermal space

fibrin

perichondrial fibrosis

degenerated cartilage

FIG. 13-4. Chondrodermatitis nodularis helicis. In an active lesion, such as is pictured here, fibrin is found within subepidermal space, around which is degenerated cartilage or perichondrial fibrosis and granulation tissue. (× 74.)

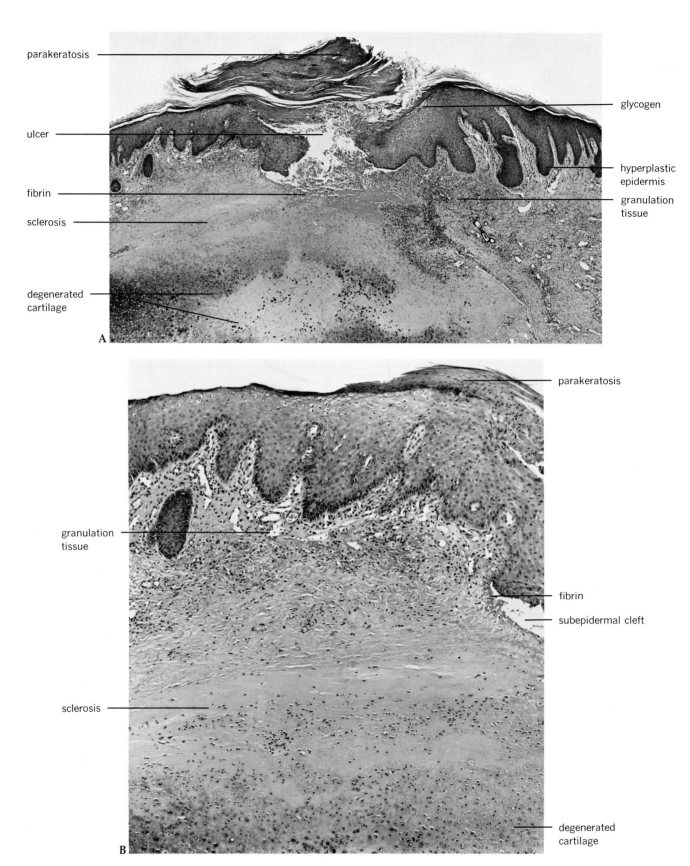

FIG. 13-5. Chondrodermatitis nodularis helicis. A, Diagnostic features are all present in this photomicrograph: parakeratotic mound, ulcer with epidermal hyperplasia to the sides and fibrin beneath, granulation tissue, perichondrial sclerosis, and degenerated cartilage. The diagnosis may be suspected if biopsy specimen includes merely the portion of lesion from the fibrin up. (× 29.) B, Higher power view permits better appreciation of just how extensive sclerosis may be. (× 76.)

Chondrodermatitis nodularis helicis usually is characterized histologically by ulceration beneath which, in descending order, there are fibrin, sclerosis, perichondrial fibrosis, and varying degrees of degeneration of the underlying cartilage. Contiguous to the zones of dermal fibrin and sclerosis there is granulation tissue associated with large fibroblasts that resemble chondrocytes. Episodically, the ulcer re-epithelizes, and the restored epidermis is then often surmounted by a mound of orthokeratotic and parakeratotic horn. This exophytic cornified spike may play a role in the pathogenesis of this process.

Usually only the surface of a lesion of chondrodermatitis nodularis helicis is submitted to the pathologist because in most instances the ulcerated or keratotic nodule is removed by shave excision as a presumed basal cell carcinoma or solar keratosis. The correct diagnosis of chondrodermatitis nodularis helicis can be suspected histologically even in superficial specimens by the presence of an ulcer, fibrin, and sclerosis in linear array and granulation tissue containing chondrocyte-like fibroblasts to the sides.

Chondrodermatitis probably results from prolonged and persistent trauma to the ear, e.g., from earphones in telephone operators and wimples in certain orders of nuns. The lesion appears as a small tender papule or nodule on the helix or the antehelix.

Pressure Papules from Prostheses (Fig. 13-6)

—Focal erosion or ulceration
—Cup-shaped depression in epidermis containing mounds of parakeratosis
—Hyperplasia of the spinous and granular layers to the sides of the thinned, cup-shaped epidermis
—Collarette of epidermis at the periphery of the lesion
—Coarse collagen bundles in the upper part of the dermis
—Superficial perivascular mixed-cell infiltrate around telangiectases

Papules from pressure of prostheses such as form on weight-bearing stumps of amputated legs are tender keratotic lesions. In such places they develop secondary to persistent pressure, especially in the popliteal area over the tendons of the hamstring muscles and over the distal femoral condyles. Papules from pressure of prostheses have many histologic features in common with chondrodermatitis nodularis helicis, and they are virtually indistinguishable from the keratotic papules, known as surfer's knots, that arise from similar influences on the knees of surfboard riders.

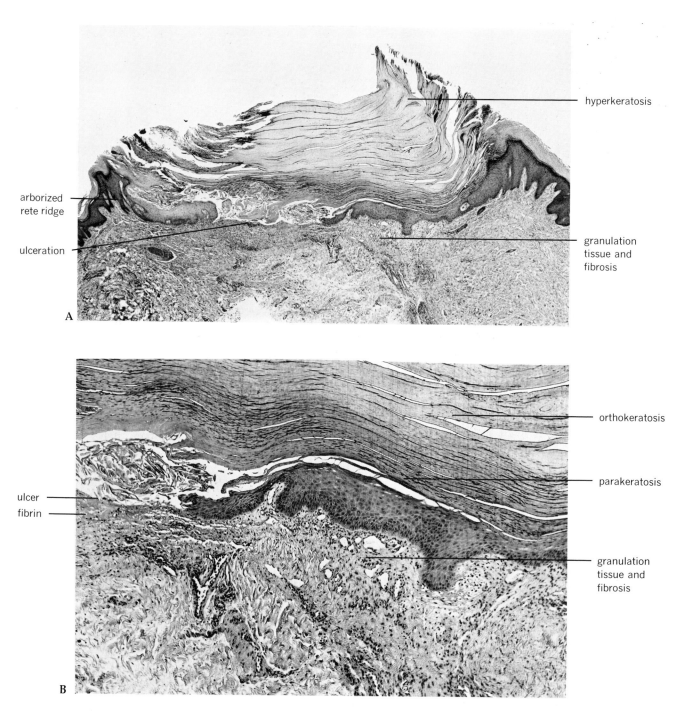

hyperkeratosis

arborized
rete ridge

ulceration

granulation
tissue and
fibrosis

A

orthokeratosis

parakeratosis

ulcer

fibrin

granulation
tissue and
fibrosis

B

FIG. 13-6. Pressure papule from prosthesis. Changes pictured in this keratotic lesion induced by pressure of prosthesis against amputation stump closely resemble those of chondrodermatitis nodularis helicis, and the mechanism of formation of both lesions probably is similar. The result is ulceration, granulation tissue, and fibrosis as shown here. (A, × 23; B, × 88.)

Vascular Proliferations

An increase in the number of capillaries and venules is a prelude in the reparative process of the skin to eventual fibrosis and sclerosis. Manifestations of this exuberant vascular response are granulation tissue and pyogenic granuloma.

—Highly vascular (capillaries and venules) edematous connective tissue
—Mixed cellular infiltrate including fibroblasts, neutrophils, lymphocytes, histiocytes, plasma cells, eosinophils, and mast cells, in addition to endothelial cells

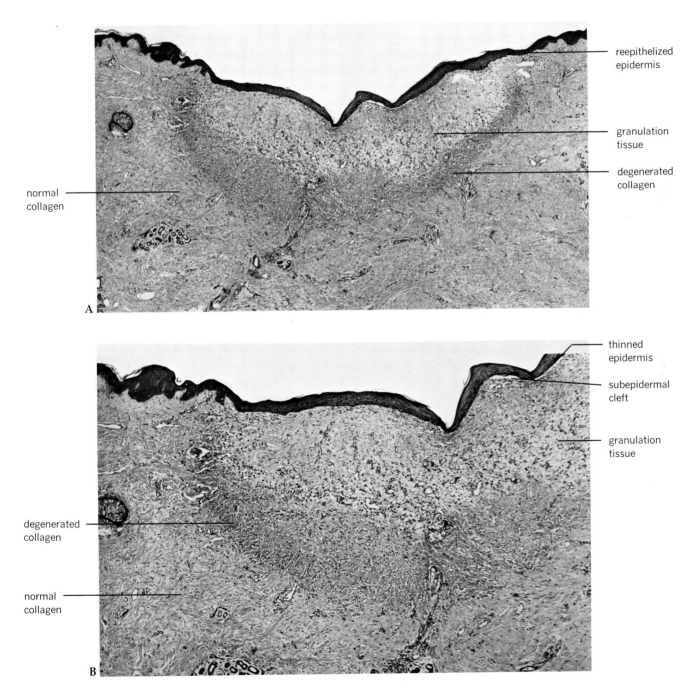

FIG. 13-7. Granulation tissue 10 days after surgical procedure. Typical features pictured are highly vascular, edematous connective tissue within which there is sparse infiltrate of scattered, mixed inflammatory cells. (A, × 28; B, × 50.)

Granulation tissue is a prominent feature of the reparative process. Capillaries and venules lined by plump endothelial cells are increased in number. Granulation tissue acts as a scaffolding for fibroblasts, which transform the granulation tissue into fibrous tissue. Granulation tissue is seen beneath all cutaneous ulcers in which significant portions of the papillary dermis have been damaged. It is also seen in other conditions ranging from acutely ruptured follicular cysts to pyogenic granulomas.

Pyogenic Granuloma, Acute (Fig. 13-8)

—Exophytic ulcerated granulation tissue
—Epidermal collarette at base

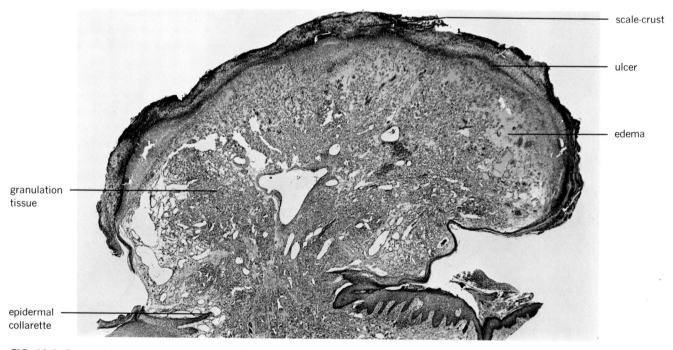

scale-crust

ulcer

edema

granulation tissue

epidermal collarette

FIG. 13-8. Pyogenic granuloma, acute stage. Early stage is nothing more than development of ulcerated exophytic granulation tissue (clinically proud flesh) as shown here. Note characteristic collarette of elongated epidermal rete ridges on both sides that point toward center of lesion. ($\times$ 22.)

Pyogenic Granuloma, Subacute (Fig. 13-9)

—Exophytic hemangioma, often with scale-crust
—Fibrous trabeculae often intersecting the angiomatous elements
—Edematous stroma
—Collarette of epidermis beneath the angiomatous tissue

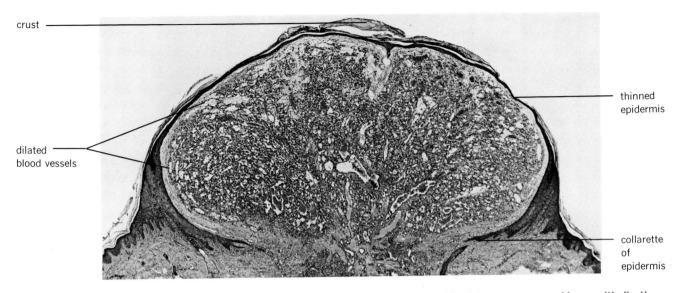

crust

dilated
blood vessels

thinned
epidermis

collarette
of
epidermis

FIG. 13-9. Pyogenic granuloma, subacute stage. Early exuberant and ulcerated proud flesh becomes covered by reepithelization, edema is gradually resorbed, and inflammatory-cell infiltrate wanes to produce lesion that resembles hemangioma but is distinctive by its prominent epidermal collarette. (× 29.)

Pyogenic Granuloma, Chronic (Fig. 13-10)

—Exophytic angiofibroma
—Epidermal collarette

The term *pyogenic granuloma* is a misnomer. The lesion is not related to bacterial infection, nor is it granulomatous, except for a brief period during the late acute stage (Fig. 13-11). In fact, pyogenic granuloma initially is a type of granulation tissue, proud flesh, that usually results from a penetrating injury to skin such as a puncture wound (Fig. 13-8). Following injury, there is formation

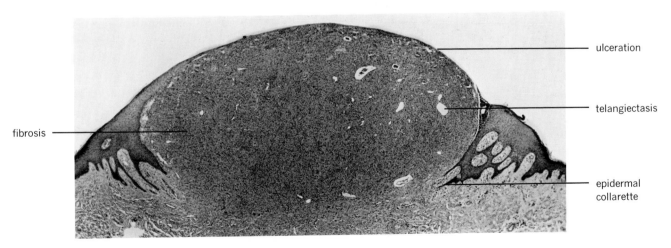

fibrosis

ulceration

telangiectasis

epidermal
collarette

FIG. 13-10. Pyogenic granuloma, chronic stage. During resolution, granulation tissue of its early stage is replaced by fibrosis. Finding fibrosis is uncommon because lesion is usually treated before fibrosis supervenes. (× 56.)

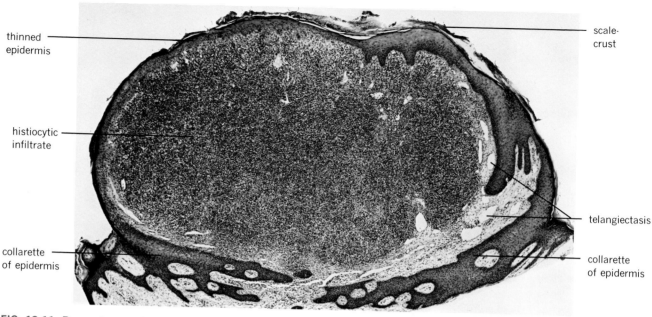

thinned epidermis

histiocytic infiltrate

collarette of epidermis

scale-crust

telangiectasis

collarette of epidermis

FIG. 13-11. Pyogenic granuloma, granulomatous stage. In this brief phase histiocytes come to predominate in highly vascular stroma. Note collarette of epidermis. (× 41.)

of exuberant granulation tissue that is seen histologically as a sessile, ulcerated mass of edematous, highly vascularized connective tissue containing a mixed inflammatory-cell infiltrate. As in all types of granulation tissue, the increased number of capillaries and venules have plump endothelial cells. A rather constant histologic feature of pyogenic granuloma is the peripheral epidermal collarette that extends beneath the granulation tissue.

In time, the granulation tissue is transformed. The ulcerated surface is covered by epidermis. The endothelial cells lining the vascular channels become smaller and more elongated; the edema and inflammatory-cell infiltrate diminish and disappear. At this stage, pyogenic granuloma resembles hemangioma (Fig. 13-12).

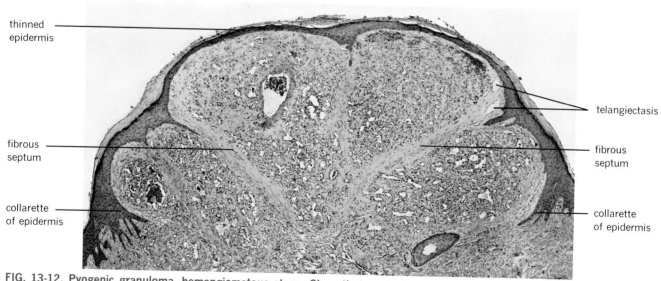

thinned epidermis

fibrous septum

collarette of epidermis

telangiectasis

fibrous septum

collarette of epidermis

FIG. 13-12. Pyogenic granuloma, hemangiomatous stage. Clues that mark this lesion as truly pyogenic granuloma and not hemangioma are trabeculation by fibrous septa and collarette of epidermis. (× 48.)

If the lesion remains untreated, fibrosis progresses, and eventually the angiofibroma shrinks.

Clinically early pyogenic granuloma is identical to proud flesh, being composed of exuberant granulation tissue that has a beefy glistening appearance. Later, pyogenic granuloma may be indistinguishable clinically from a hemangioma.

Fibroses

Alterations in the formation of fibrous tissue are confined principally to the dermis, although they may involve the subcutaneous fat. Fibroses may be classified as hypertrophic or atrophic, depending upon whether the scarring process rises above or dips below the surface of the skin. The prototype of the hypertrophic fibrosis is a hypertrophic scar; that of atrophic fibroses is an atrophic scar.

Hypertrophic Fibroses

Hypertrophy results mainly from an overgrowth of fibroblasts, accompanied by excessive production of collagen, and is seen in some scars, in keloid, and in dermatofibroma. Keloids, scars, and dermatofibromas are merely different ways that fibroblasts respond to injuries.

Scar, Hypertrophic (Fig. 13-13)

—Fibrillary collagen oriented parallel to the skin surface
—Increased fibroblasts also aligned parallel to the skin surface
—Increased number of dilated blood vessels generally arranged perpendicular to the skin surface
—Epidermis usually thin with a diminished pattern of epidermal rete and dermal papillae
—Decreased number of adnexal epithelial structures

In early scars, there may be stellate fibroblasts and mucin as well as a predominantly perivascular mixed inflammatory-cell infiltrate. In older scars, the fibroblasts are thin and elongated, the amount of mucin is negligible, and the inflammatory cells are gone. In all scars, the normal collagen bundles are replaced by fibrillary collagen. Within a scar there are usually no remnants of pilosebaceous units. Eccrine sweat glands and ducts are apparently more persistent, but if the scarring process is sufficiently severe they, too, will be obliterated. Elastic fibers, as evidenced by special

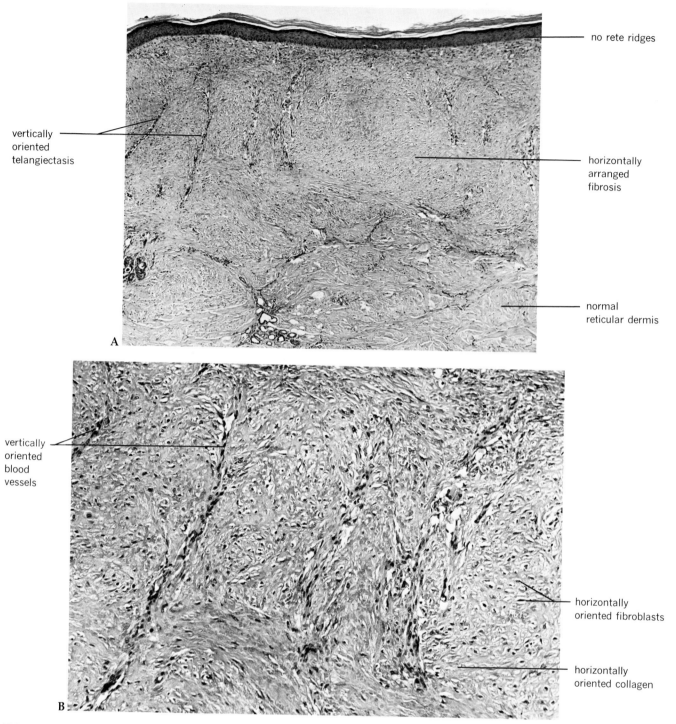

no rete ridges

vertically oriented telangiectasis

horizontally arranged fibrosis

normal reticular dermis

vertically oriented blood vessels

horizontally oriented fibroblasts

horizontally oriented collagen

FIG. 13-13. Scar. Note that fibroblasts and collagen fibers are oriented roughly parallel to skin surface, whereas dilated blood vessels run perpendicularly to it. The epidermis is thinned and devoid of rete ridges. (A, × 49; B, × 167.)

stains, are not present in a scar (Fig. 13-14). Scars in skin commonly result from rupture of hair follicles and follicular cysts. Histologically, squames within macrophages, remnants of follicular epithelium, or fragments of hair surrounded by histiocytic giant cells are evidence of a follicular role in the scarring process (Fig. 13-15).

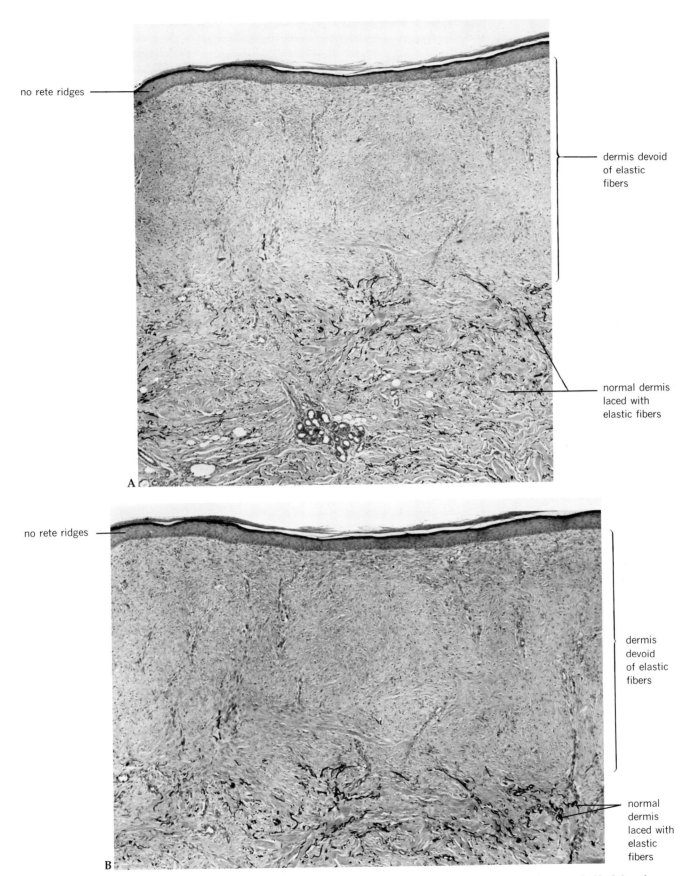

no rete ridges —

dermis devoid of elastic fibers

normal dermis laced with elastic fibers

no rete ridges —

dermis devoid of elastic fibers

normal dermis laced with elastic fibers

A

B

FIG. 13-14. Scar. In these sections of Fig. 13-13 specially stained for elastic tissue, the scarred area in upper half of dermis can be seen to be devoid of elastic fibers, whereas normal reticular dermis below has normal complement of elastic tissue. (A, × 51; B, × 69.)

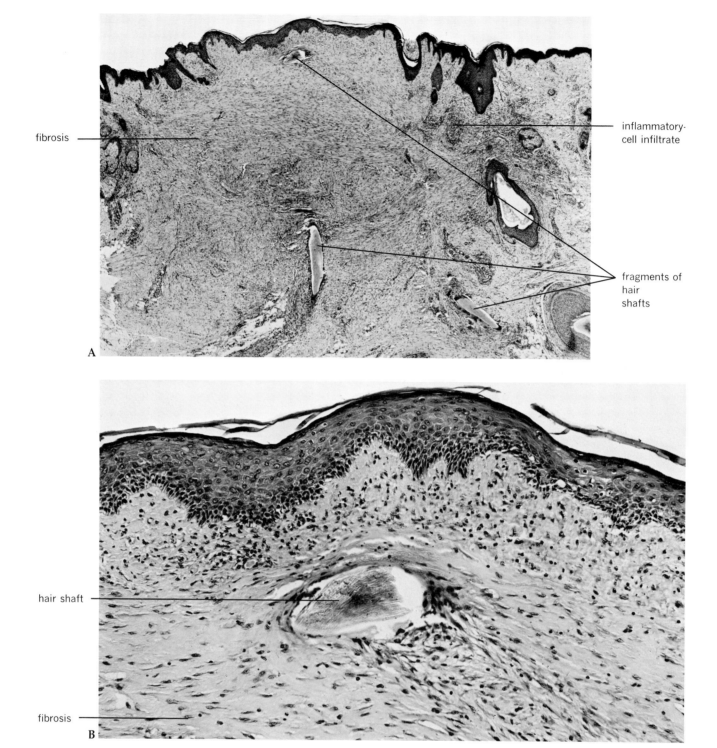

FIG. 13-15. Scar secondary to rupture of hair follicles. Tell-tale signs of follicular role are fragments of hair, three of which may be seen, each surrounded by histiocytic giant cells. (A, × 32; B, × 170.)

The factors that control fibroplasia, as well as removal and restructuring of collagen, are not known. Many scars tend to be hypertrophic, extending above the skin surface (Fig. 13-16). Clinically, neither hairs, sebum, nor sweat appear in scarred skin. The surface of scars is usually smooth, shiny, and telangiectatic.

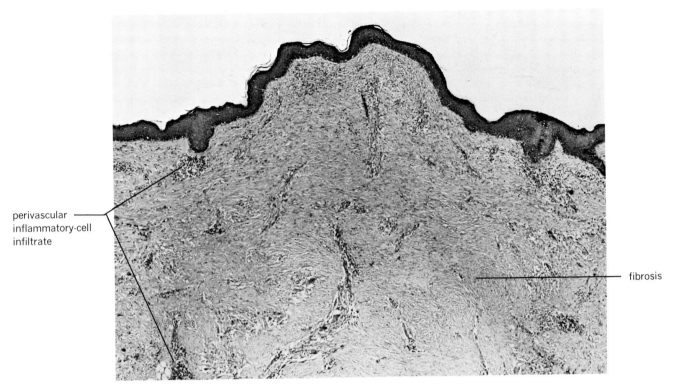

perivascular inflammatory-cell infiltrate

fibrosis

FIG. 13-16. Hypertrophic scar. Except for elevation above skin the histologic attributes of an ordinary scar can be seen: fibroblasts and fibrillary collagen oriented roughly parallel to skin surface and blood vessels vertical to surface. Note inflammatory-cell infiltrate around each blood vessel in this still progressing scar. (× 60.)

Keloid (Fig. 13-17)

—Thickened collagen bundles in haphazard array
—Fibroblasts contiguous with and parallel to the thick collagen bundles
—Decreased adnexal structures

A keloid is distinguished histologically from a scar by the presence of thickened, homogeneous, brightly eosinophilic-staining collagen bundles. Arranged parallel to these thickened collagen bundles are plump fibroblasts. In the spaces between the keloidal collagen bundles there is abundant mucin. In addition to this random arrangement of thick collagen bundles that is histologically diagnostic of a keloid, there also may be collagen fibrils arranged like those in a scar (Fig. 13-18). This should not be surprising because both keloids and scars are inflammatory, primarily fibroblastic, responses to dermal injury. Early lesions are accompanied by an inflammatory-cell infiltrate. No elastic fibers are present in either a keloid or a scar.

Keloids are easily recognized clinically as firm nodules and plaques at obvious sites of injury such as where earlobes have

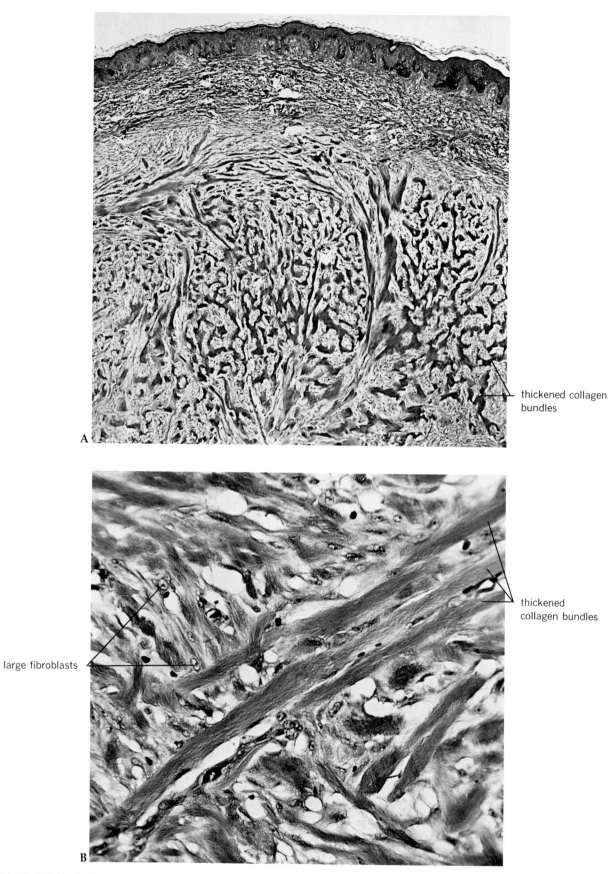

thickened collagen
bundles

large fibroblasts

thickened
collagen bundles

FIG. 13-17. Keloid. A, Note thickened collagen bundles in haphazard array. (× 56.) B, In this higher magnification large plump fibroblasts are seen to align themselves roughly parallel to thickened collagen bundles. (× 341.)

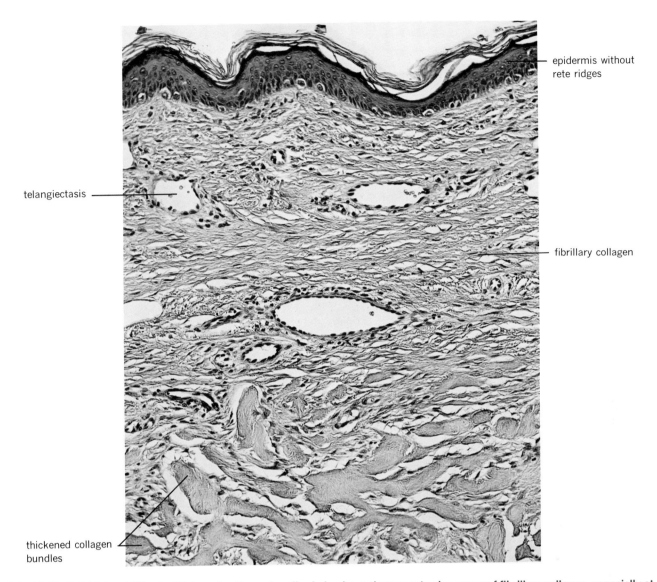

epidermis without rete ridges

telangiectasis

fibrillary collagen

thickened collagen bundles

FIG. 13-18. Keloid. In addition to thickened collagen bundles in haphazard array note also zones of fibrillary collagen, especially at periphery. (× 108.)

been pierced, "cysts" of acne have resolved, pseudofolliculitis of the beard has occurred, or the skin has been burned. Events, such as ruptured hair follicles, that induce scars also cause keloids (Fig. 13-19). Keloids are never spontaneous. They occur frequently in black people, in whom they may be disfiguring.

Dermatofibroma (Fig. 13-20)

—Haphazard arrangement of increased fibroblasts, some histiocytes, and associated coarse collagen (Fig. 13-21)
—Fibroblasts at periphery of the lesion appearing to wrap around thickened collagen bundles
—Epidermal hyperplasia and hyperpigmentation
—Decreased or absent epithelial adnexal structures

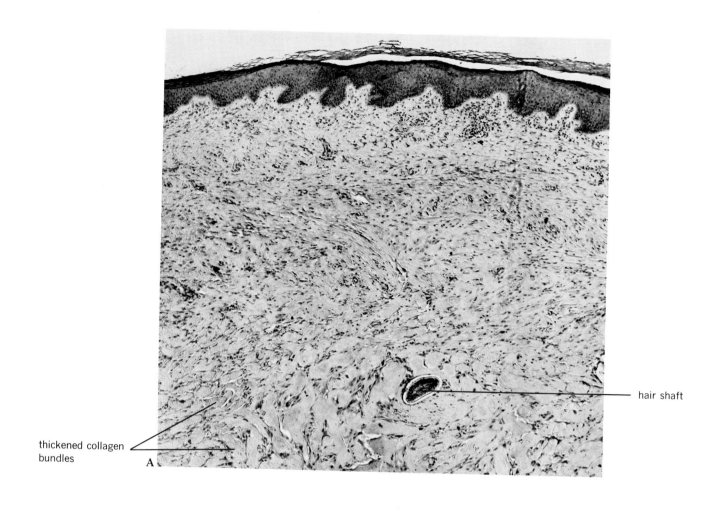

thickened collagen bundles

hair shaft

A

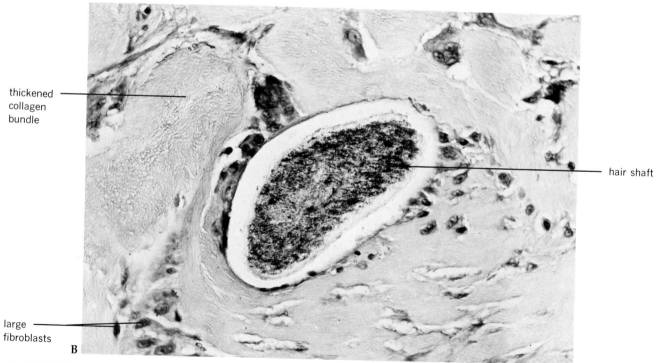

thickened collagen bundle

hair shaft

large fibroblasts

B

FIG. 13-19. Hair shaft within keloid. A, Shown is only a remnant of follicle that may have been responsible for this exuberant form of fibroplasia. (× 456.) B, Fragment of hair is embedded in bundles of collagen that are thickened, typical of a keloid. (× 64.)

The term *dermatofibrosis* would be preferable to dermatofibroma, because it suggests that this lesion is a type of fibrosing dermatitis, a reactive rather than a neoplastic fibroblastic process. There are several synonyms for dermatofibroma, namely, histiocytoma, subepidermal nodular sclerosis, nodulus cutaneous,

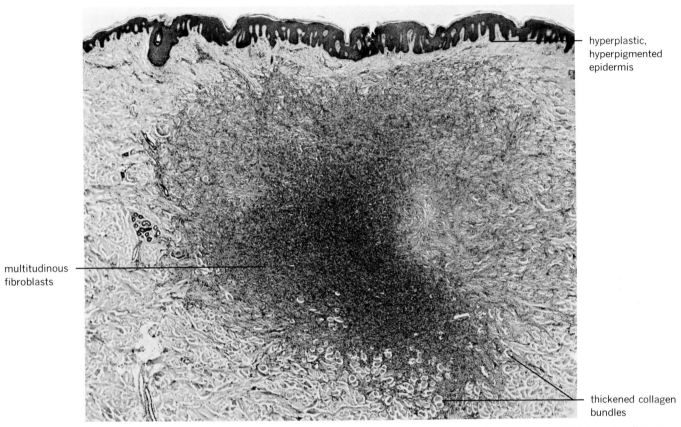

FIG. 13-20. Dermatofibroma. Highly cellular infiltrates of fibroblasts and histiocytes tend to wrap around thickened collagen bundles at periphery of nodule, and overlying epidermis is hyperplastic and hyperpigmented. (× 26.)

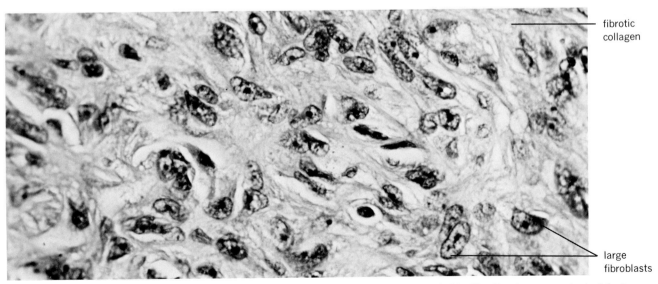

FIG. 13-21. Dermatofibroma. Numerous large fibroblasts in disorderly array embedded in fibrotic stroma are typical features. (× 832.)

fibroma durum, and sclerosing hemangioma. These terms emphasize differences of what is fundamentally a single pathologic process. Dermatofibroma, like scar and keloid, probably results from traumas to the skin that range from insect bites to rupture of hair follicles with expulsion of follicular contents into the dermis and subsequent reactive fibroplasia (Fig. 13-22). Fibroblasts are responsible for the reparative processes of dermatofibroma, just as they are for those of scar and keloid (Fig. 13-23). However, the histologic pattern formed by fibroblasts in dermatofibroma is different from that of scar and keloid. In dermatofibroma, the fibroblasts are increased in number, arranged haphazardly, and associated with coarse collagen. At the periphery of the fibrosis, the fibroblasts appear to encircle thickened collagen bundles that then merge with the normal dermal collagen.

Epidermal hyperplasia, which is sometimes found above the lateral margins of the fibroma, is an almost invariable accompaniment of dermatofibroma. The formation of hyperplastic epidermis in a dermatofibroma depends upon the site of the fibrohistiocytic process which when high in the reticular dermis promotes epidermal hyperplasia but when low does not. It seems as though epidermal hyperplasia in this condition is a reaction to influences from the underlying fibrohistiocytic abnormality. It is not unusual to see epidermal changes that resemble buds of basal

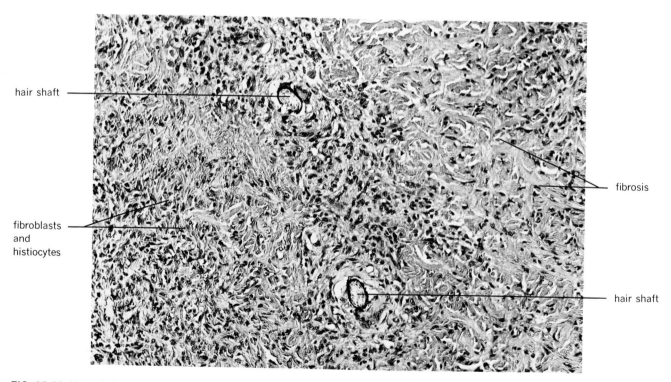

hair shaft

fibroblasts
and
histiocytes

fibrosis

hair shaft

FIG. 13-22. Hair shafts within dermatofibroma. Naked fragments of hairs bear testimony to role of follicle in development of this lesion. Note histiocytic giant cells in propinquity to each hair. ($\times$ 207.)

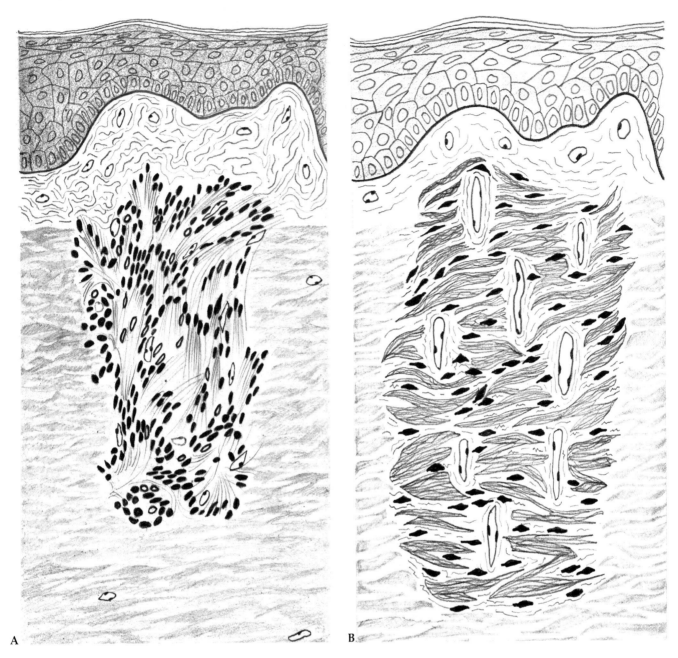

FIG. 13-23. A, Dermatofibroma. B, Scar.

cell carcinoma (Fig. 13-24). These changes are best interpreted as faulty epidermal attempts at follicular differentiation resulting in aggregates of small basaloid cells whose peripheral nuclei form a palisade. In some instances a hair bulb and papilla develop above the fibroma (Fig. 13-25). Aggregates of basal cells with the biologic potential of basal cell carcinoma occur, although rarely, in dermatofibroma (Fig. 13-26). Other epidermal changes that may be seen above dermatofibroma include focal acantholytic dyskeratosis (Fig. 13-27), epidermolytic hyperkeratosis (Fig. 13-28), simulators of seborrheic keratosis (Fig. 13-29), and pale cell acanthoma (Fig. 13-30). In exceptional cases, when the fibrohisti-

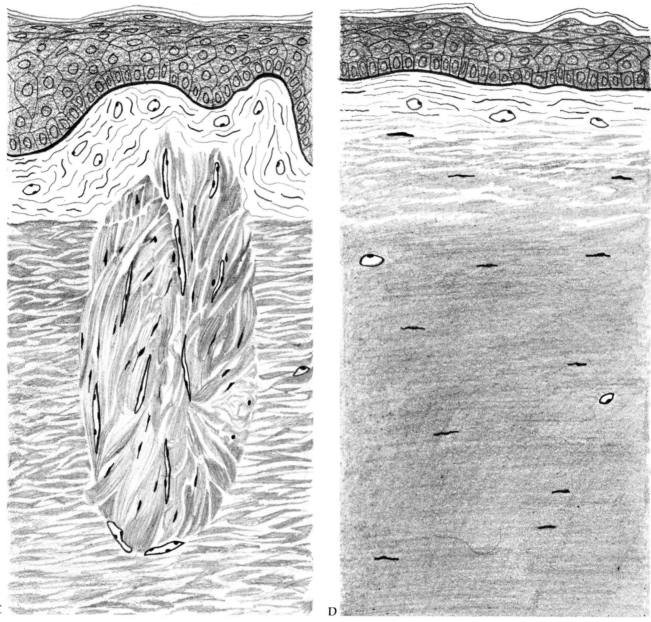

FIG. 13-23. C, Keloid. D, Sclerosis.

ocytic process extends upward to fill much of the papillary dermis, the epidermis above the dermatofibroma is thinned. In almost all instances the epidermis above dermatofibroma is hyperpigmented. Some dermatofibromas involve the mid or lower reticular dermis rather than the upper portion. In such instances, there may be no alteration of the overlying epidermis.

In a dermatofibroma, in addition to the characteristic arrangement of fibroblasts and collagen, there may be histologic features that resemble those of keloids (Fig. 13-31) or dermatofibrosarcoma protuberans (Fig. 13-32). There may also be a large circumscribed zone of sclerosis (Fig. 13-33) and even ossification (Fig. 13-34).

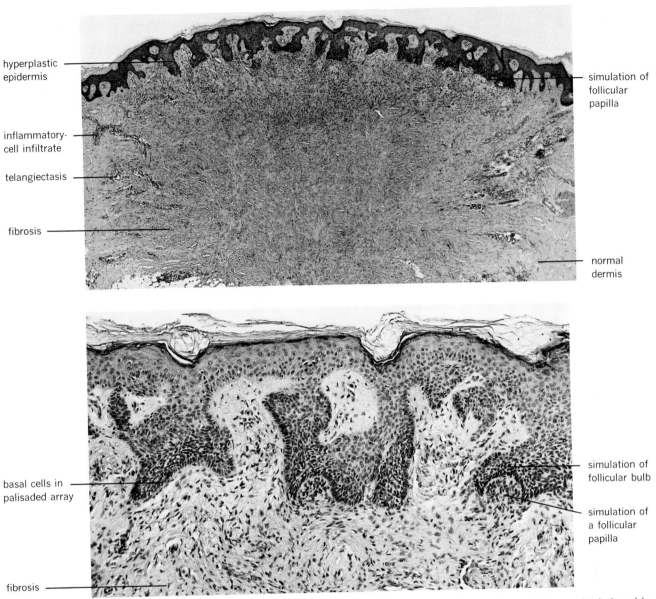

Labels on figure (clockwise from upper left):
hyperplastic epidermis
inflammatory-cell infiltrate
telangiectasis
fibrosis
simulation of follicular papilla
normal dermis
basal cells in palisaded array
fibrosis
simulation of follicular bulb
simulation of a follicular papilla

FIG. 13-24. Dermatofibroma with induction of follicular structures. A, Among more common patterns that may be induced in overlying epidermis is the one shown here, i.e., follicular differentiation that seems to reflect development of hair follicles from surface ectoderm during embryogenesis. ($\times$ 32.) B, In this higher magnification, two well-circumscribed collections of plump fibroblasts resembling those of papillae of hair follicles are seen to be partially enclosed by epidermal epithelium with differentiation toward hair matrix. The entirety resembles the beginnings of a hair bulb. ($\times$ 175.)

Dermatofibroma may also extend into the subcutaneous fat (Fig. 13-35). Like other fibrosing processes, dermatofibroma is associated with an increased number of capillaries and venules and with destruction of epithelial adnexal structures. In addition to deposition of lipid as a consequence of bleeding, hemosiderin is often found within macrophages (Fig. 13-31B). These macrophages arrive on the scene to ingest the breakdown products of extravasated blood which results from traumatic injury.

Clinically, dermatofibroma is a firm tannish-brown hairless papule or nodule, usually on the lower extremities.

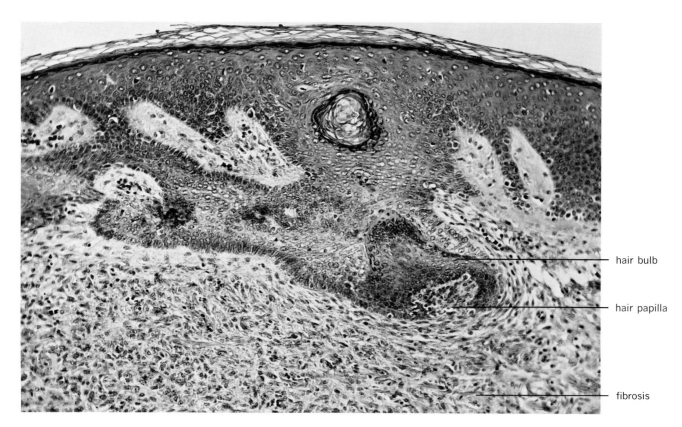

hair bulb

hair papilla

fibrosis

FIG. 13-25. Hair bulb and papilla in dermatofibroma. Hair bulbs are usually situated well within midportion of dermis or in subcutaneous fat, not immediately beneath epidermis as in this dermatofibroma. Note that this hair bulb is not only associated with a well-formed papilla, but also with a pale outer root (trichilemmal) sheath and trichohyalin granules of inner root sheath. (× 212.)

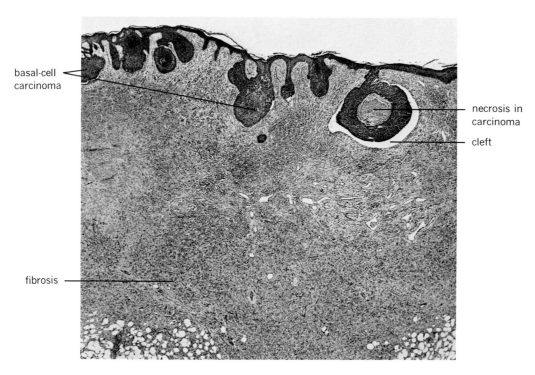

basal-cell carcinoma

necrosis in carcinoma

cleft

fibrosis

FIG. 13-26. Basal cell carcinoma in dermatofibroma, an unusual phenomenon. Necrosis can be seen within aggregate of carcinoma. Basal-cell hyperplasia at surface of dermatofibroma is common; true basal-cell carcinoma is rare. (× 21.)

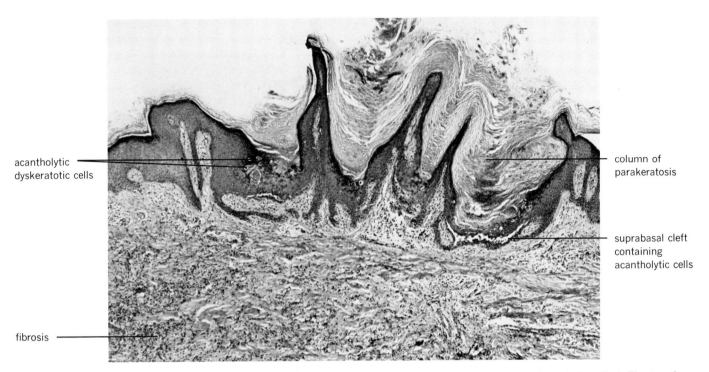

acantholytic
dyskeratotic cells

column of
parakeratosis

suprabasal cleft
containing
acantholytic cells

fibrosis

FIG. 13-27. Focal acantholytic dyskeratosis upon dermatofibroma. Among many changes that fibrohistiocytic infiltrate of dermatofibroma is occasionally associated with in epidermis are those of focal acantholytic dyskeratosis, shown here in digitate configuration. (× 61.)

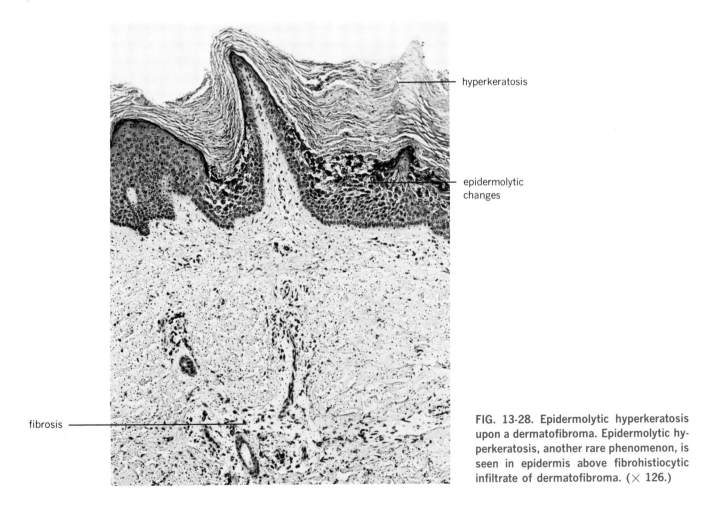

hyperkeratosis

epidermolytic
changes

fibrosis

FIG. 13-28. Epidermolytic hyperkeratosis upon a dermatofibroma. Epidermolytic hyperkeratosis, another rare phenomenon, is seen in epidermis above fibrohistiocytic infiltrate of dermatofibroma. (× 126.)

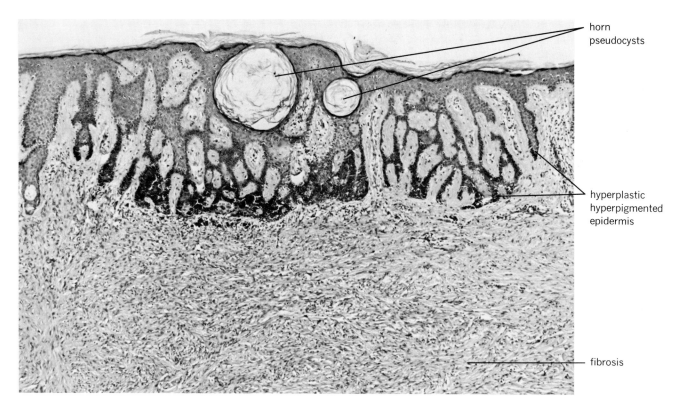

horn
pseudocysts

hyperplastic
hyperpigmented
epidermis

fibrosis

FIG. 13-29. Dermatofibroma with epidermal features like adenoid seborrheic keratosis. Hyperpigmented, interweaving cords of epidermis associated with horn pseudocysts pictured in this dermatofibroma closely simulate findings of adenoid type of seborrheic keratosis. (× 86.)

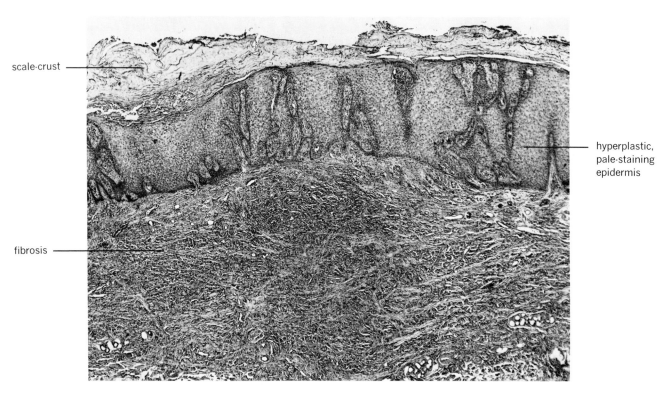

scale-crust

hyperplastic,
pale-staining
epidermis

fibrosis

FIG. 13-30. Dermatofibroma with features of pale cell acanthoma. Pale-staining cytoplasm of cells in hyperplastic epidermis above dermatofibroma shown here contained glycogen. It first took PAS stain which was then completely removed by diastase. (× 30.)

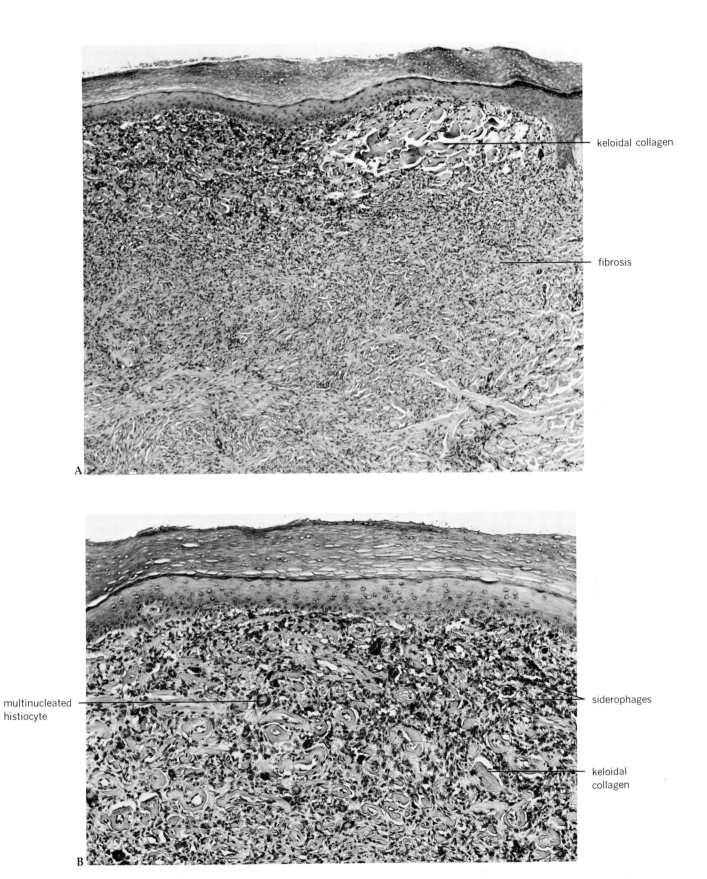

keloidal collagen

fibrosis

multinucleated
histiocyte

siderophages

keloidal
collagen

FIG. 13-31. Dermatofibroma with keloidal features. A, Among many histologic variations of dermatofibroma is one seen here, distinctively characterized by thickened collagen bundles that resemble those of a keloid. (× 70.) **B,** In this higher magnification of upper left hand portion one sees collagen bundles of keloidal character, fibroblasts, and also histiocytes containing hemosiderin. (× 175.)

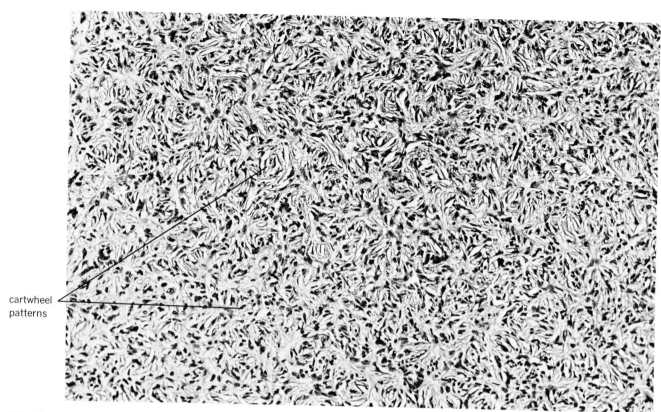

cartwheel
patterns

FIG. 13-32. Dermatofibroma resembling dermatofibrosarcoma protruberans. Cartwheel, whirligig, or storiform arrangement of fibroblasts is usually associated with dermatofibrosarcomas protruberans, but may sometimes be seen, as in this instance, in dermatofibroma. (× 178.)

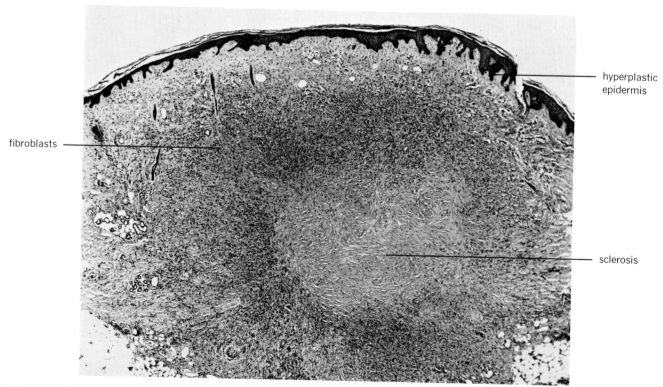

hyperplastic
epidermis

fibroblasts

sclerosis

FIG. 13-33. Dermatofibroma with sclerosis. Center of fibromatous nodule shown here is impressively sparse of fibroblasts compared with periphery. Central sclerotic zone doubtless is oldest portion of this scarring process. (× 32.)

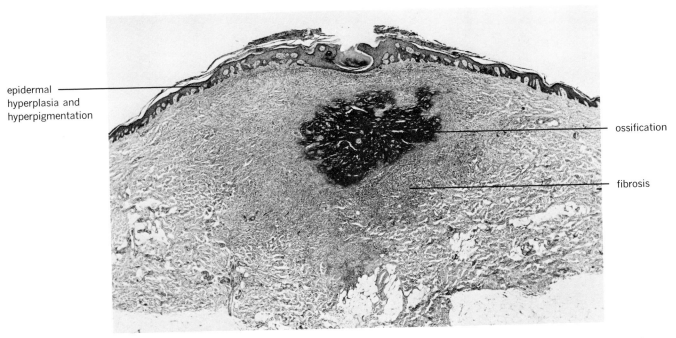

FIG. 13-34. Ossification in dermatofibroma. This rare occurrence of bone formation in midst of dermatofibroma resulted from versatile fibroblasts behaving like osteoblasts. (× 22.)

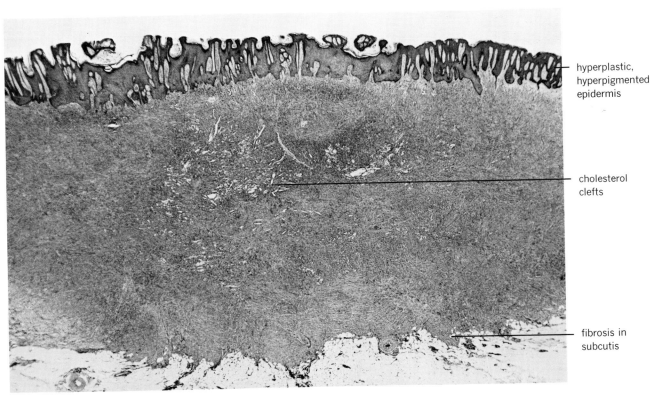

FIG. 13-35. Dermatofibroma. Numerous cholesterol clefts pictured result from antecedent extravasation of blood into dermis following sudden injury to skin. Note extension of fibrosis into subcutaneous fat. (× 14.)

Chronic Lymphedema (Fig. 13-36)

—Multiple knobby protuberances on the skin surface
—Fibrillary collagen and numerous fibroblasts oriented parallel to the skin surface and involving most of the dermis
—Dilated, thick-walled lymphatics and venules increased in number and aligned perpendicular to the skin surface
—Papillated epidermal hyperplasia with hyperkeratosis

Chronic lymphedema, as in elephantiasis, is a process that may proceed for decades. Early in the course of lymphedema, there is prominent edema in the reticular dermis and little papillomatosis or epidermal hyperplasia (Fig. 13-37).

The most common clinical manifestation of chronic lymphedema in skin is elephantiasis affecting the lower extremities. There is often a verrucous pattern to the surface of the skin caused by the fibrotic protuberances and the hyperplastic, hyperkeratotic epidermis. However, chronic lymphedema can also be found around the orbit and in other areas where there is prolonged brawny edema.

Chronic lymphedema is distinguished from the other types of hypertrophic fibroses by the increased number of thick-walled lymphatic and blood vessels throughout the dermis. These vessels

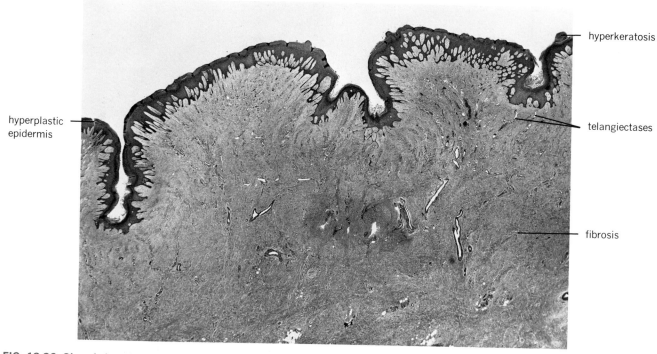

FIG. 13-36. Chronic lymphedema. A, Coarse, verrucous surfaces of legs of patients with elephantiasis are actually reflections of hypertrophic scarring, as illustrated, that results from persistent lymphedema in tissues. Dilated vessels shown are both thick-walled lymphatics and blood vessels. (× 17.)

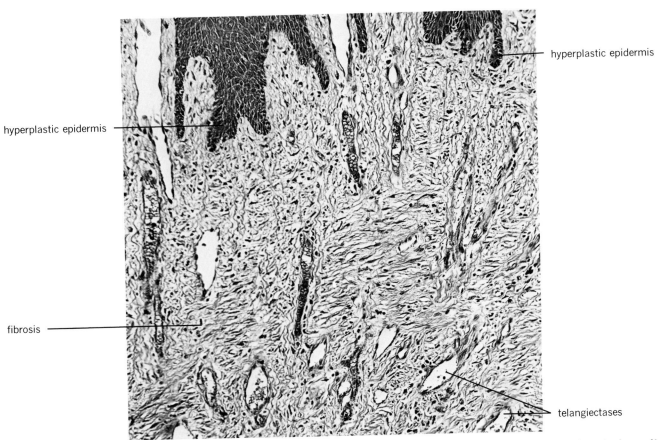

hyperplastic epidermis

hyperplastic epidermis

fibrosis

telangiectases

FIG. 13-36. Chronic lymphedema. B, This higher magnification shows highly angiomatous scarring of chronic lymphedema. It is difficult to determine with certainty which of altered vessels carried lymph and which circulated blood. (× 173.)

tend to be oriented perpendicular to the surface of the specimen. The fibrillary collagen is associated with an increased number of fibroblasts at all levels of the dermis. The changes of chronic

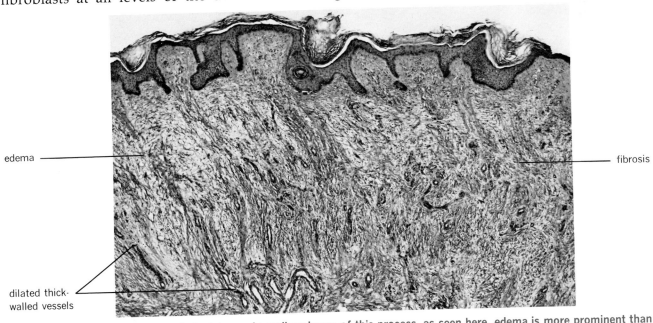

edema

fibrosis

dilated thick-walled vessels

FIG. 13-37. Chronic lymphedema in incipience. In earlier phases of this process, as seen here, edema is more prominent than fibrosis. (A, × 53; B, × 169.)

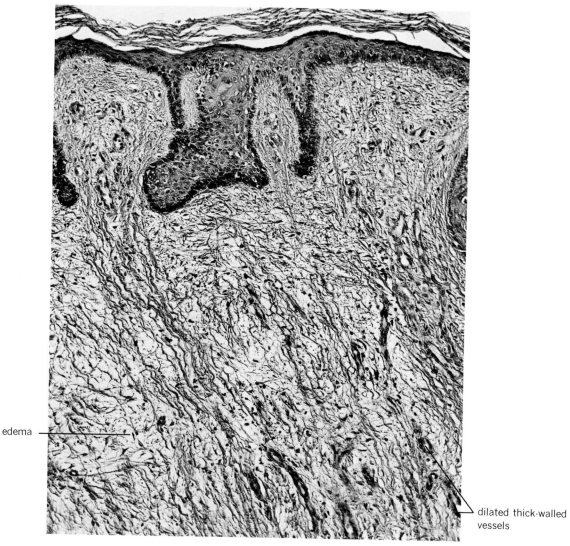

edema

dilated thick-walled vessels

FIG. 13-37. Chronic lymphedema in incipience. B.

lymphedema most closely resemble those of a scar, except for the increased number of lymphangiectases. No elastic fibers are present in the scars of chronic lymphedema.

Atrophic Fibroses

Clinically, cutaneous atrophy is characterized by shininess, whiteness, loss of surface markings of normal skin, easy wrinkling, and loss of cutaneous adnexa, especially hair follicles. Atrophy results primarily from changes in the papillary dermis, and not the epidermis. Fibrosis and sclerosis of the papillary dermis with the accompanying diminution or absence of the normal configuration of the epidermal rete and dermal papillae are major contributors to the clinical appearance of atrophy. The slight thinning of the epidermis makes a negligible contribution to the clinical constellation that constitutes atrophy.

Scars can be atrophic as well as hypertrophic. These distinctions are made primarily on clinical grounds. Hypertrophic scars are raised above the skin surface, whereas atrophic scars are depressed below it. Atrophic scars are also easily wrinkled when compressed between the thumb and first finger. Histologically, atrophic and hypertrophic scars are similar. A major difference between them lies in the total thickness of the scar compared to the surrounding normal dermis, well exemplified for atrophic variety by the pitted scars of acne vulgaris (Fig. 13-38). Subtle degrees of atrophy can result from alterations in the papillary dermis only. A subepidermal cleft or blister may form above an atrophic scar (Fig. 13-39).

With time, atrophic scars may become sclerotic histologically. Squamous cell and basal cell carcinomas may develop in the sclerotic scars of such dissimilar conditions as chronic discoid lupus erythematosus, chronic radiodermatitis, and granuloma inguinale. It may be theorized that the altered collagen in the papillary dermis of atrophic scars telegraphs faulty messages to the epidermal basal cells which respond by becoming neoplastic. Curiously, neoplasms do not develop in atrophic scars caused by surgical incisions or in striae distensae.

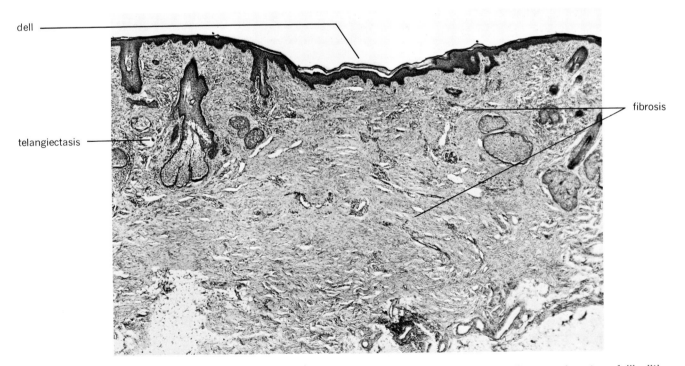

FIG. 13-38. Pitted scar of acne vulgaris. An ''ice-pick'' scar of acne results from severe suppurative granulomatous folliculitis that eventuates in well-circumscribed but extensive fibrosis. Note complete absence of adnexal epithelial structures in zone of fibrosis that extends from beneath delled epidermis to subcutaneous fat. ($\times$ 32.)

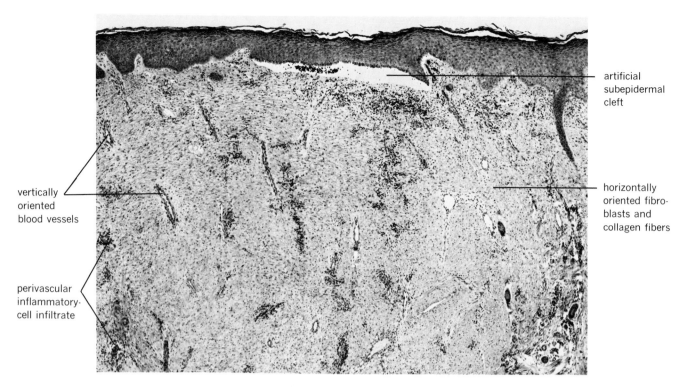

vertically oriented blood vessels

perivascular inflammatory-cell infiltrate

artificial subepidermal cleft

horizontally oriented fibro-blasts and collagen fibers

FIG. 13-39. Subepidermal cleft above scar. Faulty adhesion between connective tissue and epithelium in scar is revealed by formation in histologic processing of subepidermal cleft as illustrated. When this happens in vivo from friction or other trauma, tissue fluid accumulates within cleft and a subepidermal blister is formed. ($\times$ 63.)

Striae Distensae—Acute, Elevated Plethoric Stage (Fig. 13-40)

—Skin surface slightly domed
—Sparse, predominantly lymphocytic infiltrate around telangiectatic blood vessels of the superficial plexus
—Edema of the papillary and reticular dermis
—Elastic fibers fragmented throughout the reticular dermis (revealed in sections stained specially for elastic tissue) (Fig. 13-41)

Striae Distensae—Chronic, Depressed Whitened Stage (Fig. 13-42)

—Skin surface slightly bowed
—In the upper part of the dermis, increased numbers of closely packed elastic fibers arranged parallel to one another and to the surface of the skin in sections stained for elastic tissue (Fig. 13-43)
—Thinned collagen bundles in the zone of altered elastic fibers, associated with decreased numbers of thin fibroblasts
—Telangiectases and fibroblasts aligned parallel to the skin surface in the upper half of the dermis

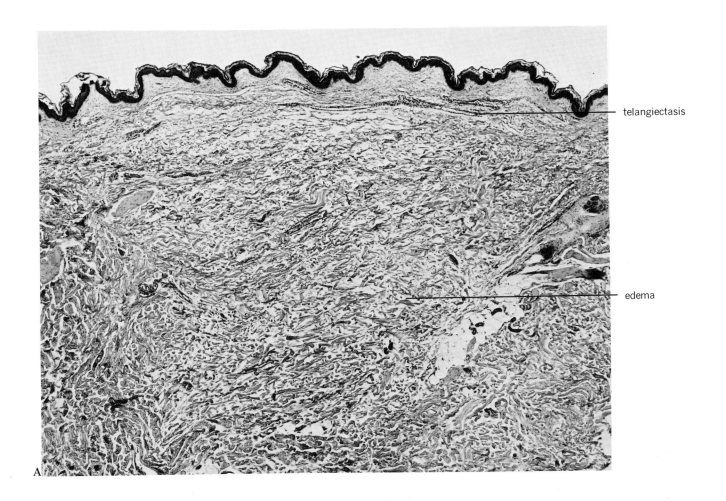

telangiectasis

edema

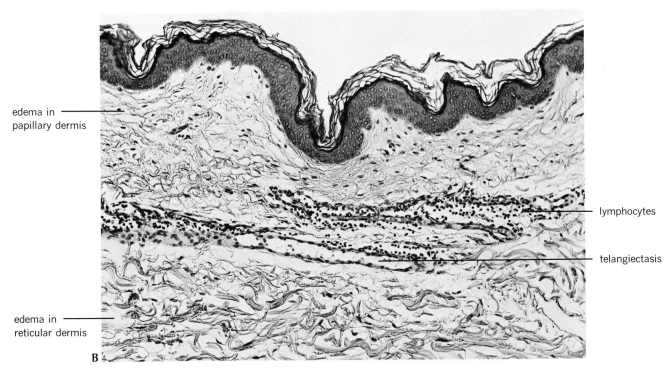

edema in
papillary dermis

lymphocytes

telangiectasis

edema in
reticular dermis

FIG. 13-40. Stria distensa, acute stage. In early stages of development pictured, collagen bundles in reticular dermis become widely separated from one another by edema, and a sparse lymphocytic infiltrate surrounds telangiectatic vessels of superficial plexus. (A, × 28; B, × 174.)

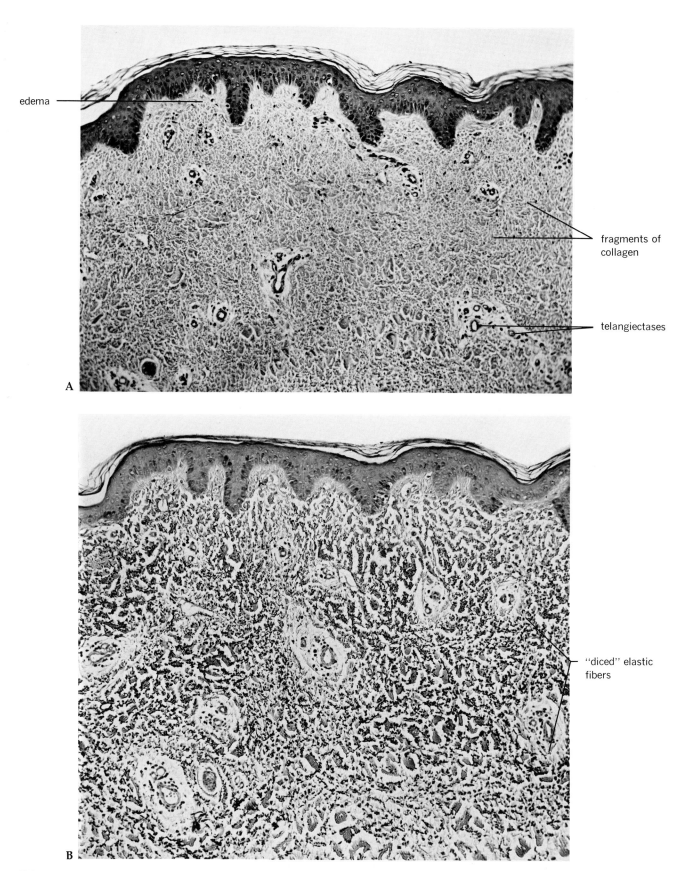

edema

fragments of
collagen

telangiectases

"diced" elastic
fibers

A

B

FIG. 13-41. Stria distensa, acute plethoric stage, elastic tissue stain. In these specimens both collagen and elastic fibers are seen
to be severely damaged. Instead of being normally elongated and wiry, elastic fibers appear to be fragmented into short, stubby
pieces as if they had been diced. Moreover, fragmented collagen bundles are separated by edema. (A, × 182; B, × 172.)

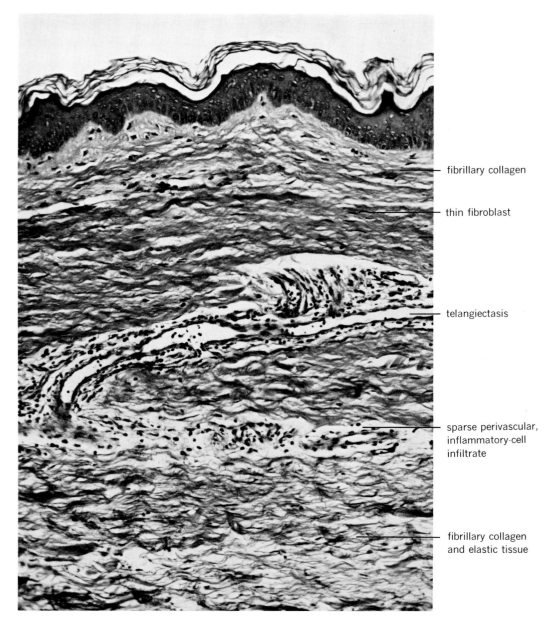

— fibrillary collagen

— thin fibroblast

— telangiectasis

— sparse perivascular, inflammatory-cell infiltrate

— fibrillary collagen and elastic tissue

FIG. 13-42. Stria distensa, atrophic stage. Abnormal features seen in fibrous tissue in reticular dermis include collagen not arranged in bundles in an orthogonal pattern, but rather as fibrils oriented parallel to skin surface and elastic tissue rather than collagen comprises much of the fibrillary material shown. Note telangiectases which are so prominent they may be visualized clinically. ($\times$ 182.)

The development of striae can be divided roughly into two clinical phases: elevated plethoric and depressed atrophic. During the acute phase, there is a sparse, mostly lymphohistiocytic infiltrate around widely dilated capillaries and venules in the edematous upper dermis. These telangiectases, engorged with erythrocytes, give early striae their livid hue. Stains for elastic tissues show severe fragmentation of the fibers in acutely distended striae. Rather than being normally long and straight, the elastic fibers in the reticular dermis are then only tiny bits that look as if they had been diced.

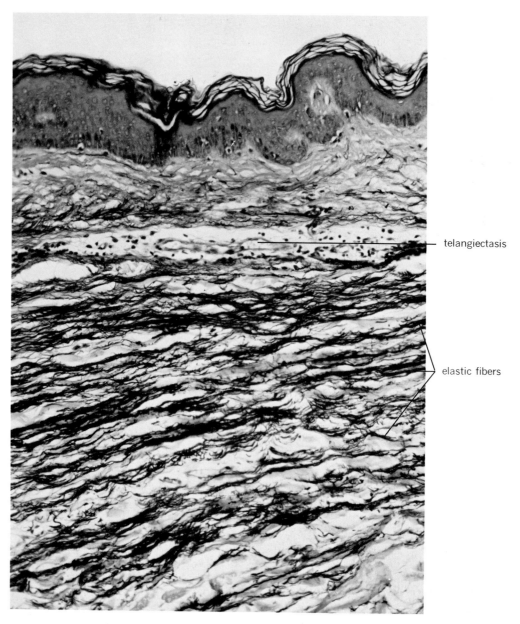

FIG. 13-43. Stria distensa, atrophic stage. Higher magnification of specimen illustrated in Fig. 13-42 stained for elastica reveals abundance of newly formed elastic fibers in an atrophic stria. Note paucity of collagen, which largely disappears during progression from plethoric to atrophic stage. (× 187.)

In atrophic striae, in contrast to earlier moments in the history of striae, there is alteration of both collagen and elastic tissue in the upper portion of the reticular dermis. Elastic tissue stains reveal a striking increase of presumably newly formed elastic fibers which are oriented parallel to the skin surface, as are the fibroblasts and dilated blood vessels. In sections stained by hematoxylin and eosin, atrophic striae can be differentiated from atrophic scars by the alignment of the blood vessels (horizontal in striae, vertical in scars), the number of fibroblasts (fewer in striae), and the amount of elastic tissue in the upper dermis (greater in striae).

Striae are caused by many factors, among them mechanical stretching of the skin and the effects of corticosteroids (topically or systemically) upon fibroblasts.

Macular Atrophies (including Anetodermas) (Fig. 13-44)

Macular atrophies are variously sized, well-circumscribed out-pouchings of thinned, soft, easily wrinkled skin. They occur secondary to a number of identifiable inflammatory skin diseases (secondary macular atrophy) that resolve with atrophic scars such as the conglobate lesions of acne vulgaris, particularly those on the chest and back, and also as a consequence of some diseases that cannot be identified with certainty (primary macular atrophy), either because no active lesions remain or those that do cannot be recognized with precision.

The term *anetoderma* applies to a variety of atrophic scars that tend to be raised as relatively large outpouchings above the skin surface. Finger pressure into the pouch reduces it back under the skin surface.

Histologically, macular atrophies possess all the features of an atrophic scar. Fibrillary collagen and fibroblasts parallel the skin surface and, most important, no elastic fibers can be demonstrated with stains for elastic tissues. Macular atrophies are gravestones of previous severe inflammatory reactions.

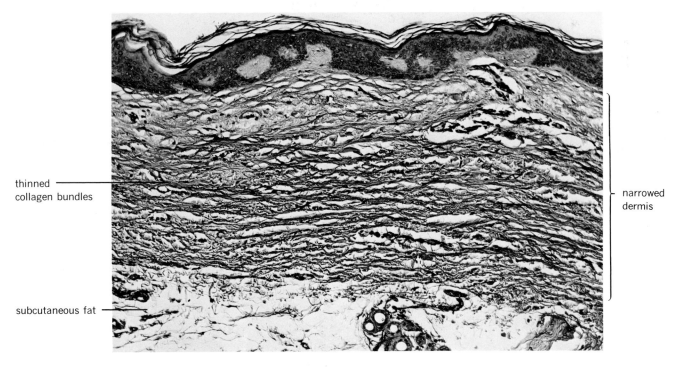

FIG. 13-44. Anetoderma. Characteristic changes pictured are narrowing of entire dermis, thinning of individual collagen bundles, and loss of elastic fibers. (× 180.)

Acrodermatitis Chronica Atrophicans

Acrodermatitis chronica atrophicans, a rare condition of the extremities, has a long inflammatory phase that eventuates in atrophy. Histologically, early lesions show a dense, bandlike lymphohistiocytic infiltrate in the upper middle portion of the edematous dermis; late lesions show a sclerotic superficial dermis, vacuolar alteration at the dermoepidermal junction, a thin epidermis with loss of the rete, and orthokeratosis. The atrophic dermis is reduced to approximately one half of its former thickness.

Clinically, acrodermatitis chronica atrophicans is a disease that affects middle-aged European women mostly. It begins on one or more limbs as dusky erythema that gradually resolves with atrophy. Carcinomas may develop in the atrophic patches.

Poikiloderma (Fig. 13-45)

The term *poikiloderma* refers to a constellation of clinical findings, namely, atrophy, mottled hyperpigmentation and hypopigmentation, and telangiectases. Poikiloderma represents an end stage of various pathologic (usually inflammatory) processes.

Histologically, the atrophy in poikiloderma, regardless of the underlying disease, results from alterations in the papillary dermis. Instead of the normal delicate collagen fibrils and the normal pattern of epidermal rete and dermal papillae there are thickening and homogenization of the collagen in the papillary dermis and a flat dermoepidermal interface. Additionally, there are usually melanophages and telangiectases in the papillary dermis and foci of epidermal hypopigmentation and hyperpigmentation.

Nonetheless, histologic distinctions can be made among some of the poikilodermas, such as of solar poikiloderma (Civatte), poikilodermatomyositis, poikiloderma vasculare atrophicans, and poikiloderma associated with chronic radiodermatitis. Differentiation is accomplished on the basis of critical histopathologic changes coincident with those of poikiloderma such as solar elastosis in poikiloderma of Civatte, vacuolar alteration and thickening of the basement membrane zone in dermatomyositis, a bandlike mononuclear cell infiltrate in the papillary dermis with mononuclear cells solitarily and in nests within the epidermis of poikiloderma vasculare atrophicans, and large bizarre fibroblasts in the sclerotic dermis of poikiloderma caused by excessive radiation therapy. Fluorinated corticosteroids, which have high potency when applied topically for long periods, can cause poikilodermatous changes. Some inflammatory processes resolve with clinical features of poikiloderma, but histologic examination gives no clue as to their cause.

In rare instances, such as pictured in Figure 13-45, it may be impossible to determine the exact nature of a poikilodermatous process, just as it may be futile to identify precisely the cause of a scar or a dermatofibroma. However, in most instances the word *poikiloderma* should be joined with other explanatory terms such as *vasculare atrophicans* or *of Civatte,* just as the words *parapsoriasis* and *porokeratosis* should always be modified and not used unmodified.

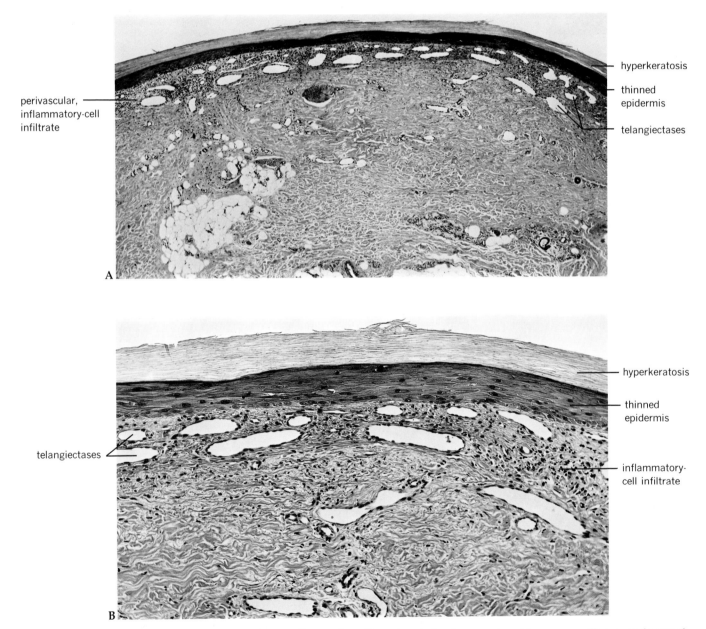

FIG. 13-45. Poikiloderma. The normally delicate collagen of papillary dermis has been replaced by coarse collagen, and normal pattern between dermal papillae and epidermal rete ridges has been effaced. Prominent telangiectases contribute to poikilo-dermatous appearance of lesion clinically. (A, × 52; B, × 175.)

Disseminated Superficial Porokeratosis

Disseminated superficial porokeratosis, which was discussed previously in Chapter 6, resolves with small atrophic patches that are sharply marginated by slightly raised keratotic rims. The atrophic center consists of fibrotic papillary dermis overlain by a thin epidermis (Fig. 13-46A). The usual pattern of rete and papillae is missing. These histologic features are second-

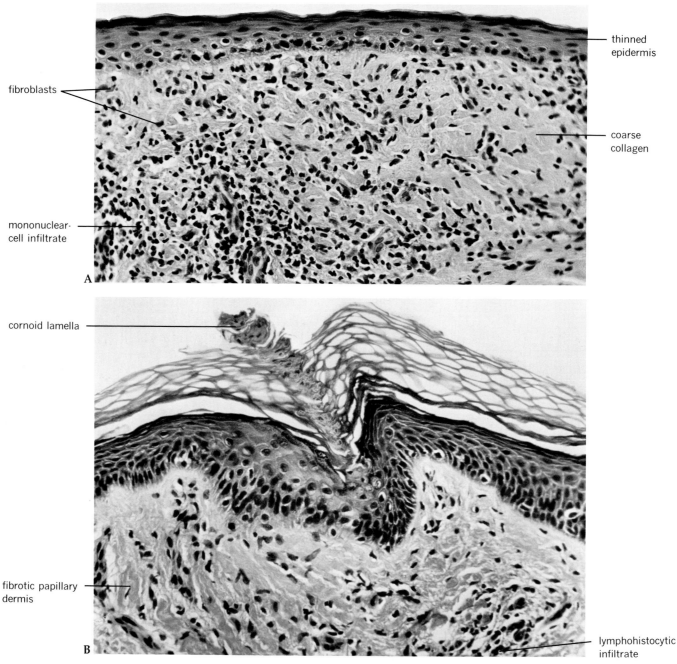

FIG. 13-46. Disseminated superficial porokeratosis. A, Atrophic center in lesion shown results from thickening of papillary dermis, coarseness of collagen bundles, obliteration of normal pattern of dermal papillae and rete ridges, and, to a lesser extent, thinning of epidermis. (× 352.) B, A diagnostic feature is cornoid lamella that leans toward center of lesion. (× 382.)

ary to a long-standing inflammatory-cell infiltrate in the papillary dermis that also leaves melanophages and telangiectases as residua. Stain for elastic tissues reveals decreased elastic fibers in the altered papillary dermis. The thin keratotic rim is represented histologically by a cornoid lamella (Fig. 13-46B).

Lichen Planus, Atrophic (Fig. 13-47)

Some lesions of lichen planus resolve with clinical features of atrophy as has been discussed previously (Chapter 6). As in other inflammatory processes that end atrophically, the papillary dermis in old lesions of lichen planus is extensively altered. The normal delicate collagen fibers are replaced by coarse ones, and the normal undulating pattern between dermal papillae and epidermal rete ridges is effaced. The long-standing superficial bandlike inflammatory-cell infiltrate in lichen planus doubtlessly influences fibroblasts in the papillary dermis to manufacture altered collagen, just as it influences keratinocytes and melanocytes in the epidermal basal layer to release melanin to macrophages.

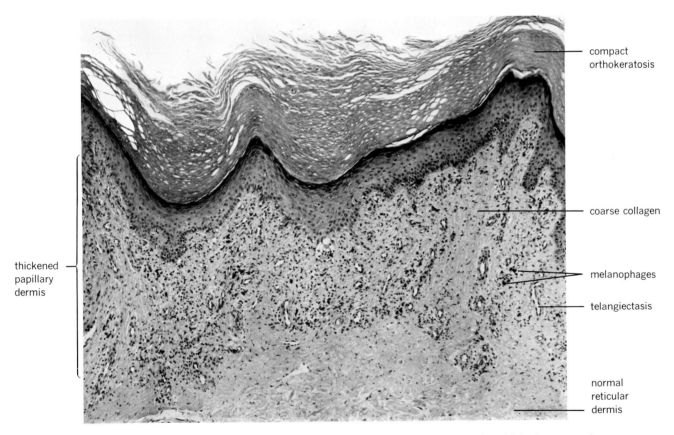

FIG. 13-47. Lichen planus, resolving lesion. Note fibrotic thickening of papillary dermis in which there are also numerous telangiectases and melanophages. Combination of fibrosis in papillary dermis plus alteration of normal pattern between epidermal rete ridges and dermal papillae gives rise to clinical features of atrophy, despite prominent cornified layer which is normal for volar aspect of wrist, from which this biopsy came. ($\times$ 88.)

Scleroses

Scleroses, like fibroses, may be hypertrophic or atrophic. The prototype of hypertrophic sclerosis is scleroderma, and that of atrophic sclerosis is lichen sclerosus et atrophicus.

Hypertrophic Scleroses

Scleroderma (Fig. 13-48)

—Thickened homogenized collagen bundles throughout the dermis
—Spaces between thickened collagen bundles narrowed or absent
—Sclerosis often in the subcutaneous fat
—Decreased number of fibroblasts
—Decreased epithelial adnexal structures
—Melanophages often in upper dermis
—Foci of epidermal hyperpigmentation and hypopigmentation
—Lymphangiectases occasionally in upper dermis

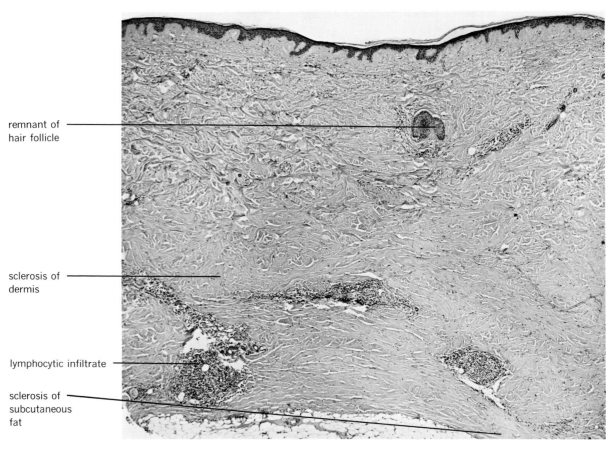

remnant of hair follicle

sclerosis of dermis

lymphocytic infiltrate

sclerosis of subcutaneous fat

FIG. 13-48. Scleroderma. A, Note extensive sclerosis in lower portion of reticular dermis and upper portion of subsutaneous fat. (× 45.)

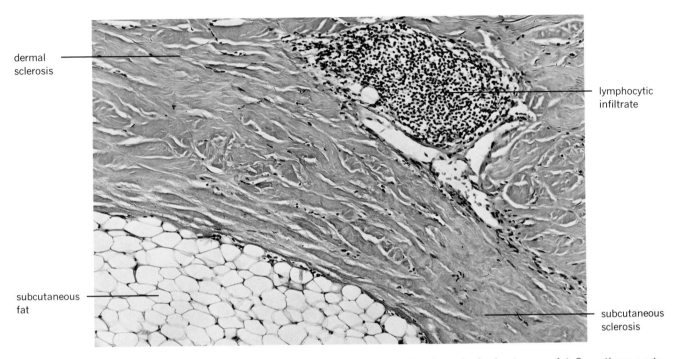

dermal
sclerosis

lymphocytic
infiltrate

subcutaneous
fat

subcutaneous
sclerosis

FIG. 13-48. Scleroderma. B, Higher magnification shows that sclerosis has replaced much of subcutaneous fat. Sometimes septa are preserved but are thickened by sclerosis. ($\times$ 167.)

The earliest histologic change in scleroderma is inflammatory, i.e., a predominantly lymphocytic infiltrate around the blood vessels of both the superficial and deep plexuses in conjunction with a panniculitis in which lymphocytes, plasma cells, and eosinophils predominate. In time the inflammatory-cell infiltrate diminishes, and prominent thickening of the collagen bundles occurs throughout the dermis. There are diminished numbers of fibroblasts associated with the thickened collagen bundles in the reticular dermis and also replacement of adnexal epithelium, especially pilosebaceous units, by sclerosis. Stains for elastic tissues reveal no destruction of elastic fibers in the reticular dermis (Fig. 13-49), but elastic tissue is absent in the zone of sclerosis that replaces the subcutaneous fat following panniculitis.

Similar histologic changes are seen in all forms of scleroderma. The atrophoderma of Pasini and Pierini is probably best interpreted as an atrophic stage of morphea.

Clinically, the induration of scleroderma results from thickened collagen bundles, especially in the reticular dermis. Sclerosis of the subcutis and fascia gives it its "hidebound" consistency. Pigmentary alterations are common in scleroderma, the mottled hyperpigmentation and hypopigmentation ("salt and pepper") being due to contiguous foci of increased and decreased melanin within the epidermis coupled with melanophages in the papillary dermis. Hairs are usually absent in sclerodermatous skin as a result of replacement of follicular units by the altered collagen.

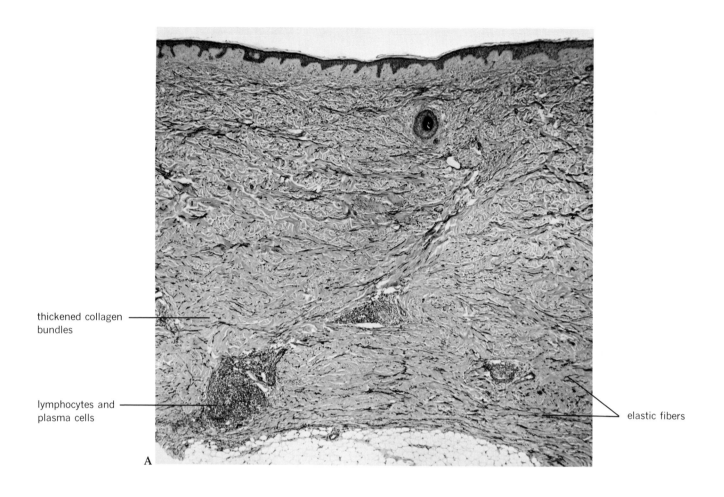

thickened collagen bundles

lymphocytes and plasma cells

elastic fibers

A

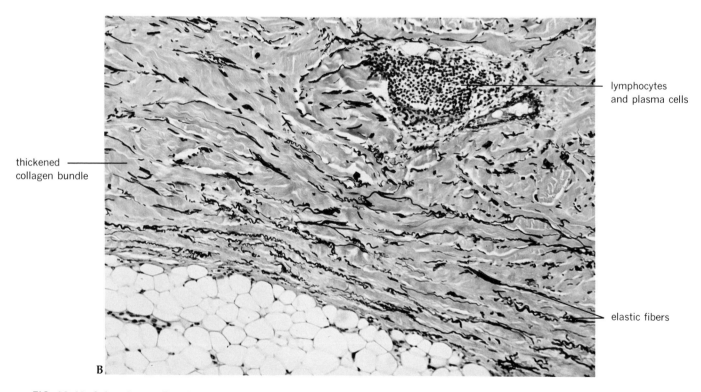

lymphocytes and plasma cells

thickened collagen bundle

elastic fibers

B

FIG. 13-49. Scleroderma. Despite dramatic alteration in dermal (and subcutaneous) collagen, a hallmark of scleroderma, elastic fibers throughout dermis are apparently unaffected, as is well shown here. (A, × 42; B, × 163.)

Lichen Sclerosus et Atrophicus (Fig. 13-50)

—Thickened sclerotic papillary dermis
—Telangiectases in sclerotic zone
—Melanophages in upper dermis
—Vacuolar alteration at dermoepidermal junction
—Thin epidermis with diminished pattern of epidermal rete and dermal papillae
—Decreased epidermal melanin
—Orthokeratosis
—Adnexal plugging (infundibular and acrosyringeal) by orthokeratotic cells

Unlike scleroderma, in which the dominant pathologic process involves the reticular dermis, lichen sclerosus et atrophicus involves only the papillary dermis. The papillary dermis initially is prominently thickened by edema and later by the sclerotic collagen that replaces it. Beneath the thickened papillary dermis is a moderately dense lymphohistiocytic perivascular infiltrate. The density of the inflammatory cells is greater during the edematous, than during the sclerotic, stage of the disease. Above the thick-

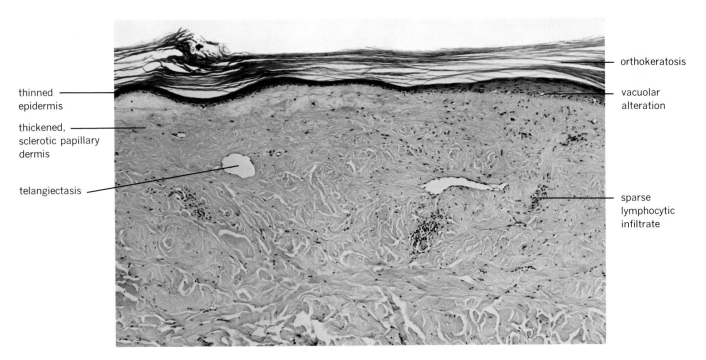

FIG. 13-50. Lichen sclerosis et atrophicus. That this is a long-standing lesion is indicated by thinned epidermis, thickened sclerotic papillary dermis, and scant inflammatory-cell infiltrate. That lesion is atrophic clinically may be inferred from complete reorganization of collagen pattern in papillary dermis and complete effacement of usual undulations between rete ridges and dermal papillae. ($\times$ 92.)

ened, sclerotic papillary dermis there are vacuolar alteration at the dermoepidermal interface, a thin epidermis with a diminished pattern of rete and papillae, and plugging of adnexal orifices by orthokeratotic cells. In long-standing lesions, the vacuolar alteration may extend to become dermoepidermal separation. When extravasated erythrocytes from telangiectatic vessels in the sclerotic dermis enter the subepidermal space, a hemorrhagic bulla develops. Elastic tissue stain of the sclerotic papillary dermis reveals few, if any, elastic fibers (Fig. 13-51).

The clinical lesions of lichen sclerosus et atrophicus are white and atrophic. Whiteness is due to sequestration of epidermal pigment in dermal melanophages and to dermal sclerosis. Atrophy results from alteration of the dermoepidermal interface by papillary dermal sclerosis and from thinning of the epidermis. Lichen sclerosus et atrophicus in the vulvar and perianal regions is intensely pruritic, and superimposition of lichen simplex chronicus is a common happening.

Two uncommon occurrences in lichen sclerosus et atrophicus merit mention. One is the finding, in a single biopsy specimen, of morphea in both the reticular dermis and subcutis and lichen sclerosus alone in the thickened papillary dermis. The other is the possibility of development of squamous cell carcinoma in atrophic lesions of lichen sclerosus situated on the vulva.

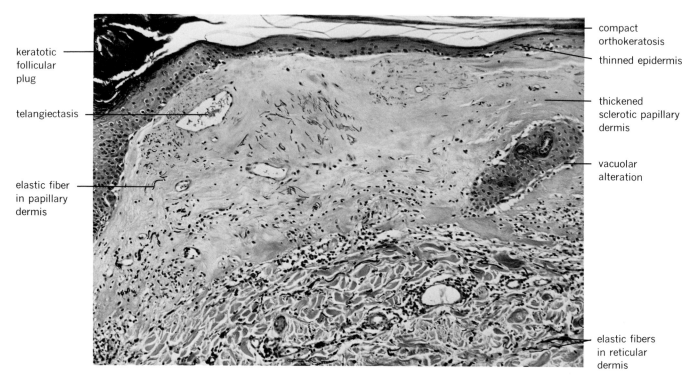

FIG. 13-51. Lichen sclerosis et atrophicus. Only a few bits of elastic tissue are seen in thickened sclerotic papillary dermis. Note relatively normal pattern of elastic fibers in reticular dermis, alteration of arrangement of collagen in papillary dermis, and obliteration of pattern between rete ridges and dermal papillae. ($\times$ 158.)

—Sclerosis throughout the upper dermis
—Bizarre fibroblasts with atypical nuclei and stellate cytoplasm in the sclerotic area
—Subepidermal fibrin often
—Vacuolar alteration at the dermoepidermal interface
—Epidermal hyperplasia with hyperkeratosis
—Fibrin thrombi in superficial, and sometimes deep, capillaries and venules
—Fibrin in walls of some superficial blood vessels
—Some vessels obliterated by sclerosis
—Melanophages and a mixed inflammatory-cell infiltrate, especially around blood vessels in the upper dermis

In many ways, the histologic changes of chronic radiation sclerosis resemble those of lichen sclerosus et atrophicus. In radiation sclerosis, however, the edema in the thickened papillary dermis is often associated with subepidermal fibrin. A mixed inflammatory-cell infiltrate of lymphocytes, histiocytes, plasma cells, eosinophils, and neutrophils occurs around increased numbers of dilated blood vessels throughout the dermis. Many of the blood vessels are rimmed and thrombosed by fibrin. Similar vasculature changes occur in late lesions of atrophie blanche. Eventually, the edematous papillary dermis of radiodermatitis is replaced by sclerotic collagen in which there are numerous melanophages, telangiectases, and large stellate fibroblasts with bizarre, and often multiple, nuclei. These fibroblasts are often so atypical that they resemble the cells of a sarcoma. The epidermis in long-standing radiation sclerosis is often hyperplastic and hyperkeratotic. Elastic tissue stains of radiation sclerosis show practically no elastic fibers in the thickened sclerotic dermis (Fig. 13-53).

The clinical lesions of chronic radiodermatitis are often poikilodermatous, the atrophy resulting from the sclerotic papillary dermis, the telangiectases from the increased number of dilated blood vessels throughout the papillary dermis, and the pigmentary alterations from focal loss of epidermal melanin into dermal macrophages.

Ironically, the sclerotic, barren dermis of chronic radiodermatitis is fertile soil for the development of neoplasms such as basal cell carcinoma, squamous cell carcinoma, malignant melanoma, radiation sarcoma, and atypical fibroxanthoma. Of these neoplasms, basal cell carcinoma occurs with greatest frequency.

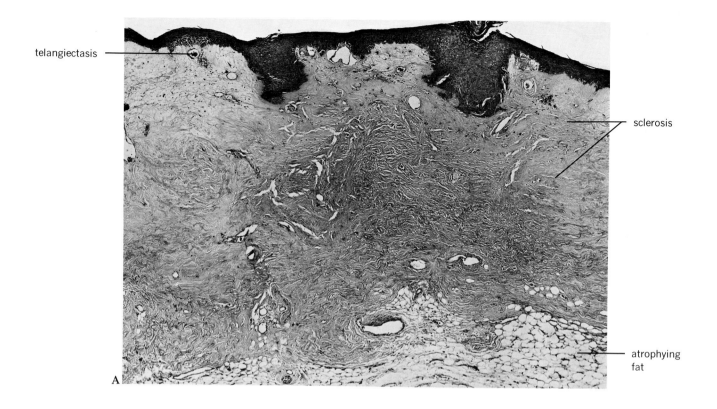

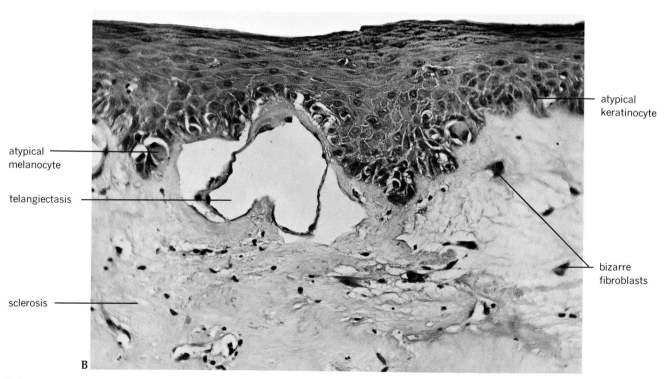

FIG. 13-52. Chronic radiodermatitis. A, Entire thickness of dermis is involved by sclerosis. Note that all adnexal epithelial structures have been destroyed in the process of sclerosis. (× 56.) B, Diagnostic features shown are large, bizarre fibroblasts associated with sclerosis and telangiectases. Note that there are both atypical keratinocytic and melanocytic hyperplasia in overlying epidermis which in time and in some instances may transform to carcinoma and even malignant melanoma. (× 374.)

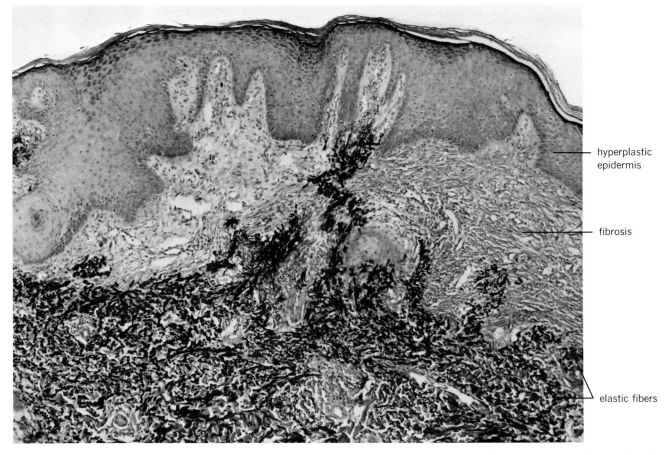

hyperplastic epidermis

fibrosis

elastic fibers

FIG. 13-53. Chronic radiodermatitis. Scarring may occur in upper part of the dermis only and is accompanied by destruction of elastic fibers in that zone as illustrated here. (Elastic tissue stain; × 85.)

Necrobiosis Lipoidica (Fig. 13-54)

—Sclerosis, especially of the lower half of the dermis
—Thickened sclerotic septa in the subcutis
—Diminution or absence of epithelial adnexal structures
—Telangiectases in the upper dermis
—Thin epidermis with a muted pattern at the interface between rete and papillae
—Sparse, predominantly perivascular infiltrate of histiocytes and plasma cells

The sclerotic stage of necrobiosis lipoidica, a cutaneous manifestation of diabetes mellitus, involves the entire dermis, but especially the mid and lower reticular dermis. Irregularly-shaped zones of sclerotic collagen are interspersed throughout the dermis at sites of previous collagen degeneration. The subcutaneous fibrous septa are usually thickened and sclerotic. A sparse granulomatous infiltrate may also be present around blood vessels and

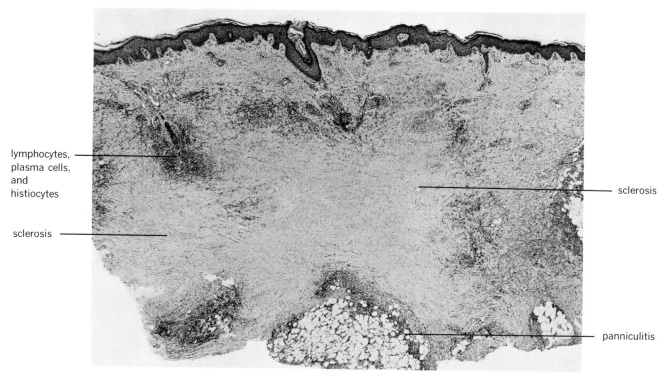

lymphocytes, plasma cells, and histiocytes

sclerosis

sclerosis

panniculitis

FIG. 13-54. Necrobiosis lipoidica, sclerosing stage. As is illustrated here, sclerosis tends to affect especially lower half of reticular dermis and subcutaneous fat. That process is still progressing is evidenced by a moderately dense infiltrate of inflammatory cells, many of which seem to be arranged in palisade around zone of sclerosis. (× 28.)

between collagen bundles at all levels of the dermis during the early sclerotic stage (Fig. 13-55). In end-stage lesions, however, there is only a desert of sclerosis. Elastic tissue stains reveal no elastic fibers in the sclerotic areas of necrobiosis lipoidica.

Clinically, the long-standing lesion of necrobiosis lipoidica is a shiny, yellowish, indurated, atrophic patch stippled with telangiectasis and containing no hairs. The yellow color results from lipid deposited in the papillary dermis. The induration is a manifestation of the dermal sclerosis; the atrophy, of obliteration of the usual relationship between rete and papillae; and the telangiectases, of dilated blood vessels in the papillary dermis.

Other atrophic and sclerotic lesions that occur in diabetics, especially on the legs, have been termed diabetic dermopathy and are reputed to be analogous to lesions of diabetic neuropathy, retinopathy, and nephropathy. Rather than resulting from occlusion of small blood vessels, however, dermopathy in diabetics probably simply represents atrophic scarring following physical trauma. A contrary view holds that dermopathy is really specific for diabetes and has diagnostic histologic signs, namely, thickening of the basal lamina of small blood vessels. These findings are best appreciated by electronmicroscopy.

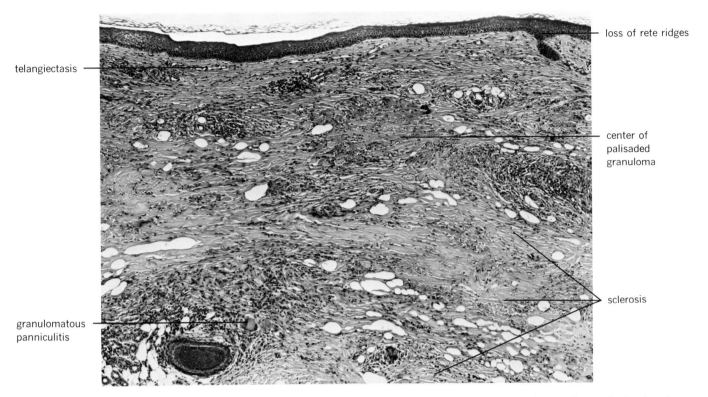

telangiectasis

loss of rete ridges

center of
palisaded
granuloma

sclerosis

granulomatous
panniculitis

FIG. 13-55. Necrobiosis lipoidica, early sclerosing stage. Earliest sclerotic changes, as are pictured here, affect reticular dermis and progress *pari passu* as granulomatous phase resolves. (× 79.)

Chronic Discoid Lupus Erythematosus (Fig. 13-56)

—Sclerosis of at least the upper third of the dermis
—Obliteration of adnexal epithelial structures, especially hair follicles, often with fibrotic tracts at sites of former follicles
—Infiltrate of variable density of lymphocytes and plasma cells around the blood vessels of the deep plexus
—Thickened basement membrane
—Thinned epidermis with diminished or absent rete ridges
—Orthokeratosis, often with plugging of dilated follicular infundibula

The indisputable sign that enables differentiation of the sclerotic dermis of chronic discoid lupus erythematosus from all other scleroses is prominent thickening of the epidermal basement membrane. When the scarring process results in permanent alopecia, as it so often does, hair erector muscles and fibrotic tracts may be the only testaments to the earlier presence of hair follicles.

Unlike most scars that are comparable to graves that lack identifying tombstones, the scars of chronic discoid lupus erythematosus are readily recognized because of the thickened basement membranes. Besides discoid lupus erythematosus, only poikilodermatous lesions of dermatomyositis have thickened basement membranes. The thickening results from reduplication of the basal lamina.

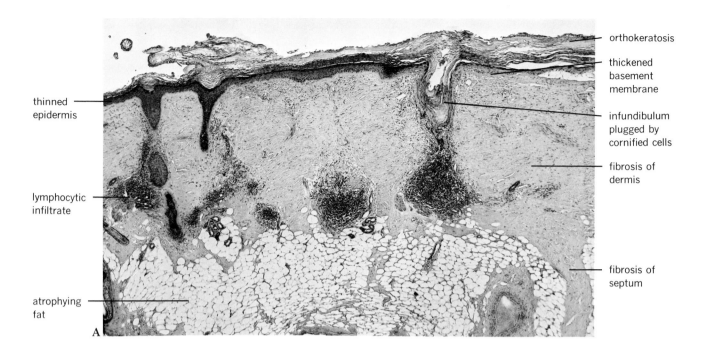

orthokeratosis

thickened basement membrane

infundibulum plugged by cornified cells

fibrosis of dermis

fibrosis of septum

thinned epidermis

lymphocytic infiltrate

atrophying fat

A

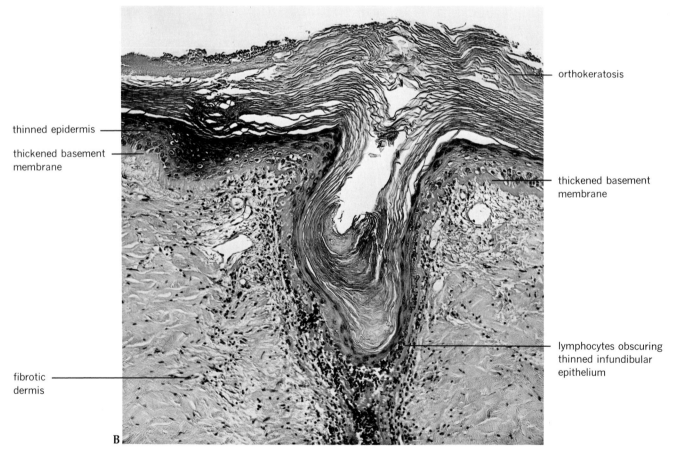

orthokeratosis

thinned epidermis

thickened basement membrane

thickened basement membrane

lymphocytes obscuring thinned infundibular epithelium

fibrotic dermis

B

FIG. 13-56. Chronic discoid lupus erythematosus. A, This long-standing lesion from scalp marred by alopecia is marked by fibrosis throughout dermis and even in subcutis. Inflammatory-cell infiltrate of lymphocytes and some plasma cells is confined mostly to regions around blood vessels of deep plexus. Clinching diagnostic feature is thickened basement membrane at interface between fibrotic dermis and thinned epidermis. ($\times$ 47.) B, In this higher magnification, note that basement membrane is thickened at interface between dermis and follicular epithelium as well as between dermis and epidermis. ($\times$ 142.)

Many inflammatory processes resolve with fibrosis and on the way to fibrosis, histiocytes and fibroblasts may predominate. A consummate example is the "woody" induration in culminating lesions of actinomycosis. Examples that will be described in more detail are histiocytoma, histoid leprosy, and xanthogranulomas. Other examples are resolving lesions of granuloma faciale (Fig. 13-57), juxta-articular nodes of syphilis (Fig. 13-58), and xanthomas (Fig. 13-59).

The presence of prominent fibrosis in the various fibrohistiocytic proliferations tends to obscure the diagnostic histologic signs of the underlying pathologic process. Each of these long-standing conditions is more easily diagnosable histologically at an earlier stage in its evolution when it is uncomplicated by fibrosis, but it can be suspected even then. Therefore, it is important to consider the possibilities of diseases like lepromatous leprosy and syphilis in what at first seems to be nothing more than a banal fibrohistiocytic proliferation and proceed to do a Fite stain to confirm the former disease and a serologic test for the latter.

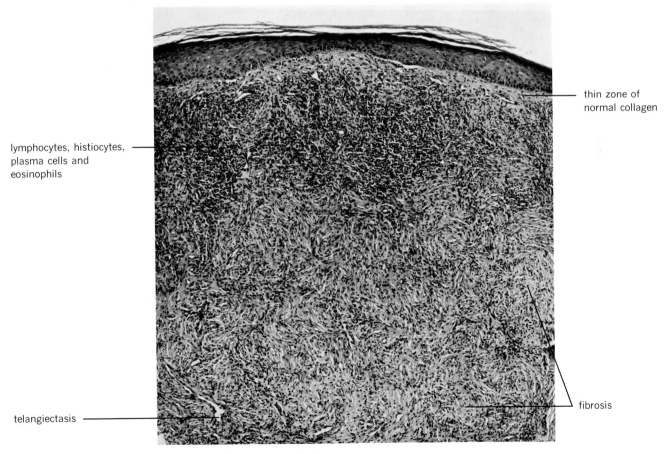

lymphocytes, histiocytes, plasma cells and eosinophils

thin zone of normal collagen

fibrosis

telangiectasis

FIG. 13-57. Granuloma faciale, fibrosing stage. Early in the evolution there is persistent leukocytoclastic vasculitis, which evolves into dense, diffuse, mixed-cell infiltrate. Then in months, or years, the process ends in fibrosis, as is beginning here. (× 82.)

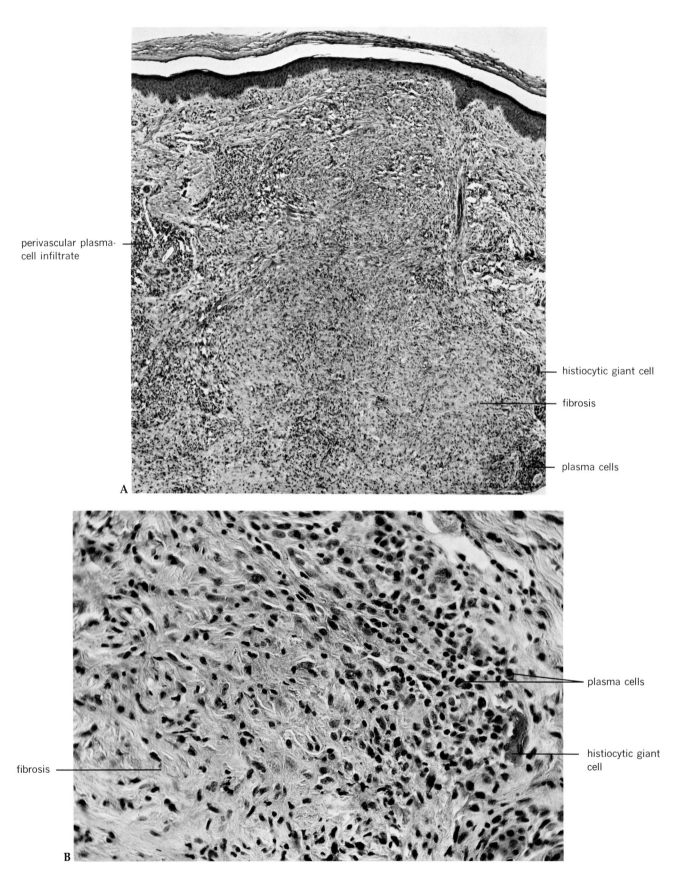

FIG. 13-58. Juxta-articular node of syphilis, a late secondary or early tertiary lesion. Center consists of fibrosis sprinkled with plump fibroblasts and histiocytes, and periphery is marked by perivascular infiltrates of lymphocytes and plasma cells. Under scanning power, a slight resemblance to palisaded granuloma is discernible. (A, × 53; B, × 352.)

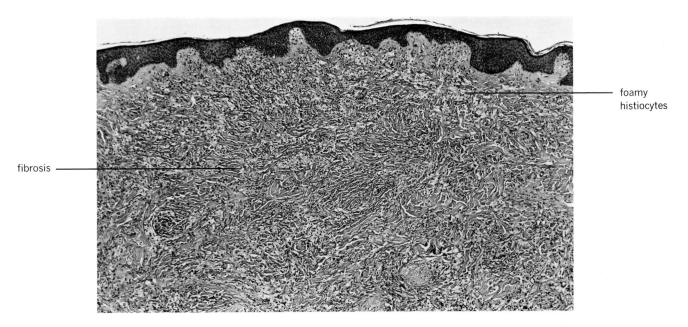

fibrosis

foamy
histiocytes

FIG. 13-59. Xanthoma resolving with fibrosis. Long-standing lesions of several types of xanthomas show fibrosis interspersed between islands of foamy histiocytes throughout the dermis as pictured here. ($\times$ 70.)

Histiocytoma (Fig. 13-60)

—Dense, diffuse, predominantly histiocytic infiltrate throughout the dermis
—Often numerous foam cells and siderophages (Plate 1)
—Many fibroblasts and endothelial cells within the infiltrate
—Hyperplastic and hyperpigmented epidermis

Just as dermatofibroma is a kind of dermatofibrosis, histiocytoma is really a histiocytosis, a reactive inflammatory process. These two conditions, histiocytoma and dermatofibroma, are related in the sense that both presumably follow local trauma, both are nodules that eventuate in fibrosis, and both are associated with overlying epidermal hyperplasia and hyperpigmentation. However, whereas fibroblasts and fibrosis are clearly the dominant histologic features of dermatofibroma, histiocytes predominate in histiocytoma. Hemosiderin and lipid are often present within the cytoplasm of histiocytes (siderophages and foam cells). The iron and fat derive from vessels during the original traumatic event. With time, the histiocytic component of histiocytoma decreases, the fibrocytic component increases, and eventually histiocytomas evolve into dermatofibromas.

It is impossible to distinguish clinically between histiocytoma and dermatofibroma, and the two conditions should be thought of as parts of the same pathologic spectrum. (Histiocytoma is discussed at greater length in Chapter 9.)

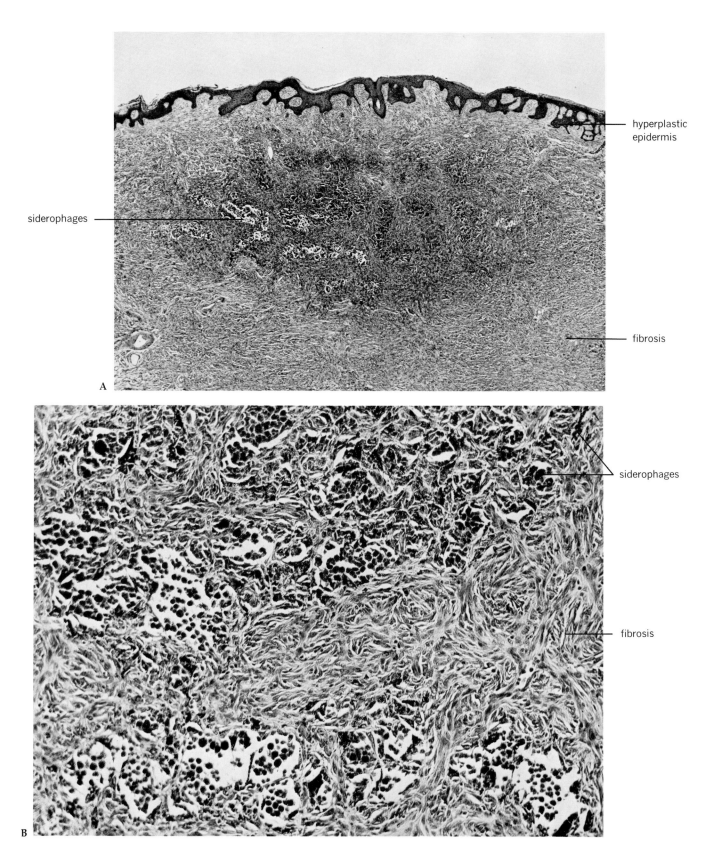

hyperplastic epidermis

siderophages

fibrosis

siderophages

fibrosis

A

B

FIG. 13-60. Histiocytoma with siderophages. A, Center of lesion in dermis consists mostly of histiocytes, many containing hemosiderin, whereas periphery of lesion pictured consists mainly of fibroblasts. These findings stem from severe, sharply targeted trauma, to a point in dermis with hemorrhage, phagocytosis of extravasated erythrocytes consequently, and fibrosis eventually. (× 31.) B, Intermingling of histiocytes containing hemosiderin and fibroblasts in this higher magnification illustrates interrelationship between histiocytoma and dermatofibroma, the former simply being a forerunner of the latter. (× 175.)

In histoid leprosy, a manifestation of lepromatous leprosy, fibroplasia partly replaces the dense nodular or diffuse infiltrate of foam cells which causes the lesion to resemble histologically a histiocytoma. Fite stain reveals the true nature of the lesion by coloring the countless lepra bacilli red. (Fig. 13-61C; Plate 3).

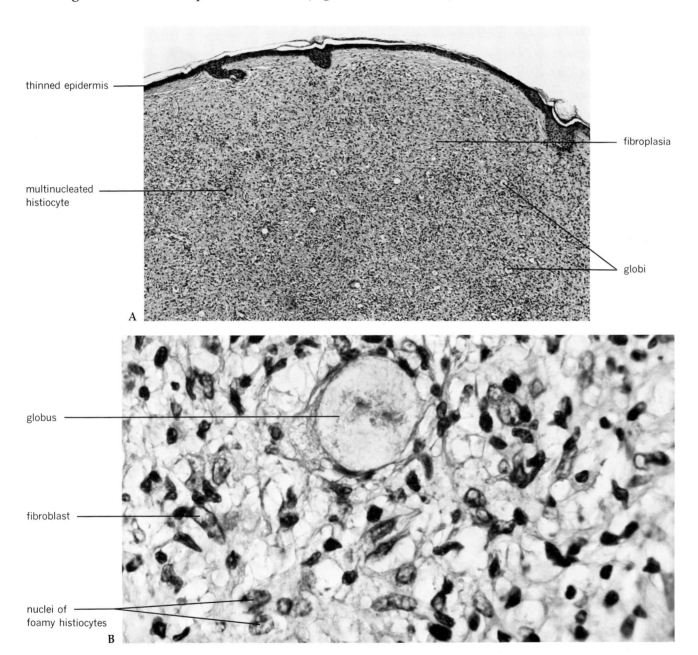

thinned epidermis

fibroplasia

multinucleated histiocyte

globi

A

globus

fibroblast

nuclei of foamy histiocytes

B

FIG. 13-61. Histoid leprosy. A, Diagnostic features illustrated are dense, diffuse, fibrohistiocytic infiltrate in which there are many foam cells containing lepra bacilli. Under scanning magnification, as in this photomicrograph, lesion could be confused with histiocytoma, but unlike that condition there is no epidermal hyperplasia, rather epidermal thinning instead. (× 64.) B, In this higher magnification many foam cells such as are common in lepromatous leprosy are pictured. Large foam cell in the center, called a globus, contains innumerable lepra bacilli. Even in this section stained by hematoxylin and eosin the diagnosis of leprosy, rather than simple xanthoma, may be suspected because of presence of granular gray-staining material within foam cells. Granules represent bacilli of leprosy. (× 916.)

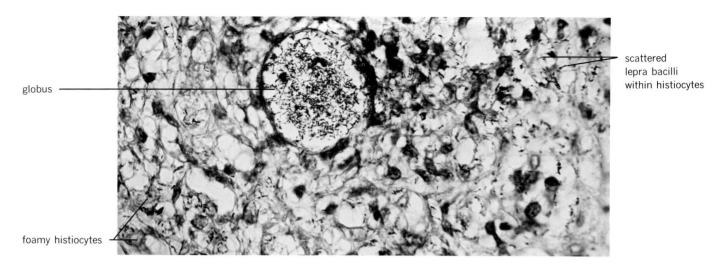

globus

scattered lepra bacilli within histiocytes

foamy histiocytes

FIG. 13-61. Histoid leprosy. C, In this Fite-stained section contiguous to that of B, lepra bacilli are clearly revealed. (× 893.)

Xanthogranulomas, Juvenile and Adult (Fig. 13-62)

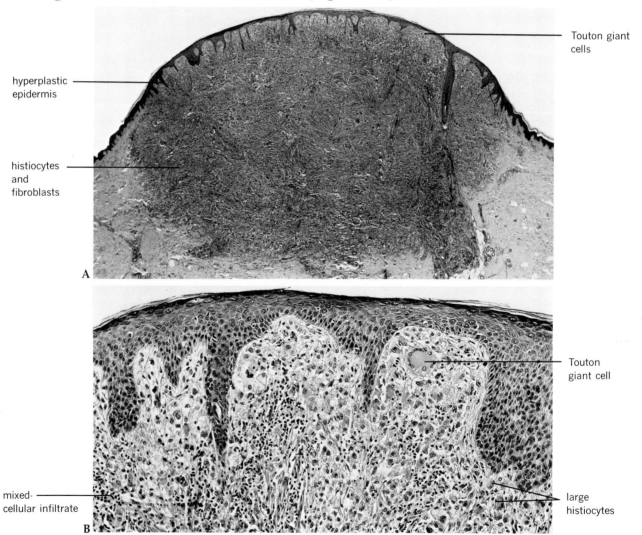

Touton giant cells

hyperplastic epidermis

histiocytes and fibroblasts

A

Touton giant cell

mixed-cellular infiltrate

large histiocytes

B

FIG. 13-62. Xanthogranuloma, fibrosing stage. A characteristic is tendency to undergo spontaneous resolution by gradual fibrosis, some of which is illustrated here. Because scarring process is still early, diagnostic histologic features to be seen are dense, diffuse, mixed-cell infiltrate composed mostly of histiocytes, many of which are multinucleated and have foamy cyto-plasm, i.e., Touton giant cells. (A, × 20; B, × 48.)

Xanthogranulomas are characterized by dense diffuse dermal infiltrates composed predominantly of histiocytes with foamy cytoplasm, characteristic multinucleated histiocytes with foamy cytoplasm (Touton giant cells), and other scattered inflammatory cells such as lymphocytes, plasma cells, and eosinophils. With time, fibroblasts join the granulomatous infiltrate, which gradually, but progressively, is replaced by fibrosis (Fig. 13-60).

Xanthogranulomas that are histologically indistinguishable occur in both children and adults (see Chapter 9). Spontaneous resolution, the result of fibrous replacement of the granulomatous infiltrate, occurs predominantly in juvenile xanthogranuloma, but may occur in the adult form as well.

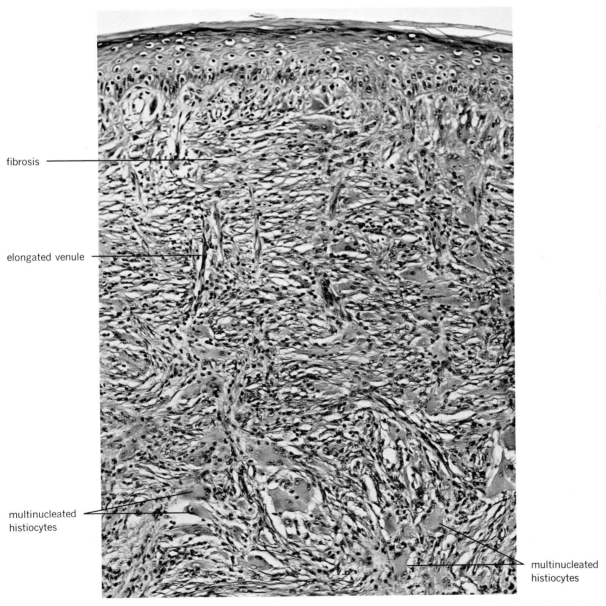

FIG. 13-63. Xanthogranuloma, resolving with fibrosis. At first glance, changes in upper part of dermis are those of scar: fibrillary collagen and fibroblasts oriented parallel to surface of specimen and blood vessels arranged perpendicular to it. ($\times$ 176.)

Panniculitis

Septal Panniculitis

With vasculitis
  Small vessel
    Leukocytoclastic vasculitis
  Large vessel
    Subcutaneous polyarteritis nodosa
    Scleroderma, acute lesions
    Thrombophlebitis
      Multiple segmental (migratory) thrombophlebitis
      Varicose thrombophlebitis
Without vasculitis
  Erythema nodosum
  Necrobiosis lipoidica
  Scleroderma, chronic lesions
  Fasciitis with eosinophilia

Lobular Panniculitis

With large vessel vasculitis
  Nodular vasculitis
  Erythrocyanosis with nodules and pernio
Without vasculitis
  Sclerema neonatorum
  Subcutaneous fat necrosis of the newborn
  Poststeroid panniculitis
  Weber-Christian syndrome
  Subcutaneous sarcoidosis
  Subcutaneous granuloma annulare
  Lipodystrophy
  Infections (e.g., with fungi or bacteria)
  Lupus erythematosus profundus
  Pancreatic panniculitis
  Physical (thermal, mechanical, chemical)
    and factitial panniculitis
  Lymphomatous and leukemic "panniculitis"

Panniculitis

14

THE SUBCUTANEOUS fat is an integral part of the skin. Fat cells are frequently present in the lower dermis, the vasculature of the fat is continuous with that of the dermis, and the fibrous trabeculae of the fat are extensions of the dermis. Thus the three major components of the subcutis—lipocytes, blood vessels, and fibrous trabeculae—are continuous with the dermis.

The basic unit of the subcutaneous fat, the primary microlobule, is composed of a microscopic collection of lipocytes. The primary microlobule measures approximately 1 mm in diameter. An aggregate of primary microlobules, termed the secondary lobule, is approximately 1 cm in diameter. The secondary lobule is surrounded by an easily discernible fibrous cloak, seen as septa in microscopy. Thin collagen fibers extend from the fibrous septa to surround each primary microlobule. These thin septa between microlobules may be impossible to discern in sections routinely stained with hematoxylin and eosin, but they become evident with the reticulin stain or when india ink has been injected into the blood vessels of the subcutaneous fat.

The arteries and veins of the panniculus are housed within the major septa (Fig. 14-1). The arteries are small (0.5 mm to 20 μ) and muscular, whereas the veins are slightly larger (20 μ to 1 mm). In sections stained with hematoxylin and eosin it is not always possible to differentiate between these septal vessels. However, the veins, in addition to their larger size, tend to be oval in transverse section rather than round and have thinner, less muscular walls. Internal elastic laminae, better visualized with stains for elastic tissue, are usually present in the subcutaneous arteries, but not in the veins.

Smaller vessels branch from the large blood vessels to supply portions of the secondary lobule (Fig. 14-2). One arteriole and one venule supply each primary microlobule. The arteriole occupies a central position within the microlobule, whereas the venule courses along the periphery. Between the arteriole and the venule is a capillary system. Each fat cell is surrounded by a capillary network. The vascular supply of each microlobule is terminal in the sense that there are no capillary connections between adjacent microlobules. Furthermore, although the same large blood vessels supplying the panniculus continue on to nourish the dermis, there are no capillary connections between the dermis and the subcutaneous fat. In addition to the blood vessels within the fibrous septa, there are also lymphatics and nerves.

The importance of proper biopsy of the subcutaneous fat in the histologic diagnosis of panniculitis cannot be too strongly emphasized. Because the inflammatory process often decreases the adhesion of the subcutis to the dermis, a punch biopsy frequently fails to deliver the fat. A scalpel incisional biopsy is imperative. It should extend broadly and deeply to include sufficient fatty tissue for study. For diagnostic purposes, it is important to examine microscopically the most "active" lesion, i.e., one that is red, indurated, and perhaps tender or painful. There is clearly a need

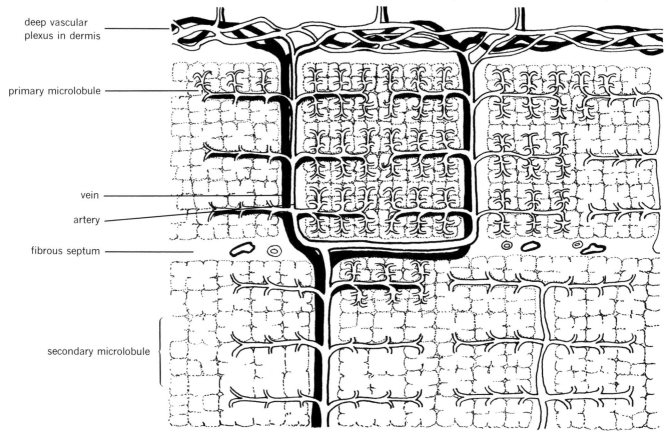

deep vascular plexus in dermis

primary microlobule

vein

artery

fibrous septum

secondary microlobule

FIG. 14-1. Architecture of the subcutaneous fat and its vasculature.

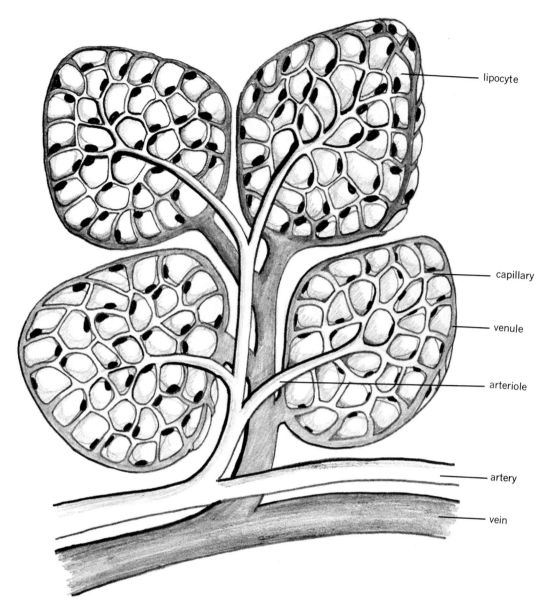

FIG. 14-2. Vascular supply to four microlobules.

for more biopsies of panniculitides because so much fundamental information is still lacking. In addition, the panniculitides would be better understood, if when feasible, clinicians consulted pathologists before the biopsy so that the tissue could be specially processed for immunofluorescent and chemical studies.

In the pathology laboratory, the specimen must be properly fixed to enable proper tissue sectioning. Step sections should be done to ensure that areas containing diagnostic changes are not overlooked. For example, when pathologic changes in large blood vessels are essential for diagnosis, a single histologic section, which may not contain large vessels, would be inadequate. In large-vessel disease, special stains may be indicated, e.g., stain for elastic tissue to distinguish an artery from a vein by the presence or absence of an internal elastic lamina. In some granulomatous panniculitides, the PAS stain should be used to search for deep fungi, and the acid-fast stain for mycobacteria. Polarized light should be utilized to detect foreign bodies.

Diagnosis of inflammatory diseases of the fat, like diagnosis of inflammatory diseases in the dermis, is based on patterns perceived with the scanning objective. The two major patterns of panniculitis are septal and lobular, depending on where most of the inflammatory cells are found (Fig. 14-3). The terms *lobular* and *lobule* hereafter refer to the secondary lobule. Although most panniculitides can clearly be separated into either septal or lobular types, in some instances these patterns overlap. In rare cases, such as when the inflammatory cells from a septal panniculitis occasionally spill over to involve large portions of lobules, it may be impossible to make a decisive judgment as to whether the process is predominantly septal or lobular.

It is important to emphasize that many lobular panniculitides involve large blood vessels coursing within the septa. Thus, in lobular panniculitis, pathologic changes may also occur in the septa. The term *lobular panniculitis,* however, does not imply that entire lobules are necessarily involved. Only portions of some lobules may be affected. In almost all panniculitides there is some dermal involvement, but it is extensive in but a few. At the least, this involvement is manifested by a sparse perivascular inflammatory-cell infiltrate around dilated dermal blood vessels. Conversely, panniculitis may follow pathologic events in the dermis, such as rupture of follicular cysts or pilonidal sinuses.

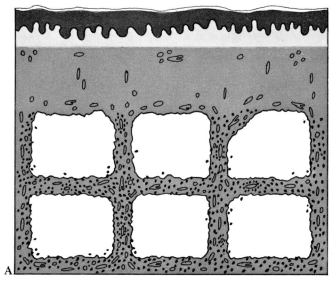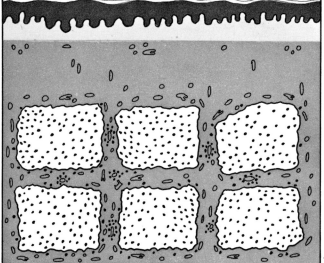

FIG. 14-3. A, Septal panniculitis. B, Lobular panniculitis.

Unlike most dermatitides, which tend to be short-lived, most panniculitides are persistent, lasting for weeks and even months and years. Depending on when the biopsy is taken in these long-standing processes, different histologic features will be found. In most panniculitides, the sequence of cells that dominate the site of injury is first the neutrophils, then the lymphocytes, the histiocytes, and eventually the fibroblasts. Frequent final changes of panniculitis are either septal or lobular fibrosis.

Because panniculitis tends to be long-standing, each panniculitis has different diagnostic features at different stages in its course. For this reason, no attempt has been made in this chapter to capture in telegraphic capsular form the sometimes great histologic variability in the course of panniculitis.

Septal Panniculitis (Fig. 14-3A)

Panniculitides with predominantly septal involvement may be classified into those with vasculitis and those without.

With Vasculitis

Vasculitic changes in septal panniculitis may occur either in small vessels (leukocytoclastic vasculitis) or in large vessels (subcutaneous polyarteritis nodosa, acute lesions of scleroderma, and thrombophlebitis). These vasculitides were discussed more fully in Chapter 8.

Small-vessel Vasculitis

Leukocytoclastic Vasculitis. This condition involving the capillaries and venules in the septa of the subcutis is nearly always associated with similar changes involving the blood vessels of both dermal plexuses. Inflammatory cells are often present at the periphery of contiguous lobules secondary to vasculitic changes within the septa.

Large-vessel Vasculitis

Subcutaneous Polyarteritis Nodosa. This condition begins as a neutrophilic vasculitis involving the muscular arteries of the panniculus. Secondary to these vascular changes, there is circumscribed, rather than diffuse, panniculitis in the vicinity of the affected blood vessel.

Scleroderma, Acute Lesions. As has previously been mentioned in Chapter 8, neutrophilic infiltrates within the walls of small and medium-sized arteries in the subcutaneous fat are among the earliest histologic changes in acute lesions of scleroderma. Concurrent with this neutrophilic vasculitis are perivascular nodular infiltrates of lymphocytes and plasma cells around small blood vessels at the junction of fat septa and lobules.

Thrombophlebitis. Panniculitis may be seen in two types of thrombophlebitis: multiple segmental thrombophlebitis and varicose thrombophlebitis. In *multiple segmental (migratory) thrombophlebitis,* a disease of the superficial veins of the arms and legs, a consistent finding is thrombosis, and the inflammatory-cell infiltrate varies from sparse to profuse. Initially, neutrophils are present within the vessel walls. Later they are joined by lymphocytes and histiocytes, some multinucleated. Since there is but slight panniculitis, multiple segmental thrombophlebitis is discussed in greater detail in Chapter 8.

In patients with chronic venous insufficiency secondary to stasis and with varicosities in the subcutis, a *varicose thrombophlebitis* may result. In these circumstances, severe panniculitis develops as a consequence of the phlebitis. The clinical manifestations of this combined vasculitis and panniculitis are plaquelike areas of indurated erythema of the skin and subcutaneous tissue. Ulceration is common. Varicose thrombophlebitis tends to involve the lower third of the legs.

Without Vasculitis

Erythema Nodosum. This disease is the prototype of septal panniculitis. The earliest stage of erythema nodosum is characterized by a sparse infiltrate of neutrophils and, episodically, of eosinophils around an increased number of capillaries and venules within edematous septa (Fig. 14-4). In time, the infiltrate becomes predominantly lymphohistiocytic, and eventually histiocytic giant cells appear. During this evolution from granulation tissue to granulomatous inflammation, the inflammatory-cell infiltrate extends progressively from the septa into the adjacent lipocytes at the periphery of the lobule (Fig. 14-5). Slight fat necrosis and foam cells may then be seen. Granulomatous inflammation, in which histiocytic giant cells are often conspicuous, occurs between the granulation tissue and the fibrosis in the thickened trabeculae. In some foci within the septa, there are dense collections of lymphocytes, and in others, collections of histiocytes (tubercles). All of these changes, ranging from granulation tissue with neutrophils

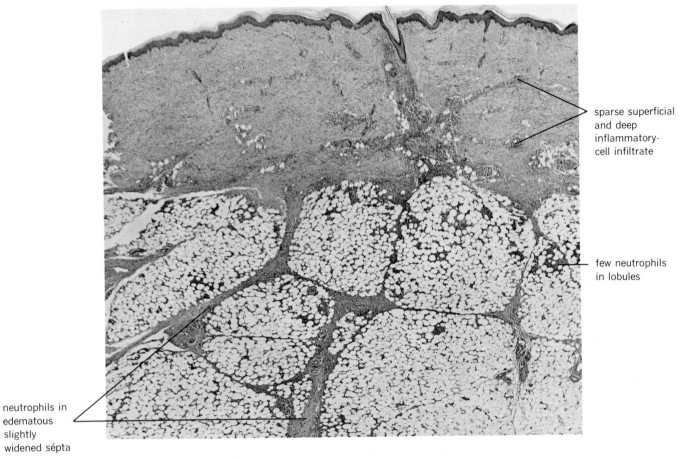

sparse superficial and deep inflammatory-cell infiltrate

few neutrophils in lobules

neutrophils in edematous slightly widened sépta

FIG. 14-4. Erythema nodosum, early lesion. Note widening of septa of subcutaneous fat caused by transudate and neutrophils. (× 23.)

and eosinophils to granulomatous inflammation to fibrosis, may be present in a single histologic section of erythema nodosum. In time, the acute inflammatory changes wane, and only thickened fibrotic septa remain. Older lesions of erythema nodosum exhibit thick fibrotic septa, and as a consequence fat lobules become reduced in size and even obliterated (Fig. 14-6).

The absence of large-vessel involvement (Fig. 14-7), i.e., vasculitis, significant lobular involvement, and necrosis is what distinguishes erythema nodosum from nodular vasculitis. However, in exceptional cases of erythema nodosum, the extent of lobular involvement may be comparable with that in mild cases of nodular vasculitis. Rarely, if ever, is there phlebitis.

Although the major changes of erythema nodosum are in the subcutaneous fat, there is always some involvement of the overlying dermis. A sparse lymphohistiocytic infiltrate surrounds blood vessels throughout the dermis. Capillaries and venules of the superficial plexus are widely dilated.

Classically, erythema nodosum begins as bright-red, shiny, warm, exquisitely tender, symmetrical patches, usually in the skin

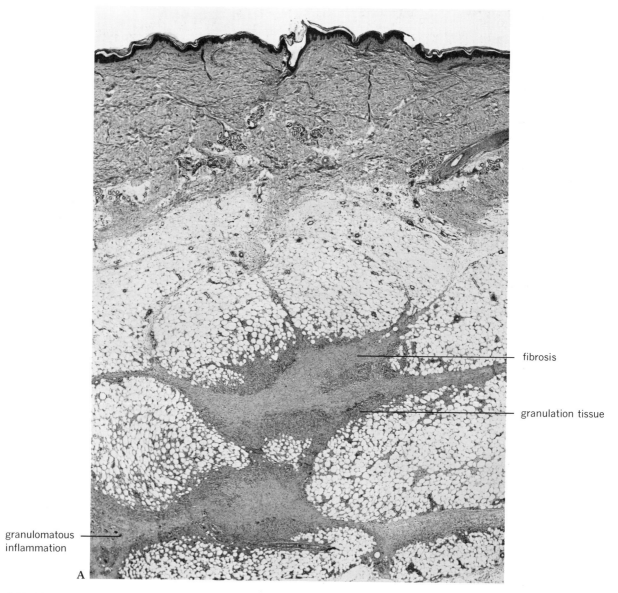

fibrosis

granulation tissue

granulomatous
inflammation

A

FIG. 14-5. Erythema nodosum. A, Diagnostic features pictured are those of granulomatous septal panniculitis in which widened septa also have granulation tissue at their peripheries and fibrosis in their centers. (× 17.)

overlying the anterior aspect of the tibiae. With time, the lesions become increasingly nodose and violaceous. Eventually, the lesions resolve without sequellae, save for hyperpigmentation and on rare occasions slight depressions below the surface of the skin. Indeed, a critical clinical feature of erythema nodosum is the absence of ulceration. For much of its life span, the typical lesion of erythema nodosum resembles a bruise, and for this reason the condition was formerly termed "erythema contusiformis."

Lesions of erythema nodosum are not necessarily confined to the lower extremities but may develop anywhere in the subcutaneous tissue. Young women are affected more commonly than men, and there may be associated fever and arthralgia.

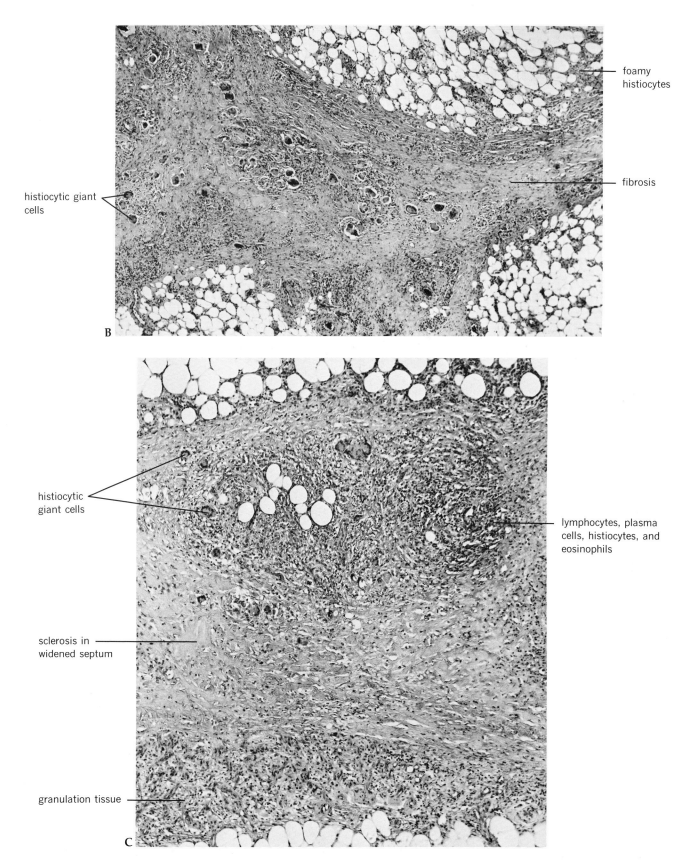

foamy
histiocytes

fibrosis

histiocytic giant
cells

histiocytic
giant cells

lymphocytes, plasma
cells, histiocytes, and
eosinophils

sclerosis in
widened septum

granulation tissue

Fig. 14-5. Erythema nodosum. B, Granulomatous inflammation and fibrosis are better seen in this higher magnification. Note that slight lobular panniculitis is also present, especially at peripheries of lobules. (× 60.) C, Stages seen are granulation tissue at junction between widened septum and constricted fat lobule, granulomatous and mixed-cell infiltrates scattered throughout septum, and fibrosis toward center of septum. (× 74.)

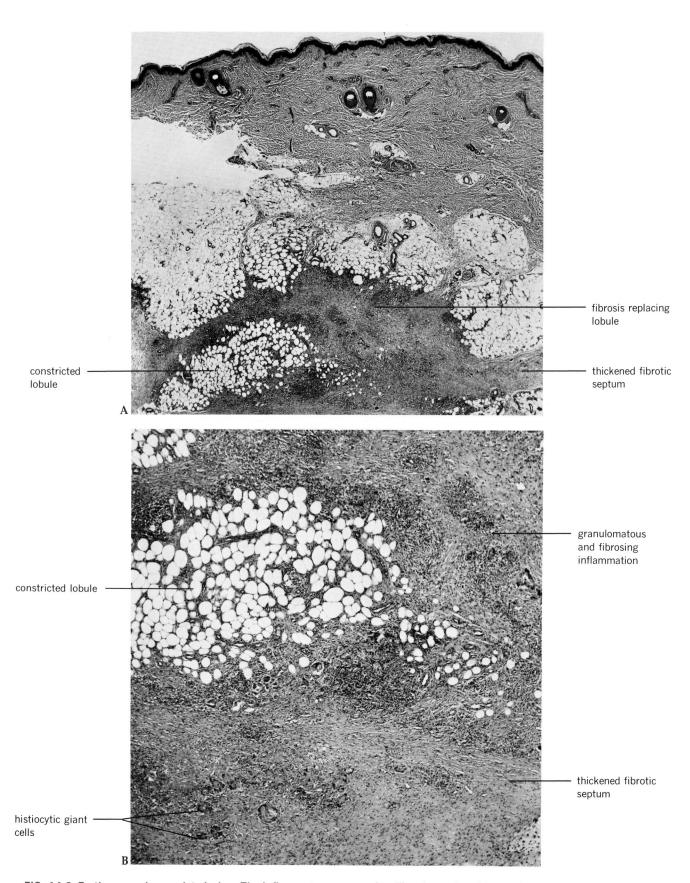

FIG. 14-6. Erythema nodosum, late lesion. The inflammatory process is still active as is evidenced by persistence of granulomatous changes within thickened fibrotic septa. However, lesion is a long-standing one as is told by extent of fibrosis that has partially obliterated a fat lobule. (A, × 21; B, × 44.)

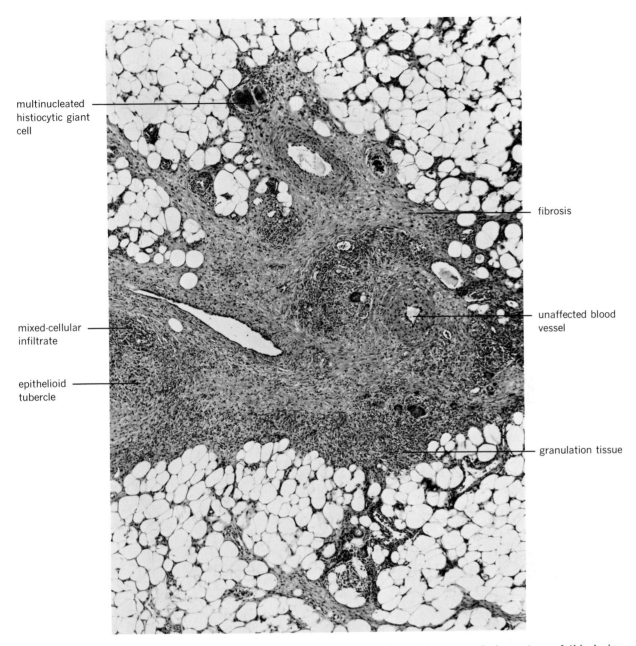

multinucleated
histiocytic giant
cell

fibrosis

mixed-cellular
infiltrate

unaffected blood
vessel

epithelioid
tubercle

granulation tissue

FIG. 14-7. Erythema nodosum. This photomicrograph shows clearly that large blood vessels in septum of this lesion are completely spared by intense inflammatory reaction, that is, there is no vasculitis, only perivascular inflammatory-cell infiltration. (× 53.)

In most instances, individual lesions of erythema nodosum last approximately for 3 to 6 weeks, but in exceptional cases they persist for many months. Erythema nodosum can recur. Regardless of duration of the lesions, the basic pathologic process is the same. The subacute nodular migratory panniculitis of Vilanova and Piñol is histologically indistinguishable from erythema nodosum, but clinically there are fewer, less tender, asymmetrically distributed lesions that migrate centrifugally and persist longer. I consider subacute nodular migratory panniculitis to be a variant of erythema nodosum.

Erythema nodosum is thought to be a reaction of delayed hypersensitivity involving the subcutaneous fat. In the United States, erythema nodosum is most frequently associated with streptococcal infection, sarcoidosis, coccidioidomycosis, histoplasmosis, and drugs such as oral contraceptives.

The clinical and histologic features of erythema nodosum are fundamentally the same, regardless of cause. Erythema nodosum is a pathologic process wholly different from erythema nodosum leprosum, which is a leukocytoclastic vasculitis associated with lepromatous leprosy.

Necrobiosis Lipoidica. In necrobiosis lipoidica, the dominant pathologic process involves the dermis where there is palisaded

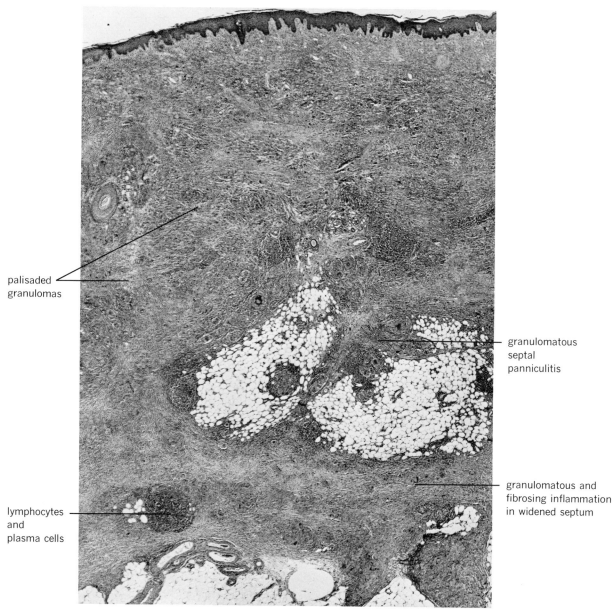

palisaded
granulomas

granulomatous
septal
panniculitis

granulomatous and
fibrosing inflammation
in widened septum

lymphocytes
and
plasma cells

FIG. 14-8. Necrobiosis lipoidica. All early lesions are marked by granulomatous panniculitis as shown here. Note similarity of changes in subcutis to those of erythema nodosum. (A, × 24; B, × 59.)

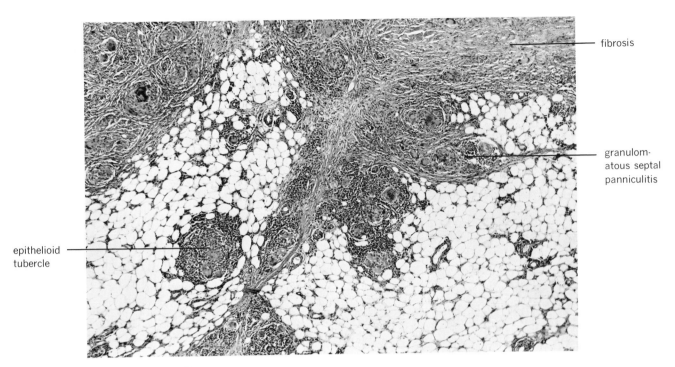

FIG. 14-8. Necrobiosis lipoidica. B.

granulomatous dermatitis. Usually there is concurrent involvement of the subcutaneous fibrous septa and the periphery of the fat lobule by granulomatous panniculitis (Fig. 14-8). Granulomatous septal panniculitis in necrobiosis lipoidica closely resembles that of erythema nodosum.

Scleroderma. In both localized (guttate, morphea, linear) and systemic (progressive systemic sclerosis, acrosclerosis) forms of scleroderma, the pathologic changes involve not only the dermis, but the subcutaneous fat as well so that the active inflammatory stage is both a dermatitis and a panniculitis. The earliest histologic change is a moderately dense predominantly lymphocytic perivascular and sometimes interstitial infiltrate throughout the dermis and in the thickened fibrous septa. In time, histiocytes, plasma cells, and eosinophils join the lymphocytic infiltrate in both the dermis and the subcutaneous fat (Fig. 14-9). The nodular infiltrate of inflammatory cells within the septa extends into the peripheries of the fat lobules. Eventually there are fat necrosis and replacement of the fat by sclerotic collagen. The end stage of sclerodermatous involvement in the dermis is thickened collagen bundles with narrowing of the spaces between them and obliteration of adnexal structures, and in the fat there is partial replacement of lobules by sclerotic collagen and thickening and sclerosis of the septa (Fig. 14-10). Some deep dermal and subcutaneous arterioles

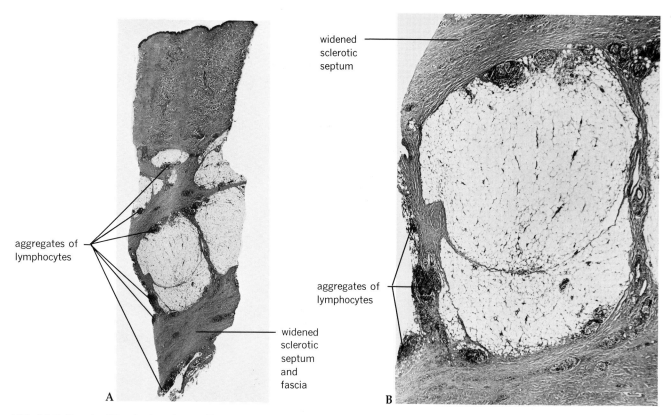

widened
sclerotic
septum

aggregates of
lymphocytes

aggregates of
lymphocytes

widened
sclerotic
septum
and
fascia

A

B

FIG. 14-9. Panniculitis of scleroderma. This scanning magnification of a well-advanced lesion shows the characteristic localization of lymphocytic aggregates at peripheries of the fat lobules, contiguous with thickened and sclerotic septa. (A, × 8; B, × 25.)

may be obliterated by sclerosis. In sum, there is a notable increase in the collagen content of skin and a consequent thickening and sclerosis of the dermis owing to these dermal and subcutaneous changes. (Scleroderma is also discussed in Chapters 7 and 13.)

Fasciitis with Eosinophilia. This inflammatory process of the fascia may also involve the septa of the subcutaneous fat and the deep reticular dermis. It occurs in conjunction with eosinophilia of the circulating blood and of the bone marrow and with hypergammaglobulinemia. The inflammatory-cell infiltrate within the fascia consists of lymphocytes, histiocytes, and plasma cells, but usually not of eosinophils. For this reason, the term *eosinophilic fasciitis,* as it is sometimes called, is inexact. In time, there is thickening of the fascia by sclerosis, a phenomenon that may also occur in the septa of the subcutis.

Whether fasciitis with eosinophilia is part of the spectrum of scleroderma or a disease sui generis is not yet resolved. Visceral involvement is unusual in fasciitis with eosinophilia, but the cutaneous changes clinically resemble those of acrosclerosis or diffuse scleroderma. Histologically, fasciitis with eosinophilia appears to be a deep form of scleroderma, analogous to lupus erythematosus profundus.

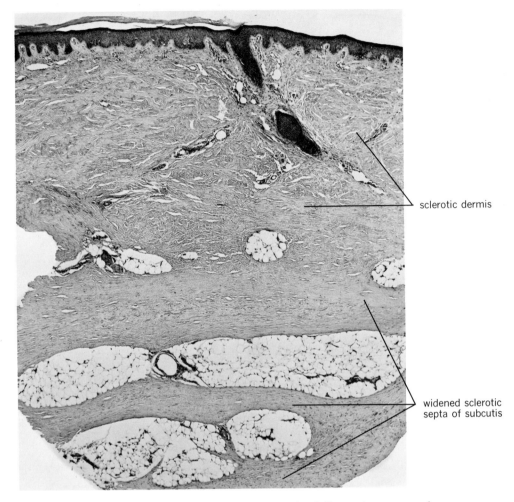

sclerotic dermis

widened sclerotic
septa of subcutis

FIG. 14-10. End stage of panniculitis of scleroderma. After inflammatory process has subsided, scleroderma consists of prominent sclerosis that affects entire dermis (but expecially lower half), and septa in subcutaneous fat, which are widened by sclerosis shown here. The fascia is also affected in most instances. ($\times$ 40.)

Lobular Panniculitis (Fig. 14-3B)

Fat necrosis of different kinds tends to develop in the lobular panniculitides. One type of fat necrosis, commonly found in nodular vasculitis, among others, begins with lysis of membranes of lipocytes (Fig. 14-11). Contiguous lipocytes so affected en masse become micropseudocysts within the lobules (Fig. 14-12). Another type of fat necrosis, typified by pancreatic panniculitides, begins with basophilic-staining, granular changes within the cytoplasm of lipocytes and in time progresses to extensive lobular necrosis (Fig. 14-13). When fatty acids are split from neutral fats normally present within lipocytes, for any reason, ranging from trauma to enzyme reaction, they are likely to combine with calcium. Calcification of fat, therefore, is not an uncommon sign of prior panniculitis. Hyalinized sclerosis is often the end stage of necrotizing panniculitides.

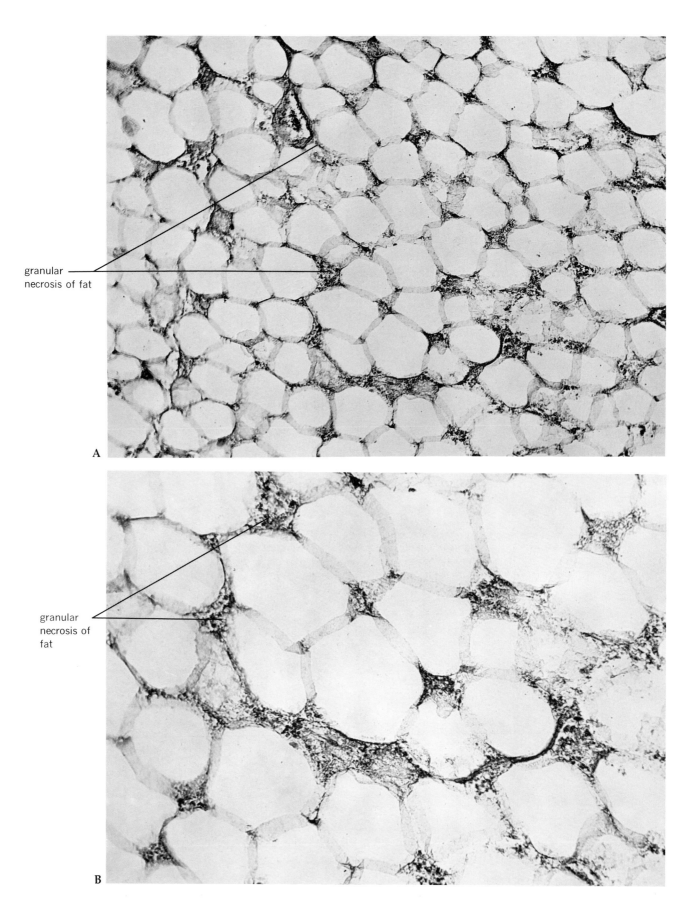

granular
necrosis of fat

granular
necrosis of
fat

A

B

FIG. 14-11. Early stage of fat necrosis. Among earliest histologic changes are basophilic granules, such as shown here, at peripheries of lipocytes. (A, × 192; B, × 365.)

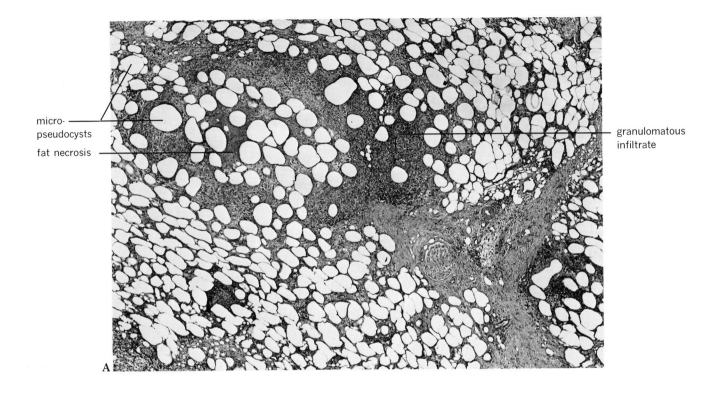

micro-
pseudocysts

fat necrosis

granulomatous
infiltrate

A

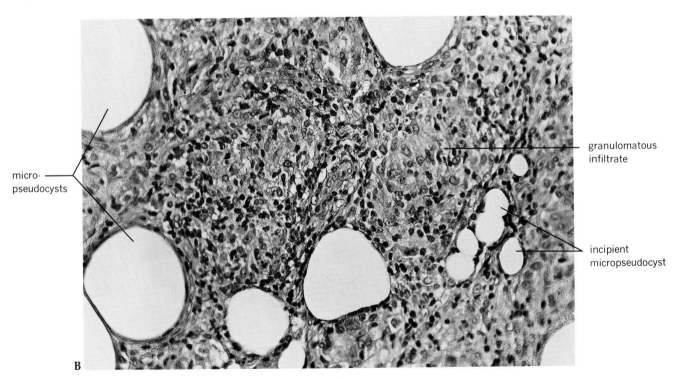

granulomatous
infiltrate

micro-
pseudocysts

incipient
micropseudocyst

B

FIG. 14-12. Micropseudocysts in nodular vasculitis. The character of subcutaneous fat has been altered by inflammation, and fat cells now have different sizes and shapes. Most of lipocytes pictured are much larger than normal fat cells as a result of confluence. (× 65.) B, In this higher magnification the progression from confluence of relatively normal-sized lipocytes on the right side of the photomicrograph to larger-sized micropseudocysts on the left may be better appreciated. (× 400.)

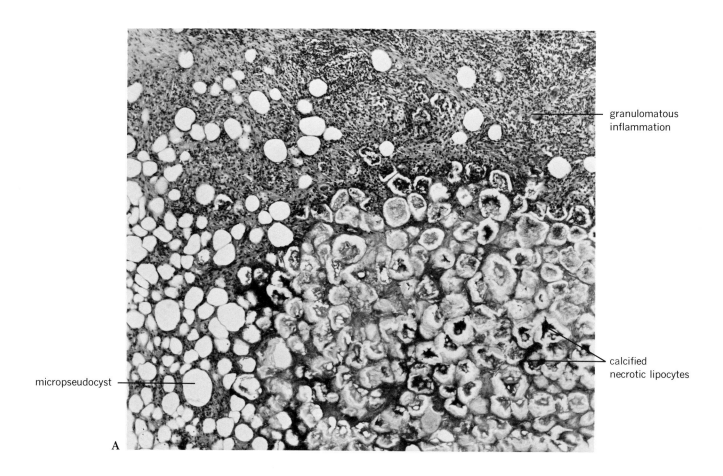

granulomatous
inflammation

calcified
necrotic lipocytes

micropseudocyst

A

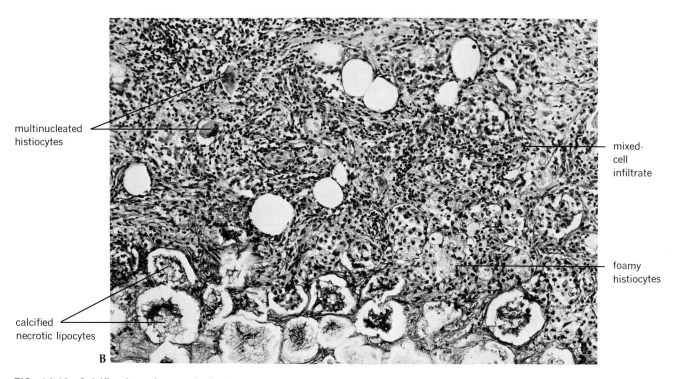

multinucleated
histiocytes

mixed-
cell
infiltrate

foamy
histiocytes

calcified
necrotic lipocytes

B

FIG. 14-13. Calcification of necrotic fat in pancreatic panniculitis. Characteristic changes caused by lipases released from diseased pancreas are extensive calcification of individual necrotic lipocytes. Entire process is surrounded first by suppuration, later by granulomatous inflammation as shown here, and finally by fibrosis. (A, × 72; B, × 171.)

Nodular Vasculitis. Nodular vasculitis is so named because clinically the lesion is a nodule, and microscopically it is an arteritis. This severe vasculitis, in which neutrophils, lymphocytes, and histiocytes participate, involves a muscular artery and eventuates in ischemic changes within the lobule or portions of the lobules supplied by the affected artery (Fig. 14-14). Other lobules,

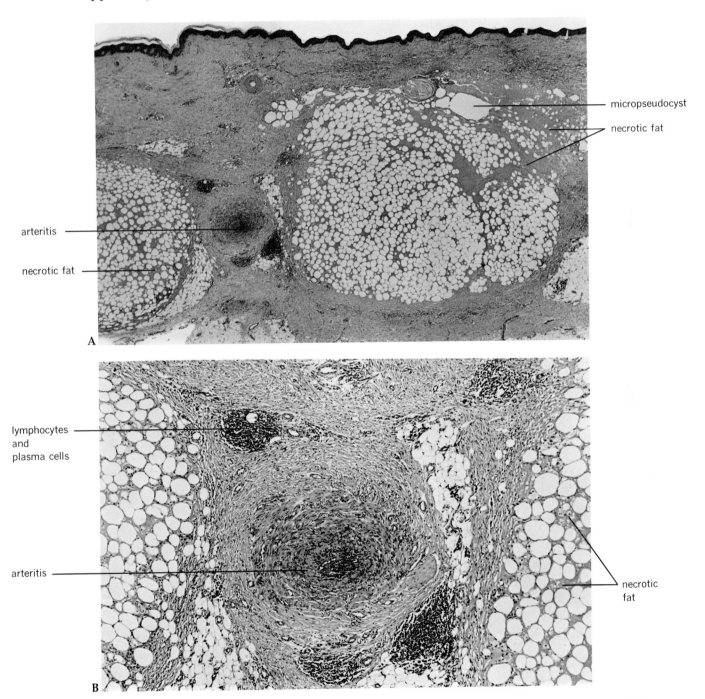

FIG. 14-14. Nodular vasculitis. Severe arteritis so well seen between two large lobules of fat accounts for subsequent changes. (A, × 23; B, × 70.)

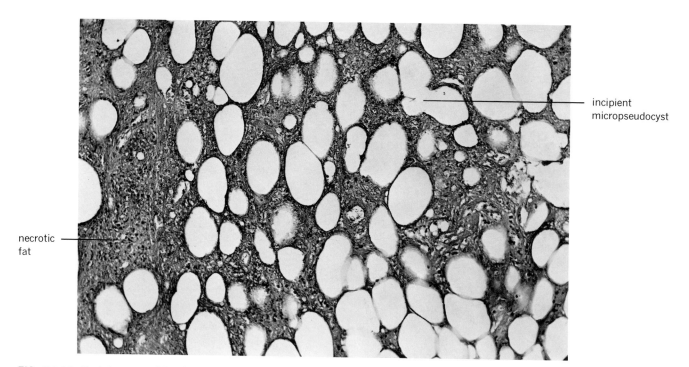

incipient
micropseudocyst

necrotic
fat

FIG. 14-14. Nodular vasculitis. C. (× 178.)

or portions thereof, having their own independent vascular supply, are spared. The ischemia results in coagulation necrosis (Fig. 14-15), and the necrotic material in turn is chemotactic for neutrophils whose lysosomal enzymes further contribute to destruction of fat cells. Release of fat substances then calls forth histiocytes that ingest the lipids and assume a foamy appearance. In addition to these foam cells, numerous multinucleated histiocytes are often present, as are accumulations of epithelioid cells. All or part of the lobule is eventually replaced by fibrosis.

Nodular vasculitis is both an arteritis and a lobular panniculitis. Because the dominant pathologic alteration is in the fat lobule, nodular vasculitis is included in this chapter on panniculitis, rather than in the chapter on vasculitis. Nodular vasculitis is also partly a septal panniculitis because the major vessel involved resides within a fibrous trabeculum.

In addition to the presence of a mixed inflammatory-cell infiltrate within the wall of the artery, there are prominent thickening of the intima and widening of the spaces between the muscle bundles (Fig. 14-16A, B). Stains for elastic tissue reveal severe fragmentation of elastic fibers in the internal and external laminae (Fig. 14-16C).

It must be emphasized that it is not possible to make an unequivocal diagnosis of nodular vasculitis in the absence of large-vessel vasculitis. In suspected cases of nodular vasculitis, step sections must be cut through the tissue block in search of this critical diagnostic feature.

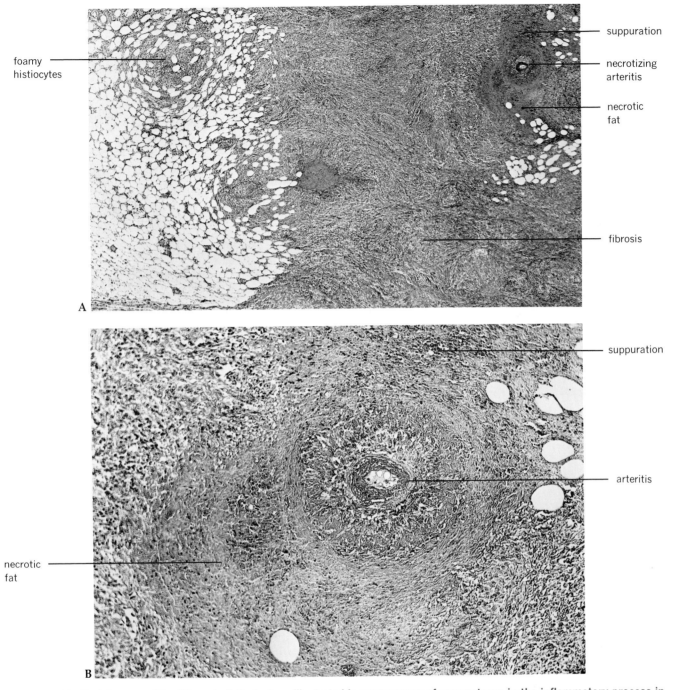

foamy
histiocytes

suppuration

necrotizing
arteritis

necrotic
fat

fibrosis

A

suppuration

arteritis

necrotic
fat

B

FIG. 14-15. Nodular vasculitis. Characteristic feature illustrated is concurrence of many stages in the inflammatory process in a single histologic section: necrotizing arteritis, necrosis of fat, suppuration, granulomatous infiltrate of foamy histiocytes, and fibrosis. (A, × 34; B, × 174.)

Clinically, nodular vasculitis consists of dull-red, variably tender nodules asymmetrically distributed on the calves of young and middle-aged women. Depending upon the degree of fat necrosis, ulceration may occur. The lesions frequently heal with scarring. The clinical features of nodules that are slightly tender, usually situated on the calves, often ulcerated, and replaced by scar distinguish nodular vasculitis from erythema nodosum. His-

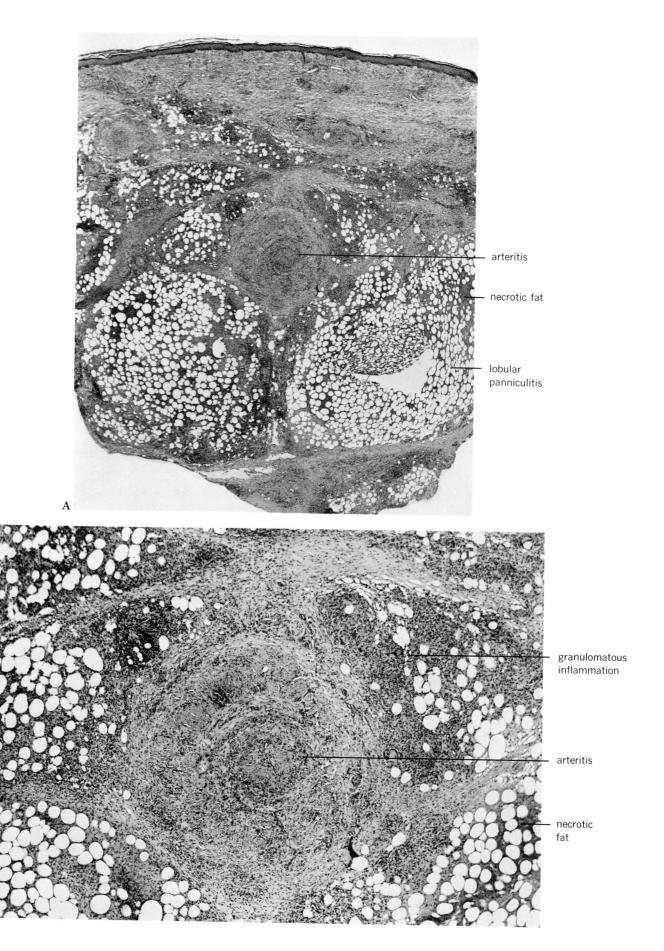

arteritis

necrotic fat

lobular
panniculitis

granulomatous
inflammation

arteritis

necrotic
fat

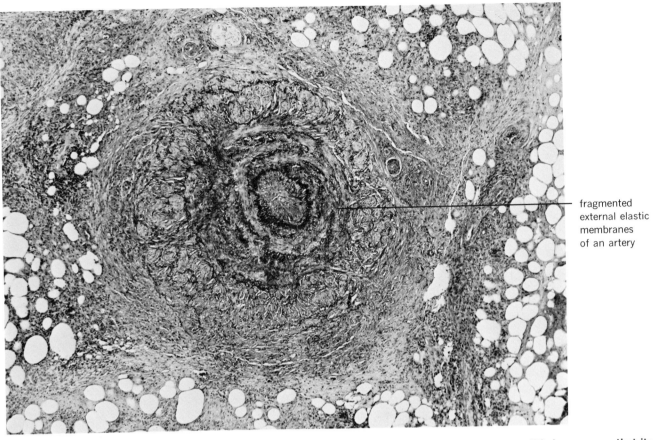

fragmented
external elastic
membranes
of an artery

FIG. 14-16. Nodular vasculitis. Arteritis of vessel pictured in center of this specimen of nodular vasculitis is so severe that its lumen appears to be totally occluded. As a result of this vascular compromise, fat lobules have undergone necrosis, followed by suppuration, granulomatous inflammation, and fibrosis. (A, × 17; B, × 44.) C, This specimen stained for elastic tissue demonstrates fragmentation of elastic membranes in a subcutaneous artery, evidences of severe arteritis. Note that intima is so thickened that lumen appears to be completely occluded. (× 58.)

tologically, nodular vasculitis is readily differentiated from erythema nodosum by the large-vessel vasculitis and the predominantly lobular involvement.

The term *nodular vasculitis* is used synonymously with erythema induratum. When tuberculosis really involves the fat, it can cause both nonliquefying and liquefying forms of panniculitis, such as scrofuloderma, but these granulomatous panniculitides are not associated with an arteritis. The cause of nodular vasculitis is not known.

Erythrocyanosis with Nodules; Pernio. Histologically, the nodules that occur in patients with erythrocyanosis and pernio are indistinguishable from nodular vasculitis. Clinically, erythrocyanosis and pernio are characterized by reddish discolorations on the buttocks, thighs, and legs of girls and young women. These lesions are precipitated by cold. In some instances, nodules develop, which, like those of nodular vasculitis, not uncommonly ulcerate and heal with scarring.

Sclerema Neonatorum. The histologic changes of sclerema neonatorum are distinctive. Diffusely distributed throughout the lobules in the subcutaneous fat are adipose cells containing needle-shaped clefts in radial array (Fig. 14-17). The clefts represent the former sites of crystals composed of triglycerides with an increased ratio of saturated to unsaturated fatty acids. These crystals were dissolved out during histologic processing. Neutrophils, eosinophils, and histiocytes, some multinucleated, may be sprinkled in the affected lobules. Whereas some clefts are present within histiocytic giant cells, most are within fat cells. Older lesions may show calcification and thickened septa.

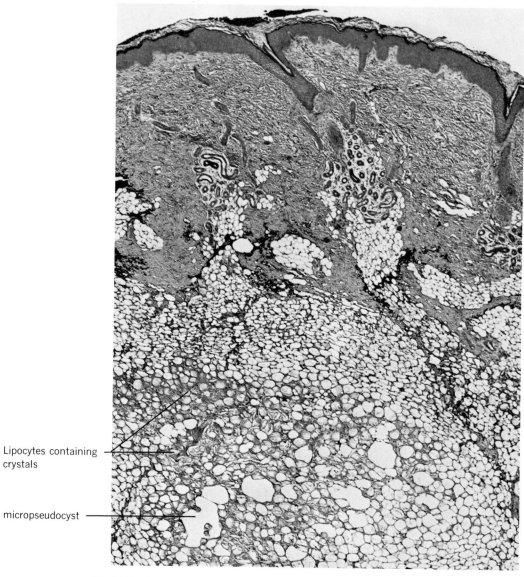

Lipocytes containing crystals

micropseudocyst

FIG. 14-17. Sclerema neonatorum. A, Critical diagnostic feature is presence of crystals within nearly all lipocytes in affected lobules. ($\times$ 45.)

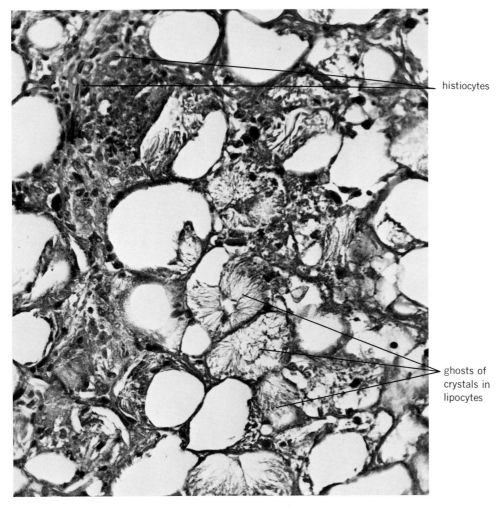

histiocytes

ghosts of crystals in lipocytes

FIG. 14-17. Sclerema neonatorum. B, This higher magnification shows feathery appearance of lipocytes that contained crystals before this specimen was processed in solutions which removed them. Note sparseness of inflammatory-cell infiltrate. (× 363.)

Sclerema neonatorum begins at or within a few days after birth in debilitated neonates. The skin looks and feels waxy. Hard nodules and plaques begin on the buttocks and rapidly extend to the thighs and calves, and then to the rest of the body.

Although no cause has yet been established for sclerema neonatorum, the condition always develops in infants with severe, often fatal, underlying diseases such as respiratory or gastrointestinal infections or developmental defects. At birth, most of these infants are weak and cyanotic and have difficulty maintaining body temperature.

Subcutaneous Fat Necrosis of the Newborn. In contrast with sclerema neonatorum, subcutaneous fat necrosis consists histologically of multiple foci of fat necrosis associated with striking granulomatous panniculitis (Fig. 14-18A, B). Needle-shaped clefts are present in many foamy and multinucleated histiocytes (Fig. 14-18C, D). Eventually, fibrosis supervenes. Clinically, subcuta-

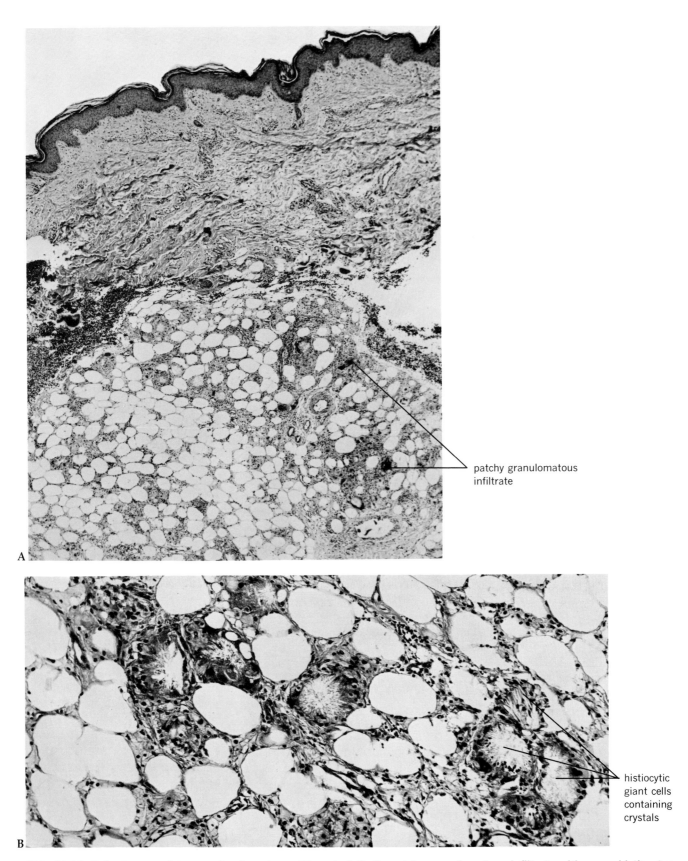

patchy granulomatous
infiltrate

histiocytic
giant cells
containing
crystals

FIG. 14-18. Subcutaneous fat necrosis of newborn. Characteristically patchy granulomatous infiltrate with many histiocytes containing crystals within their cytoplasms is typical also of panniculitis induced by systemic adrenocorticosteroids. Crystals are associated with both subcutaneous fat necrosis of newborn and sclerema neonatorum, but they are found within histiocytes in the former and lipocytes in the latter. (A, × 45; B, × 177; C, × 547; D, × 547.)

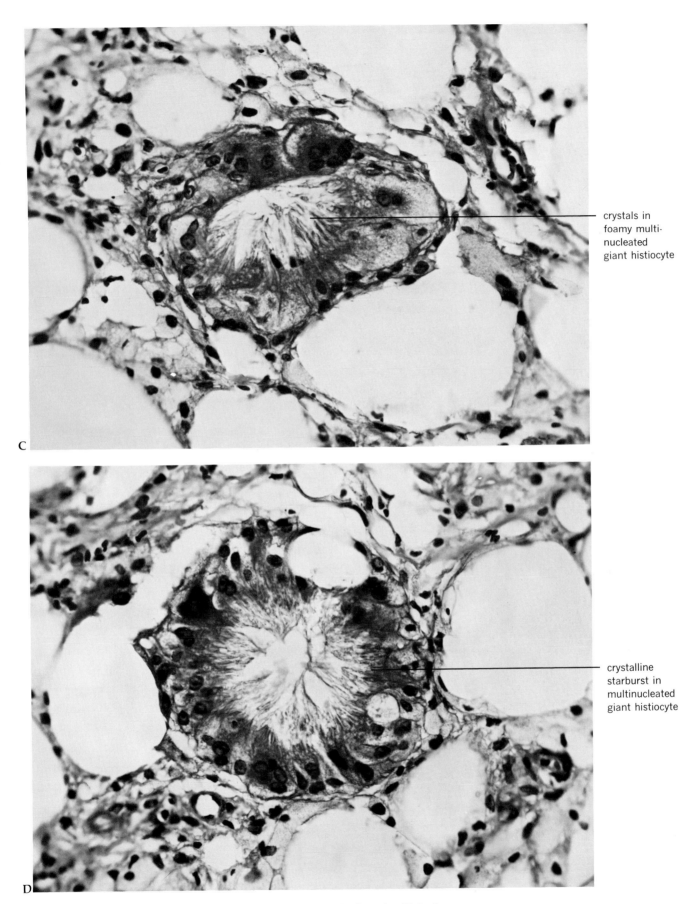

crystals in
foamy multi-
nucleated
giant histiocyte

crystalline
starburst in
multinucleated
giant histiocyte

FIG. 14-18. Subcutaneous fat necrosis of newborn. C and D. See also Plate 4.

neous fat necrosis occurs in healthy full-term newborns as one or more firm, dusky-red nodules on the buttocks, thighs, shoulders, back, or arms. The nodules often become fluctuant and discharge an oily liquid. Spontaneous resolution occurs within a few weeks to months. The lesions of subcutaneous fat necrosis of the newborn are thought by some to result from obstetrical trauma, anoxemia, or exposure to cold.

Histologically, subcutaneous fat necrosis may be indistinguishable from poststeroid panniculitis.

Poststeroid Panniculitis. This exceptionally rare panniculitis has histologic features resembling those of subcutaneous fat necrosis of the newborn. There is patchy, rather than diffuse, lobular panniculitis that spares the interlobular septa. Needle-shaped clefts are found within lipocytes and histiocytes, some of which have foamy cytoplasm (foam cells) and others many nuclei (giant cells). The cleft-containing fat cells are often surrounded by histiocytic giant cells. The needle-shaped clefts represent former sites of fatty-acid crystals dissolved by tissue processing.

Fat cells containing clefts are also seen in subcutaneous fat necrosis and sclerema neonatorum. The latter disease lacks foam cells and has diffuse, rather than focal, involvement of the lobules.

Poststeroid panniculitis develops in children 1 to 14 days after sudden discontinuation of systemic corticosteroids that had been given in large doses for long periods for a variety of conditions, including acute rheumatic fever, nephrosis, and leukemia. The subcutaneous nodules, located primarily on the cheeks, arms and trunk can be both pruritic and painful. The nodules usually disappear spontaneously. When the systemic corticosteroid is reinstituted, the subcutaneous nodules always wane.

Relapsing Febrile Nodular Nonsuppurative Panniculitis (Weber-Christian Syndrome). Despite the numerous case reports of relapsing febrile nodular nonsuppurative panniculitis (Weber-Christian syndrome) in the first half of the twentieth century, its exact nosologic status is still unclear. It is not even certain that this syndrome exists as a distinct clinicopathologic entity. Classically, relapsing febrile nodular nonsuppurative panniculitis was described as an evolution through suppurative, macrophagic, and fibrotic stages. The macrophagic stage is reputedly diagnostic because of the countless foamy histiocytes (Fig. 14-19). The clinical concomitants of these histologic changes are recurrent crops of subcutaneous nodules, especially on the thighs, buttocks, and lower part of the trunk of women. The nodules are usually nonsuppurative, but occasionally they liquefy and heal with atrophic scars. Fever was considered a constant accompaniment of these cutaneous changes.

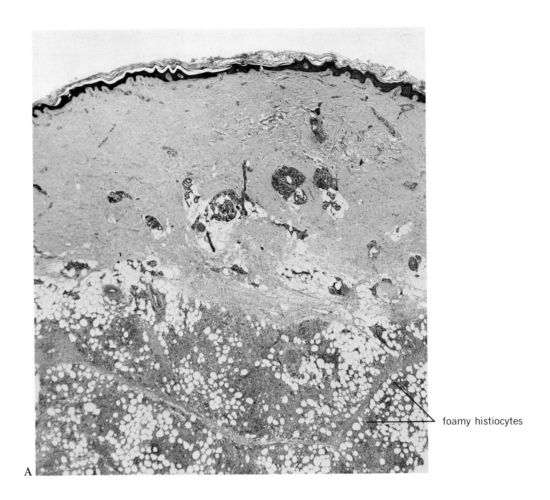

foamy histiocytes

A

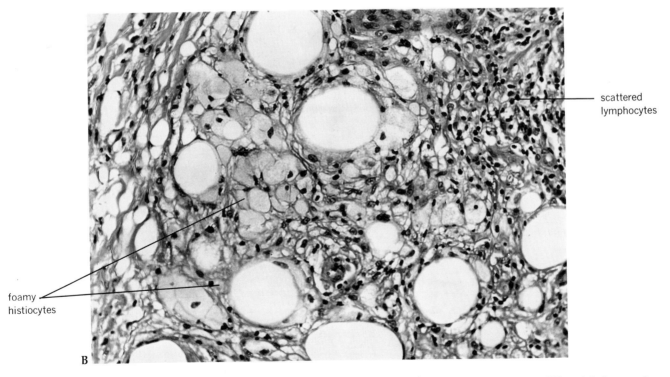

scattered
lymphocytes

foamy
histiocytes

B

FIG. 14-19. Relapsing febrile nodular nonsuppurative panniculitis (Weber-Christian syndrome). A, Dense diffuse lobular panniculitis composed of foamy histiocytes, as pictured, is typical of macrophagic stage. ($\times$ 17.) B, Foamy histiocytes with lipid-laden cytoplasm diffusely distributed throughout fat lobule are easily seen in this higher power view. ($\times$ 360.)

Lipogranulomatosis subcutanea (Rothmann-Makai syndrome) is said to be a nonfebrile and nonrecurrent variant of Weber-Christian syndrome. Sometimes there is only a solitary subcutaneous nodule. Tuberculoid granulomas with microcysts are found within the fat lobules of Rothmann-Makai syndrome (Fig. 14-20).

Certainly, there are lobular panniculitides that are predominantly foam-cell granulomas devoid of large-vessel involvement. Whether these cases truly represent a specific syndrome, the Weber-Christian syndrome, is yet to be determined. The same is true for the lipogranulomatosis subcutanea of Rothmann and Makai.

Subcutaneous Sarcoidosis. Sarcoidosis may involve the subcutaneous fat both directly and indirectly. Direct involvement of the fat by sarcoidosis is seen histologically as epithelioid tubercles distributed throughout the fat lobules (Fig. 14-21). Similar tubercles may also be present in the dermis. Sarcoidosis may involve the fat indirectly by inducing erythema nodosum. In these instances, the erythema nodosum is indistinguishable clinically and histologically from erythema nodosum of other causes.

Subcutaneous Granuloma Annulare. Rarely will granuloma annulare involve primarily the deep dermis and the subcutis, in which cases palisaded granulomatous infiltration initially involves the septa, but the process soon spills into the lobules which often become obscured by it (Fig. 14-22). There is abundant mucin deposition, a feature that differentiates granuloma annulare from necrobiosis lipoidica. Many lesions labeled pseudorheumatoid nodules are actually examples of subcutaneous granuloma annulare. In the centers of the palisaded granulomas mostly fibrin is deposited in rheumatoid nodules, whereas mostly mucin is deposited in granuloma annulare. (The palisaded granulomas are discussed more extensively in Chapter 9.)

Lipodystrophy. The earliest histologic changes in progressive lipodystrophy are neutrophils around septal blood vessels and within the fat lobules, followed by lymphocytes, histiocytes, multinucleated histiocytes, and, eventually, destruction of the subcutaneous fat. Clinically, there is gradual disappearance of the subcutaneous fat, in some cases on the face, neck, and upper trunk and in others predominantly on the lower part of the torso and lower extremities. If the biopsy is performed during the atrophic stage of the disease, the pathologist will find loss of only subcutaneous fat. On the other hand, if the biopsy is done during an earlier, more active phase, a suppurative or granulomatous lobular panniculitis will be discerned.

Infections. Lobular panniculitis that is suppurative and/or granulomatous can result from various infectious agents (e.g.,

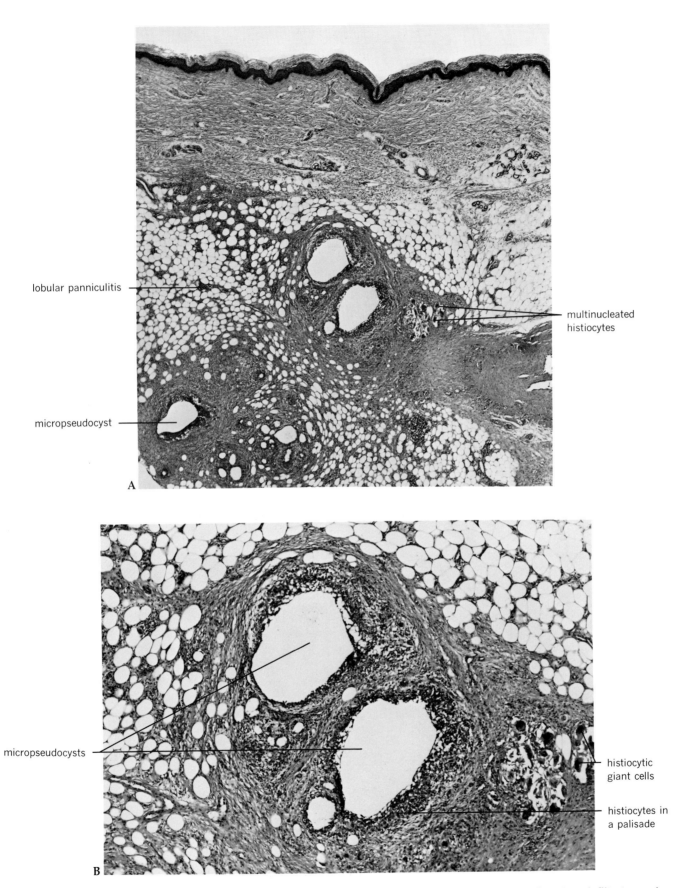

lobular panniculitis

multinucleated
histiocytes

micropseudocyst

A

micropseudocysts

histiocytic
giant cells

histiocytes in
a palisade

B

FIG. 14-20. Lipogranulomatosis subcutanea of Rothmann and Makai. Typical features are patchy granulomatous infiltrates and micropseudocysts within fat lobules. (A, × 22: B, × 69.)

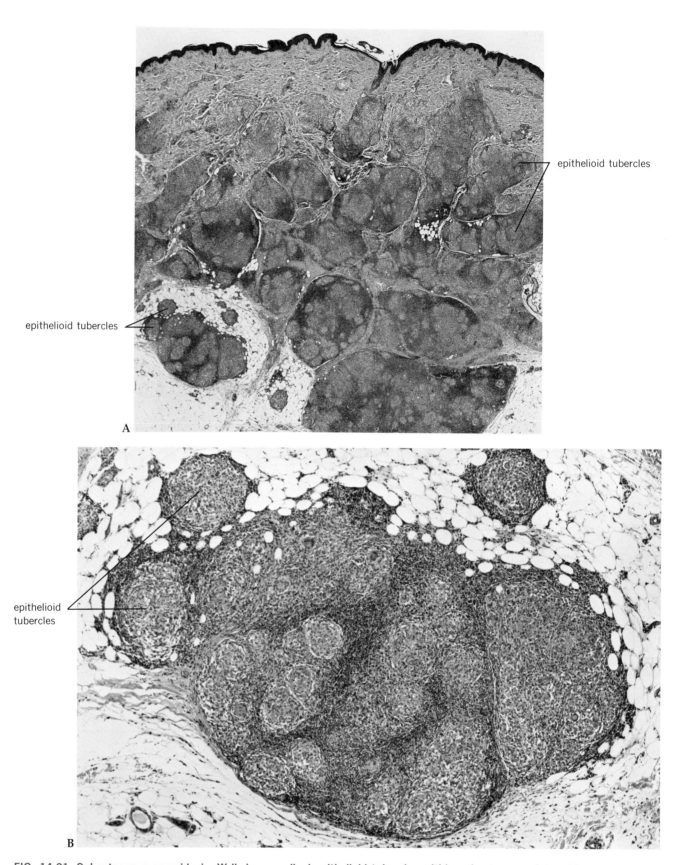

FIG. 14-21. Subcutaneous sarcoidosis. Well-circumscribed epithelioid tubercles within subcutaneous fat and lower portion of dermis are one histologic expression. Although sarcoidosis is typically attended in microscopy by "naked" tubercles, i.e., without enveloping mantles of lymphocytes, that is not always the case, as is well illustrated in these photomicrographs. (A, × 13; B, × 68.)

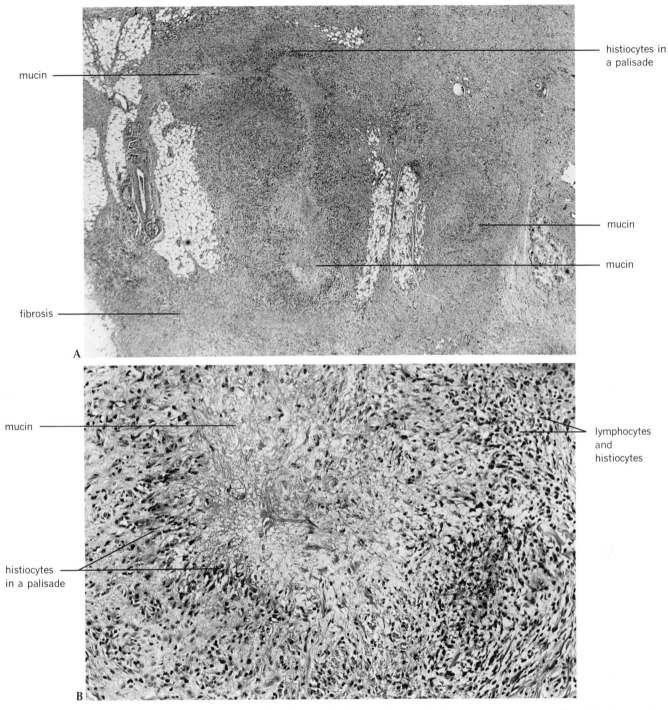

mucin

histiocytes in
a palisade

mucin

mucin

fibrosis

A

mucin

lymphocytes
and
histiocytes

histiocytes
in a palisade

B

FIG. 14-22. Subcutaneous granuloma annulare. Lobular panniculitis, palisaded and granulomatous as pictured, is diagnostic because of abundant mucin within centers of aggregations of histiocytes. (A, × 25; B, × 170.)

fungi or bacteria), most of which have already been considered in Chapter 9. Diseases such as mycetoma, chromomycosis, sporotrichosis, actinomycosis, and scrofuloderma may be seated in the subcutis, as well as within the dermis. The yeasts of cryptococcosis may fill the fat lobules nearly completely where they are associated with fat necrosis and a sparse predominantly mononuclear-cell infiltrate (Fig. 14-23).

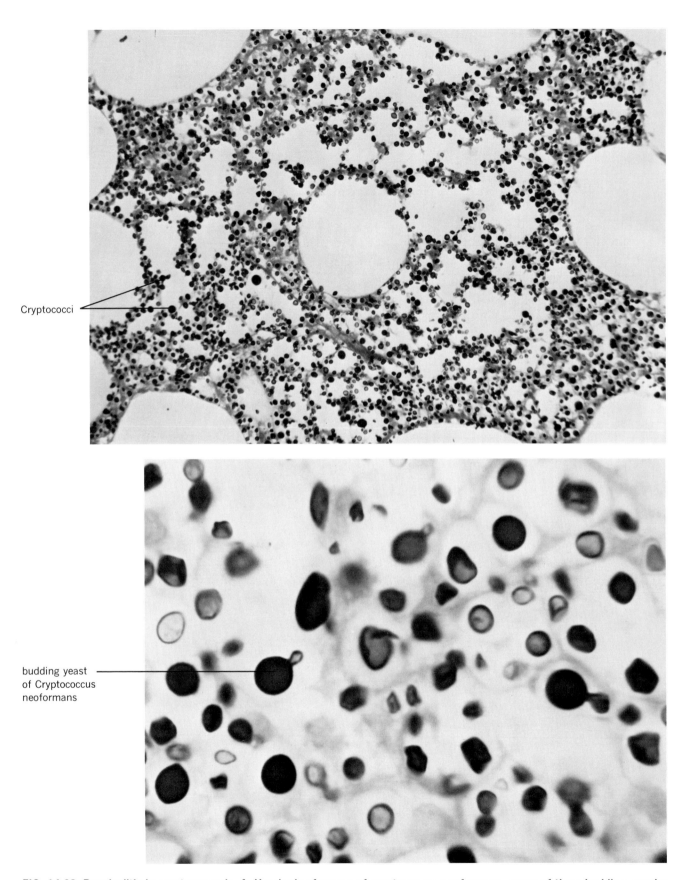

Cryptococci

budding yeast
of Cryptococcus
neoformans

FIG. 14-23. Panniculitis in cryptococcosis. A, Hundreds of spores of cryptococcus neoformans, many of them budding, can be seen. (× 403.) B, Numerous yeasts of Cryptocococcus neoformans, some of them budding, are distributed diffusely throughout subcutaneous fat in this specimen from a patient who also suffered from an immunodeficiency disease. (× 1201.)

Lupus Erythematosus Profundus. This rare variant of cutaneous lupus erythematosus primarily involves the deep reticular dermis and the subcutaneous fat (Fig. 14-24). The dense infiltrate of lymphocytes, plasma cells, and histiocytes within the fat septa gradually extends into the fat lobule with resultant necrosis that resolves with feathery hyalinization of lipocytes and sclerosis (Fig. 14-25). Small blood vessels in the deep dermis and fibrous septa in the subcutis may be obliterated by sclerosis.

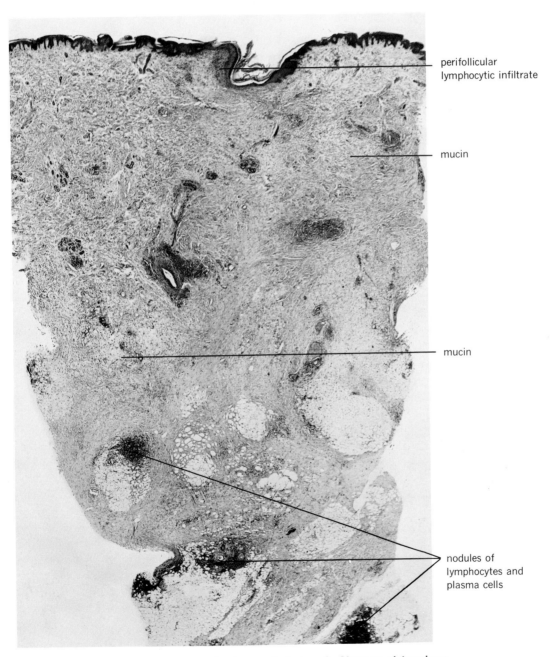

perifollicular lymphocytic infiltrate

mucin

mucin

nodules of lymphocytes and plasma cells

FIG. 14-24. Lupus erythematosus profundus, early lesion. A, Changes pictured are basically those of deep form of discoid lupus erythematosus, namely, dense, predominantly lymphocytic infiltrate around blood vessels at all levels of dermis and in septa of fat, coupled with abundant deposition of mucin. ($\times$ 15.)

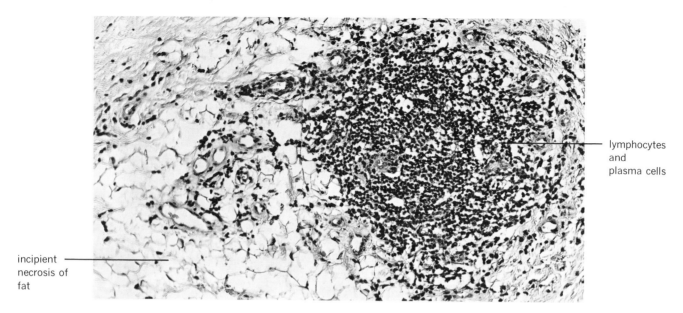

incipient
necrosis of
fat

lymphocytes
and
plasma cells

FIG. 14-24. Lupus erythematosus profundus, early lesion. B, Higher magnification shows dense infiltrate of lymphocytes and plasma cells within septum and encroachment of infiltrate upon lobules whose lipocytes are already beginning to shrink. (× 182.)

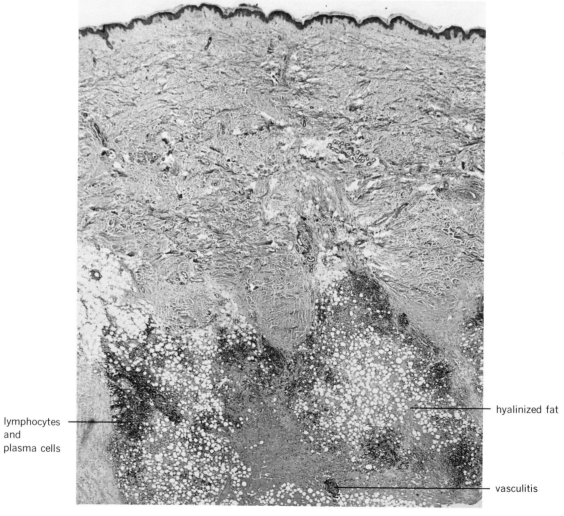

lymphocytes
and
plasma cells

hyalinized fat

vasculitis

FIG. 14-25. Lupus erythematosus profundus, late lesion. Characteristic features are dense infiltrate of lymphocytes and plasma cells throughout fat lobules, necrosis of fat, and hyalinized sclerosis. (A, × 20; B, × 188.)

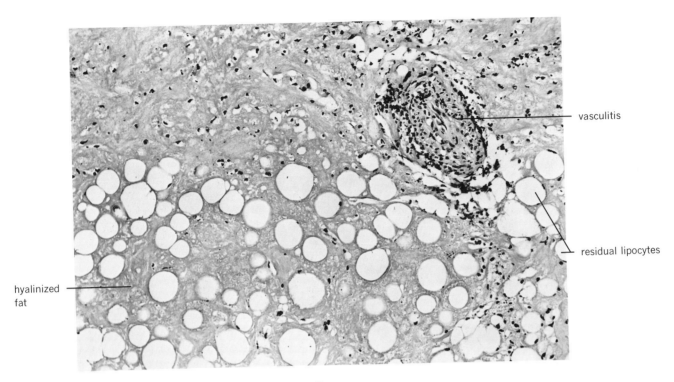

FIG. 14-25. Lupus erythematosus profundus, late lesion. B.

In some instances of lupus erythematosus profundus, there is no dermal or epidermal abnormality. In other cases, in addition to the panniculitis, the typical histologic changes of acute or chronic discoid lupus erythematosus are found in the epidermis and dermis, and at the dermoepidermal junction. These include vacuolar alteration, a thickened basement membrane, increased mucin, and sclerosis within the dermis (Fig. 14-26).

Clinically, lupus erythematosus profundus consists of well-circumscribed, firm, nontender, subcutaneous nodules. Depending upon the histologic changes in the dermis and the epidermis, there may be overlying clinical features of discoid lupus erythematosus. Lupus erythematosus profundus may occur in association with other typical lesions of discoid lupus erythematosus. Just as discoid lupus erythematosus may be found independent of systemic lupus erythematosus, so, too, lupus erythematosus profundus may develop in the absence of systemic connective tissue disease.

The subcutaneous nodules of lupus erythematosus profundus usually do not ulcerate but often resolve with depressed scarring.

Cutaneous lupus erythematosus, like other inflammatory processes such as granuloma annulare, sarcoidosis, and scleroderma, ordinarily affects the dermis primarily, but occasionally may affect deeper tissues. The characteristic features of each of these diseases are retained irrespective of whether they are in the dermis, the subcutaneous fat, or the fascia, or in a combination of these.

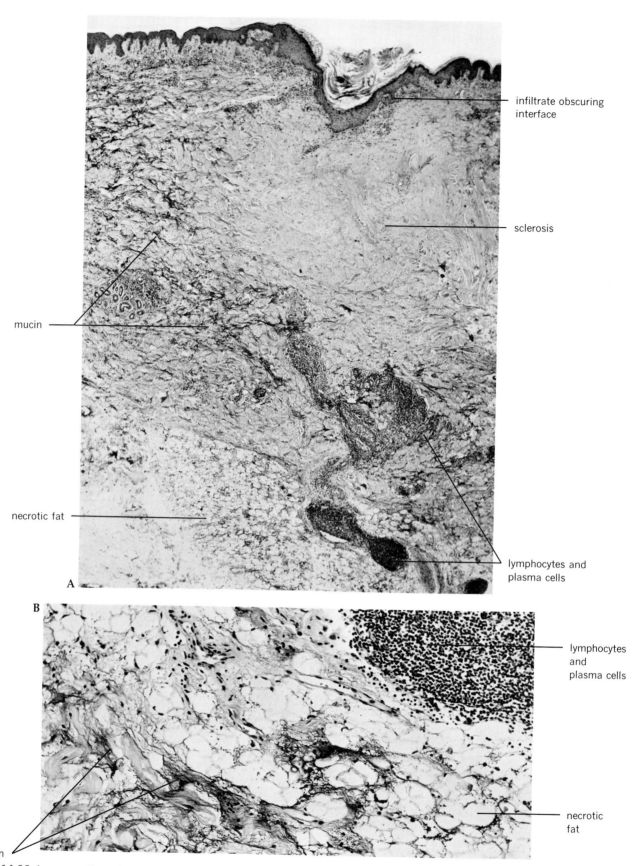

infiltrate obscuring
interface

sclerosis

mucin

lymphocytes and
plasma cells

necrotic fat

A

B

lymphocytes
and
plasma cells

necrotic
fat

mucin

FIG. 14-26. Lupus erythematosus profundus. Presence of abundant mucin throughout dermis (and even in fat) in association with nodular inflammatory-cell infiltrates in deep reticular dermis and subcutis are cogent clues to diagnosis. (A, × 26; B, × 210.)

Pancreatic Panniculitis. The histologic features of pancreatic panniculitis are unique. The initial changes are those of fat necrosis involving portions of the fat lobule. Lipases are responsible for these changes. The characteristics of pancreatic fat necrosis are granular basophilic alteration of lipocytes (coagulation necrosis), loss of nuclear staining, and ghosts of fat cells with varying degrees of calcification (Fig. 14-27). Areas of these diagnostic changes are often contiguous to other foci within the lobule that are completely spared. Peripheral to areas of fat necrosis, there is a sparse inflammatory-cell infiltrate ranging from neutrophils and nuclear dust to multinucleated histiocytes (Fig. 14-28). The varying hues of basophilia reflect the degree of saponification of fat by calcium salts. These histologic changes are identical with those caused by acute pancreatitis in the peripancreatic fat and in adipose tissues throughout the body.

Pancreatic panniculitis is manifested clinically by crops of reddish-violet, painful, tender subcutaneous nodules from which occasionally drains an oily substance. Presumably, the nodules result from the action of lipase carried to the skin hematogenously from a pancreas diseased by inflammation (pancreatitis) or a lipase-producing acinar adenocarcinoma.

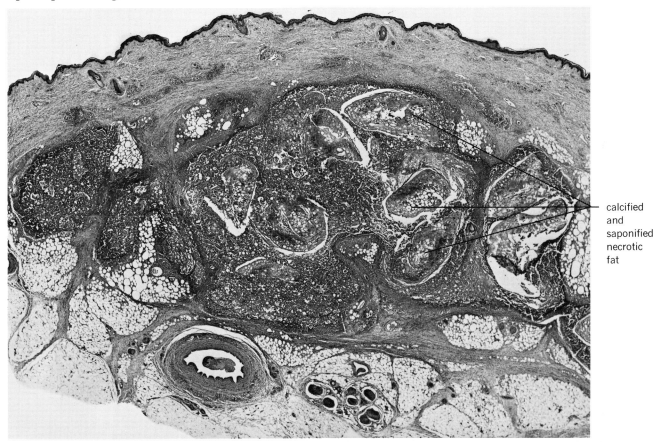

calcified and saponified necrotic fat

FIG. 14-27. Pancreatic panniculitis. Diagnostic features illustrated—necrosis of fat and calcific saponification of necrotic fat—are induced by lipases released from pancreas diseased by inflammatory or neoplastic changes. (A, × 9; B, × 197.)

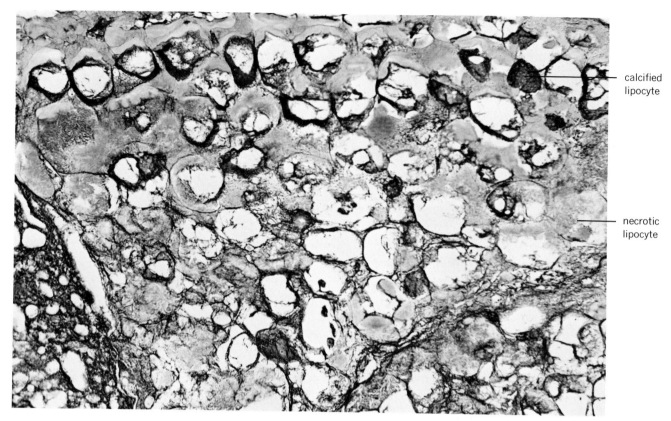

calcified
lipocyte

necrotic
lipocyte

FIG. 14-27. Pancreatic panniculitis. B.

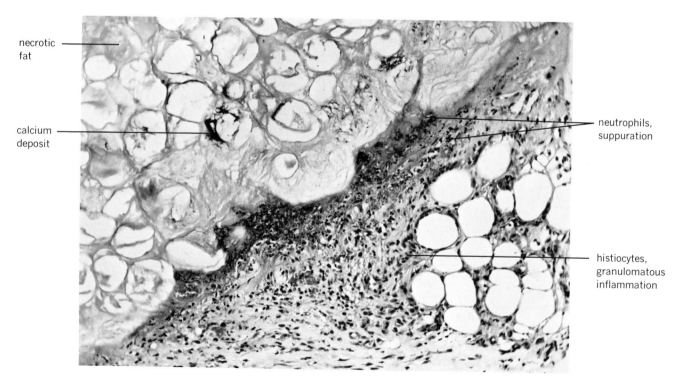

necrotic
fat

calcium
deposit

neutrophils,
suppuration

histiocytes,
granulomatous
inflammation

FIG. 14-28. Pancreatic panniculitis. From left to right are three zones of reaction: necrosis of fat, incipient suppuration, and incipient granulomatous inflammation indicating the progression of this pathologic process. (× 187.)

Physical and Factitial Panniculitis. Numerous panniculitides result from physical effects of a thermal, mechanical, or chemical nature. These include cold (e.g., from sucking on popsicles), pressure (e.g., secondary to focal compression), trauma (e.g., following a blow with a fist or cudgel), and injections of medicines (e.g., insulin, morphine, and corticosteroids). Whenever a panniculitis, or any inflammatory disease of the skin, does not histologically resemble a well-described condition, one must consider the possibility of factitial cause.

There is wide histologic variation in this group of physical and factitial panniculitides, depending upon the modality and material involved, as well as the stage of the pathologic process at the time of biopsy. For example, rupture of contents of follicular cysts can result in lobular panniculitides that range from suppurative (Fig. 14-29) to granulomatous (Fig. 14-30) and, depending upon the chronicity, may resolve with fibrosis. The same may be said for the effects of trauma on the panniculus (Figs. 14-31, 14-32).

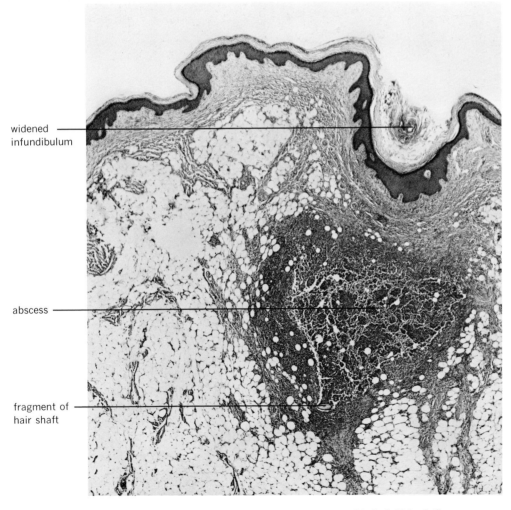

widened infundibulum

abscess

fragment of hair shaft

FIG. 14-29. Suppurative lobular panniculitis following rupture of hair follicle. Inflammation was response to extruded contents of follicle, which includes fragment of hair shaft pictured. If cause is microbial, the process then is a small furuncle. (× 27.)

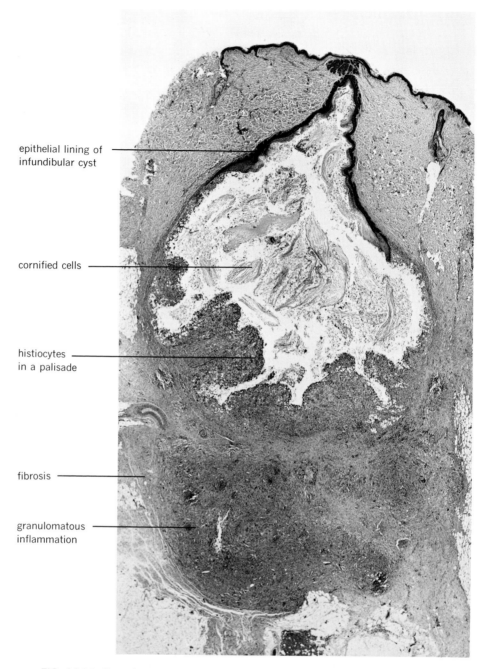

epithelial lining of
infundibular cyst

cornified cells

histiocytes
in a palisade

fibrosis

granulomatous
inflammation

FIG. 14-30. Granulomatous lobular panniculitis following rupture of follicular (infun-dibular) cyst. Spewing of follicular contents, especially cornified cells, into dermis and subcutis led to granulomatous inflammation and fibrosis. (× 12.)

Cold panniculitis usually occurs within hours following exposure to cold and is more common in infants than in adults. Histologically, the process involves the fat lobules where there are necrosis of lipocytes, fat microcysts, and a moderately dense, patchy mixed-cellular infiltrate of neutrophils, lymphocytes, and histiocytes. Clinically, cold panniculitis appears as firm, warm, reddish plaques that reach their zenith in about 72 hours and wane spontaneously in about 2 weeks. Infants with the condition tend to outgrow it before they are of school age.

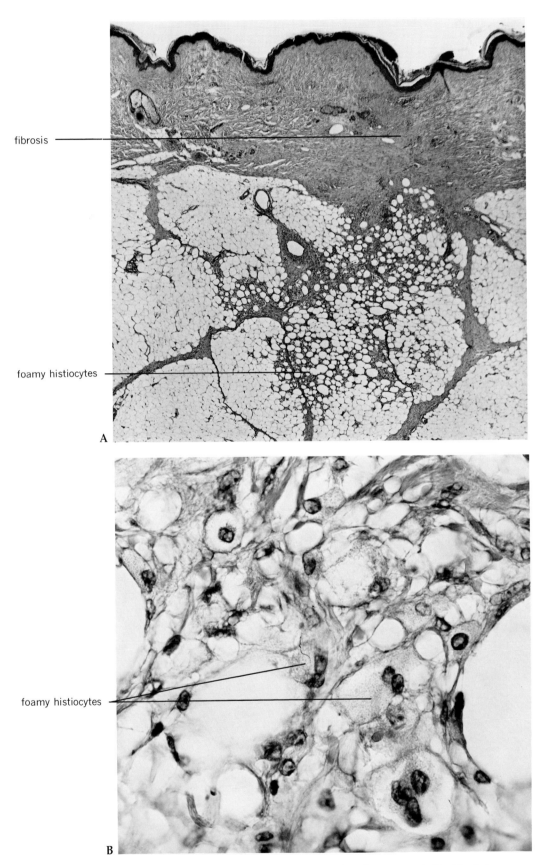

FIG. 14-31. Traumatic panniculitis (three weeks after surgery). Residual changes are linear scar in dermis and well-circumscribed, granulomatous, lobular panniculitis. (A, × 18; B, × 612.)

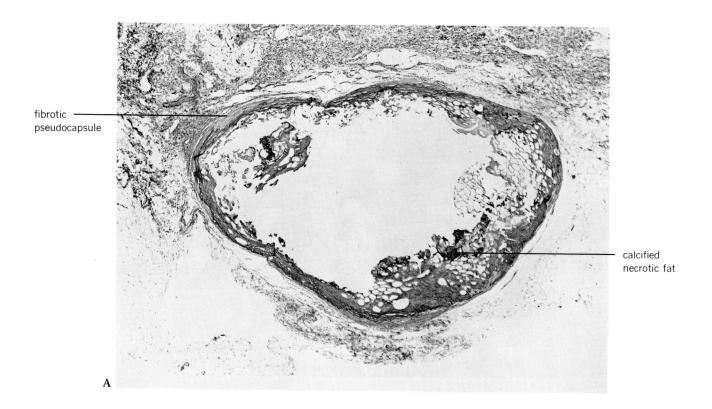

fibrotic
pseudocapsule

calcified
necrotic fat

A

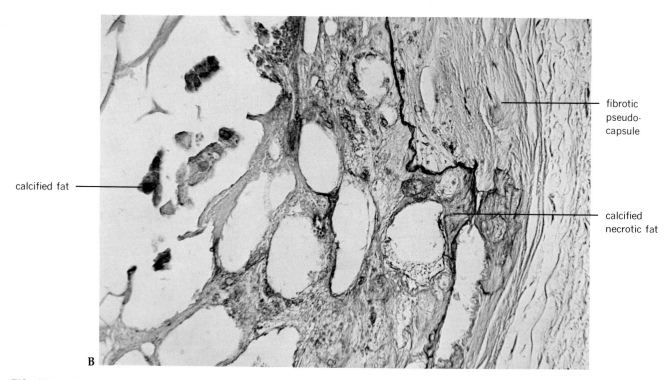

fibrotic
pseudo-
capsule

calcified fat

calcified
necrotic fat

B

FIG. 14-32. Calcification in old lesion of traumatic necrosis of fat. A, This old lesion that resulted from a blow shows circumscription by fibrosis and calcification of fat that earlier was necrotic. (× 26.) B, Note that calcified fat at left is in form of spicule. (× 384.)

Sclerosing lipogranuloma is a panniculitis (and dermatitis) induced by injections of oily materials, such as by plastic surgeons for restorative purposes and by psycopaths for masochistic or other disordered purposes. Other factitial panniculitides result from injections of milk, acids, and even feces. Among the earliest histologic responses to such injections is a suppurative lobular panniculitis.

In panniculitides not conforming to well-described pathologic processes, a factitial cause must be suspected. Other helpful clues are large, variously sized and shaped vacuoles in oil panniculitides, such as in paraffinoma, and obvious evidences of other foreign material, such as can be demonstrated by polarized light. Spectroscopic and chromatographic techniques can sometimes be helpful in identifying the causative agent.

Lymphomatous and Leukemic "Panniculitis." The infiltrates

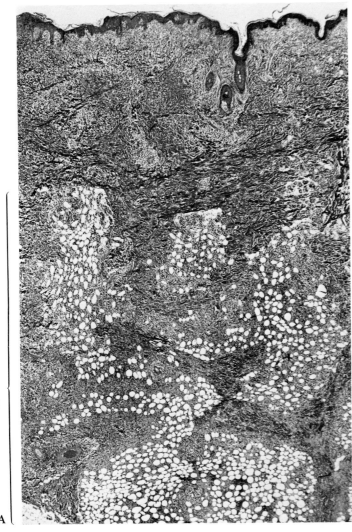

dense diffuse infiltrate of atypical mononuclear cells

A

FIG. 14-33. Lymphomatous panniculitis. In nodular lesion of mycosis fungoides, atypical mononuclear cells may be seen to infiltrate not only the dermis, but also the subcutaneous fat. This is representative of what may happen in malignant lymphomas in general. (A, × 18; B, × 1728.)

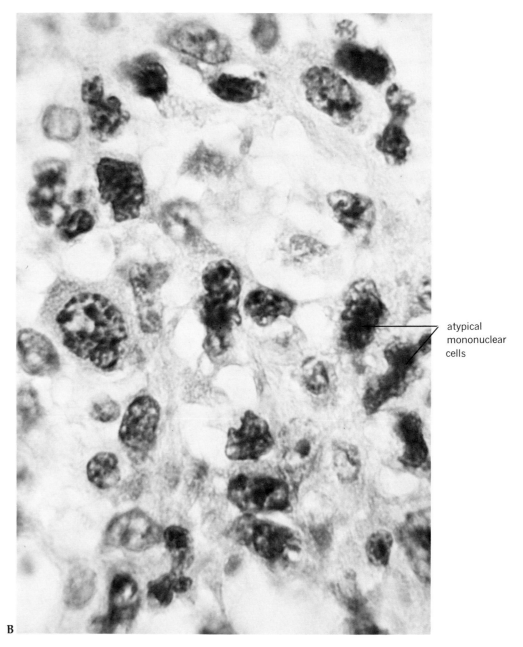

atypical
mononuclear
cells

FIG. 14-33. Lymphomatous panniculitis. B.

of malignant lymphomas and leukemias (lymphocytic and mye-
locytic types) may diffusely involve the fat lobules, giving the
impression —under scanning magnification—of a lobular panniculitis (Fig. 14-33). Atypical mononuclear cells within these
infiltrates indicate their truly neoplastic natures. Clinically, these
lesions are often misdiagnosed as erythema nodosum.

Probably no aspect of the inflammatory diseases of the skin has received as little attention from histologists as the panniculitides. By the time of the second edition of this book, I hope much more will have been learned about inflammatory processes in the subcutaneous fat.

When You See—Think!

Changes in the Epidermis

Changes at the Dermoepidermal Junction

Changes in the Dermis

Changes in and around Follicular Epithelium

Changes in the Subcutaneous Fat

When You See— Think!

A MAXIM that could apply to morphologists in general and to anatomic pathologists in particular enjoins one to "look with the eyes, see with the brain." The brief hints that follow are designed to aid in viewing and interpreting histologic sections of inflammatory diseases in skin with greater optical and mental discrimination. They are proffered in the same spirit as those of the physician Sir Arthur Conan Doyle who, in THE ADVENTURES OF SHERLOCK HOLMES, has his characters articulate his thoughts as follows:

> "Quite so," he answered, lighting a cigarette, and throwing himself down into an armchair. "You see but you do not observe."

> "By George!" cried the inspector. "How ever did you see that?"
> "Because I looked for it."

> "I can see nothing," said I, handing it back to my friend."
> "On the contrary, Watson, you can see everything. You fail, however, to reason from what you see. You are too timid in drawing your inferences."

> "You know my method. It is founded upon the observation of trifles."

> "To remember it—to docket it. We may come on something later which will bear upon it."

Changes in the Epidermis

✓ When you see neutrophils within parakeratosis ("neuts in the horn") over a superficial perivascular dermatitis, think of psoriasis (plaque lesions when neutrophils are layered in parakeratotic tiers, guttate lesions when neutrophils are confined to parakeratotic mounds).

✓ When you see neutrophils within parakeratosis over a superficial and deep perivascular dermatitis, think of pityriasis lichenoides et varioliformis acuta (Mucha-Habermann disease).

✓ When you see neutrophils in parakeratotic mounds at the margins of infundibular ostia, think of seborrheic dermatitis.

✓ When you see neutrophils in the cornified layer of a lesion that is surely not psoriasis, seborrheic dermatitis, or pityriasis lichenoides et varioliformis acuta, think of superficial fungus infections and do a special stain for hyphae and spores.

✓ When you see compact orthokeratosis over a psoriasiform dermatitis, think of a superficial fungus infection and do special stains for fungal elements.

✓ When you see wedge-shaped hypergranulosis in association with a lichenoid infiltrate, think of lichen planus.

✓ When you see psoriasiform dermatitis covered by alternating orthokeratosis and parakeratosis (and often associated with follicular plugging), think of pityriasis rubra pilaris.

✓ When you see focal erosion or ulceration over a scant inflammatory-cell infiltrate within the dermis, think of an excoriated lesion.

✓ When you see necrosis of the upper, outer portion of the epidermis only, think of external injury to the skin such as is caused by physical trauma or ultraviolet light and also of pityriasis lichenoides et varioliformis acuta.

✓ When you see confluent pallor of cells in the upper spinous and granular layers, think of vitamin deficiencies such as of nicotinic acid in pellagra, mineral deficiencies as of zinc in acrodermatitis enteropathica, and deficiencies of serum amino acids such as are associated with a pancreatic neoplasm (glucagonoma) in the form of necrolytic migratory erythema.

√ When you see focal acantholytic dyskeratosis, think of keratosis follicularis (Darier's disease), transient acantholytic dermatosis (Grover's disease), certain epidermal nevi, some solitary keratoses, an incidental finding secondary to a variety of inflammatory and neoplastic processes, and, if in the lining of a follicular (infundibular) cyst, of warty dyskeratoma.

√ When you see acantholytic cells in spongiotic foci, especially in association with other foci having features of keratosis follicularis (Darier's disease), familial benign chronic pemphigus (Hailey-Hailey disease), and superficial and deep forms of pemphigus, think of transient acantholytic dermatosis (Grover's disease).

√ When you see numerous necrotic and ballooned keratinocytes (not multinucleated as in infections with herpesvirus) and spongiosis, think of erythema multiforme (including toxic epidermal necrolysis), pityriasis lichenoides et varioliformis acuta, acute fixed drug eruption, irritant contact dermatitis, and phototoxic dermatitis, and look at the composition and depth of the inflammatory-cell infiltrate to differentiate among them.

√ When you see multinucleated epithelial giant cells, especially in acantholytic separation, think of the herpesvirus infections, namely, herpes simplex, herpes zoster, and varicella, but not of poxvirus infections such as vaccinia or variola.

√ When you see spongiosis around acrosyringia, think of miliaria rubra.

√ When you see psoriasiform lichenoid dermatitis, think of secondary syphilis and the plaque stage of mycosis fungoides and look for histiocytes and plasma cells in the infiltrate of the former and lymphocytes, singly and/or in conglomerations, within the epidermis of the latter.

√ When you see a biopsy specimen from a nail, think of the possibility of a superficial fungus infection among other things and always do a special stain for fungal elements in the cornified cells.

Changes at the Dermoepidermal Junction

√ When you see vacuolar alteration, necrotic keratinocytes, and an inflammatory-cell infiltrate obscuring the dermoepidermal interface, think of erythema multiforme, pityriasis lichenoides et varioliformis acuta, and acute fixed-drug eruption and look for a superficial perivascular lymphohistiocytic infiltrate in erythema multiforme, a superficial and deep perivascular lymphohistiocytic infiltrate in pityriasis lichenoides et varioliformis acuta, and a superficial and deep perivascular and interstitial mixed-cell infiltrate containing many neutrophils and eosinophils in acute fixed-drug eruption.

√ When you see a thickened zone of basement membrane, think of discoid lupus erythematosus (and, less likely, of dermatomyositis).

Changes in the Dermis

√ When you see a subepidermal blister above solar elastosis in a dermis that is practically devoid of an inflammatory-cell infiltrate, think of porphyria cutanea tarda.

√ When you see a subepidermal blister with numerous eosinophils in the upper part of the dermis, think of pemphigoid.

√ When you see extraordinary edema of the papillary dermis, think of polymorphous light eruption, erysipelas, some reactions to insect bites, acute febrile neutrophilic dermatosis (Sweet's syndrome), and early lichen sclerosus et atrophicus and scrutinize the composition and distribution of the inflammatory-cell infiltrate that may permit differentiating them.

√ When you see sclerosis and telangiectases in the upper part of the dermis, think of chronic radiodermatitis and look for large bizarre fibroblasts indicative of sclerosis caused by radiotherapy.

√ When you see a thickened edematous or sclerotic papillary dermis sandwiched between a thinned epidermis and a mononuclear-cell infiltrate, think of lichen sclerosus et atrophicus.

√ When you see a sclerotic reticular dermis with a diminished number of adnexal epithelial structures, think of scleroderma.

√ When you see collagen arranged in coarse vertical streaks within a thickened papillary dermis, think of lichen simplex chronicus and its pruritic variants (prurigo nodularis and picker's nodule) and look further for signs of an underlying cause for the pruritus, such as contact dermatitis, nummular dermatitis, and mycosis fungoides.

✓ When you see numerous melanophages in the papillary dermis as in postinflammatory pigmentary alterations, think also of macular and lichenoid amyloidosis and look for pink globules of amyloid in the dermal papillae.

✓ When you see a specimen of skin that in cursory examination appears histologically normal, think of urticaria and look between collagen bundles in the reticular dermis for spaces that are widened by edema and for a sparse perivascular, predominantly lymphocytic infiltrate.

✓ When you see telangiectases in the upper part of the dermis surrounded by sparse mononuclear cell infiltrates, think of urticaria pigmentosa (telangiectasia macularis eruptiva perstans), look for mast cells, and stain specifically for them to confirm or deny the diagnosis.

✓ When you see inflammatory cells in the dermis arranged in a V-shape with the point toward the subcutis, think of reactions to arthropod assaults and pityriasis lichenoides et varioliformis acuta, and then examine the composition of cellular infiltrates that may permit distinction between them, namely, eosinophils in arthropod reactions, but not in pityriasis lichenoides et varioliformis acuta (Mucha-Habermann disease).

✓ When you see numerous eosinophils scattered among collagen bundles, think of reaction to arthropod assaults and look in the cornified layer for the mite of scabies, its ova, or its wastes.

✓ When you see histiocytes scattered here and there between collagen bundles, think of granuloma annulare and look for mucin between the collagen bundles.

✓ When you see mucin surrounded by histiocytes arrayed in a palisade, think of granuloma annulare.

✓ When you see what looks like granuloma annulare in a specimen from the face, think of granulomatosis disciformis chronica et progressiva (Miescher) and look for asteroid bodies in the histiocytes.

✓ When you see degenerated collagen surrounded by histiocytes arranged in a palisade, think of necrobiosis lipoidica.

✓ When you see fibrin surrounded by histiocytes in palisaded array, think of rheumatoid or pseudorheumatoid nodule.

✓ When you see crystals or homogeneous basophilic material surrounded by histiocytes in palisaded array, think of gout and examine the specimen by polarized light in an attempt to demonstrate rainbow-colored urate crystals.

✓ When you see germinal centers (lymphoid follicles) in a dense nodular or diffuse infiltrate, think of pseudolymphoma.

✓ When you see mononuclear inflammatory cells in small dermal nerves, think of leprosy and do a Fite stain for acid-fast bacilli.

✓ When you see a suppurative granulomatous dermatitis covered by pseudocarcinomatous hyperplasia, think of deep mycoses and infections with atypical mycobacteria, and look for microorganisms with PAS and acid-fast stains.

✓ When you see neutrophils, nuclear dust, and fibrin in the walls of small blood vessels, think of leukocytoclastic (allergic) vasculitis.

✓ When you see neutrophils in the walls of small blood vessels and thrombi within their lumina, think of septic vasculitis (e.g., gonococcal, meningococcal).

✓ When you see neutrophils, nonsegmented neutrophils (bands), and nuclear dust in a basophilic-staining papillary dermis, think of dermatitis herpetiformis.

✓ When you see thrombi within superficial, small blood vessels and a scant inflammatory-cell infiltrate often accompanied by epidermal necrosis, think of a consumptive coagulopathy.

✓ When you see necrosis of sweat glands, think of barbiturate intoxication, carbon monoxide poisoning, certain diseases of the central nervous system, and occlusive diseases of deeper arteries and seek corroboration by the medical history of the patient.

✓ When you see under scanning power magnification in sections stained by hematoxylin and eosin black-staining inflammatory cells, think of lymphocytes; larger, paler cells, of histiocytes; ovoid cells that stain intermediately between lymphocytes and histiocytes, of plasma cells; cells with a reddish cast, of eosinophils; and smaller cells that look like salt and pepper, of neutrophils.

Changes in and around Follicular Epithelium

√ When you see spongiosis near the base of dilated infundibula plugged by cornified cells, think of Fox-Fordyce disease.

√ When you see suppurative folliculitis, think of infectious agents, among them dermatophytic fungi (e.g., in Majocchi's granuloma) and look for hyphae in the cornified cells of hair follicles (hair shafts, internal root sheaths, and infundibular squames).

√ When you see pustules within the epidermis or follicular epithelium, think of diseases caused by infectious agents such as dermatophytosis, candidiasis, and rupial syphilis and then do appropriate special stains in an attempt to identify causative organisms.

√ When you see trichomalacia (pleated hair shafts containing irregular clumps of melanin) in association with follicles in catagen and telogen (and rarely everted follicles), think of trichotillomania.

√ When you see a predominantly lymphocytic infiltrate around hair bulbs in association with some catagen and telogen hairs, think of alopecia areata.

Changes in the Subcutaneous Fat

√ When you see an arteritis accompanied by necrosis of fat, suppuration, granulomas, and fibrosis, think of nodular vasculitis.

√ When you see crystals in subcutaneous fat cells, think of sclerema neonatorum, subcutaneous fat necrosis of the newborn, and poststeroid panniculitis and look for histiocytes (some may be multinucleated) containing similar crystals, as is the case in the latter two conditions.

√ When you see nodules of lymphocytes (and sometimes plasma cells) at the junction of fat lobules and sclerotic widened septa, think of scleroderma.

√ When you see calcific saponification of necrotic lipocytes, think of pancreatic panniculitis and look for evidences of pancreatitis or pancreatic carcinoma.

Burns (*Continued*)
  first-degree, 592
  keloids and, 733
  malignant neoplasms and, 716
  "scalded" skin in, 550
  second degree, 583, 591–593, *592, 593*
  third-degree, 592
Burrow, definition of, 142
  of scabies, 297–298, *299, 301*
"Butterfly" blush, in systemic lupus erythematosus, 316

Cactus, 440, *440, 441*
Calcification, dystrophic, 442
  in deep folliculitis, 660
  in fat necrosis, 793, *796*
    traumatic, *822*
  in pancreatic panniculitis, 817, 833
  in sclerema neonatorum, 802
  metastatic, 442
Calcific "gout," 442
Calcinosis, pseudotumoral, 442
Calcium, 415, 440, *441,* 442
  in granulomatous slack skin, 483, 485
Calymmatobacterium granulomatis, 488
Candida, in folliculitis, 663
  in granuloma, 454, 457, *459, 461*
  in Janeway lesions and Osler's nodes, 360
Candida albicans, 489, Plates *1, 2*
Candidiasis, 457, *459, 461,* 569, *569, 570,* 578, *579,* 833, Plate *2*
  scaling lesions in, 266–268, *267*
  subcorneal pustules in, 574, *574*
Cantharidin, 548
Cantharis vesicatoria, 548
Capillary(ies), 24
  structure of, 23
Carbon, 439, *439*
Carbon monoxide intoxication, 596
Carbon monoxide poisoning, 832
Carbuncle, 673, *673*
Carcinoma(s). *See also* specific names
  disseminated intravascular coagulation and, 382
Caseation necrosis, 122, 397, 398, 400
  differentiation of, from gummatous necrosis, 404
Catagen, 60, *61*
Catagen follicle, *62*
Catagen hairs, in alopecia areata, 696
  in trichotillomania, 702, 703
Caterpillar dermatitis, 301
Cellulitis, 291–292
  dissecting, of scalp, 391, 465, 679
Cercaria, Plate *2*
Cercarial dermatitis, 295, 301, *303,* 327
C-fibers, 32
Chancre, of syphilis, 485–488, *486*

  tuberculous, 397, 398, 399
Chancroid, 485, 486, 487, 488
Chemical burn, 592
Chemotaxis, for eosinophils, 94
  for neutrophils, 91–93
Chlorpromazine, photoallergic dermatitis and, 226
Chlorthiazides, lichenoid photodermatitis and, 321
Cholesterol, 469
Cholesterol clefts, in atheroemboli, 382
Chondrodermatitis nodularis helicis, 718–721, *719, 720*
  similarities to pressure papules from prostheses, 721
Chromate, "dermal" contact dermatitis and, 226
Chromium, chronic contact dermatitis and, 261
Chromomycosis, *456, 457, 460,* Plate *3*
  panniculitis in, 811
Chronic bullous erythema multiforme. See Pemphigoid
Chronic urticaria, *182*
Churg-Strauss syndrome, 371–372, 373, 374
Cicatricial pemphigoid, 633–635, *634,* 717
  scars in, 599
Civatte, poikiloderma of, 756, 757
Civatte bodies, 122
  in lichen planus, 204, 609
Cleft(s), *124*
  definition of, 123
  subepidermal, above atrophic scar, 749, *750*
Clostridium in gas gangrene, 596
Clotting system, 92
  in leukocytoclastic vasculitis, 337
Club hair, 60, 61, 63
Coagulation necrosis, 122
  in nodular vasculitis, 798
  in pancreatic panniculitis, 817
Coccidioidomycosis, 457, *458, 461*
  erythema nodosum and, 790
Cold panniculitis, 819, 820
Collagen, *20*
  in vertical streaks, *127,* 256, 257, *257, 258, 259*
    definition of, 125
    in chronic contact or nummular dermatitis, 260
    in lichen simplex chronicus, 830
  lamellated, definition of, 125–126
  laminated, in angiofibromas, 260
  types of, 20–21
Collagen degeneration, 416, 831
  definition of, 125
  in acute febrile neutrophilic dermatosis, 388
  in allergic granulomatosis, 372
  in granuloma annulare, 418
  in hyperparathyroidism with calcification and gangrene, 380
  in malignant atrophic papulosis, 375
  in necrobiosis lipodica, 415, 424, 425, 428, 433
  in spirochetal vasculitis of secondary syphilis, 361

Dermatophytic infections, vesiculopustules in, 555, *555*

Dermatophytic vesicular dermatitis, 499–500, 502

Dermatophytosis(es), 569, 578, 833, Plate *2*
  abscesses in, 391, 393, 505, 532
  as cause of id reaction, 502
  differentiation from erythema annulare centrifugum, 232
  scaling lesions, 266–268, *266, 268*
  subcorneal pustules in, 574, *575*
  vesicular lesions, 229–231, *229, 230, 231*

Dermatosis(es), a confusing term, 145
  acute febrile neutrophilic, 292, 388–390, *389, 390,* 830
    classification of, 344
  distinctive exudative discoid and lichenoid chronic, 276, 506
  persistent acantholytic, *540,* 543
  subcorneal pustular, 255, 497, 571, *572*
  transient acantholytic, 497, 537, 538–543, *538–543,* 829

Dermis, adventitial, *18*
    anatomy of, 18, 19, 23, 26, 28
    in granuloma faciale, *448*
  papillary, 17, *17, 18,* 19, 21, 28, 31, 42
  periadnexal, 17, *18,* 52
  reticular, 17, *17,* 19, 21
  structure and function of, 13–29

Dermoepidermal interface, in embryogenesis, 5

Dermolytic bullous dermatosis, 583, 585–588, *586, 587*
  acquired type, 587, *587*
  dominant type, 585, *586*
  recessive type, 586, 587
  scars in, 599

Desmosomes, 40, *40, 41,* 77

Diabetes insipidus, in xanthoma disseminatum, 470
  in necrobiosis lipoidica, 767

Diabetic dermopathy, 768

Diapedesis, 338

Diastase, for demonstration of sporotrichosis, 457

Dichroism, in amyloidosis, 599

Diffuse dermatitis, 447–495
  definition of, 385, *386*

Diffuse scleroderma, 792, 833

Digitate dermatosis, *236*

Dilantin, discoid lupus erythematosus and, 316

Dimorphous leprosy, 402, *404*

Diphenylhydantoin, discoid lupus erythematosus and, 316

Discoid lupus erythematosus, 306–315, *307–315,* 641, 648, 653–655, *654, 656,* 712, *712, 713,* 769, *770,* 830, Plate *1*
  acute, 195, *195,* 306, 307–308, *307, 308*
  chronic, 306, 308–310, *309, 310,* 588, 769–770, *770*
  differentiation of, from dermatomyositis, 194

from lichen planus, 204
from morbilliform drug eruptions, 197
from pityriasis lichenoides et varioliformis acuta, 319
from polymorphous light eruption, 291
forerunner of malignant neoplasms, 716, 749
in systemic lupus erythematosus, 341
lichenoid, 315, *315*
relationship to lupus erythematosus profundus, 815
subacute, 306, 310, *311, 312,* 313
tumid form of, *314,* 315

Disease(s). *See* specific names

Dissecting cellulitis of scalp, 391, 465, 679

Disseminated intravascular coagulation, 356, 380–382, *381, 382*
  in acute septicemias, 360

Donovan bodies, 481, 487, 488

Down's syndrome: elastosis perforans serpiginosa in, 688

Drug eruption(s), dermatitis herpetiformis–like, 626–627, *627*
  fixed, 323, 327, 497, 516, *517, 518,* 829, 830
  inadequate designation, 323
  leukocytoclastic vasculitis as, 344
  lichen-planuslike, 210–211, *210, 211*
  morbilliform, 196, *196*
  pustular, 256
  types of, 196–197

Drugs, as causes of pseudolymphomas, 446

Dyshidrotic dermatitis, 499, *500,* 500
  acute, 227, *228*

Dyskeratoma, warty, 537, 829

Dyskeratosis, focal acantholytic, 535, *536,* 537, 829
  above dermatofibroma, 737, *741*
    analogous to follicular mucinosis, 706

Dyskeratosis follicularis, 537

Dyskeratotic cells, *122*
  definition of, 121
  in acrodermatitis enteropathica, 274
  in disseminated superficial porokeratosis, 218
  in lichenoid photodermatitis, 321
  in lichen planus, 204, 609
  in lichen striatus, 241, 415
  in verrucous lesions of incontinentia pigmenti, 272, *273*

Ecchymoses, definition of, 135

Eccrine dark cells, functions of, 79

Eccrine ducts, 77–78, *77*

Eccrine gland(s); distribution of, 75
  electron-microscopic features of, *79*
  embryogenesis of, 7
  histogenesis of, *9*
  histology of, 75, 76, *76, 77*
  innervation of, 77
  role in thermoregulation, 80

Hyperglobulinemic purpura (Waldenström), leukocytoclastic vasculitis in, 344
Hypergranulosis, *116*
  in lichen planus, 828
Hyperkeratosis, *114, 116*
  definition, of, 113
  epidermolytic. *See* Epidermolytic hyperkeratosis
Hyperkeratosis follicularis et parafollicularis in cutem penetrans, 685, *686,* 687
Hyperlipoproteinemia, 469, 471
Hypermelanosis in porphyria cutanea tarda, 589
Hyperparathyroidism with calcification and gangrene, 375, 380, 442
Hyperpigmentation, postinflammatory, 46
Hyperplasia, cutaneous lymphoid. *See* Pseudolymphomas
  definition of, 117
  irregular, *118*
    definition of, 117
  papillated, 118
    definition of, 117
  pseudocarcinomatous, *118,* 485
    definition of, 117
  psoriasiform, *118*
    definition of, 117
Hypersensitivity angiitis. *See* Leukocytoclastic vasculitis
Hypertrichosis, in porphyria cutanea tarda, 589
Hypertrophic lichen planus, 204, *207,* 260
Hypertrophic scar, 727–731, *728–731,* 749
Hypertrophy, definition of, 119
Hypervitaminosis D, calcification in, 442
Hypogranulosis, *116*
  definition of, 117
Hypoplasia, definition of, 119
Hyposensitization injections, as cause of pseudolymphomas, 446
Hypoxemia, blisters from, 583, 595–596, *595*

Ichthyosis, lamellar, 270, *270*
Ichthyosis hystrix, 537
Ichthyosis vulgaris, differentiation from lamellar ichthyosis, 270
  keratosis pilaris in, 649, *650*
Idiopathic atrophoderma of Pasini and Pierini, 287
Id reaction, 499, 500, 502
  acute, 227
IgG, in leukocytoclastic vasculitis, 337
IgM, in leukocytoclastic vasculitis, 337
  in polyarteritis nodosa, 354
Immune complexes, in leukocytoclastic vasculitis, 337, 338
  in polyarteritis nodosa, 351
Immunity, cell-mediated, in diffuse lepromatous leprosy, 344
Immunofluorescent findings, in benign familial

chronic pemphigus, 534
  in bullous disease of childhood, 629
  in cicatricial pemphigoid, 635
  in dermatitis herpetiformis, 626
  in herpes gestationis, 616–617
  in leukocytoclastic vasculitis, 337
  in pemphigoid, 591, 615
  in pemphigus vegetans, 532
  in pemphigus vulgaris, 526, 532
  in superficial pemphigus, 550
  in transient acantholytic dermatosis, 543
Impetiginized spongiotic dermatitis, vesiculopustules in, 556, *556*
Impetigo, 497, 573
  bullous, 548, 550, *551, 552,* 573
    differentiation of, from superficial pemphigus, 571
    similarities to staphylococcal scalded-skin syndrome, 606
  in chronic granulomatous disease of childhood, 574
  of Bockhart, 663, 673
Impetigo herpetiformis, 562, 563, 571
  variant of pustular psoriasis, 256
Incontinentia pigmenti, 585, 586
  differentiation from toxic erythema of the newborn, 576
  eosinophilic spongiosis in, 248, *249,* 502
  verrucous lesions, 272–273, *273*
Indeterminate leprosy, 287–288, *288*
Infarction, in allergic granulomatoses, 372
  in hyperparathyroidism with calcification and gangrene, 380
  in malignant atrophic papulosis, 375, 376
Infectious granulomatous dermatitis, 454, 456
Infectious mononucleosis, interface dermatitis in, 163, 197
Inflammatory cells, comparative cytology, *90*
Inflammatory linear verrucous epidermal nevus, 271–272
Infundibular cyst, 437
  beneath a nevus, 438, *438*
Infundibulofolliculitis, 691, *692*
Infundibulum of hair follicle, histology of, 51, 57
Insect bites. *See* Arthropod reactions
Intercellular edema, definition of, 119
Intercellular substance, 40
Interface dermatitis, 187–219
  lichenoid, 203–219
  superficial, *170*
  superficial and deep, 306–327, *306*
  vacuolar, 188–203
Intermembranous space, 581
Intracellular edema, definition of, 119
Intracorneal pustular dermatitis, 577–579
Intracorneal pustules, 498

Intracorneal pustules (*Continued*)
  in psoriasis, *252, 253, 254, 255*
Intraepidermal pustular dermatitis, 561–579
Intraepidermal vesiculopustular dermatitis, 553, 555–560
Invasion, a confusing term, 146
Iodides, 463
Irritant contact dermatitis, 243–245, *244, 245, 829*
  ballooning in, 516
    spongiosis with keratinocytic necrosis in, 505
    vesiculopustules in, 556
Isthmus, *58*
  of hair follicle, histology of, 51, 57
Itching: mechanism of, 32
"Itchy red bump" disease, 184

Janeway lesions, 360
Jessner's lymphocytic infiltration, 282–283, *283*, 291
Junctional bullous epidermatosis, 583, 584–585, *584*
Juxta-articular node(s), 405
  of syphilis, 436, 771, *772*
Kala-azar, 489
Kaposi's varicelliform eruption, Tzanck smear in, 524
Karyolysis, 122
Karyorrhexis, 122
Keloid, 19, 585, 586, 727, 731–733, *732, 733, 734, 736, 738, 738*
  resemblance to dermatofibroma, 738, *743*
Keratin, 7, 38
  relation to sebum, 68
Keratinocytes, 7
  necrotic, in bullous lichen planus, 581, 585
    in blister beetle dermatitis, 548
    in blistering diseases, 581
    in dermatitis herpetiformis, 618
    in discoid lupus erythematosus, 307
    in erythema dyschromicum perstans, *198*
    in erythema multiforme, 188, 516, 581, 601
    in fixed drug eruption, 323, 516
    in herpes gestationis, 616
    in herpesvirus infections, 544
    in irritant contact dermatitis, 556
    in junctional bullous epidermatosis, 584
    in measles, 240
    in necrolytic migratory erythema, 512
    in photoallergic contact dermatitis, 500
    in pityriasis lichenoides et varioliformis acuta, 316
    in toxic epidermal necrolysis, 581, 605, 606
  of epidermis, 33, *34–37*
Keratoderma blenorrhagicum, 562, 563, 571
  variant of pustular psoriasis, 256
Keratohyaline granules, *39*
  in acrosyringeal cells, 77
  in embryonic epidermis, 5
Keraolysis, pitted, *177*, 178

Keratoses, lichen-planuslike, 208–210, *209*
  lichen-planuslike solar, *201*
  seborrheic, above dermatofibroma, 737, *742*
Keratosis follicularis, 534–537, *535*, 538, 642, *646, 829*
Keratosis pilaris, 648–650, *649, 650*
  relation to perforating folliculitis, 687
  similarities to pityriasis rubra pilaris, 263
Keratotic-crusted scabies, 298–299, *300*, 328, *328*, 561
Kerion, 454, 663, 678
Kinin system, 92
Klebsiella rhinoscleromatis, 488
Koplik's spots, 241
Kraurosis vulvae, a confusing term, 147
Kveim test site, histologic features of sarcoidosis, 412
Kyrle's disease, 685, *686*, 687
  differentiation from elastosis perforans serpiginosa, 688
Kogoj spongiform pustules, 254

Lamellar ichthyosis, 270, *270*
Lamina lucida, 42, *42*
Langerhans' cells, 49, *49*
Langerhans' granules, 49, *49*, 470
  in histiocytosis-X, 493
Langhans' giant cell, 386, 397, 398
Lanugo hairs, 50
  in vernix caseosa, 69
LE cells, in bullous systemic lupus erythematosus, 629
Leishman-Donovan bodies, 387, 481
Leishmania braziliensis, 482
Leishmania tropica, 481, 482, Plate *3*
Leishmaniasis, 488–489, Plate *3*
  acute, 485, 486
  cutaneous, 488
    acute, 481–482, *481, 482*
    chronic, *397*, 400, 482
    disseminated anergic, 481–482, *481, 482*
  mucocutaneous, 488
  post-kala-azar, 489
Leishmaniasis recidivans, 482
Lepra bacillus(i), 287, 344, Plate *3*
  in histoid leprosy, 775
Lepromas, 480
Leprosy, 832
  dimorphous, 402, *404*
  indeterminate, 287–288, *288*
  lepromatous, 465, 469, 476, 479–480, *479, 480*, 771, 775, 790
    diffuse, 344
  in reaction, leukocytoclastic vasculitis in, 344
  tuberculoid and dimorphous, 400–403, *401, 402, 403*
Leptomonad, 481
Letterer-Siwe disease, 256, 492
Leukemia, lymphocytic, 283
  chronic, 282

Microabscesses, Munro, 254
  Pautrier's, 492
Microfibrils, definition of, 20
Microlobule, primary, of subcutaneous fat, 779, *780,* 780, 781
Micropseudocysts, in cold panniculitis, 820
  in lipogranulomatosis subcutanea, 808, *809*
  in panniculitis, 793, *795, 797, 798*
  in sclerema neonatorum, *802*
Microscopic polyarteritis nodosa, 337
Microsporum canis, 230
Microsporum canis, in kerion, 678
Miescher's granuloma, 431, 432, *431, 432,* 831
Mikulicz cells, 488
Milia, 437, 642, *645*
  in epidermolysis bullosa, 588, *588*
  in porphyria cutanea tarda, 589
Miliaria crystallina, 572, *572*
Miliaria rubra, 242–243, *242, 243,* 499, 829
Miliary tuberculosis, 400
Milker's nodule, 508, *509, 510*
Milonig's fixative, 155
Mixed cellular infiltrate, definition of, 124
Mixed cryoglobulinemia, leukocytoclastic vasculitis in, 344
Mondor's disease, 362
Mongolian spots, relation to dermal melanocytes, 44
Monomorphous cellular infiltrate, definition of, 124
Mononuclear cells, atypical, in actinic reticuloid, 330
  in arthropod reactions, 297, 298
  in halogenodermas, 463, *464,* 568
  in lymphomatoid granulomatosis, 379
  in lymphomatoid papulosis, 319, *320,* 321, *321*
  in mycosis fungoides, 324
  in pseudolymphomas, 442
Mono- pentasymptom complexes, 337
Montgomery's tubercles, 66
Morbilliform drug eruptions, 196, *196*
Morbilliform viral eruptions, 197
Morphea, 286, 287, 716, 791, 833
  with lichen sclerosus et atrophicus, 764
Mosquito bites, 295
  contrasted with tick bites, 294
Moths, as causes of dermatitis, 301
Mucha-Habermann disease, 316–319, *317, 318,* 519–521, *519, 520,* 828, 831
  epidermal changes in, 191
  vasculitis in, 369
Mucin, as clue to differentiation of Jessner's lymphocytic infiltration from polymorphous light eruption, 291
  in acute discoid lupus erythematosus, *307, 308, 314,* 315
  in bullous systemic lupus erythematosus, 629
  in dermatomyositis, 193, 195, 315
  in discoid lupus erythematosus, 195, 307, 653

  in follicular mucinosis, 705, 706
  in granuloma annulare, 415, 416, 418, 420, 421, 428, 433, 831, Plate *1*
  in keloids, 731
  in lupus erythematosus profundus, 815, *813, 816*
  in lymphocytic infiltration (Jessner), 282, 283, 291
  in subcutaneous granuloma annulare, 808
  in young scars, 727
  stains for, 418, 428, 438
Mucinosis, follicular, 706
Mucopolysaccharides, acid. *See* Acid mucopolysaccharides
  neutral, 23
  in basement membrane, 40
Mucous membranes, histology of, *13*
Multinucleated epithelial giant cells, in pityriasis rosea, 235, *235*
Multiple myeloma, 489
Multiple segmental thrombophlebitis, 362, *363,* 784
Munro microabscesses, 254
Mycetoma, 391, 454, 457, 462, Plate *3*
  panniculitis in, 811
Mycobacteria, as cause of abscesses, 391
  atypical, acid-fast stains for, 832
    contrasted to tubercle bacilli, 457
Mycobacterial infections, atypical, 454, 457
Mycobacterium marinum, 457
Mycoses, deep, 832
Mycosis fungoides, 216, 217, 247, 248, *215–217, 248,* 829, 830
  differentiation of, from actinic reticuloid, 330–331
    from lymphomatoid papulosis, *320*
    from secondary syphilis, 324
  follicular mucinosis in, 706
  lichen simplex chronicus superimposed upon, 260
  resemblance to histiocytosis-X, 492
  relationship to parapsoriasis variegata, 271
  spongiotic simulant of, 238, *238,* 247–248, *247*
Myoepithelial cells, around apocrine glands, 70, 74
  of eccrine glands, 76
Myxedema, 23

Nail(s), abnormalities of, in alopecia areata, *699*
  embryogenesis of, 7
  histogenesis of, *8*
  structure and function of, 80–84
Nail matrix, epithelial kinetics of, 82–83
Nail plate, diseases of, 83–84
Nail unit, analogies to hair follicle, 83
  architecture of, *81*
  histology of, 82
"Naked tubercle," 408
  in granuloma annulare, 421, *423*
Necrobiosis, a confusing term, 145, 416
Necrobiosis lipoidica, 415, 424–431, *424–427, 429,* *430,* 716, 767–769, *768, 769,* 790–791, *790,*

Osteogenesis imperfecta, elastosis perforans serpiginosa in, 688

Pachyonychia congenita, 512
Pacini's corpuscles, 4, 32
"Palpable purpura," 341
Panartertis nodosa. *See* Polyarteritis nodosa
Panniculitis, acid-fast stains in, 782
    actinomycosis with, 811
    biopsy of, 151, 780
    chromomycosis in, 811
    cold, 819, 820
    factitial, 819, 823
    from injections, 819
    granulomatous, in necrobiosis lipoidica, 425, 428
    in nodular vasculitis, 356, 364
    in scleroderma, 285, 791–792, *792*, 793
    infectious, 808, 811, *812*
    lobular, 782, *782*, 793–825
    migratory, 789
    pancreatic, 793, *796*, 817–818, *817*, *818*, 833
    physical, 819–823
    poststeroid, 806, 833
    pressure, 819
    relapsing febrile nodular nonsuppurative, 806–808, *807*
    septal, 782, *782*, 783–793
    traumatic, 819, *821*, *822*
Papanicolaou stain, for Tzanck smears, 524
Papillary dermis, *17, 18*
    anatomy of, 17, 19, 21, 28, 31, 42
Papilloma, *133*
    definition of, 132
Papillomatosis, *127*
    definition of, 126
Papular eruption of pregnancy, 185, 246
Papule(s), *129*
    definition of, 128
    pressure, from prostheses, 721
Papulosis, lymphomatoid, 319–321, *319–321*
    vasculitis in, 369
    malignant atrophic, 375–376, 715
Papulosquamous lesions, 130
Paracoccidioidomycosis, 457, *458*
Paraffin, 476, *477, 477*
Paraffinoma, 823
Parakeratosis, *115*
    definition of, 114
    of pityriasis lichenoides et varioliformis acuta, 828
    of psoriasis, 828
    of seborrheic dermatitis, 828
Paraproteinemias, in association with pyoderma gangrenosum, 454
Parapsoriasis, 757
    a confusing term, 143–145
    guttate. *See* Guttate parapsoriasis

Parapsoriasis en plaques, 215–217, *215, 217*
    similarity to granulomatous slack skin, 485
Parapsoriasis variegata, 271
Paroxysmal nocturnal hemoglobinuria, 380, 381
PAS stain, Plate *1*
    for basement membrane, 40, *41*
        in chronic discoid lupus erythematosus, *314*
    for candida, 267, *267*, 569, Plate *2*
    for deep mycoses, 832
    for dermatophytes, 230, 267, *267*, 569
    for fungi, 387, 391, 412
        deep, 457
        superficial, 569, 576, 578
    for lesions with neutrophils in epidermis, 230
    for sporotrichosis, 391
    for Sporotrichum schenckii, Plate *3*
    in erythropoietic protoporphyria, 293, *293*
    in folliculitis, 663
        dermatophytic, 674, *674, 675*
    in mycetoma, Plate *3*
    in panniculitis, 782
    in pustular dermatitides, 230
    in tinea versicolor, 177
Pasini and Pierini, idiopathic atrophoderma of, 761
Patch, *129*
    definition of, 128
Patterns of inflammatory skin diseases, 158–162
Pautrier's microabscesses, 492
Pellagra, 269, *269*, 512, 828
Pemphigoid, 603, 629, 717, 830, Plate *6*
    benign mucous membrane, 633–635, *634*
    cell-poor, 583, 585, 590–591, *590*
    cell-rich, 591, 613–615, *613–615*
    cicatricial, 599, 633–635, *634*, 717
    differentiation of, from cicatricial pemphigoid, 635
        from erythema multiforme, 191
    eosinophilic spongiosis in, 248, 250, 502, 503, 591, 614
    neutrophils in, 203, 250, 613, 614, 635
    similarity to herpes gestationis, 616
    urticarial lesions, 203, *203*, 248, 250
        misinterpretation of, 604
        similarities to herpes gestationis, urticarial lesions, 303
Pemphigus, 629
    acantholysis in, 623
    benign familial chronic. *See* Benign familial chronic pemphigus
    similarities of, to transient acantholytic dermatosis, 541–542, *542*
    superficial, 571, *571*
        similarities of, to bullous impetigo, 573
        to staphylococcal scalded-skin syndrome, 606
Pemphigus erythematosus, 548, 549, *549, 550, 571*
Pemphigus foliaceus, 548, 549, *549*, 550, 571, *571*
Pemphigus neonatorum, "scalded" skin in, 550

Protozoa, as cause of abscesses, 391
Prurigo nodularis, 258, *259*, 260, 830
Prussian blue stain, in Schamberg's disease, 172
Pseudofolliculitis, 669, *671*, 672, *672*
  forerunner of keloids, 733
Pseudolymphomas, 442–447, *443–447*, 494–495, *494*, *495*, 832
  in arthropod assault, 296–297
  in nodular scabies, 298
  in pityriasis lichenoides et varioliformis acuta, 319
Pseudomonas pseudomycetoma, 391, *394*
Pseudomonas septicemia, as cause of disseminated intravascular coagulation, 382
Pseudomycelia, in candidiasis, 457, *459*, *461*
Pseudopelade, 652, *711*
Pseudorheumatoid nodule, 433, 808, 831
Pseudoxanthoma elasticum, perforating, 688
Psoriasiform dermatitis, 250–275
  spongiotic, *222*, 274–279, *275*, 506
  superficial, *170*, *222*
  superficial and deep, *328*, 328–331
Psoriasiform lichenoid dermatitis, 829
  in secondary syphilis, *329*
Psoriasis, 251–256, *251–255*, 577–578, *577*, 828
  active zone at periphery, 305
  analogy to discoid lupus erythematosus, 316
  differentiation from pityriasis rubra pilaris, 264
  guttate lesions, early, *252*
    neutrophilic spongiosis in, 505
  intermediate lesions, *253*, *254*, *255*
  long-standing plaque, *251*
  mitoses in, 33
  pustular, 254, 255, 557, 562–565, *563*, *564*, 576–577, *576*
Psoriasis-like lesions in secondary syphilis, 324
Punch biopsy, disadvantages of, 151, *151*, 780
Purpura, *136*
  anaphylactoid. *See* Leukocytoclastic vasculitis
  definition of, 135
  in allergic granulomatosis, 372
  lichenoid, 211, *211*, *212*
  thrombotic thrombocytopenic, 380
Purpura fulminans, 380, 381
Purpura rheumatica, 337
Purpuric lesions, in systemic lupus erythematosus, 316
Pustule, *135*
  definition of, 135
  spongiform, *123*, 254, 498
    definition of, 121
    in condyloma latum, 324
    in guttate psoriasis, 252
    in halogenodermas, 256, 465
    in Letterer-Siwe disease, 256
    in necrolytic migratory erythema, 512
    in psoriasis, 253–255, *254*, 256

  in pustular drug eruptions, 256
  in pyoderma gangrenosum, 256
  in rupial secondary syphilis, 256, 324
  in secondary syphilis, 324
  subcorneal, 498
    in psoriasis, 252, *252*, 255, 256
Pyknosis, 122
Pyoderma gangrenosum, 256, 451, 452, 454, *451*, *452*, *453*
  in rheumatoid arthritis, 343, 454
  spongiform pustules in, 568, 576
  subcorneal blisters in, 552
  subcorneal pustules in, 568, 576
Pyogenic granuloma, 722, 724–726, *724–726*

Radiation, as cause of alopecia, 709
Radiodermatitis, *379*
  acute, 593
    alopecia in, 707
  chronic, 201–202, *201*, *202*, 756, 765–767, *766*, 830
    neoplasms in, 765
  forerunner of malignant neoplasms, 716, 749
Raynaud's phenomenon, in systemic lupus erythematosus, 316
Reactions, to arthropods. *See* Arthropod reactions
  to bee sting, 296–297
Recalcitrant vesiculopustular dermatitis of palms and soles, 556–557, *557*
Reepithelization, beneath blisters, 150
  of subepidermal blisters, 582, *582*
Reiter's disease. *See* Keratoderma blenorrhagicum
Relapsing febrile nodular nonsuppurative panniculitis, 806–808, *807*
Reticular dermis, *17*, 17, 19, 21
Reticulin, 21
Reticulin fibers, 4, 23
Reticuloendothelial system, 96
Reticulohistiocytoma, 472–473, *473*
Reticuloid, actinic, 330–331, *330*, *331*
Reticulum cells, 96
Rheumatic nodule, 433
Rheumatoid arthritis, leukocytoclastic vasculitis in, 341, 343
  with pyoderma gangrenosum, 343, 454
Rheumatoid factor, high titers of, 343
Rheumatoid neutrophilic dermatitis, 449, 451, *450*
Rheumatoid nodule(s), 341, 343, 415, 416, 433, *434*, 831
  leukocytoclastic vasculitis in, 348
Rhinophyma, 659, 685
Rhinoscleroma, 482, 485, 486, 488
Rhinosporidiosis, 457, *458*
Rickettsia rickettsii, in Rocky Mountain spotted fever, 180
Ringworm, 663

Rocky Mountain spotted fever, 179–180
    disseminated intravascular coagulation and, 382
Rosacea, 406–407, 648, 658–659, *658, 659,* 683–685,
        683, 684
    superficial folliculitis in, 669
Rothmann-Makai syndrome, 808–809, *809*
Rothmund-Thomson syndrome, 202
Rupial syphilis, 562, 565–566, *565–567,* 667, 833
Ruptured follicular unit, in pyoderma gangrenosum,
        452
Russell bodies, 104, 487, *487*

Sandfly, carrier of leishmaniasis, 481
Saponification of fat, in pancreatic panniculitis, 817
Sarcoidal, definition of, 408
Sarcoid-like lesions in secondary syphilis, 324
Sarcoidosis, 387, 409–412, *409–411*
    alopecia in, 709
    as cause of erythema nodosum, 790, 808
    calcification in, 442
    differentiation from tuberculoid leprosy, 402
    similarities to rosacea, 658
    subcutaneous, 808, *810*
Sarcoptes scabiei, 297, Plate *2*
Scabies, 297–299, *297–301,* 327, 831, Plate *2*
    eosinophilic spongiosis in, 250, 505, *505*
    keratotic-crusted, 298–299, *300,* 328, *328,* 561
    nodular, 298, 446–447, *447*
    Norwegian, 298–299, *300,* 328, *328,* 562, *562*
    similarity to insect bite, 184
    vasculitis in, 369, *370, 371*
Scabietic bite, 295
    contrasted with tick bites, 294
"Scalded" skin, in erythema multiforme, 550
    in toxic epidermal necrolysis, 606
Scalded-skin syndrome, staphylococcal, 548, 550, 571
    contrasted with toxic epidermal necrolysis, 606
        differentiation from bullous impetigo, 550–551
        similarity to bullous impetigo and superficial
            pemphigus, 573, 606
Scale, *137*
    definition of, 136
Scale-crust, *116*
    definition of, 115
    in acral papular eruption of childhood (Gianotti-
        Crosti syndrome), 238
    in guttate parapsoriasis, 236
    in guttate psoriasis, 252
    in irritant contact dermatitis, 243
    in lichenoid photodermatitis, 321
    in reactions to arthropods, 295
    in seborrheic dermatitis, 239, 278
Scalpel biopsy, for panniculitis, 780
Scar(s), *140,* 727, 736, *737*
    atrophic, 19, 727, 749–750, *749, 750*
    blisters over, 583, 598–599, *598*

definition of, 139
    hypertrophic, 727, *727–731, 728–731*
    in pityriasis lichenoides et varioliformis acuta, 318
Scarring inflammatory alopecias, 707–713
Scarring pemphigoid, 633–635, *634*
Schamberg's disease, 172, *173*
Schistosomes, as cause of swimmer's itch, 301
Scleredema, 19
Sclerema neonatorum, 802–803, *802, 803,* 833
    differentiation of, from poststeroid panniculitis, 806
        from subcutaneous fat necrosis of the newborn,
            803
Scleroderma, 760–762, *760–762,* 830, 833
    acrosclerosis, 791
    alopecia in, 708, *708*
    differentiation from lichen sclerosus et atrophicus,
        763
    diffuse, 792, 833
    fibrous replacement of fat in, 29
    guttate, 791
    in porphyria cutanea tarda, 589
    inflammatory stage, 283, 285–287, *285, 286*
    linear, 286, 791, 833
    morphea, 791
    panniculitis in, 285, 791–792, *792, 793*
    progressive systemic sclerosis, 791
    vasculitis in, 366, *368, 369,* 783–784
Sclerodermoid lesions, 287
Sclerosis(es), *126, 736,* 760–770
    atrophic, 763–770
    definition of, 125, 140
    in dermatofibroma, 738, *744*
    progressive systemic, 287, 791
    subepidermal nodular, 735
    systemic, calcification in, 442
Scrofuloderma, 400, 801
    panniculitis in, 811
Scurvy, 648, 655, 657, *657*
Sebaceous cyst, a misnomer, 438
Sebaceous duct, 51, 57, 68
    architecture of, *66*
    embrogenesis of, 7
Sebaceous follicles, 12, *14, 66,* 642, *642, 643*
Sebaceous gland(s), architecture of, *66*
    distribution of, 65
    electron microscopy of, *68, 69*
    embryogenesis of, 7
    histogenesis of, *6*
    histology of, 67, *67*
    structure and function, 65–69
Sebaceous secretion, absence of neural influences on,
        32
Seborrheic dermatitis, 499, 828
    acute, 239–240, *239*
    chronic, 262, *262*
    subacute, 278–279, *279*

Ulcer(s) (*Continued*)
in spirochetal vasculitis of secondary syphilis, 361
in subcutaneous polyarteritis nodosa, 356
in syphilitic chancre, 487
in systemic lupus erythematosus, 316, 341
in third-degree burns, 592
in transient acantholytic dermatosis, 543
in varicose thrombophlebitis, 784
in venereal diseases, 485, *485*
in Wegener's granulomatosis, 373
scarring alopecias, and, 707, 709
Ulcerative colitis, with pyoderma gangrenosum, 454
Urates, 440
in gout, 415, 433, *435*, Plate *5*
Uroporphyrin, 589
Urtica, *131*
definition of, 130–131
Urticaria, 180–181, *181, 831*
chronic, *182*
papular, 296
eosinophilic spongiosis in, 505
Urticaria pigmentosa, 831, Plate *1*
bullous, 490, 638
differentiation from xanthogranulomas, 472
macular and papular lesions, 185–186, *186*
nodular type, 490–491, *490, 491*
Urticarial allergic eruptious, active zones at the peripheries, 305
deep, 305, *305*
relation to urticarial vesiculobullous allergic eruption, 636
superficial, 181–183, *182*
Urticarial drug eruptions, misinterpretation of, 604
Urticarial vasculitis, 337
Urticarial vesiculobullous allergic eruption, 636–637, *636*

Vaccination, as cause of pseudolymphoma, 446
scars from, forerunners of malignant neoplasms, 716
Vaccinia, 506, *507*
Vacuolar alteration, *124*
definition of, 122–123
in discoid lupus erythematosus, 312
Valves, in larger lymphatics, 29
Varicella, 497, 508, 544–548, *545–547*, 829
differentiation from variola, 508
Varicella septicemia, disseminated intravascular coagulation and, 382
Varicose thrombophlebitis, 362, 784
Varicose veins, phlebothromboses in, 383
Variola, 508
Vasculature, of skin, *334*
of subcutaneous fat, 779, 780, *780, 781*
Vasculitis, arterial, *335*
arteriolar, *335*
capillary-venular, *334*

classification of, 332, 336
definition of, 333, 338
differentiation from perivascular inflammatory-cell infiltrates, 336
granulomatous, 371–375
in arthropod reactions, 369, *370, 371*
in granuloma annulare, 420, 421, *420, 421*
in lymphomatoid granulomatosis, 379
in necrobiosis lipoidica, 424, 427, *428*
in pyoderma gangrenosum, 452
in scleroderma, 285
in secondary syphilis, 324
large vessel type, 338
leukocytoclastic. *See* Leukocytoclastic vasculitis
lymphocytic, 336, 369
in pityriasis lichenoides et varioliformis acuta, 347
neutrophilic, 336, 337–369
nodular. *See* Nodular vasculitis
pseudomonas, 360
septic, 356, 358, 561, 632–633, *632, 633, 832*
arthritis in, 360
vesiculopustules in, 558, *560*
small vessel type, 338
spirochetal, 360–362
venous, *336*
with panniculitis, 366, *368, 369*, 783–784
Vegetations, definition of, 137
Vellus follicles, 642, *642, 643*
Vellus hairs, 12, 50
on ear, *15*
Venule(s), postcapillary, in leukocytoclastic vasculitis, 338
structure of, 23–24
Vernix caseosa, 69
Verrucous, definition of, 132
Vesicle, *134*
definition of, 133–134
intraepidermal, ruptured, 582, *582*
Vesicular dermatitis, ballooning, 506–522
Vesiculation, intraepidermal, 497–498
Vesiculopustule, in septic vasculitis, 358
Viral eruptions, morbilliform, 197
Viral exanthems, 174
similarities to moribilliform drug eruptions, 197
Vitiligo, Langerhans' cells increased in, 49
with alopecia areata, 699
Von Zumbusch pustular psoriasis, 563
V-shaped infiltrate, in pityriasis lichenoides et varioliformis acuta, 316
in reactions to arthropods, 795

Waldenström's macroglobulinemia, 380, 381
Warthin-Starry stain, for granuloma inguinale, 486
for spirochetes, 327, 387
for syphilis, 412, 486, 487, Plate *1*
Warty dyskeratoma, 537, 829

This edition of Histologic Diagnosis of Inflammatory Skin Diseases by A. Bernard Ackerman, M.D. was designed by Howard N. King. The type is Palatino and Modern Number Twenty and was set by York Graphic Services, Inc. Printed by William J. Dornan, Inc. Bound by Murphy-Parker, Inc. The paper is P. H. Glatfelter's 70 lb. Velvetlith.

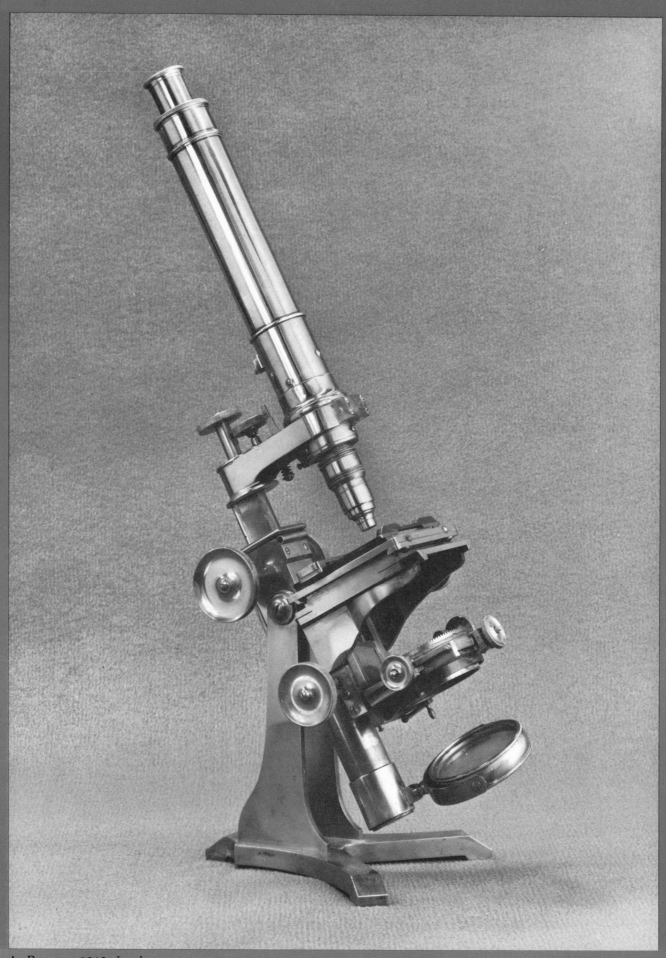

A. Ross, c. 1840, *London*

From the collection of A. Bernard Ackerman, M.D.